The Complete Diagnosis Coding Solution

Third Edition

Shelley C. Safian, PhD, RHIA

MAOM/HSM, CCS-P, CPC-H, CPC-I,

AHIMA-Approved ICD-10-CM/PCS Trainer

Mary A. Johnson, CPC

Central Carolina Technical College

Mc
Graw
Hill
Education

THE COMPLETE DIAGNOSIS CODING SOLUTION, THIRD EDITION

Published by McGraw-Hill Education, 2 Penn Plaza, New York, NY 10121. Copyright © 2016 by McGraw-Hill Education. All rights reserved. Printed in the United States of America. Previous editions © 2012 and 2009. No part of this publication may be reproduced or distributed in any form or by any means, or stored in a database or retrieval system, without the prior written consent of McGraw-Hill Education, including, but not limited to, in any network or other electronic storage or transmission, or broadcast for distance learning.

Some ancillaries, including electronic and print components, may not be available to customers outside the United States.

This book is printed on acid-free paper.

2 3 4 5 6 RMN 19 18 17 16

ISBN   978-0-07-802070-4
MHID   0-07-802070-0

Senior Vice President, Products & Markets: *Kurt L. Strand*
Vice President, General Manager, Products & Markets:
Marty Lange
Vice President, Content Design & Delivery: *Kimberly Meriwether David*
Managing Director: *Chad Grall*
Brand Manager: *William Mulford*
Director, Product Development: *Rose Koos*
Senior Product Developer: *Michelle Flomenhoft*
Executive Marketing Manager: *Roxan Kinsey*

Market Development Manager: *Kimberly Bauer*
Digital Product Analyst: *Katherine Ward*
Director, Content Design & Delivery: *Linda Avenarius*
Program Manager: *Faye M. Herrig*
Content Project Managers: *Jane Mohr, Brent dela Cruz, and Judi David*
Buyer: *Susan K. Culbertson*
Design: *Studio Montage, St. Louis, MO*
Content Licensing Specialist: *Lorraine Buczek*
Compositor: *SPi Global*
Printer: *R. R. Donnelley*

All credits appearing on page or at the end of the book are considered to be an extension of the copyright page. All figures referenced in the product as "Booth et al., MA, 5e" come from Booth et al., *Medical Assisting: Administrative and Clinical Procedures with Anatomy and Physiology,* 5e. McGraw-Hill Education, 2013. Copyright © 2013 by McGraw-Hill Education. All rights reserved. Used with permission. ISBN 007340232X

Library of Congress Cataloging-in-Publication Data

Safian, Shelley C.
    The complete diagnosis coding solution.—Third edition / Shelley C.
Safian, PhD, RHIA, MAOM/HSM, CCS-P, CPC-H, CPC-I, AHIMA-Approved ICD-10-CM/PCS
trainer, Mary A. Johnson, CPC, Central Carolina Technical College.
        pages cm
Includes index.
ISBN 978-0-07-802070-4 (alk. paper)
1. Medicine—Terminology—Code numbers. I. Johnson, Mary A. (Medical record
coding program manager) II. Title.
R123.S18 2016
610.1'4—dc23

2014045722

The Internet addresses listed in the text were accurate at the time of publication. The inclusion of a website does not indicate an endorsement by the authors or McGraw-Hill Education, and McGraw-Hill Education does not guarantee the accuracy of the information presented at these sites.

All brand or product names are trademarks or registered trademarks of their respective companies. CPT five-digit codes, nomenclature, and other data are © 2015 American Medical Association. All rights reserved. No fee schedules, basic unit, relative values, or related listings are included in the CPT. The AMA assumes no liability for the data contained herein. CPT codes are based on CPT 2015. All references to ICD-10-CM codes, guidelines, or related data are based on the International Classification of Diseases, Tenth Revision, Clinical Modification (ICD-10-CM) 2015. All references to CMS HCPCS codes, guidelines, or related data are based on the Centers for Medicare and Medicaid Services (CMS), Healthcare Common Procedure Coding System (HCPCS) Level II 2015. All names, situations, and anecdotes are fictitious. They do not represent any person, event, or medical record.

mheducation.com/highered

ABOUT THE AUTHORS

Shelley C. Safian

Shelley Safian has been teaching medical coding and health information management for more than a decade, at both on-ground and online campuses. In addition to her regular teaching responsibilities at Herzing University and Berkeley College Online, she often presents seminars sponsored by AHIMA and AAPC, writes regularly about coding for the *Just Coding* newsletter, and has written articles published in AAPC *Healthcare Business Monthly, SurgiStrategies,* and *HFM* (Healthcare Financial Management) magazine. Safian is the course author for multiple distance education courses on various coding topics, including ICD-10-CM, ICD-10-PCS, and HCPCS Level II coding.

Safian is a Registered Health Information Administrator (RHIA) and a Certified Coding Specialist–Physician-based (CCS-P) from the American Health Information Management Association and a Certified Professional Coder–Hospital (CPC-H), and a Certified Professional Coding Instructor (CPC-I) from the American Academy of Professional Coders. She is also a Certified HIPAA Administrator (CHA), and has earned the designation of AHIMA-Approved ICD-10-CM/PCS Trainer.

Safian completed her Graduate Certificate in Health Care Management at Keller Graduate School of Management. The University of Phoenix awarded her Master of Arts/Organizational Management degree. She earned her Ph.D. in Health Care Administration with a focus in Health Information Management.

Mary A. Johnson

Mary Johnson is currently the Medical Record Coding Program Director at Central Carolina Technical College, Sumter, South Carolina. Her background includes corporate training as well as on-campus and online platforms. Johnson also designs and implements customized coding curricula. Johnson received her Bachelor of Arts dual degree in Business Administration and Marketing from Columbia College, Columbia, South Carolina. Johnson is a Certified Professional Coder (CPC) credentialed through the American Academy of Professional Coders and is ICD-10-CM proficient.

Acknowledgements

—This book is dedicated to *Joshua* and *Roxie*, without whose love and support I could not accomplish all that I do - *Shelley*.

—This book is dedicated in loving memory of my parents, *Dr. and Mrs. Clarence J. Johnson, Sr.* and to my Aunt Wanda for their love and support. Also, to those students that I have had the privilege to work with and to those students who are beginning their journey into the world of medical coding - *Mary*

BRIEF CONTENTS

CONTENTS

Welcome to *The Complete Diagnosis Coding Solution!* This product is part of a three-part series that instructs students on how to become proficient in medical coding—a health care field that continues to be in high demand. The Bureau of Labor Statistics notes the demand for health information management professionals (which includes coders) will continue to increase incredibly through 2018 and beyond.

This series was written to speak directly to the medical coding student, using step-by-step instructions and conversational language to maximize understanding. Built into the structure of these solutions are many opportunities for students to practice coding and apply what they have learned. Students will also have the chance to practice abstracting with real-world health professionals' documentation and accurately translating these facts into the best, most accurate codes.

To the Student

Your medical coding classes introduce you to the skills you will need to work in the health information management field. A fundamental role of an insurance coding and medical billing specialist's job is to work with the insurance companies that will reimburse the health care facility for the services and treatments provided to patients. You may be employed by a hospital, clinic, doctor's office, health maintenance organization, mental health care facility, insurance company, government agency, or long-term care facility. Your career will be challenging, interesting, and one of the top 10 fastest-growing Allied Health professions.

Before you begin your adventure, here are some tips to help you succeed:

- First, take a deep breath. Coding is complex and is not like anything else you have tackled before. Remember that you are learning a new skill! Give yourself some time to become proficient.
- Second, *never* code directly from the Alphabetic Index. *Always* look the code up in the Tabular List before deciding on a code. If you remember this rule, you will always head in the right direction.
- Third, when you encounter a word or abbreviation that you don't understand, stop and look it up in your medical dictionary.
- Fourth, after you finish coding the case studies, scenarios, or whatever you are coding, put it all aside. Then, later or the next day, go back and do "back coding." In the Tabular List, look up each code you came up with and match the code description carefully with the case study or scenario words. Remember the importance of documentation by the health care provider—this is more important than ever with the implementation of ICD-10-CM! This process is a very effective way to double-check your answers. Your fresh eyes will enable you to see words and notations you may have missed before.
- Finally, reevaluate your work by checking each and every question to make certain you understand how you found your answer. When you find you have gotten an exercise, test question, or other activity wrong, try to figure out what happened. Make sure you ask your instructor for help when you need it!

Good luck on your medical coding journey!

To the Instructor

The Safian/Johnson Medical Coding series includes three products:

The Complete Diagnosis Coding Solution, 3e
The Complete Procedure Coding Solution, 3e
You Code It! Abstracting Case Studies Practicum, 2e (Third edition coming soon!)

These solutions are designed to give your students the medical coding experience they need in order to pass their first medical coding certification exams, such as the CCS/CCS-P or CPC/CPC-H. The products offer students a variety of practice opportunities by reinforcing the learning outcomes set forth in every chapter. The chapter materials are organized in short bursts of text followed by practice—keeping students active and coding!

In addition to providing innovative approaches to learning medical coding, McGraw-Hill Education knows how much effort it takes to prepare for a new course. Through focus groups, symposia, reviews, and conversations with instructors like you, we have gathered information about the materials you need in order to facilitate successful courses. We are committed to providing you with high-quality, accurate instructor support.

Digital Resources

Knowing the importance of flexibility and digital learning, McGraw-Hill Education has created multiple assets to enhance the learning experience no matter what the class format: traditional, online, or hybrid. This product is designed with digital solutions to help instructors and students be successful.

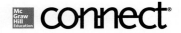

Learn Without Limits: McGraw-Hill Connect

Today's learning extends beyond the classroom, beyond one format, beyond a singular style. That's why we deliver everything instructors and students need directly to your fingertips, integrating education seamlessly into your lives. We don't just improve results, we make the everyday a little smoother by providing intuitive technology that enables learning and simplifies life.

Students at the Center

To design a powerful learning experience that makes a palpable difference, we went straight to the source. Collecting and mining millions of data points, we partnered closely with students and educators globally, compiling feedback that revealed deep insights to inform the construction of each facet within this revolutionary learning environment. The result? An innovative synthesis of adaptive technology and learning resources perfectly calibrated to guide each student on a personalized path toward better grades.

Activate Learning

Learning doesn't just happen. To encourage achievement and evoke curiosity, it's essential to shift learning from a passive experience to one that is energetic and engaged—in and outside the classroom. By immersing students in their course content and prompting them to interact with key concepts, while continually adapting to their individual needs, Connect activates learning and empowers students to take control, raising grades and increasing retention and raising grades. Connect makes digital teaching and learning personal, easy, and effective. Learn more at **www.mcgrawhillconnect.com!**

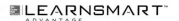

Learning at the speed of you: the LearnSmart Advantage Suite

Connect's Superior Adaptive Technology 'Fills the Knowledge Gap' and Empowers Students Outside of Class for a More Engaging and Interactive Experience in Class. Connect builds student confidence outside of class with adaptive technology that pinpoints exactly what a student knows and what they don't, and then seamlessly offers up learning resources within the platform that are designed to have the greatest impact on that specific learning moment. With SmartBook, reading is an interactive and dynamic experience in which content is tailor-made for each student. Built with the unique LearnSmart adaptive technology, it focuses not only on addressing learning in the moment, but empowers students by helping them retain information over time, so that they are more prepared and engaged in class.

- **LearnSmart Advantage:** More than 2 million students have answered more than 1.3 billion questions in LearnSmart since 2009, making it the most widely used and intelligent adaptive study tool available on the market today. LearnSmart is proven to strengthen memory recall, keep students in class, and boost grades—students using LearnSmart are 13% more likely to pass their classes, and 35% less likely to dropout.

- **SmartBook [New Capabilities]:** SmartBook makes study time as productive and efficient as possible. It identifies and closes knowledge gaps through a continually adapting reading experience that provides introduces personalized learning resources at the precise moment of need. This ensures that every minute spent with SmartBook is returned to the student as the most value-added minute possible. The result? More confidence, better grades, and greater success.

Go to **www.LearnSmartAdvantage.com** for more information!

Record and distribute your lectures for multiple viewing: My Lectures—Tegrity

McGraw-Hill Tegrity records and distributes your class lecture with just a click of a button. Students can view it anytime and anywhere via computer, tablet, or other mobile device. It indexes as it records your PowerPoint presentations and anything shown on your computer, so students can use key words to find exactly what they want to study. Tegrity is available as an integrated feature of **McGraw-Hill *Connect* Medical Coding** and as a stand-alone product.

A single sign-on with Connect and your Blackboard course: McGraw-Hill Education and Blackboard—for a premium user experience

Blackboard, the web-based course management system, has partnered with McGraw-Hill Education to better allow students and faculty to use online materials and activities to complement face-to-face teaching. Blackboard features exciting social learning and teaching tools that foster active learning opportunities for students. You'll transform your closed-door classroom into communities where students remain connected to their educational experience 24 hours a day. This partnership allows you and your students access to McGraw-Hill's *Connect* and *Create* right from within your Blackboard course—all with a single sign-on. Not only do you get single sign-on with *Connect* and *Create,* but you also get deep integration of McGraw-Hill Education content and content engines right in Blackboard. Whether you're choosing a book for your course or building *Connect* assignments, all the tools you need are right where you want them—inside Blackboard. Gradebooks are now seamless. When a student completes an integrated *Connect* assignment, the grade for that assignment automatically (and instantly) feeds into your Blackboard grade center. McGraw-Hill Education and Blackboard can now offer you easy access to industry leading technology and content, whether your campus hosts it or we do. Be sure to ask your local McGraw-Hill Education representative for details.

Still want a single sign-on solution and using another Learning Management System?

See how **McGraw-Hill Campus** makes the grade by offering universal sign-on, automatic registration, gradebook synchronization, and open access to a multitude of learning resources—all in one place. MH Campus supports Active Directory, Angel,

Blackboard, Canvas, Desire2Learn, eCollege, IMS, LDAP, Moodle, Moodlerooms, Sakai, Shibboleth, WebCT, BrainHoney, Campus Cruiser, and Jenzibar eRacer. Additionally, MH Campus can be easily connected with other authentication authorities and LMSs. Visit **http://mhcampus.mhhe.com/** to learn more.

Create a textbook organized the way you teach: McGraw-Hill Education *Create*

With *Create,* you can easily rearrange chapters, combine material from other content sources, and quickly upload content you have written, such as your course syllabus or teaching notes. Find the content you need in *Create* by searching through thousands of leading McGraw-Hill Education textbooks. Arrange your book to fit your teaching style. *Create* even allows you to personalize your book's appearance by selecting the cover and adding your name, school, and course information. Order a *Create* book and you'll receive a complimentary print review copy in 3 to 5 business days or a complimentary electronic review copy (eComp) via e-mail in minutes. Go to **www.mcgrawhillcreate.com** today and register to experience how *Create* empowers you to teach *your* students *your* way.

Best-in-Class Digital Support

Based on feedback from our users, McGraw-Hill Education has developed Digital Success Programs that will provide you and your students the help you need, when you need it.

- *Training for Instructors:* Get ready to drive classroom results with our **Digital Success Team**—ready to provide in-person, remote, or on-demand training as needed.
- *Peer Support and Training:* No one understands your needs like your peers. Get easy access to knowledgeable digital users by joining our Connect Community, or speak directly with one of our **Digital Faculty Consultants,** who are instructors using McGraw-Hill Education digital products.
- *Online Training Tools:* Get immediate anytime, anywhere access to modular tutorials on key features through our **Connect Success Academy.**

Get started today. Learn more about McGraw-Hill Education's Digital Success Programs by contacting your local sales representative or visiting **http://connect .customer.mheducation.com/start**.

Need help? Contact the McGraw-Hill Education Customer Experience Group (CXG)

Visit the CXG website at **www.mhhe.com/support**. Browse our FAQs (frequently asked questions) and product documentation and/or contact a CXG representative. CXG is available Sunday through Friday.

Additional Instructor Resources

The following resources are available in the Instructor Resources located under the Library tab in Connect:

- **Instructor's Manual and Tools to Plan Course** pages with course overview, lesson plans, and answers for end-of-chapter exercises, as well as competency correlations, sample syllabi, conversion guide (from second edition to third edition), asset map, and more. Answer keys are updated annually.
- **PowerPoint Presentations** for each chapter correlated to learning outcomes. Each presentation seeks to reinforce key concepts and provide an additional visual aid for students.

- **Test Bank** and answer key for use in class assessment. The comprehensive test bank includes a variety of question types, with each question linked directly to a learning outcome from the text. Questions are also tagged with relevant topic, Bloom's Taxonomy level, difficulty level, and competencies, where applicable. The test bank is available in *Connect;* Word and EZ Test versions are also available.

What's New in Our Third Edition

The Complete Diagnosis Coding Solution, third edition, has been revised to include a greater number of realistic scenarios and case studies for students to gain hands-on learning with the popular **Let's Code It!** scenarios and **You Code It!** case studies. **Guidance Connection** boxes—a new feature for this edition—make it easier for students to connect learning concepts and specific official guidelines to critical thinking. **Coding Tips** also include additional helpful information to support students' learning. Throughout the text, more anatomy and physiology descriptions, as well as more information on inclusive signs and symptoms, enhance students' comprehension of the diagnosis coding process.

Several brand-new chapters have been added to ensure complete coverage of all body systems and provide relevant information students need in order to learn diagnosis coding.

The entire text has been updated using 2015 ICD-10-CM codes. The new instructor's manual features a 2015-compliant answer key to all end-of-chapter tests: **Chapter Review** (matching, short-answer, and multiple-choice questions), **You Code It! Practice** (short scenarios), and **You Code It! Application** (full physician's notes/operative reports). Answer keys are also updated annually for the newest diagnosis codes and are made available in the password-protected Instructor Resources within *Connect.*

Chapter-by-Chapter Updates

Chapter 1: Introduction to Diagnostic Coding
- Key Terms include additional ICD-10-CM key terms
- The new Guidance Connection feature points readers directly to the applicable Official Guidelines
- Updated explanations of risk factors, signs, symptoms, and resources to support accurate coding
- New addition of anatomy basics, including medical terminology, organ systems, body areas, anatomical positions and directions, and more

Chapter 2: Introduction to ICD-10-CM
- The new Guidance Connection feature points readers directly to the applicable Official Guidelines
- Updated section on format of the ICD-10-CM
- Updated section on co-morbidities, manifestations, and sequelae (late effects)

Chapter 3: General Guidelines and Notations
- The new Guidance Connection feature points readers directly to the applicable Official Guidelines
- Updated section on notations and placeholder characters
- Updated section on multiple and additional codes

Chapter 4: Coding Infectious Diseases
- The new Guidance Connection feature points readers directly to the applicable Official Guidelines
- New section on pathogens, communicable diseases, and sepsis

Chapter 5: Coding Neoplasms
- The new Guidance Connection feature points readers directly to the applicable Official Guidelines
- New section on screenings and other diagnostic testing

New! Chapter 6: Coding Diseases of the Blood and Immune Mechanism
- The new Guidance Connection feature points readers directly to the applicable Official Guidelines
- New sections cover the anatomy of the blood and blood-forming organs, different types of anemias, coagulation defects, and disorders involving the immune mechanism

Chapter 7: Coding Conditions of the Endocrine and Metabolic Systems
- Additional key terms
- The new Guidance Connection feature points readers directly to the applicable Official Guidelines
- New section on the anatomy of the endocrine system
- Expanded sections on diabetic manifestations

New! Chapter 8: Coding Mental and Behavioral Disorders
- The new Guidance Connection feature points readers directly to the applicable Official Guidelines
- New sections cover the anatomy of brain function, physiology of mental and behavioral disorders and underlying causes, and stress-related disorders, including PTSD

New! Chapter 9: Coding Nervous System Conditions
- The new Guidance Connection feature points readers directly to the applicable Official Guidelines
- New sections cover the anatomy and physiology of the central and peripheral nervous systems; neurologic disorders, including diagnostic testing such as the Glasgow coma scale; and various treatments for various conditions
- New section dedicated to pain management

New! Chapter 10: Coding Diseases of the Eye and Adnexa
- The new Guidance Connection feature points readers directly to the applicable Official Guidelines
- New sections cover the anatomy and physiology of the optical system, including a listing of optical-related abbreviations

New! Chapter 11: Coding Diseases of the Auditory System (Ears)
- The new Guidance Connection feature points readers directly to the applicable Official Guidelines
- New sections cover the anatomy and physiology of the auditory system, underlying causes, diagnostic testing, and treatment options

Chapter 12: Coding Circulatory Conditions
- The new Guidance Connection feature points readers directly to the applicable Official Guidelines
- New section added to cover anatomy and physiology details, as well as signs and symptoms

Chapter 13: Coding Respiratory Conditions
- The new Guidance Connection feature points readers directly to the applicable Official Guidelines
- New section added to cover anatomy and physiology of the respiratory system

- New section added to cover tobacco use, abuse, dependence, and use history
- New section on external cause coding
- Additional You Code It! exercises

New! Chapter 14: Coding Diseases of the Digestive System
- The new Guidance Connection feature points readers directly to the applicable Official Guidelines
- New sections cover the anatomy and physiology of the digestive system, as well as health conditions connected to poor oral hygiene

New! Chapter 15: Coding Diseases of the Integumentary System
- The new Guidance Connection feature points readers directly to the applicable Official Guidelines
- New sections cover the anatomy and physiology of the integumentary system and various types of lesions and ulcers, including pressure ulcers

Chapter 16: Coding Muscular Conditions
- The new Guidance Connection feature points readers directly to the applicable Official Guidelines
- New sections on the anatomy and physiology of the muscular system, as well as diseases of the muscles
- Updated information on external cause coding
- Additional Let's Code It! and You Code It! exercises

New! Chapter 17: Coding Skeletal Conditions
- The new Guidance Connection feature points readers directly to the applicable Official Guidelines
- New sections cover the anatomy and physiology of the axial and appendicular skeletal systems, types of fractures, and sequelae of fractures

New! Chapter 18: Coding Diseases of the Urinary System
- The new Guidance Connection feature points readers directly to the applicable Official Guidelines
- New sections cover the anatomy and physiology of the urinary system and conditions affecting the prostate

Chapter 19: Coding for Obstetrics and Gynecology
- The new Guidance Connection feature points readers directly to the applicable Official Guidelines
- New section on the anatomy of the female reproductive system
- New case in You Code It! Application

Chapter 20: Coding Congenital and Pediatric Conditions
- The new Guidance Connection feature points readers directly to the applicable Official Guidelines
- Additional Let's Code It! exercise
- New case in You Code It! Application

New! Chapter 21: Coding Injuries, Poisonings, and Certain Other Consequences of External Causes
- The new Guidance Connection feature points readers directly to the applicable Official Guidelines
- New sections cover traumatic wounds, burns, poisonings, adverse effects, abuse and neglect, and complications of care; administration of pharmaceuticals; use of the Table of Drugs and Chemicals; and external cause codes

New! Chapter 22: Factors Influencing Health Status and Contact with Health Services
- The new Guidance Connection feature points readers directly to the applicable Official Guidelines
- New sections on preventive care, genetics, and all subsections of this ICD-10-CM chapter

Chapter 23: Hospital (Inpatient) Diagnosis Coding
- The new Guidance Connection feature points readers directly to the applicable Official Guidelines

Chapter 24: You Code It! Practice and Application
- Expanded cases
- New and additional exercises included to increase practice opportunities.
- 30 You Code It! Practice scenarios and 20 You Code It! Application case studies.
- All exercises also available in Connect

CodeitRightOnline™: Your Online Coding Tool

So that your students can gain experience with the use of an online coding tool, they will have access for a 29-day period to CodeitRightOnline, produced by Contexo Media, a division of Access Intelligence. CodeitRightOnline offers a comprehensive search function for CPT, HCPCS Level II, and ICD-10-CM/PCS code sets. It includes helpful tools like search indexing for easy reference and offers newsletter articles and other coding resources. For more information about the features of CodeitRightOnline and how to sign up for a trial, visit the Instructor Resource center or talk to your local McGraw-Hill Education representative.

ACKNOWLEDGMENTS

Reviews

Many instructors reviewed the manuscript while it was in development and provided valuable feedback that directly affected the product's development. Their contributions are greatly appreciated.

Geanetta J. Agbona, CPC, CPC-I, CBCS
South Piedmont Community College

Katherine Baus, RHIA, CCS-P
Southern Technical College

Pamela Harris-Brown, MBA, CPC,
CMAS, CAHI
Saint Louis College of Health Careers

Dawn Kantz, MAEd, CPC-A
Lenoir Community College

Loreen MacNichol, CMRS, RMC, CCS-P
Southern Maine Community College

Jane Mansell, CPC
Living Arts College

Jenny Roberts, CPC
Beckfield College

Irma Rodriguez, MEd, RHIA, CCS
South Texas College

Loretta Swan, BS
Tyler Junior College

Amy Tabak, MBA/HR, CPC, CMAA,
CBCS
Antonelli College

Suzanne Thorpe, AOS, CPC
Elmira Business Institute

Technical Editing/Accuracy Panel

A panel of instructors completed a technical edit and review of all content in the page proofs to verify its accuracy.

Eleonora Alvarado, RN, MHA, CPC
Nashville State Community College

Leathecia Arnold-Jackson, MHA, RHIA,
CCS, CHTS-TR, Approved AHIMA
ICD-10-CM/PCS Trainer
Peak Health Solutions

Kristi Couch, RHIA, CPC, CCA, CHP,
CHA
Jefferson Community and Technical
College

Angelia Hamilton, MHA, RHIA, CCS,
CPC
South Suburban College

Susan Hawkins, M.S., M.B.A., M.H.A,
CPC, CHTS-TR
Nashville State Community College

Digital Tool Development

Special thanks to the instructors who helped with the development of *Connect* and SmartBook. An expanded acknowledgments list is available in the Instructor Resources section of Connect.

GUIDED TOUR

The Complete Diagnosis Coding Solution was developed with student success in mind!

Chapter Openers

Each chapter begins by clearly identifying the **Learning Outcomes** students need to master along with the **Key Terms** they need to remember.

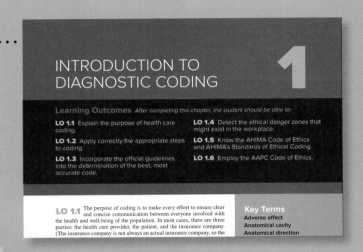

INTRODUCTION TO DIAGNOSTIC CODING 1

Learning Outcomes *After completing this chapter, the student should be able to:*

LO 1.1 Explain the purpose of health care coding.

LO 1.2 Apply correctly the appropriate steps to coding.

LO 1.3 Incorporate the official guidelines into the determination of the best, most accurate code.

LO 1.4 Detect the ethical danger zones that might exist in the workplace.

LO 1.5 Know the AHIMA Code of Ethics and AHIMA's Standards of Ethical Coding.

LO 1.6 Employ the AAPC Code of Ethics.

LO 1.1 The purpose of coding is to make every effort to ensure clear and concise communication between everyone involved with the health and well-being of the population. In most cases, there are three parties: the health care provider, the patient, and the insurance company. (The insurance company is not always an actual insurance company, so the

Key Terms
Adverse effect
Anatomical cavity
Anatomical direction

Coding Tips

These helpful tips appear periodically throughout the text to provide students with useful insights for ensuring their success and to illuminate strategies for avoiding the most common mistakes. These features also walk students through the critical thinking process required to make the necessary evaluations and determine the necessary specificities to code accurately.

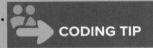

CODING TIP

Why the health care professional is providing services, procedures, and/or treatments to this patient is translated into the diagnosis code or codes.

Examples and Let's Code It! Scenarios

These features establish the connection between medical coding concepts and real-world application! Students experience guided practice and step-by-step examples that mirror situations they will most likely encounter in their professions.

LET'S CODE IT! SCENARIO

Louise Jorgensen, a 61-year-old female, came to see Dr. Mulkey. Earlier in the day, she was lightheaded and a little dizzy. In addition, she complained that her heart was beating so wildly that she thought she may have had a heart attack. Due to her previous diagnosis of type 1 diabetes, Dr. Mulkey ordered a blood glucose test. He also performed an electrocardiogram (ECG or EKG) to check her heart. After getting the results of the tests, Dr. Mulkey determined that Louise's lightheadedness and dizziness were a result of her glucose being too high. He spoke with Louise about how to bring her diabetes under control. He also told her that her EKG was negative and that there were no signs of a heart attack.

Let's Code It!

Dr. Mulkey confirmed that Louise's *type 1 diabetes mellitus* was out of control and this was the reason she felt lightheaded and dizzy. This tells you that these two symptoms are included in the confirmed diagnosis of diabetes mellitus. It seems that the diabetes is the only confirmed diagnosis in Dr. Mulkey's notes. However, the doctor performed an EKG. A diagnosis of diabetes mellitus does not provide any medical necessity for performing an EKG. In addition, the test was negative and, therefore, provided no diagnosis.

You still need a diagnosis code to report that there was a medically valid reason to run the EKG. Why did Dr. Mulkey perform the EKG? Because Louise complained of a *rapid heartbeat*. Therefore, you will report the code for rapid heartbeat to justify the EKG.

For this encounter, you have one confirmed diagnosis (type 1 diabetes mellitus) and one symptom that is unrelated to the confirmed diagnosis (rapid heartbeat). The guidelines state that the code for a confirmed diagnosis should precede the code for a sign or symptom, so you will report the diabetes code first and then the code for the tachycardia (the medical term for rapid heartbeat).

Guidance Connections

Each of these boxes connects the concepts students are learning about in the chapter to ICD-10-CM Official Guidelines to further students' knowledge and understanding of coding resources.

GUIDANCE CONNECTION

Review the ICD-10-CM Coding Guidelines: Section I.C. 18, Chapter 18: **Symptoms, signs, and abnormal clinical and laboratory findings, not elsewhere classified (R00–R99)**, Subsection b, **Use of a symptom code with a definitive diagnosis code.**

End-of-Chapter Reviews

Every chapter ends with Using Terminology (matching), Checking Your Understanding (multiple-choice), and Applying Your Knowledge (short-answer) questions that reinforce the chapter learning outcomes.

CHAPTER 1 REVIEW
Introduction to Diagnostic Coding

connect

Using Terminology

Part I
Match each key term to the appropriate definition.

____ 1. LO 1.3 Objective evidence of a disease or condition.
____ 2. LO 1.1 The acronym for International Classification of Diseases, Ninth Revision, Clinical Modification.
____ 3. LO 1.4 The paperwork in the patient's file that corroborates the codes presented on the claim form for a particular encounter.
____ 4. LO 1.4 Using a code on a claim form that indicates a higher level of service, or a more severe aspect of disease or injury, than that which was actual and true.
____ 5. LO 1.1 The determination that the health care professional was acting according to standard practices in providing a particular procedure for an individual with a particular diagnosis.
____ 6. LO 1.1 The acronym for International Classification of Diseases, Tenth Revision, Clinical Modification.
____ 7. LO 1.4 Coding the individual parts of a specific diagnosis or procedure rather than one combination or bundle that includes all of those components.
____ 8. LO 1.4 Choosing a code on the basis of what the insurance company will cover (pay for) rather than accurately reflecting the truth.
____ 9. LO 1.1 A subjective sensation or departure from the norm as related by the patient.
____ 10. LO 1.4 Sending a claim for the second time to the same insurance company for the same procedure or service, provided to the same patient on the same date of service.
____ 11. LO 1.1 A physician's determination of a patient's condition, illness, or injury.

A. Diagnosis
B. Sign
C. Symptom
D. ICD-9-CM
E. ICD-10-CM
F. Medical necessity
G. Supporting documentation
H. Coding for coverage
I. Upcoding
J. Unbundling
K. Double billing

Part II
Match each key term to the appropriate definition.

____ 1. LO 1.4 Medical terminology used to provide the location of a health problem or an approach for a surgical procedure.
____ 2. LO 1.4 Medical terminology that describes the patient's position (on the surgical or examination table).
____ 3. LO 1.4 The structure of the human body.
____ 4. LO 1.4 Medication (drugs).
____ 5. LO 1.4 The study of physiological processes of disease.
____ 6. LO 1.4 The study of the causes of disease.
____ 7. LO 1.4 The study of disease.
____ 8. LO 1.4 A space or area that is hollow and often houses organs and vessels.
____ 9. LO 1.4 A specific location within the anatomy (body).

A. etiology
B. pathology
C. pathophysiology
D. pharmaceuticals
E. anatomy
F. anatomical site
G. anatomical cavity
H. anatomical direction
I. anatomical position

Real Abstracting Practice with You Code It!

Gain real-world experience by using actual patient records (with names and other identifying information changed) to practice ICD-10-CM, ICD-10-PCS, CPT, and HCPCS Level II coding for both inpatient and outpatient! Exercises can be found at the end of each chapter. Plus, Chapter 24 consists solely of these activities.

You Code It! Practice

Practice diagnosis or procedure coding with these short coding scenarios.

YOU CODE IT! Practice
Chapter 12: Coding Circulatory Conditions

Using the techniques described in this chapter, carefully read through the case studies and determine the most accurate ICD-10-CM code(s) and external cause code(s), if appropriate, for each case study.

1. Sarah Linscott, a 37-year-old female, was diagnosed with benign hypertension due to a brain tumor.

2. David Nguyen, a 53-year-old male, is diagnosed with unspecified hypertension due to renal artery stenosis.

3. Dr. Sirianni diagnosed Gordon Baxa with secondary malignant hypertension due to Cushing's disease.

4. Robert Hall, a 61-year-old male, was diagnosed with accelerated hypertension.

You Code It! Application

Using physicians' notes documenting realistic patient encounters, students gain experience with abstracting and coding.

YOU CODE IT! Application
Chapter 12: Coding Circulatory Conditions

The following exercises provide practice in abstracting physicians' notes and learning to work with SOAP notes from our health care facility, *Taylor, Reader, & Associates*. These case studies (SOAP notes) are modeled on real patient encounters. Using the techniques described in this chapter, carefully read through the case studies and determine the most accurate ICD-10-CM code(s) and external cause code(s), if appropriate, for each case study.

TAYLOR, READER, & ASSOCIATES
A Complete Health Care Facility
975 CENTRAL AVENUE • SOMEWHERE, FL 32811 • 407-555-4321

PATIENT: CHEN, MELONIE
ACCOUNT/EHR #: CHENME001
DATE: 08/11/18

Attending Physician: Willard B. Reader, MD

S: Pt is an 81-year-old female who suffered a stroke last week. Her daughter is concerned about the patient's dysphasia. Evidently her speech has been impaired as a result of the stroke. The daughter notes that the patient has been unable to speak properly, having trouble forming sentences and finding the right word.

O: Ht 5'1" Wt. 135 lb. R 19. T 98.6. BP 145/93 Physical examination: unremarkable.

A: Dysphasia, late effect of a CVA.

P: 1. Pt to return PRN
   2. Referral to physical therapist

Willard B. Reader, MD

WBR/pw D: 08/11/18 09:50:16 T: 08/13/18 12:55:01

Determine the most accurate ICD-10-CM code(s).

INTRODUCTION TO DIAGNOSTIC CODING

1

Learning Outcomes *After completing this chapter, the student should be able to:*

LO 1.1 Explain the purpose of health care coding.

LO 1.2 Apply correctly the appropriate steps to coding.

LO 1.3 Incorporate the official guidelines into the determination of the best, most accurate code.

LO 1.4 Detect the ethical danger zones that might exist in the workplace.

LO 1.5 Know the AHIMA Code of Ethics and AHIMA's Standards of Ethical Coding.

LO 1.6 Employ the AAPC Code of Ethics.

LO 1.1 The purpose of coding is to make every effort to ensure clear and concise communication between everyone involved with the health and well-being of the population. In most cases, there are three parties: the health care provider, the patient, and the insurance company. (The insurance company is not always an actual insurance company, so the broader term *third-party payers* is used most of the time.) Codes are more precise than words, as you will find out as you venture through this material. Generally, the communication enables the third-party payer to clearly understand exactly what occurred between the provider and the patient and why, so the payer can feel comfortable paying for this encounter.

Additionally, the government uses coding information to direct research activities and funding into particular areas of concern. For these and other purposes, including the continuity of care for each and every individual, every health care encounter must be documented in complete detail.

When a person goes to see a health care provider, he or she must have a reason—a health-related reason. After all, as much as you might like your physician, you probably wouldn't make an appointment, sit in the waiting room, and go through all the paperwork just to say "hello." Whether the reason is a checkup, a flu shot, or something more serious, there is always a reason *why*. The physician will create notes (documentation), typed into an electronic health record, handwritten, or dictated, recounting the events of the encounter. The **diagnosis,** or diagnostic statement, in these notes will explain *why* the patient was seen and treated.

The notes may include a diagnosis that identifies a specific condition or illness, the **signs** or **symptoms** of an unnamed problem, or another reason for the encounter. As a coding specialist, it is your job to translate these reasons into a diagnosis code (or codes), so that everyone involved will clearly understand the issues of a particular patient at a particular time.

Key Terms

Adverse effect
Anatomical cavity
Anatomical direction
Anatomical position
Anatomical site
Body areas
Coding for coverage
Diagnosis
Double billing
Etiology
ICD-9-CM
ICD-10-CM
Medical necessity
Organ system
Pathology
Pathophysiology
Pharmaceuticals
Risk factor
Sign
Supporting documentation
Symptom
Unbundling
Upcoding

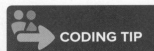
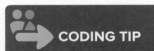
EXAMPLE

Hypertension is a diagnosis: The physician has determined the specific condition of a patient.

Feeling tired is a symptom: It is subjective, because it's based on the patient's opinion.

Fever is a sign: It is objective, because it's measurable.

The National Center for Health Statistics (NCHS) put together a committee to create the International Classification of Diseases, Ninth Revision, Clinical Modification **(ICD-9-CM)** in February 1977. The members of the committee represented a wide variety of organizations, including the American Hospital Association, the American College of Physicians, and the American Psychiatric Association. The ninth revision was designed to be a system to categorize information relating to diseases and to establish a more complete picture of patient care. ICD-9-CM is a directory of every diagnosis, sign, symptom, or other valid reason that could possibly be identified by a health care provider with regard to a patient encounter.

Recently, the U.S. health care industry implemented the International Classification of Diseases, Tenth Revision, Clinical Modification **(ICD-10-CM).** This update provides professional coding specialists with more codes from which to choose to report diagnoses, signs, and symptoms with even more specificity. Whereas the codes themselves look different from those used in ICD-9-CM, the process used for finding the most accurate code is the same.

Medical Necessity

The diagnosis codes that you assign justify the procedure, service, or treatment the health care professional provided to the patient during the encounter. Every time a health care professional provides treatment or service to a patient, there must be a valid medical reason. Certainly everyone would agree that health care professionals must have a good reason to perform procedures on a patient. This is referred to as **medical necessity.** Requiring medical necessity helps ensure that the health care provider is not performing tests and giving injections without a good medical reason. Diagnosis codes explain *why* the individual came to see the physician and support the physician's decision about *what* procedures to provide (i.e., the WHY justifies the WHAT).

Medical necessity is one of the reasons it is so very important to code the diagnosis accurately and with all the specifics possible. If you are one number off, you could accidentally cause the claim to be denied because the diagnosis identified by the incorrect code does not justify the procedure the doctor performed.

EXAMPLE

Caring Insurance Company received a claim form for patient Miranda Polichek, a 17-year-old female. The claim was seeking reimbursement for taking an MRI (magnetic resonance imaging) of her brain. An MRI costs $2,000, and the insurance company is not going to pay for the procedure without knowing that there was a valid medical reason for the patient to have it done.

Miranda had a *concussion with less than 30 minutes loss of consciousness* (S06.0x1A) that was caused by her *falling from a ladder* (W11.xxxA) while *working on her hobby* (Y99.8). These three diagnosis codes explain to the insurance company that it was *medically necessary* for the doctor to perform the MRI and that the claim should be paid.

However, the coder made a mistake when entering the code for the diagnosis and keyed in S60.011A instead of S06.0x1A. Caring Insurance Company had no choice but to deny the claim. Code S60.011A reports that Miranda had *contusion of right thumb without damage to nail.* You can see that it would not make any sense to perform an MRI of her brain when the problem was with her thumb. A simple error and the claim was denied.

In addition to ensuring that the code is correct, you are also responsible for making certain the codes you report tell the *whole story* about this patient's condition. Omitting a detail may seem like no big deal; however, that detail may be the portion of the story that is the key to supporting the medical necessity for the physician's decisions about treatment.

EXAMPLE

Isaac, a 31-year-old male, has had mild, persistent asthma since he was 10 years old. He always carries an inhaler in his pocket, and it has always worked before. However, today, the inhaler is not making any improvement. Actually, his wheezing is getting worse. His wife takes him to the emergency department (ED), and the doctor gives him a shot of epinephrine. It doesn't help, and he is immediately admitted into the hospital with a diagnosis of status asthmaticus.

J45.30 Mild persistent asthma, uncomplicated
J45.31 Mild persistent asthma with (acute) exacerbation
J45.32 Mild persistent asthma with status asthmaticus

Just the difference of the fifth character in the diagnosis code will determine whether Isaac's hospital bill will be paid for by his insurance company because this one number provides the explanation of why there was medical necessity for this admission in the hospital.

Uncomplicated asthma can be treated with medication, such as an inhaler, a nebulizer, or an injection. Acute exacerbation explains that the signs/symptoms are very severe but can still be treated with medication. This diagnosis (acute exacerbation) would support a visit to the ED, but it is not a reason to admit a patient into the hospital. Status asthmaticus, however, is a severe episode of asthma that is not responding to other treatments. Status asthmaticus is responsible for approximately 50,000 deaths a year in the United States. This is a serious condition, from which the patient could die, and does support admission into an acute care facility (a hospital).

Risk Factors

There are many **risk factors** that can be at the root of a health concern (an underlying cause) or be an aggravating factor. These may be documented during counseling, an annual preventive checkup, or other health care encounter. Professional coders need to understand the various causes and components of the condition being treated because these factors may affect the code or codes reported.

risk factor
A characteristic that increases a person's susceptibility to a disease or injury.

Lifestyle factors, particularly involvement in activities that may affect one's health, are also important for the physician to know about a patient and may require an additional code or codes, determined by the involvement of that activity in regard to the patient's condition. For example, long-term (current) use of nonsteroidal anti-inflammatory drugs (NSAIDs), ICD-10-CM code Z79.1, might be the underlying cause of a bleeding stomach ulcer, or tobacco use, ICD-10-CM code Z72.0, might be the underlying cause of chronic bronchitis.

Environmental factors can also be involved with a patient's health. Often it is important to report the external causes of injury, poisoning, underdosing, or **adverse effect,** using codes from ICD-10-CM code range V00–Y99. However, there may be other issues that require a coder's attention; for example, smoke inhalation from a building fire, ICD-10-CM code X02.1xxA, causing respiratory distress, or accidental submersion while in a swimming pool, ICD-10-CM code W67xxxA, causing anoxia.

Preexisting conditions, known as *personal history,* may also require additional codes to report the complete story of this patient's condition. For example, reporting ICD-10-CM code Z85.820, Personal history of malignant melanoma of skin, would support more frequent dermatologic screenings. Reporting ICD-10-CM code Z87.11, Personal history of peptic ulcer disease, may support alternative treatments for the patient's arthritis because the standard care (NSAID) may aggravate the ulcerative condition and cause hemorrhaging.

Stress can also be a negative factor to one's health, as you probably already know. Professional coders must discern from the documentation when this warrants additional coding; for example, ICD-10-CM code Z56.6, Work-related mental stress, to support a prescription or a disability claim, and ICD-10-CM code Z63.4, Family disruption due to bereavement, to support a referral for counseling.

Signs and Symptoms

One of the reasons you, as a professional coding specialist, must learn about pathology and physiology is to be able to distinguish between signs and symptoms that are included in a confirmed diagnosis and those that are not. Signs and symptoms that are integral as a part of a confirmed diagnosis are *not* separately reported, whereas those that are not included are coded separately.

A *sign* is an indication of an abnormal state that can be measured. A fever is a good example, because a patient's temperature can be measured with a thermometer. High blood pressure is another sign because it can be measured with a sphygmomanometer (commonly referred to as a *blood pressure cuff*).

A *symptom* is an indication of an abnormal state as described by the patient. When patients complain of pain, health care professionals must accept their word. There is no way to measure this. Or, if a patient complains of feeling achy or dizzy, again, there is no way to measure this concern.

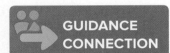

GUIDANCE CONNECTION

Review the ICD-10-CM Coding Guidelines: Section I.C. 18, Chapter 18: **Symptoms, signs, and abnormal clinical and laboratory findings, not elsewhere classified (R00–R99),** Subsection a, **Use of symptom codes.**

EXAMPLE

John comes to see Dr. Finch complaining of chest congestion, runny nose, sneezing, headaches, and being achy all over. Dr. Finch examines John, does a quick lab test, and tells John he has the flu.

As the coding specialist, you must know that *"chest congestion, runny nose, sneezing, headaches, being achy all over"* are signs and symptoms of the flu. Therefore, when you report the code for the flu, there is no reason to also code the signs and symptoms—doing so would be redundant.

LET'S CODE IT! SCENARIO

Louise Jorgensen, a 61-year-old female, came to see Dr. Mulkey. Earlier in the day, she was lightheaded and a little dizzy. In addition, she complained that her heart was beating so wildly that she thought she may have had a heart attack. Due to her previous diagnosis of type 1 diabetes, Dr. Mulkey ordered a blood glucose test. He also performed an electrocardiogram (ECG or EKG) to check her heart. After getting the results of the tests, Dr. Mulkey determined that Louise's lightheadedness and dizziness were a result of her glucose being too high. He spoke with Louise about how to bring her diabetes under control. He also told her that her EKG was negative and that there were no signs of a heart attack.

Let's Code It!

Dr. Mulkey confirmed that Louise's *type 1 diabetes mellitus* was out of control and this was the reason she felt lightheaded and dizzy. This tells you that these two symptoms are included in the confirmed diagnosis of diabetes mellitus. It seems that the diabetes is the only confirmed diagnosis in Dr. Mulkey's notes. However, the doctor performed an EKG. A diagnosis of diabetes mellitus does not provide any medical necessity for performing an EKG. In addition, the test was negative and, therefore, provided no diagnosis.

You still need a diagnosis code to report that there was a medically valid reason to run the EKG. Why did Dr. Mulkey perform the EKG? Because Louise complained of a *rapid heartbeat*. Therefore, you will report the code for rapid heartbeat to justify the EKG.

For this encounter, you have one confirmed diagnosis (type 1 diabetes mellitus) and one symptom that is unrelated to the confirmed diagnosis (rapid heartbeat). The guidelines state that the code for a confirmed diagnosis should precede the code for a sign or symptom, so you will report the diabetes code first and then the code for the tachycardia (the medical term for rapid heartbeat).

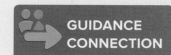

GUIDANCE CONNECTION

Review the ICD-10-CM Coding Guidelines: Section I.C. 18, Chapter 18: **Symptoms, signs, and abnormal clinical and laboratory findings, not elsewhere classified (R00–R99),** Subsection b, **Use of a symptom code with a definitive diagnosis code.**

Procedures and Services

The other part of the story you, as a professional coding specialist, will need to tell with codes is *what* was done for the patient. You will report procedures, treatments, and services provided to a patient using codes from either the Current Procedural Terminology (CPT) code set or ICD-10-PCS. Which code set you use will depend upon where you work.

When coding inpatient services for the facility, those services provided by the hospital while a patient is admitted in the hospital, you will probably use ICD-10-PCS (International Classification of Diseases, Tenth Revision, Procedure Coding System).

For services provided in an outpatient setting, such as a physician's office, a clinic, or an ambulatory care center, you will probably use CPT.

Remember: When you are coding diagnoses or procedures using any of the code sets, each set of numbers and letters is so specific that a code number just one character off could mean something totally different. That difference could cause the claim to be rejected, resulting in your patient being labeled with a disease he or she does not have and/or your facility not being paid for the work it provided. This is why it is very critical to be careful and accurate when coding and always *double-check* your codes.

These procedure code sets are mentioned here so you will be familiar with their names and what they represent. This volume, however, focuses solely on the diagnosis coding portion of a professional coding specialist's job.

LO 1.2 Seven Steps to Accurate Coding

Here is a seven-step process that you can follow to code a health care encounter in the approved manner. As you gain experience, it will take you less time to go through these steps. However, remember that time is not the number one consideration when coding—no matter what anyone says, *accuracy* is the most important factor.

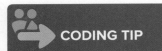

1. Read completely through the superbill and the physician's notes (see Figure 1-1) for the encounter, from beginning to end.

2. Reread the physician's notes and highlight key words regarding diagnoses and procedures directly relating to the encounter. Pulling out the key words is also called *abstracting* physician's notes. You will need to evaluate the key words and distinguish between diagnostic statements and procedural statements.

3. Make a list of any questions you have regarding unclear or missing information necessary to code the encounter. Query, or confer with, the health care provider who treated the patient. Never assume or try to guess. Code only what you know from actual documentation. If it is not written down, it did not happen, and you cannot code it!

EXAMPLE

Dr. Mandell diagnosed Ilona with malignant neoplasm of the brain (brain cancer). The code category for this is C71, Malignant neoplasm of the brain. However, you need a fourth character. As you read down the list of code descriptions for the four-character codes in this category, you will notice that each one identifies WHERE in the brain the tumor (the neoplasm) is located. Rather than report code C71.9, Malignant neoplasm of the brain, unspecified, you need to query the physician to add this specific information to the patient's documentation.

Why go through all this effort when you have heard that the insurance company has paid the claim with a diagnosis code of C71.9 (or other unspecified code)? Two reasons:

1. Next week, Dr. Mandell may want to perform a procedure on Ilona that would *not* be supported for medical necessity with an unspecified code.

2. Often, the physician does not include additional information because he or she does not know what specific piece of information is needed for coding. You know; the doctor, typically, does not.

4. Code each diagnosis and/or appropriate signs or symptoms describing *why* the health care provider treated this patient during this encounter, as documented in his or her notes. Use the best, most accurate code available based on that documentation.

  a. Look key terms up in the Alphabetic Index.

  b. Read the complete code description in the Tabular List.

  c. Read all notations and symbols.

  d. Read the guidelines in the front of the book.

  e. Assign codes to the greatest specificity (highest level of detail) of confirmed diagnoses, signs, symptoms, and other conditions that are connected to, or related to, services and procedures provided at this visit.

  f. Code only those documented conditions that require or influence treatment at this encounter.

  g. Include as many codes as necessary to report the reasons *why* completely (to tell the whole story).

5. Code each procedure, as stated in the notes, describing *what* the provider did for the patient. Use the best, most accurate codes available based on the documentation. There are similar steps to determining the procedure code to report.

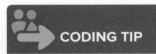

Family Doctors Associates
123 Main Street • Anytown, FL 32711
(407) 555-1200

Date: September 16, 2018   Attending Physician: J. Healer, MD

Patient Name: George Willows

This patient is a 74-year-old patient of mine for the past 20 years. He is a retired construction worker who now lives at home alone after his wife's recent death. He has COPD from years of smoking, but quit 12 years ago. I asked the patient how he is doing with the diuretic I had prescribed, and he good-naturedly responded that he hasn't been able to keep track of it real well now that his wife isn't there nagging him all the time. I explain to him that it is important for him to take his medication. He states, "Hey, doc, come on, I'm 74 already and haven't had any health problems! What's the big deal anyways?" I patiently stress further to Mr. Willows the importance of this medication. He agrees to try harder to stay on schedule with his HCTZ. "It'll be just like punchin' the clock, doc; no problem."

PAST MEDICAL HISTORY: He had an appendectomy as a child and three inguinal hernia repairs during his working life. He has long-standing HTN, and that has never been well-controlled. We tried him on clonidine, methyldopa, and prazosin back when those were the choice drugs. I recently switched him to hydrochlorothiazide (25 mg) from clonidine to see if it couldn't make an impact on his BP.

FAMILY HISTORY: He can't remember what his parents died from, but thinks it was "old age."

VITAL SIGNS: BP 176/104.

DX: Essential hypertension

RX: Nifedipine

Jerrome Healer, MD

FIGURE 1-1 An Example of Physician's Notes

These are reviewed at length in the companion volume *The Complete Procedure Coding Solution*.

6. Link each and every procedure code to at least one diagnosis code to verify medical necessity.

7. Double-check your codes. Go back into the books you have used, and reread the code descriptions of the codes you have assigned and match them with the notes— one more time.

Following these steps will help you code precisely, resulting in a greater number of your claims getting paid quickly. That is much better than having the claims rejected or denied and dealing with the same case again.

Coding from Physician's Notes

As mentioned earlier in this chapter, you, as the professional coding specialist, will need all of the details and specifics about what occurred between the health care professional and the patient during an encounter, and why. The best way to gather this information is to review the physician's notes, lab reports, superbill/encounter form, and *all* documentation for that encounter. When you read *exactly* what the physician thought, heard, and observed in his or her own words, you will have more specific information to help you determine the most accurate code. The more complete the communication between the providing professional and the professional coding specialist, the more accurate the codes will be—ensuring optimal reimbursement.

CODING TIP

Use a medical dictionary to learn the true meaning of a medical term or abbreviation. If you don't know what the term means, you will have a problem interpreting it into an accurate code.

CODING TIP

A great way to help ensure you have all the necessary diagnosis codes to tell the whole story: Take a look at all of the procedures, services, and treatments (WHAT was done for the patient), and confirm that you have at least one diagnosis code to support providing each procedure. This works well even when you are not responsible for coding procedures.

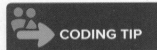
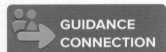
Your diagnosis codes will be more accurate and will report medical necessity for the procedures, services, and treatments provided when you access all the documentation. After all, how can you report the *whole story* if you don't know the *whole story?*

EXAMPLE

Janelle's facility has her use information from the office's preprinted encounter form rather than waiting for the doctor to dictate his notes from the encounter. However, that superbill only offers one choice for a diagnosis of hypertension and one code for heart disease, to save room on the one-page encounter form:

> I10 Essential (primary) hypertension
>
> I51.9 Heart disease, unspecified

After reading the notes, Janelle discovered that the actual diagnosis written by the physician was hypertensive heart disease, changing the correct code to:

> I11.9 Hypertensive heart disease, without heart failure

The difference between these two codes could dramatically affect whether or not the facility gets paid for the procedures provided.

LO 1.3 Official ICD-10-CM Guidelines for Coding and Reporting

In the front of your ICD-10-CM book, you will find the Official Guidelines for Coding and Reporting as issued by the Centers for Medicare and Medicaid Services (CMS) and the National Center for Health Statistics (NCHS), two departments within the U.S. government's Department of Health and Human Services (HHS). You will learn all about them as you study this material. The guidelines will literally guide you toward the best, most accurate code and make coding decisions easier.

The guidelines are divided into four sections and an appendix:

I. Conventions, General Coding Guidelines, and Chapter-Specific Guidelines
II. Selection of Principal Diagnosis
III. Reporting Additional Diagnoses
IV. Diagnostic Coding and Reporting Guidelines for Outpatient Services
V. Appendix I. Present on Admission Reporting Guidelines

The guidelines are the same for, and are applicable to, both inpatient (those patients admitted into the hospital) and outpatient (outpatient departments, same-day surgical centers, physicians offices, etc.) coding with a few exceptions. The exceptions are important.

Section II, Selection of Principal Diagnosis, Subsection H, Uncertain diagnosis. The guidelines state that with regard to a diagnosis documented as "probable," "suspected," "likely," "questionable," "possible," or "still to be ruled out," you should "code the condition as if it existed or was established."

Now: consider the following.

Section IV, Diagnostic Coding and Reporting Guidelines for Outpatient Services, Subsection H. The guidelines state, "Do not code diagnoses documented as 'probable,' 'suspected,' 'questionable,' 'rule out,' or 'working diagnosis.' Rather, code the condition(s) to the highest degree of certainty for that encounter/visit."

The difference between these two rules is that when you are coding for a hospital inpatient, you are permitted to code those conditions stated as possible or likely, but not when you are coding for a physician or outpatient service. These guidelines are always right there, in your ICD-10-CM book, for you to reference at any time.

In the Official Guidelines, Section I, Conventions, General Coding Guidelines and Chapter-Specific Guidelines, Subsection C, lists detailed rules affecting your decisions when coding certain diseases, conditions, illnesses, and injuries. The headings, or sections, of the guidelines are very specific:

C. CHAPTER-SPECIFIC CODING GUIDELINES

1. Chapter 1: Certain infectious and parasitic diseases (A00–B99)
2. Chapter 2: Neoplasms (C00–D49)
3. Chapter 3: Disease of the blood and blood-forming organs and certain disorders involving the immune mechanism (D50–D89)
4. Chapter 4: Endocrine, nutritional, and metabolic diseases (E00–E89).
5. Chapter 5: Mental, behavioral, and neurodevelopmental disorders (F01–F99)
6. Chapter 6: Diseases of the nervous system (G00–G99)
7. Chapter 7: Diseases of the eye and adnexa (H00–H59)
8. Chapter 8: Diseases of the ear and mastoid process (H60–H95)
9. Chapter 9: Diseases of the circulatory system (I00–I99)
10. Chapter 10: Diseases of the respiratory system (J00–J99)
11. Chapter 11: Diseases of the digestive system (K00–K95)
12. Chapter 12: Diseases of the skin and subcutaneous tissue (L00–L99)
13. Chapter 13: Diseases of the musculoskeletal system and connective tissue (M00–M99)
14. Chapter 14: Diseases of the genitourinary system (N00–N99)
15. Chapter 15: Pregnancy, childbirth, and the puerperium (O00–O9A)
16. Chapter 16: Certain conditions originating in the perinatal period (P00–P96)
17. Chapter 17: Congenital malformations, deformations, and chromosomal abnormalities (Q00–Q99)
18. Chapter 18: Symptoms, signs, and abnormal clinical and laboratory findings, not elsewhere classified (R00–R99)
19. Chapter 19: Injury, poisoning, and certain other consequences of external causes (S00–T88)
20. Chapter 20: External causes of morbidity (V00–Y99)
21. Chapter 21: Factors influencing health status and contact with health services (Z00–Z99)

We review all these guidelines in the chapters to come.

LO 1.4 Rules for Ethical and Legal Coding

As a coder, you have a very important responsibility—to yourself, your patients, and your facility. The work you do results in the creation of health claim forms and other reports that are legal documents. What you do can contribute to your facility staying healthy (businesswise) or being fined and possibly shut down by the Office of the Inspector General and your state's attorney general. You might make an error that could cause a patient to be unfairly denied health insurance coverage. It is important that you clearly understand the ethical and legal aspects of your position.

1. It is very important that the codes indicated on the health claim form represent the services actually performed and the reasons why they are provided as supported by the documentation in the patient's health record. Don't use a code on a claim form without ensuring the **supporting documentation** is there in the file.

supporting documentation
The paperwork in the patient's file that corroborates the codes presented on the claim form for a particular encounter.

Stephanie Zambro's file indicates that Dr. Villa ordered a blood test to determine whether or not she is pregnant. There is no report showing the results of the test. You see Dr. Villa, and he tells you that Stephanie is pregnant and you should go ahead and code that diagnosis so the claim can be sent in. He promises to place the lab report and update the notes in her file later. Until the physician documents that the patient is pregnant, you are not permitted to code the pregnancy.

coding for coverage
Choosing a code on the basis of what the insurance company will cover (pay for) rather than accurately reflecting the truth.

2. Some health care providers may improperly encourage **coding for coverage.** This term refers to the process of determining diagnostic and procedural codes not by the accuracy of the code but with regard to what the insurance company will pay for or "cover." That is dishonest and is considered fraud. If you find yourself in an office or facility that insists you "code for coverage" rather than code to accurately reflect the documentation and the services actually performed, you should immediately discuss your situation with someone you trust. Some providers will rationalize the process by saying they are doing it so the patients can get the treatment they really need paid for by the insurance company. Altruism aside, it is still illegal and, once discovered, financial penalties and possible jail time can be assessed.

Kyle Ford wants a nose job (rhinoplasty); however, he cannot afford it. The insurance carrier will not pay for cosmetic surgery, so the coder changes the code to indicate that Kyle has a deviated septum requiring surgical correction so that the insurance carrier will pay for the procedure. That is coding for coverage and is fraud.

3. If you find yourself in an office or facility that insists that you include codes for procedures that you know, or believe, were never performed at a level of intensity or complexity as described by the code, this might be fraudulent behavior, known as **upcoding**—the process of using a code that claims a higher level of service, or a more severe illness, than is true. Upcoding is considered falsifying records. Even if all you do is fill out the claim form, you are participating in something unethical and illegal.

upcoding
Using a code on a claim form that indicates a higher level of service or a more severe aspect of disease or injury than that which was actual and true.

Tracey Mendez, a 71-year-old female, in the hospital for a broken hip, had her glucose level checked by the nurse, and it was at an abnormal level. Dr. Basso ordered additional tests to rule out diabetes mellitus. Coding that Tracey has diabetes is upcoding her condition and will fraudulently increase reimbursement from Medicare by changing the diagnosis-related group (DRG). In addition, placing a chronic disease on her health chart, when she doesn't have it, will cause her problems later on.

unbundling
Coding the individual parts of a specific diagnosis or procedure rather than one combination or bundle that includes all of those components.

4. It is not permissible to code and bill for individual (also known as *component*) elements when a comprehensive or combination (bundle) code is available. This is referred to as **unbundling** and is illegal.

Dr. Cooke's notes indicate that Sabrina was experiencing nausea and vomiting. Instead of coding R11.2, Nausea with vomiting, the coder unbundles, coding R11.0, Nausea, alone and R11.11, Vomiting, alone.

5. You must code all conditions or complications that are relevant to the current encounter. Failure to do so can be considered unethical.

6. Separating the codes relating to one specific encounter and placing them on several different claim forms over the course of several different days is neither legal nor ethical. It not only indicates a lack of organization of the office but also can cause suspicion of duplicating service claims, known as **double billing.** Even if you are reporting procedures that were actually done for diagnoses that actually exist, remember that the claim form is a legal document. All data on that claim form, including dates of service, must be accurate. Do not submit the claim form until you are certain it is complete, with all diagnoses and procedures listed. If it happens that, after you submit a claim, an additional service provided comes to light (such as a lab report with an extra charge that didn't come across your desk until after you filed the claim), then you must file an amended claim. While not illegal because you are identifying that the claim contains an adjustment, most third-party payers really dislike amended claims. You can expect an amended claim to be scrutinized.

double billing
Sending a claim for the second time to the same insurance company for the same procedure or service, provided to the same patient on the same date of service.

All the activities mentioned here are considered fraud and are against the law. The Health Insurance Portability and Accountability Act (HIPAA) created the Health Care Fraud and Abuse Control Program (HCFACP). This program, under the direction of the attorney general and the secretary of the HHS, acts in accordance with the Office of the Inspector General (OIG) and coordinates with federal, state, and local law enforcement agencies to discover those who attempt to defraud or abuse the health care system, including Medicare and Medicaid patients and programs.

By catching those who submitted fraudulent claims, approximately $723 million was returned to the Medicare Trust Fund in 2003 and another $151.6 million was reimbursed to the Centers for Medicare and Medicaid Services (CMS). The federal government deposited approximately $2.51 billion to the Medicare Trust Fund in fiscal year 2009, plus more than $441 million of federal Medicaid funds were brought into the U.S. Treasury. Since it was created in 1997, the HCFACP has collected more than $15.6 billion to the Medicare Trust Fund—money improperly received by health care professionals filing fraudulent claims. The statistics show that for every $1 spent to pay for these investigations and prosecutions, the government actually brings in about $4 in money returned.

Also, in 2003, 362 criminal indictments were filed in health care fraud cases, and 437 defendants were convicted for health care fraud-related crimes. Another 231 civil cases were filed and 1,277 more civil matters were pending during this same year. These investigations also prohibited 3,275 individuals and organizations from working with any federally sponsored programs (such as Medicare and Medicaid). Most of these were as a result of convictions for Medicare- or Medicaid-related crimes, including patient abuse and patient neglect, or as a result of providers' licenses having been revoked.

In 2009, 1,014 new investigations were started by the Fraud Section of the criminal division in conjunction with the U.S. Attorneys' offices. These investigations involve 1,786 defendants, while the federal prosecutors filed criminal charges involving 803 defendants in 481 cases and had another 1,621 health care fraud investigations involving 2,706 potential defendants. At the same time, the Department of Justice had 1,155 civil health care fraud cases pending and 886 new civil investigations opened.

When you compare the 2003 numbers with the 2009 numbers you can see that an increasing number of people are being caught trying to get money for health care

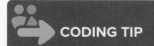

CODING TIP

Always read the complete description in the provider's notes in addition to referencing the encounter form or superbill, and then carefully find the best available code that supports medical necessity according to the documentation.

services to which they are not entitled. This is an important reminder that if individuals try to get you to participate in illegal or unethical behaviors, the question is not "Will you be caught?" but "*When* will you be caught?"

It is not worth breaking the law and being charged with any of these penalties just to hang onto a job.

Resources

Using the ICD-10-CM to identify the correct diagnosis code can be like a treasure hunt. Sometimes it is very easy to find the best, most accurate code in accordance with the physician's notes. Other times, it may seem as though the code isn't there. However, you must remember that if the health care provider can diagnose it, the code exists!

To help you in your search, use only credible references; for example:

- The ICD-10-CM Official Guidelines for Coding and Reporting will support your accurate use of the code set, and they appear right in the front of your code manual, always at your fingertips.
- A medical dictionary will help you find an alternate term that might be easier to find in the ICD-10-CM manual.
- The *Merck Manual,* along with credible websites, such as MedlinePlus and Medscape, will help you determine which signs and symptoms are included in a confirmed diagnosis and which should be coded separately.
- The *Physicians' Desk Reference* (PDR) will help you find alternate or generic names for drugs or other chemicals used in the patient's treatment that may have been prescribed by the physician, been taken incorrectly or accidentally, caused an allergic reaction, or had a toxic effect.
- Publications including the *Coding Clinic* (published by the American Hospital Association) and the *Correct Coding Initiative* (from CMS), as well as *CodeWrite,* a free electronic newsletter from the American Health Information Management Association, provide current information on coding.
- Professional and government websites, including www.ahima.org, www.cms.hhs.gov, www.aapc.com, and www.dhhs.gov, offer a variety of health and coding information.
- Of course, the health care provider who saw the patient and wrote the documentation can help answer any questions and provide additional details.

Foundational Knowledge

The health care system has its own language to refer to the various components of the human body (see Figure 1-2). Health care professionals need to communicate in the most specific and accurate manner possible when documenting a patient's various signs, symptoms, conditions, and diagnoses, as well as the procedures, treatments, and services provided. This is critical to medical decision making, continuity of care, and maximization of the effectiveness and efficiency of resources, as well as for reimbursement. This is why professional coding specialists need to have a complete understanding of medical terminology in addition to the specifics of anatomy, etiology, and pathophysiology.

Let's begin with the terms that relate to the body as a whole before the following chapters review each body system individually.

Anatomy refers to the structure of the human body, including organs, bones, muscle, tissue, and blood. The term **anatomical site,** a variation of anatomy, is referencing a specific location within the anatomy (body). **Pathology** means the study of disease, while **pathophysiology** is the study of physiological processes of disease. **Etiology** is the study of the causes of disease. Information about **pharmaceuticals,** or medication (drugs), will also be included.

anatomical site
A specific location within the anatomy (body).

pathology
The study of disease.

pathophysiology
The study of physiological processes of disease.

etiology
The study of the causes of disease.

pharmaceuticals
Medication (drugs).

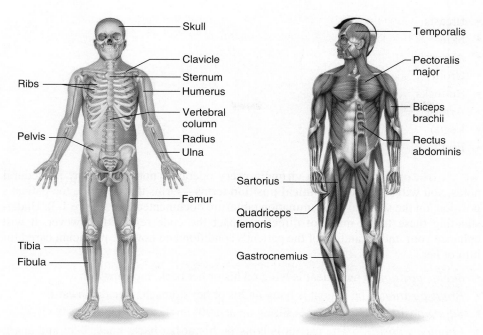

FIGURE 1-2 The Human Body

Source: Booth et al., MA, 5e. Copyright © 2013 by McGraw-Hill. Figure 22-6a, p. 478

Organ Systems As a whole, proper function of the human body is dependent upon each of the **organ systems** working correctly. In addition, some organ systems are dependent upon other organ systems to properly function. The intertwining of these functions creates the makeup of a healthy body. These systems are:

- *Integumentary system:* skin, subcutaneous tissue, accessory structures, hair, and nails.
- *Musculoskeletal system:* muscles, tendons, ligaments, cartilage, and bones.
- *Respiratory system:* nose, accessory sinuses, larynx, trachea, bronchi, lungs, and pleura.
- *Cardiovascular system:* heart, pericardium, arteries, and veins.
- *Digestive system:* mouth, palate, uvula, pharynx, adenoids, tonsils, esophagus, stomach, intestines, appendix, rectum, anus, liver, pancreas, biliary tract, abdomen, peritoneum, and omentum.
- *Urinary system:* kidneys, ureters, urinary bladder, and urethra.
- *Genital system:* penis, testes, epididymis, tunica vaginalis, scrotum, vas deferens, spermatic cord, seminal vesicles, and the prostate in the male; vulva, perineum, introitus, vagina, cervix uteri, corpus uteri, ovaries, and fallopian tubes in the female.
- *Nervous system:* the central nervous system (the brain and spinal cord) and the peripheral nervous system.
- *Sensory systems:* eyes (orbit, conjunctiva, cornea, sclera, iris, lens, retina, etc.) and ears (external ear, middle ear, inner ear).
- *Endocrine system:* pituitary gland, hypothalamus, thyroid gland, parathyroid glands, adrenal glands, and thymus.
- *Lymphatic system:* lymph nodes, spleen, and lymphatic vessels.
- *Hematologic system:* blood itself and blood-forming organs.

Body Areas There are times when physicians will document evaluation of **body areas** rather than complete systems. These references may include:

- Head, eyes, ears, nose, and throat (HEENT)
- Neck
- Torso (chest and/or back)

organ system
A group of anatomical sites working together to perform a specific bodily function.

body area
A region of the human structure.

- Breasts
- Skin
- Abdomen
- Groin
- Buttocks
- Arm(s)
- Leg(s)
- Feet

Anatomical Positions In virtually every operative note, and many procedural notes, you will see that **anatomical position** terms—terms that describe the patient's position (on the surgical or examination table) are documented (see Figure 1-3). Understanding these terms may not directly impact the code reported; however, it will enhance your understanding of the patient's condition and how the physician cared for him or her.

anatomical position
Medical terminology that describes the patient's position (on the surgical or examination table).

- *Supine position:* The patient is lying on his or her back, face upward.
- *Prone position:* The patient is lying on his or her stomach, face downward.
- *Sitting position:* The patient is sitting up at a 90° angle to the table.
- *Lithotomy position:* The patient is lying on his or her back, knees bent and apart, feet in stirrups.

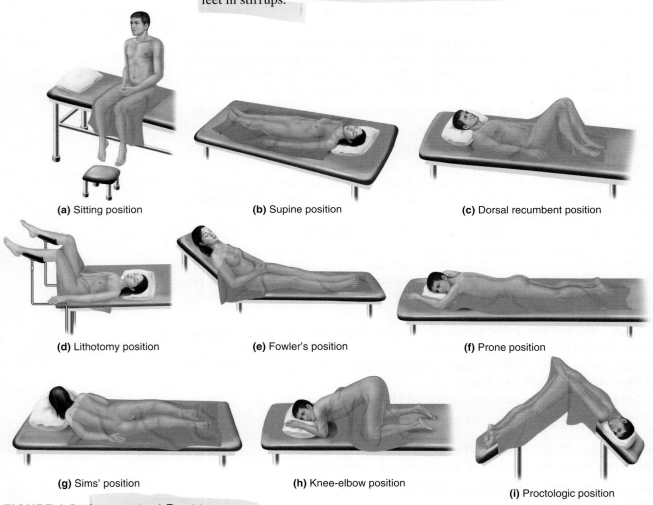

(a) Sitting position   **(b)** Supine position   **(c)** Dorsal recumbent position

(d) Lithotomy position   **(e)** Fowler's position   **(f)** Prone position

(g) Sims' position   **(h)** Knee-elbow position   **(i)** Proctologic position

FIGURE 1-3 Anatomical Positions

Source: Booth et al., MA, 5e. Copyright © 2013 by McGraw-Hill. Figure 38-1, p. 729

- *Dorsal recumbent position:* The patient is lying on his or her back, knees bent, feet flat on the table.
- *Sims' (left lateral) position:* The patient is lying on his or her stomach, right arm at side, right leg straight, left arm at right angle to head, left-leg knee bent upward toward waist (Sims' right lateral position would reverse the positions of the arms and legs).
- *Fowler's position:* The patient is lying on his or her back with a headrest bringing the head and torso up at a 45° angle.
- *Knee-elbow position:* The patient is face down on the table, arms above head, buttocks in the air with knees at right angle.
- *Proctologic position:* The patient is lying face down with table assisting an upward presentation of rectum and anus.

Anatomical Directions Medical terminology allows health care professionals to be very specific as to the **anatomical direction** of a health concern, location of a health problem, or approach for a surgical procedure (see Figure 1-4). In fact, you might find more than one word to indicate a surface or direction. You will see, though,

anatomical direction
Medical terminology used to provide the location of a health problem or an approach for a surgical procedure.

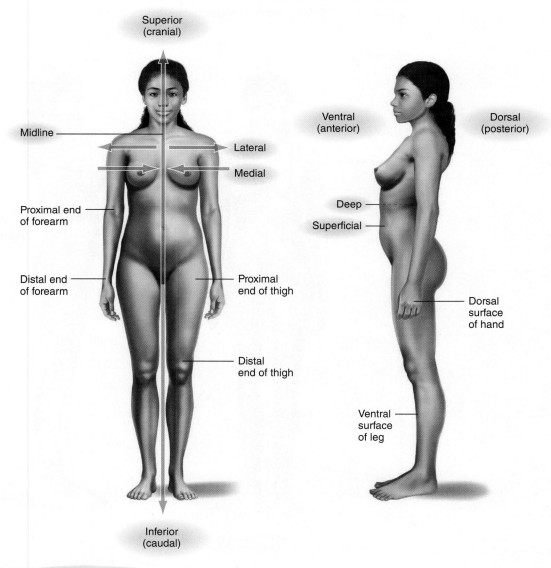

FIGURE 1-4 Anatomical Directions

Source: Booth et al., MA 5e. Copyright © 2013 by McGraw-Hill. Figure 22.7, p. 481

that each term has its purpose. There are many instances in which your understanding of these terms will enable you to determine the correct diagnosis code.

> ## EXAMPLE
>
> E84.19 Cystic fibrosis with other intestinal manifestations (Distal intestinal obstruction syndrome)
> G57.41- Lesion of medial popliteal nerve, right lower limb.

Top and Bottom   The *transverse* plane (see Figure 1-5) invisibly divides the body in half: top and bottom.

Superior	Toward the top (the head) of the body
Cephalad	Toward the head of the body
Inferior	Toward the bottom (the feet) of the body
Caudal	Toward the tail (really means tail)

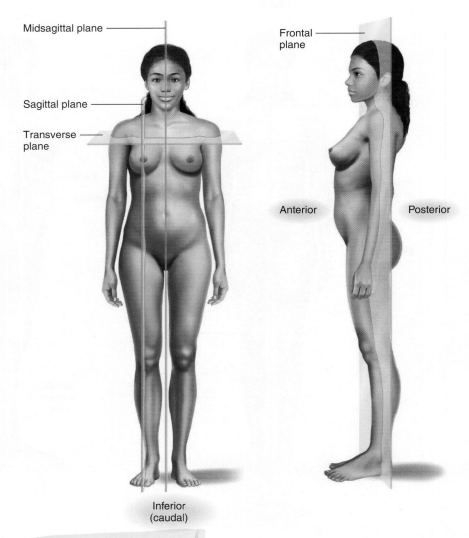

Midsagittal plane

Sagittal plane

Transverse plane

Frontal plane

Anterior   Posterior

Inferior (caudal)

FIGURE 1-5 Body Planes

Source: Booth et al., MA, 5e. Copyright © 2013 by McGraw-Hill. Figure 22-8, p. 482

| Palmar | The surface of the palm of the hand |
| Plantar | The surface of the sole of the food |

Side and Side The *sagittal* plane (see Figure 1-5) invisibly divides the body in half: right and left.

Left	Toward the left of the patient
Right	Toward the right of the patient
Lateral	Toward the side (either side)
Bilateral	Both sides
Medial	Toward the middle of the body
Proximal	Toward the point of attachment (usually applies to appendages, or extremities)
Distal	Away from the torso
Transverse	Across horizontally (side to side)

Front and Back The *frontal* plane (see Figure 1-5) invisibly divides the body in half: front and back.

Anterior	Toward the front of the body
Ventral	Toward (or along) the front (belly) of the body
Posterior	Toward the back of the body
Dorsal	Toward (or along) the back (spine) of the body

Inside and Outside

Visceral	Toward an internal organ
Deep	Toward the inside of the body
Medullary	The inner region
Parietal	Toward the outer wall of the body
Superficial	Toward the surface of the body
Cortical	The outer region

C45.1 Mesothelioma of peritoneum (parietal)(pelvic)
C90.01 Multiple myeloma (Medullary plasmacytoma), in remission

In addition to using these terms to describe the location of an organ or a symptom, you may see combinations of these terms used in identifying the direction of imaging. The most frequently used are:

- *Anteroposterior (AP):* The image was taken from front to back.
- *Lateral (lat):* The image was taken from one side to the other side.
- *Left anterior oblique (LAO):* The image was taken at an angle from the left front.
- *Left posterior oblique (LPO):* The image was taken at an angle from the left back.
- *Oblique (O):* The image was taken at an angle.
- *Posteroanterior (PA):* The image was taken back to front.
- *Right anterior oblique (RAO):* The image was taken at an angle from the right front.
- *Right posterior oblique (RPO):* The image was taken at an angle from the right back.

anatomical cavity
A space or area that is hollow and often houses organs and vessels.

Anatomical Cavities There are many pockets, or cavities, within the body (see Figure 1-6) that you will see referenced in physician documentation. An **anatomical cavity** is a space or area that is hollow. Often, this space houses organs and vessels.

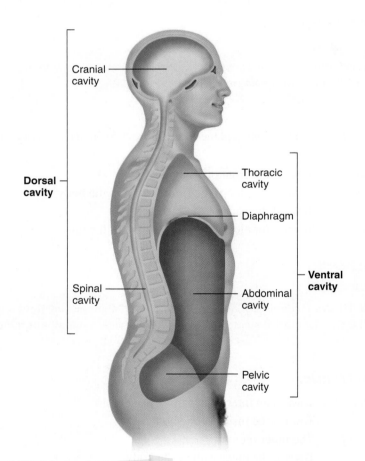

FIGURE 1-6 Anatomical Cavities

Source: Booth et al., MA, 5e. Copyright © 2013 by McGraw-Hill. Figure 22-10, p. 484

- *Cranial cavity:* The space within the skull.
- *Tympanic cavity:* The area located in the middle ear, within the temporal bone, that contains the ear ossicles.
- *Nasal cavity:* The area that lies between the base of the cranium and the roof of the mouth. The nasal septum, also known as the *vertical septum,* divides this space in two subsections.
- *Spinal cavity:* The space that lies along the dorsal line of the body and contains the spinal column and spinal cord.
- *Thoracic cavity:* Also known as the *chest cavity,* the space that is framed by the ribs and spinal column and contains the heart and lungs.
- *Oral cavity:* The medical term that references the mouth.
- *Pleural cavity:* The space between the parietal pleura and the visceral pleura in the chest cavity, between the lungs and the ribs.
- *Abdominal cavity:* The area between the diaphragm at the superior and the pelvis at the inferior.
- *Peritoneal cavity:* The area between the abdominal cavity and the pelvic cavity, below the umbilicus.
- *Pelvic cavity:* The space that is within the skeletal pelvis and contains the colon, rectum, bladder, and some of the organs of reproduction.

The Abdominopelvic Cavity   The abdominopelvic cavity is the area within the torso from the inferior aspect (bottom) of the sternum to the groin area. This section of the body may be described by one of its four quadrants or one of its nine regions. *Note:* When you see a reference to the right side or left side, such as with the four quadrants of the abdominal area, it refers to the *patient's* right side or left side.

The Nine Regions   As you can see in Figure 1-7a, to get more specific, the abdominopelvic area of the body is divided into nine regions, each named for an organ or

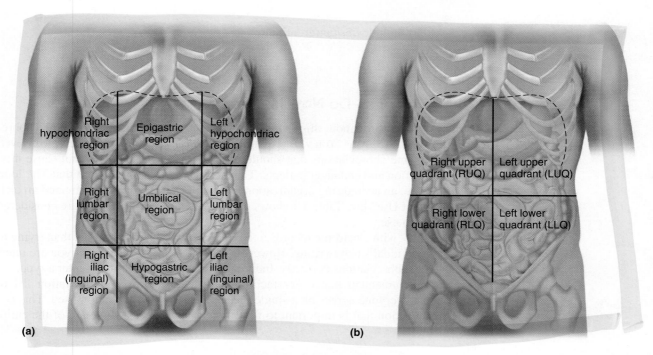

(a)

(b)

FIGURE 1-7 (a) Abdominopelvic Regions and (b) Abdominopelvic Quadrants
Source: Booth et al., MA, 5e. Copyright © 2013 by McGraw-Hill. Figure 22-10, p. 484

aspect of the body. Again, the belly button is used as the center point, and this area is known as the *umbilical region* (from the insertion point of the umbilical cord). To either side of the umbilical region, at the same level as the lumbar vertebrae, are the right lumbar region (to the patient's right of the umbilical region) and the left lumbar region (to the patient's left of the umbilical region).

Directly above the umbilical region is the epigastric region, named so because it is the area in which the stomach is located. On either side of the epigastric region are the right and left hypochondriac regions. These are the areas below the ribs.

Directly below the umbilical region is the hypogastric region. The iliac (inguinal) regions are located to the right and the left.

EXAMPLE

> K40.90 Unilateral inguinal hernia, without obstruction or gangrene, not specified as recurrent
>
> S34.5xxA Injury of lumbar, sacral and pelvic sympathetic nerves (Injury of hypogastric plexus), initial encounter

The Four Quadrants Using the belly button as the center, these areas are referred to as the left upper quadrant (LUQ), left lower quadrant (LLQ), right upper quadrant (RUQ), and right lower quadrant (RLQ) (see Figure 1-7b).

These descriptors may be used to describe the location of an organ or a symptom. For example, the appendix is located in the right lower quadrant. A patient's complaint of pain in the RLQ may indicate possible appendicitis.

EXAMPLE

> R10.31 Right lower quadrant pain

Abbreviations—Do Not Use

In many places throughout this chapter, you read about terms and the accepted abbreviations for those terms. You will see more of these as you continue reading. However, there are some abbreviations that should never be used because they can cause miscommunication and endanger patients. This has become such a concern that The Joint Commission, an accrediting organization for health care facilities, has created an official "Do Not Use" list. Table 1-1 shows some of the abbreviations that are considered dangerous to use.

Of course, with electronic records, reading typed words is more exact than trying to read an individual's handwriting. However, you still want to ensure that you are interpreting any abbreviations correctly. Individuals may still accidentally enter a typo.

It is recommended that every facility publish an approved abbreviation list to ensure that everyone agrees on a single meaning for each abbreviation used. This is a safety precaution that is important to the efficient and effective function of the entire organization.

TABLE 1-1 Do-Not-Use List

Do Not Use This Abbreviation	Potential Problem	Use This Instead
U (abbreviation for unit)	Mistaken for 0 (zero) or the number 4	Write out "unit"
IU (abbreviation for international unit)	Mistaken for IV (intravenous) or the number 10 (ten)	Write out "international unit"
Q.D. (abbreviation for daily) Q.O.D. (abbreviation for every other day)	Confused with each other	Write out "daily" or "every other day"
X.0 mg (trailing zero)	Decimal point can be missed, mistakenly multiplying the number by 10	Write "X mg"—do not include a decimal and zero
.X (missing leading zero)	Decimal point can be missed, mistakenly multiplying the number by 10	Write "0.X" mg
> (greater than symbol)	Can be confused with the number 7	Write out "greater than"
< (lesser than symbol)	Can be confused with the letter L	Write out "lesser than"
@ (at sign)	Can be confused with the number 2	Write out "at"

Source: The Joint Commission.

LO 1.5 American Health Information Management Association Code of Ethics

The American Health Information Management Association (AHIMA) is the preeminent professional organization for health information workers, including insurance coding specialists.

The AHIMA House of Delegates considers its Code of Ethics (Box 1-1) and Standards of Ethical Coding (Box 1-2) as being critical to the highest level of honorable behavior for its members.

LO 1.6 AAPC Code of Ethical Standards

American Academy of Professional Coders (AAPC) is another influential organization in the health information management industry. Its members, and its certifications, are well respected throughout the United States and the world. Its Code of Ethical Standards, shown in Box 1-3, also highlights the importance of an insurance coding and billing specialist exhibiting the most ethical and moral conduct.

Chapter Summary

It is your responsibility, as a professional in the health information management industry, to ensure that you always behave in an ethical and legal manner. Doing so will protect you, your health care facility, and your patients.

Once you assign a diagnosis or procedure code to a patient's claim form, it becomes a legal document and a permanent part of the patient's health care record. Coding is a very important part of the health care industry's process of caring.

BOX 1-1   AHIMA Code of Ethics

PREAMBLE

This Code of Ethics sets forth ethical principles for the health information management profession. Members of this profession are responsible for maintaining and promoting ethical practices. This Code of Ethics, adopted by the American Health Information Management Association, shall be binding on health information management professionals who are members of the Association and all individuals who hold an AHIMA credential.

ETHICAL PRINCIPLES

The following ethical principles are based on the core values of the American Health Information Management Association and apply to all health information management professionals. Health information management professionals:

1. Advocate, uphold and defend the individual's right to privacy and the doctrine of confidentiality in the use and disclosure of information.

2. Put service and the health and welfare of persons before self-interest and conduct themselves in the practice of the profession so as to bring honor to themselves, their peers, and to the health information management profession.

3. Preserve, protect, and secure personal health information in any form or medium and hold in the highest regard the contents of the records and other information of a confidential nature, taking into account the applicable statutes and regulations.

4. Refuse to participate in or conceal unethical practices or procedures.

5. Advance health information management knowledge and practice through continuing education, research, publications, and presentations.

6. Recruit and mentor students, peers and colleagues to develop and strengthen professional workforce.

7. Represent the profession to the public in a positive manner.

8. Perform honorably health information management association responsibilities, either appointed or elected, and preserve the confidentiality of any privileged information made known in any official capacity.

9. State truthfully and accurately their credentials, professional education, and experiences.

10. Facilitate interdisciplinary collaboration in situations supporting health information practice.

11. Respect the inherent dignity and worth of every person.

BOX 1-2   AHIMA Standards of Ethical Coding

The Standards of Ethical Coding are based on the American Health Information Management Association's (AHIMA's) Code of Ethics. Both sets of principles reflect expectations of professional conduct for coding professionals involved in diagnostic and/or procedural coding or other health record data abstraction.

A Code of Ethics sets forth professional values and ethical principles and offers ethical guidelines to which professionals aspire and by which their actions can be judged. Health information management (HIM) professionals are expected to demonstrate professional values by their actions to patients, employers, members of the health care team, the public, and the many stakeholders they serve. A Code of Ethics is important in helping to guide the decision-making process and can be referenced by individuals, agencies, organizations, and bodies (such as licensing and regulatory boards, insurance providers, courts of law, government agencies, and other professional groups).

The AHIMA Code of Ethics (available on the AHIMA web site) is relevant to all AHIMA members and credentialed HIM professionals and students, regardless of their professional functions, the settings in which they work, or the populations they serve. Coding is one of the core HIM functions, and due to the complex regulatory requirements affecting the health information coding process, coding professionals are frequently faced with ethical challenges. The AHIMA Standards of Ethical Coding are intended to assist coding professionals and managers in decision-making processes and actions, outline expectations for making ethical decisions in the workplace, and demonstrate coding professionals' commitment to integrity during the coding process, regardless of the purpose for which the codes are being reported. They are relevant to all coding professionals and those who manage the coding function, regardless of the health care setting in which they work or whether they are AHIMA members or nonmembers.

These Standards of Ethical Coding have been revised in order to reflect the current health care environment and modern coding practices. The previous revision was published in 1999.

STANDARDS OF ETHICAL CODING

Coding professionals should:

1. Apply accurate, complete, and consistent coding practices for the production of high-quality health care data.
2. Report all health care data elements (e.g. diagnosis and procedure codes, present on admission indicator, discharge status) required for external reporting purposes (e.g., reimbursement and other administrative uses, population health, quality and patient safety measurement, and research) completely and accurately, in accordance with regulatory and documentation standards and requirements and applicable official coding conventions, rules, and guidelines.
3. Assign and report only the codes and data that are clearly and consistently supported by health record documentation in accordance with applicable code set and abstraction conventions, rules, and guidelines.
4. Query provider (physician or other qualified health care practitioner) for clarification and additional documentation prior to code assignment when there is conflicting, incomplete, or ambiguous information in the health record regarding a significant reportable condition or procedure or other reportable data element dependent on health record documentation (e.g., present on admission indicator).
5. Refuse to change reported codes or the narratives of codes so that meanings are misrepresented.
6. Refuse to participate in or support coding or documentation practices intended to inappropriately increase payment, qualify for insurance policy coverage, or skew data by means that do not comply with federal and state statutes, regulations and official rules and guidelines.
7. Facilitate interdisciplinary collaboration in situations supporting proper coding practices.
8. Advance coding knowledge and practice through continuing education.
9. Refuse to participate in or conceal unethical coding or abstraction practices or procedures.
10. Protect the confidentiality of the health record at all times and refuse to access protected health information not required for coding-related activities (examples of coding-related activities include completion of code assignment, other health record data abstraction, coding audits, and educational purposes).
11. Demonstrate behavior that reflects integrity, shows a commitment to ethical and legal coding practices, and fosters trust in professional activities.

BOX 1-3   AAPC Code of Ethics

Commitment to ethical professional conduct is expected of every AAPC member. The specification of a Code of Ethics enables AAPC to clarify to current and future members, and to those served by members, the nature of the ethical responsibilities held in common by its members. This document establishes principles that define the ethical behavior of AAPC members. All AAPC members are required to adhere to the Code of Ethics and the Code of Ethics will serve as the basis for processing ethical complaints initiated against AAPC members.

AAPC members shall:

- Maintain and enhance the dignity, status, integrity, competence, and standards of our profession.
- Respect the privacy of others and honor confidentiality.
- Strive to achieve the highest quality, effectiveness and dignity in both the process and products of professional work.
- Advance the profession through continued professional development and education by acquiring and maintaining professional competence.
- Know and respect existing federal, state and local laws, regulations, certifications and licensing requirements applicable to professional work.

- Use only legal and ethical principles that reflect the profession's core values and report activity that is perceived to violate this Code of Ethics to the AAPC Ethics Committee.
- Accurately represent the credential(s) earned and the status of AAPC membership.
- Avoid actions and circumstances that may appear to compromise good business judgment or create a conflict between personal and professional interests.

Adherence to these standards assures public confidence in the integrity and service of medical coding, auditing, compliance and practice management professionals who are AAPC members.

Failure to adhere to these standards, as determined by AAPC's Ethics Committee, may result in the loss of credentials and membership with AAPC.

Source: Copyright © 2014, AAPC, ethics@aapc.com.

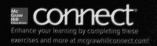

Using Terminology

Part I

Match each key term to the appropriate definition.

_____ 1. LO 1.1 Objective evidence of a disease or condition.

_____ 2. LO 1.1 The acronym for International Classification of Diseases, Ninth Revision, Clinical Modification.

_____ 3. LO 1.4 The paperwork in the patient's file that corroborates the codes presented on the claim form for a particular encounter.

_____ 4. LO 1.4 Using a code on a claim form that indicates a higher level of service, or a more severe aspect of disease or injury, than that which was actual and true.

_____ 5. LO 1.1 The determination that the health care professional was acting according to standard practices in providing a particular procedure for an individual with a particular diagnosis.

_____ 6. LO 1.1 The acronym for International Classification of Diseases, Tenth Revision, Clinical Modification.

_____ 7. LO 1.4 Coding the individual parts of a specific diagnosis or procedure rather than one combination or bundle that includes all of those components.

_____ 8. LO 1.4 Choosing a code on the basis of what the insurance company will cover (pay for) rather than accurately reflecting the truth.

_____ 9. LO 1.1 A subjective sensation or departure from the norm as related by the patient.

_____ 10. LO 1.4 Sending a claim for the second time to the same insurance company for the same procedure or service, provided to the same patient on the same date of service.

_____ 11. LO 1.1 A physician's determination of a patient's condition, illness, or injury.

A. Diagnosis
B. Sign
C. Symptom
D. ICD-9-CM
E. ICD-10-CM
F. Medical necessity
G. Supporting documentation
H. Coding for coverage
I. Upcoding
J. Unbundling
K. Double billing

Part II

Match each key term to the appropriate definition.

_____ 1. LO 1.4 Medical terminology used to provide the location of a health problem or an approach for a surgical procedure.

_____ 2. LO 1.4 Medical terminology that describes the patient's position (on the surgical or examination table).

_____ 3. LO 1.4 The structure of the human body

_____ 4. LO 1.4 Medication (drugs).

_____ 5. LO 1.4 The study of physiological processes of disease.

_____ 6. LO 1.4 The study of the causes of disease.

_____ 7. LO 1.4 The study of disease.

_____ 8. LO 1.4 A space or area that is hollow and often houses organs and vessels.

_____ 9. LO 1.4 A specific location within the anatomy (body).

A. etiology
B. pathology
C. pathophysiology
D. pharmaceuticals
E. anatomy
F. anatomical site
G. anatomical cavity
H. anatomical direction
I. anatomical position

Part III

Match each prefix or suffix to the appropriate definition.

_____ **1.** LO 1.2 meaning pain (a condition or something wrong)

_____ **2.** LO 1.2 meaning incision (an action)

_____ **3.** LO 1.2 meaning to view (an action)

_____ **4.** LO 1.2 meaning fused or stiffened (a condition or something wrong)

_____ **5.** LO 1.2 meaning seizure (a condition or something wrong)

_____ **6.** LO 1.2 meaning large (a condition or something wrong)

A. -dynia

B. -lepsy

C. -tomy

D. -scopy

E. ankyl-

F. macro-

Checking Your Understanding

Choose the most appropriate answer for each of the following questions.

1. LO 1.4 A professional coding specialist needs to have a complete understanding of

   a. medical terminology.
   b. anatomy.
   c. etiology.
   d. all of these.

2. LO 1.2 The most important factor in coding is

   a. speed of coding process.
   b. accuracy of codes.
   c. quantity of codes.
   d. level of codes.

3. LO 1.2 When you find unclear or missing information in the physician's notes, you should

   a. ask a coworker.
   b. figure it out yourself. You should know what the doctor is thinking.
   c. query the physician.
   d. place the file at the bottom of the pile.

4. LO 1.2 Diagnostic codes identify

   a. what the provider did for the patient.
   b. who the policyholder is.
   c. at which facility the patient was seen by the provider.
   d. why the provider cared for the patient.

5. LO 1.2 Procedure codes identify

   a. what the provider did for the patient.
   b. who the policyholder is.
   c. at which facility the patient was seen by the provider.
   d. why the provider cared for the patient.

6. LO 1.2 It is important to read the physician's encounter notes so you will know

   a. the deadline for filing the claim.
   b. insurance information.
   c. predetermined general codes.
   d. details to code accurately.

7. LO 1.3 ICD-10-CM Official Guidelines
   a. are generalized and do not provide details about any one section of the manual.
   b. identify specific rules for coding.
   c. apply only to hospital coders.
   d. apply only to coders working in physicians' offices.

8. LO 1.3 ICD-10-CM Official Guidelines
   a. must be memorized by professional coders.
   b. can be found in the front of every CPT-4 manual.
   c. can be found in the front of the ICD-10-CM manual.
   d. can be found in the front of the ICD-10-CM section.

9. LO 1.1 When ICD-10-CM codes support medical necessity, this means that
   a. a licensed health care professional was involved.
   b. there was a valid health care reason to provide services.
   c. the patient was seen in a hospital.
   d. a preexisting condition was treated.

10. LO 1.4 The paperwork in the patient's file that corroborates the codes presented on the claim form for a particular encounter is known as
    a. medical necessity.
    b. supporting documentation.
    c. preexisting conditions.
    d. bundling.

11. LO 1.4 Changing a code to one you know the insurance company will pay for is called
    a. coding for coverage.
    b. coding for packaging.
    c. unbundling.
    d. double billing.

12. LO 1.4 Unbundling is an illegal practice that has coders
    a. bill for services never provided.
    b. bill for services with no documentation.
    c. bill using several individual codes instead of one combination code.
    d. bill using a code for a higher level of service than what was actually provided.

13. LO 1.4 Upcoding is an illegal practice that has coders
    a. bill for services never provided.
    b. bill for services with no documentation.
    c. bill using several individual codes instead of one combination code.
    d. bill using a code for a higher level of service than what was actually provided.

14. LO 1.1/1.2 When reading the physician's notes to abstract key words with regard to diagnostic coding, you must look for
    a. confirmed diagnoses relating to why the physician is caring for the patient at this visit.
    b. signs relating to why the physician is caring for the patient at this visit.
    c. symptoms relating to why the physician is caring for the patient at this visit.
    d. all of these.

15. LO 1.2 Coding improperly on a claim form can cause that claim to be
    a. rejected.
    b. denied.
    c. published in a journal.
    d. rejected and denied.

Applying Your Knowledge

1. LO 1.1 What does a diagnosis or diagnostic statement tell us? _____

2. LO 1.1 Why is it important to tell the "whole story" of the encounter? _____

3. LO 1.1 Explain what a preexisting condition is and why it is important to the professional coder. _____

4. LO 1.2 List the seven steps to accurate coding. _____

5. LO 1.4 Explain what is meant by *unbundling*. _____

6. LO 1.5 Summarize the AHIMA Standards of Ethical Coding. _____

YOU CODE IT! Practice and Application

Chapter 1: Introduction to Diagnostic Coding

Below and on the following pages are some health care scenarios. Determine the best course of action that you, as the health information management professional for the facility, should take. Identify any legal and/or ethical issues that may need to be considered and explain how you would deal with the situation.

CIPHER, VICTORS, & ASSOCIATES
A Complete Health Care Facility
234 MAIN STREET • ANYTOWN, FL 32711 • 407-555-1234

PATIENT: HAVERLAND, JULIANNA
ACCOUNT/EHR #:   HAVEJU001
DATE: 04/05/18

Attending Physician: Valerie R. Victors, MD

This 3-year-old female is the daughter of your best friend, Sarah. Sarah comes to see you after she finishes Julianna's checkup with the doctor. Julianna has not yet begun to speak, and Dr. Victors is concerned that she may have a developmental disorder.

The correct ICD-10-CM diagnosis code for Julianna's condition is

> F80.1 Expressive language disorder, developmental aphasia

However, Sarah is very concerned about a mental disorder being placed on her daughter's chart. She is afraid of the stigma that may follow her daughter throughout her life and the things she might be denied in the future. However, with a diagnosis of

> H90.3 Sensory hearing loss, bilateral

Julianna can still get the therapy she needs to help her without the mental disorder status. Sarah begs you to change the code in Julianna's file.

     All you need to do is change the one code.

What should you do?

_____

_____

_____

CIPHER, VICTORS, & ASSOCIATES
A Complete Health Care Facility
234 MAIN STREET • ANYTOWN, FL 32711 • 407-555-1234

PATIENT: DARDEN, CONNER
ACCOUNT/EHR #:   DARDCO001
DATE: 10/15/18

Attending Physician: James I. Cipher, MD

Dr. Cipher performs a rhinoplasty on this 16-year-old male because of low self-esteem. However, cosmetic surgery is not reimbursable by the insurance carrier. So the physician writes a diagnosis of

    Deviated septum

to support medical necessity and get the insurance carrier to pay for the procedure. There is nothing at all in the rest of the documentation, including the encounter notes and lab reports, to support the diagnosis.

What should you do?

_____

_____

_____

CIPHER, VICTORS, & ASSOCIATES
A Complete Health Care Facility
234 MAIN STREET • ANYTOWN, FL 32711 • 407-555-1234

PATIENT: MAHONEY, BART
ACCOUNT/EHR #:   MAHOBA01
DATE: 11/19/18

Attending Physician: James I. Cipher, MD

The policy in your office is to create claim forms from superbills to save time and get the claims out faster. The only time coders are given the patient's chart is after a claim is rejected or denied.
The superbill presented to you for this 61-year-old male has the following codes checked off:

J11.1 URI (upper respiratory infection due to unidentified influenza virus)

81000 UA (urinalysis)

What should you do?

_____

_____

_____

CIPHER, VICTORS, & ASSOCIATES
A Complete Health Care Facility
234 MAIN STREET • ANYTOWN, FL 32711 • 407-555-1234

PATIENT: FROMAGE, LILLIAN
ACCOUNT/EHR #:   FROMLI01
DATE: 09/20/18

Attending Physician: James I. Cipher, MD

This morbidly obese 36-year-old female suffers from hypertension.

She comes in for a regular biweekly appointment, so Dr. Cipher can check her blood pressure and other vital signs and keep track of her progress on her new medications.

From previous visits, your office knows that Lillian's insurance policy will not cover any services related to her obesity. However, it will cover services related to her hypertension. With this information, Dr. Cipher has stopped including the diagnosis of morbid obesity on the encounter forms and in his notes.

What should you do?

_____

_____

_____

CIPHER, VICTORS, & ASSOCIATES
A Complete Health Care Facility
234 MAIN STREET • ANYTOWN, FL 32711 • 407-555-1234

PATIENT: KIRREN, CHARLES
ACCOUNT/EHR #:   KIRRCH01
DATE: 12/01/18

Attending Physician: Ronald Jones, DPM

This 3-year-old male presents with a diagnosis of cavus deformity. The physician's notes indicate that the deformity is acquired, leading to the code

M21.6X9 Cavus deformity of foot

The insurance policy will cover only procedures related to congenital deformities, requiring the code to be

Q66.7 Cavus foot (congenital)

The basic problem is still the same either way. Changing the code is not actually giving the patient a different condition, but it would save the family a lot of money as the surgery to correct the deformity is expensive.

What should you do?

_____

_____

_____

2

INTRODUCTION TO ICD-10-CM

Key Terms

Anatomical site

Co-morbidities

Condition

Confirmed

Eponym

External cause

Inpatient facility

Late effect

Manifestations

Outpatient services

Sequela

The ICD-10-CM book contains all of the codes you need to report the reason *why* the health care professional treated the patient during a specific encounter. This code set is available to you in print, on the Internet, and on CD-ROM.

In this chapter, as well as the rest of this textbook, all references will be made to a printed version of the code set. Let's begin by reviewing the sections of the ICD-10-CM book, to learn how to find the most accurate codes.

The Format of the ICD-10-CM Book

There are two parts in the ICD-10-CM book that contain information related to diagnostic coding:

Tabular List: Also titled "Volume 1," this part lists all ICD-10-CM codes, first in alphabetic order and then in numeric order: A00 through Z99.89 (see Table 2-1).

Alphabetic Index to Diseases: Also titled "Volume 2," this part lists all of the diagnoses, and other reasons to provide health care, by their basic description alphabetically from A to Z. Diagnostic descriptions are listed by:

- **Condition** (e.g., infections, fractures, and wounds)
- **Eponyms** (e.g., Epstein-Barr syndrome and Cushing's disease)
- Other descriptors (e.g., history, family history)

ICD-10-CM Volume 2, Section 2, contains the *Table of Drugs and Chemicals,* an Alphabetic Index of pharmaceuticals and chemicals that may cause poisoning or adverse effects in the human body.

ICD-10-CM Volume 2, Section 3, contains the *Index to External Causes,* the Alphabetic Index for the causes of injury and poisoning.

TABLE 2-1 Chapters in ICD-10-CM Tabular List

Chapter	Code Range	Title
1	A00–B99	Certain infectious and parasitic diseases
2	C00–D49	Neoplasms
3	D50–D89	Diseases of the blood and blood-forming organs and certain disorders involving the immune mechanism
4	E00–E89	Endocrine, nutritional, and metabolic diseases
5	F01–F99	Mental, behavioral, and neurodevelopmental disorders
6	G00–G99	Diseases of the nervous system
7	H00–H59	Diseases of the eye and adnexa
8	H60–H95	Diseases of the ear and mastoid process
9	I00–I99	Diseases of the circulatory system
10	J00–J99	Diseases of the respiratory system
11	K00–K95	Diseases of the digestive system
12	L00–L99	Diseases of the skin and subcutaneous tissue
13	M00–M99	Diseases of the musculoskeletal system and connective tissue
14	N00–N99	Diseases of the genitourinary system
15	O00–O99 + O9A	Pregnancy, childbirth, and the puerperium
16	P00–P96	Certain conditions originating in the perinatal period
17	Q00–Q99	Congenital malformations, deformations, and chromosomal abnormalities
18	R00–R99	Symptoms, signs, and abnormal clinical and laboratory findings, not elsewhere classified
19	S00–T88	Injury, poisoning, and certain other consequences of external causes
20	V00–Y99	External causes of morbidity
21	Z00–Z99	Factors influencing health status and contact with health services

The Coding Process

Many physicians' offices are specialized. So you will most likely end up working with a limited number of sections in the ICD-10-CM book.

condition
A health-related situation.

eponym
A condition named after a person.

EXAMPLE

If you are working for a gastroenterologist, you would rarely, if ever, use codes for mental disorders F01–F99.

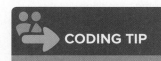

CODING TIP

In some versions of the printed ICD-10-CM, Volume 1 (the Tabular List) is located after Volume 2, Section 3.

Physician specialization makes the entire process of coding from the huge ICD-10-CM book less intimidating. However, because most of you do not know the type of health care facility you will be working in and some of you will work in a hospital or clinic that typically sees a wide range of illnesses and injuries, our learning here covers the entire array.

LO 2.1 Abstracting Physician's Notes

Determining What To Code Within Chapter 1 you learned the seven steps to coding. Remember, the first step is to read the notes completely, and then abstract the physician's notes for the encounter. Abstract (identify) the key words relating to the reason *why* the physician is caring for this patient during this visit.

EXAMPLE

Raymond went to see Dr. Langston because his throat has been scratchy and sore. After examining him and taking a throat culture, Dr. Langston determines that Raymond has strep throat and writes him a prescription.

Before Dr. Langston can determine what Raymond's problem is, he has to gather information. Talking with Raymond about his signs and symptoms in detail and examining him by looking at his eyes, ears, and throat is all part of his evaluation of Raymond's condition. Only then can he determine a course of treatment.

The ICD-10-CM Official Guidelines for Reporting state, *"The entire record should be reviewed to determine the specific reason for the encounter and the conditions treated."* As you review all of the physician's documentation, you may discover language that establishes multiple dimensions of diagnoses, and not just a straight line to a single diagnosis. You will continue to learn about all of these aspects of diagnoses. Let's begin by establishing a firm foundation of these multiple aspects.

Signs and Symptoms You began learning about signs and symptoms in Chapter 1. As a physician investigates the patient's condition for the purposes of determining what the problem is and what treatment is best, signs and symptoms can be breadcrumbs that lead to that confirmed diagnosis. In such cases, these signs and symptoms are considered integral to that confirmed diagnosis, and they are not reported with additional codes. However, sometimes the same signs and symptoms can point toward several diagnoses, and the physician needs to investigate further with more tests. While the investigation is ongoing, you will have to report the signs and symptoms to support medical necessity for those tests.

Manifestations There are some diseases that actually cause the patient to develop another condition. This second condition, directly the result of the first condition, is known as a **manifestation.** In such cases, the patient would most certainly not have the manifested disease or problem had he or she not had the first disease already present. The cause-and-effect relationship between the two conditions is known to the physician and supported by medical research.

Co-morbidities A **co-morbidity** is a condition that is present in the same body at the same time as another problem or disease, but the two conditions are unrelated. These "other diagnoses" may be referred to in the physician's documentation. However, only those conditions that the physician has specifically evaluated, treated, or ordered additional testing for or those requiring additional monitoring, nursing care, or more time in the hospital should be reported with a code.

Sequela Also known as a *late effect,* sequela is the residual impact of a previous condition or injury that may need the attention of a physician. More about sequela will be presented later on in this chapter.

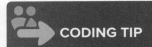

CODING TIP

Even though you might think that the Alphabetic Index (Volume 2) has provided you with the right code, you MUST confirm this code in the tabular list (Volume 1). In Volume 1, you will find additional notations, guidelines, and symbols, not provided in the Alphabetic Index, that may change your determination of the most accurate code.

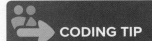

CODING TIP

Why does Dr. Langston evaluate and treat Raymond? You might think "because his throat is scratchy and sore." However, many different conditions can cause these symptoms. You have more specific information because Dr. Langston determined what the CAUSE of Raymond's symptoms (scratchy and sore throat) is: The streptococcus (strep for short) bacterium has invaded. You have the advantage of knowing the facts, and this is what you will report with codes. This is why it is important to read all the way through the notes before deciding what key terms should lead to codes.

manifestation
A condition caused or developed from the existence of another condition.

co-morbidity
A separate condition or illness present in the same patient at the same time as another, unrelated condition or illness.

More Than One Code to Tell the Whole Story When the physician treats or attends multiple conditions, you have to determine the principal or first-listed diagnosis. The Uniform Hospital Discharge Data Set (UHDDS) defines this to be "that condition established after study to be chiefly responsible for occasioning the admission of the patient to the hospital for care." For outpatient situations, the definition is very similar: "the main condition treated or investigated during the relevant episode of care."

When reading procedure or operative notes, you will typically find a preoperative diagnosis or indication and a postoperative diagnosis or findings. There may be times when preoperative and postoperative diagnoses are different. Because the notes are written *after* the physician has performed the procedure, the postoperative diagnoses or findings are considered to be more accurate; therefore, that is the information you will use to code the encounter.

In cases in which the patient has been in the hospital, you might find a difference between an admission diagnosis and the discharge diagnosis. The admission diagnosis reports the condition that prompted admitting the patient into the hospital as a medical necessity. That is important information when coding diagnoses at discharge because you may have to indicate certain conditions as being *present on admission (POA). (Learn more about coding inpatient diagnoses, including POA, in Chapter 22 in this textbook.)*

The notes may contain key words directly identified as a confirmed diagnosis, or you may need to find the patient's signs and symptoms (often called the *patient's chief complaint*).

Parsing the Diagnostic Statement Once you find it in the physician's notes, take the diagnostic statement apart and determine which word identifies the disease, illness, condition, or primary reason for the visit (also known as the "main term"). Separate this from any words that may simply describe the type of condition or the location of the condition (anatomical site).

WHY is the physician caring for the patient? Be specific. When you look at the examples below, you can see the reason the physician is seeing the patient for this visit.

EXAMPLES

1. *Arterial stenosis:* The condition is "stenosis" (narrowing); "arterial" (artery) is the anatomical site of the condition.

2. *Acute cystitis:* The condition is "cystitis" (inflammation of the bladder); the term "acute" (severe) describes what type of inflammation the patient has.

3. *Family history of heart disease:* The issue of concern is "history"—why the patient is being seen. The type of history is "family," and the secondary descriptor is "disease of the heart" to explain "a history of what?"

4. *Open fracture of the clavicle:* The condition is "fracture," "open" is the type of fracture, and "clavicle" (collarbone) is the anatomical site of the fracture.

5. *Crohn's disease:* The condition is "disease"; the eponym "Crohn's" describes the specific disease.

6. *Pulmonary necrosis:* The condition is "necrosis" (dead tissue); "pulmonary" (lungs) identifies the anatomical site of the dead tissue.

Now you know which words to look up in the ICD-10-CM's Index to Diseases, also known as the Alphabetic Index.

LO 2.2 The Alphabetic Index

Once you have identified the diagnostic-related key words abstracted from the notes, turn to the Alphabetic Index of ICD-10-CM (see Figure 2-1). You use the Alphabetic Index to guide you to the correct page or area in the Tabular List (Volume 1). Then you need to carefully read the descriptions, beginning at the top of the subheading, so you can make certain that you find the best code, to the highest level of specificity, according to the physician's notes for a particular encounter and within the directions of the book.

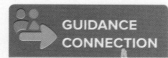
GUIDANCE CONNECTION

Refer to Official Guidelines: Sections I.B.4, **Signs and symptoms,** I.B.5, **Conditions that are an integral part of a disease process,** and I.B.6, **Conditions that are not an integral part of a disease process.**

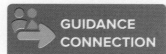
GUIDANCE CONNECTION

Refer to Official Guidelines: Section I.A.13, **Etiology/ manifestation convention** ("code first," "use additional code" and "in diseases classified elsewhere" notes).

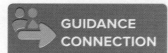
GUIDANCE CONNECTION

Refer to Official Guidelines: Section III, **Reporting Additional Diagnoses.**

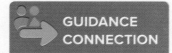
GUIDANCE CONNECTION

Refer to Official Guidelines: Section I.B.10, **Sequela (late effects).**

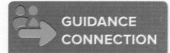
GUIDANCE CONNECTION

The Official ICD-10-CM Coding Guidelines, Section II, **Selection of Principal Diagnosis,** and Section III, **Reporting Additional Diagnoses,** can guide you when reporting multiple diagnosis codes for one encounter.

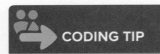
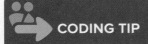
Abnormal, abnormality, abnormalities—*see also* Anomaly

acid-base balance (mixed) E87.4
albumin R77.0
alphafetoprotein R77.2
alveolar ridge K08.9
anatomical relationship Q89.9
apertures, congenital, diaphragm Q79.1
auditory perception H93.29
   diplacusis—*see* Diplacusis
   hyperacusis—*see* Hyperacusis
   recruitment—*see* Recruitment,
    auditory
   threshold shift—*see* Shift,
    auditory threshold
autosomes Q99.9
   fragile site Q95.5
basal metabolic rate R94.8
biosynthesis, testicular androgen E29.1
bleeding time R79.1
blood-gas level R79.81
blood level (of)
   cobalt R79.0
   copper R79.0
   iron R79.0
   lithium R78.89
   magnesium R79.0
   mineral NEC R79.0
   zinc R79.0
blood pressure
   elevated R03.0
   low reading (nonspecific) R03.1
blood sugar R73.09

bowel sounds R19.15
   absent R19.11
   hyperactive R19.12
brain scan R94.02
breathing R06.9
caloric test R94.138
cerebrospinal fluid R83.9
   cytology R83.6
   drug level R83.2
   enzyme level R83.0
   hormones R83.1
   immunology R83.4
   microbiology R83.5
   nonmedicinal level R83.3
   specified type NEC R83.8
chemistry, blood R79.9
   C-reactive protein R79.82
   drugs—*see* Findings, abnormal, in blood
   gas level R79.81
   minerals R79.0
   pancytopenia D61.818
   PTT R79.1
   specified NEC R79.89
   toxins—*see* Findings, abnormal, in blood
chest sounds (friction) (rales) R09.89
chromosome, chromosomal Q99.9
   with more than three X
    chromosomes, female Q97.1
   analysis result R89.8
    bronchial washings R84.8
    cerebrospinal fluid R83.8

FIGURE 2-1 Example of a Page from ICD-10-CM Alphabetic Index

When you begin, you will realize that looking for a diagnostic key word in the Alphabetic Index may not be as easy as it sounds. Sometimes, it's a snap, and you find the code right away!

For example, suppose you read that "Dr. Files diagnosed Alvira Gomez with polyphagia."

Turning to the Alphabetic Index, you find:

Polyphagia R63.2

Now look this up in the Tabular List, and find code:

R63 Symptoms and signs concerning food and fluid intake

See the indented list below with the available fourth characters, and continue reading to find:

R63.2 Polyphagia

This matches the physician's notes perfectly.

Occasionally, you have to look a little further. Suppose you read that "Dr. Farina removed a splinter from Jaleel Waters's right index finger. This is the first time Jaleel has seen Dr. Farina."

When you look in the Alphabetic Index under splinter, you discover a *see* reference:

Splinter—*see* Foreign body, superficial, by site.

Therefore, you turn to:

Foreign body
   Superficial
      Finger(s) S60.459

Put this all together and you can see it reads: "Superficial foreign body to finger(s) S60.459." Wait a minute, though. Notice that there is a list indented beneath the word "finger(s)" that shows the various, specific fingers:

index S60.45-

little S60.45-

middle S60.45-

ring S60.45-

Check back with the case scenario: In which finger was the splinter embedded? His *right index* finger. So the more accurate suggestion here in the Alphabetic Index refers you to S60.45-. (The hyphen after the last character indicates that additional characters are required. You will discover the choices when you look at this code in the Tabular List.)

Turn to the Tabular List (remember to always begin reading at the code category [three-character] code), and find:

S60 Superficial injury of wrist, hand and fingers

You can see the long, long list of codes and descriptions within this code category. Let's look at all of the choices for the required *fourth* character and see what matches the physician's documentation:

S60.0 Contusion of finger without damage to nail

S60.1 Contusion of finger with damage to nail

S60.2 Contusion of wrist and hand

S60.3 Other superficial injuries of thumb

S60.4 Other superficial injuries of other fingers

S60.5 Other superficial injuries of hand

S60.8 Other superficial injuries of wrist

S60.9 Unspecified superficial injury of wrist, hand and fingers

From the details in the physician's notes and what you read in the Alphabetic Index, the choice seems clear: S60.4 Other superficial injuries of other fingers.

Next, you will need to determine the most accurate *fifth* character. Review all of the choices:

S60.41 Abrasion of fingers

S60.42 Blister (nonthermal) of fingers

S60.44 External constriction of fingers

S60.45 Superficial foreign body of fingers

S60.46 Insect bite (nonvenomous) of fingers

S60.47 Other superficial bite of fingers

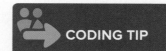

CODING TIP

Never, never, never code *only* from the Alphabetic Index (Volume 2, Alphabetic Index to Diseases). *Always check* the code in the Tabular List (Volume 1), and read the entire code description and all notations before deciding it is the most accurate code.

You can see that S60.45 is clearly in agreement with the physician's notes.

Next, you will need to determine the most accurate *sixth* character. Review all of the choices:

S60.450 Superficial foreign body of right index finger

S60.451 Superficial foreign body of left index finger

S60.452 Superficial foreign body of right middle finger

S60.453 Superficial foreign body of left middle finger

S60.454 Superficial foreign body of right ring finger

S60.455 Superficial foreign body of left ring finger

S60.456 Superficial foreign body of right little finger

S60.457 Superficial foreign body of left little finger

S60.458 Superficial foreign body of other finger

S60.459 Superficial foreign body of unspecified finger

You can tell, by matching the code description to the physician's notes, that the most accurate choice here is:

S60.450 Superficial foreign body of right index finger

Wait, you are not done yet. Did you notice the symbol next to this code that reminds you a seventh character is required? Take a look back at the S60 code at the start of this code category. Directly beneath S60, Superficial injury of wrist, hand and fingers, is a boxed-off area that reads:

The appropriate 7th character is to be added to each code from category S60

A initial encounter

D subsequent encounter

S sequela

This notation is all the way at the top of this code category because it applies to every code that begins with S60. So go back to the case scenario and find the answer to the question, "Is this the first time Jaleel Waters has seen Dr. Farina for this splinter?" If the answer is yes, then the seventh character to use is the letter "A." If this is a follow-up, then the seventh character to use is the letter "D," and if this encounter is for a sequela of the splinter (such as a scar), then the letter "S" will be the seventh character.

There may be lots of choices, but you can clearly see which code description matches the physician's notes and tells the whole story as to why Jaleel needed Dr. Farina's care:

S60.450A Superficial foreign body of right index finger, initial encounter

You can see how the ICD-10-CM book led you, step-by-step, to the correct code: from splinter to foreign body to superficial. However, not all diagnostic statements follow a straight line like this one. Sometimes, you have to really read carefully and think about what the problem really is. Other times, you may have to use alternate terms from those used in the notes to determine the correct code description. A medical dictionary will help you, so it is recommended that you keep one by your side (especially now, while you are early in your learning). Also, be certain to keep practicing and learning from your mistakes. This way, you can familiarize yourself with the terms used as well as the thinking process that is part of the coding process.

Stephan Lewis fell off his bicycle and scraped his left knee very badly, so he came to see Dr. Martinez.

Scrape is not in the Alphabetic Index. You can look in a medical dictionary to find that another term for scrape is abrasion. Turn to abrasion in the Alphabetic Index, and you will see Abrasion, knee S80.21-. Eventually you arrive at S80.212A, Abrasion, left knee, initial encounter.

Remember that accuracy is the *most* important issue here. It is not a race. You need to be careful and meticulous.

LET'S CODE IT! SCENARIO

Jerry Califon, a 47-year-old male, came to see his regular physician, Dr. Warren. Jerry has a family history of pancreatic cancer, so he is very diligent about his checkups.

Let's Code It!

As you read through the notes, you can see that Dr. Warren identified the reason for Jerry's visit. He has a "family history of pancreatic cancer."

There are four key words: *family, history, pancreas,* and *cancer.* Let's look them up in the Alphabetic Index one at a time.

Cancer: When you look up the word *cancer* in the Alphabetic Index, you find that the ICD-10-CM book refers you to *see also Neoplasm, by site, malignant.* (You may remember from your medical terminology class that *malignant neoplasm* is the proper term for what is commonly called cancer.) But be careful! Jerry does *not have* a malignant neoplasm, just a family history. If you follow this lead and go to the neoplasm listings, you will see that there is nothing that indicates a family history. You now know that this key word will not lead to the correct ICD-10-CM code for this particular encounter.

Go to the next key word.

Pancreas: Find the word *pancreas* in the Alphabetic Index, and you read the direction *see condition.* This does not mean to go to the listing for the word *condition;* it means that you should go back to the physician's notes and look for the condition of Jerry's pancreas. What is wrong with his pancreas? Well, there really isn't anything indicating that there is anything wrong with his pancreas. So this is not going to get you any closer to the correct code because the Alphabetic Index does not include code listings by **anatomical site.**

Don't get frustrated. Look at this like a treasure hunt. The correct answer is here in this book. You just have to find it. Let's go to the next key word: *family.*

Family: Next to the word *family,* the book directs us to *see also condition.* Underneath, there are codes indicated for:

Family disruption Z63.8

Family Li-Fraumeni (syndrome) Z15.01

Family planning advice Z30.09

Family problem Z63.9

anatomical site
A specific location or part of the human body.

Family problem specified circumstance NEC Z63.8

Family retinoblastoma C69.2-

None of these possibilities comes close to the reason why Jerry came to see Dr. Warren. So let's move on to the last key word.

History: Looks like you struck gold! There are over a page and a half of codes listed under *History (personal) of.* The first question you need to answer is what kind of history does this individual have: a *family* history. Look down the column at the long list of words indented under the word *history* until you reach *family.*

You will notice under the word *family* there is an indented column, in alphabetic order, of codes for different conditions. Let's go ahead and look down the list to see if the word *pancreas* appears. It does not. A person can't have a family history of having a pancreas. Everyone has one! What does the individual actually have? A *family history* of a *malignant neoplasm* of the pancreas. Aha! Let's continue down the list:

History

    Family

        Malignant neoplasm (of) NOS Z80.9

This is read as "family history of a malignant neoplasm not otherwise specified (NOS)." But that's not our situation. Let's keep going down the list indented under *malignant neoplasm.*

Pancreas is not listed. How can this be? Look at the list again, carefully. Do you remember that the pancreas is part of the digestive system? Now you can identify the potential of:

Digestive organ Z80.0

As you can see, each word or phrase indented below another word or phrase includes the one above.

Look above to *family* indented once under the heading *history.* You read this as "family history." Then *malignant neoplasm* is indented once under *family* that is indented once under *history.* So we read this as "family history of malignant neoplasm." This can get a little confusing, so use a ruler or your finger to keep track of what is indented at which level. If you let your eyes jump ahead, you might accidentally look at the next column under *history* that says "malignant neoplasm (of) Z85.9." If you look at the indentations of the columns, you will see that this means a *history of malignant neoplasm* (indicating that the patient had been previously diagnosed) but not a *family* history of a malignant neoplasm (indicating that someone in the family, not this individual, was diagnosed). A *big* difference!

Now turn to the Tabular List (Volume 1), and look for code Z80.0 to make certain this is the best, most specific code available. You read:

Z80 Family history of primary malignant neoplasm

    Z80.0 Family history of malignant neoplasm of digestive organs

        Conditions classifiable to C15–C26

But Jerry has a family history of pancreatic cancer. Is that a digestive organ? Take a look at the notation indented below the code description:

Conditions classifiable to C15–C26

This means that the original diagnosis would have come from the code range of C15 through C26. As you read through the descriptions of all the codes in that range, take a look at code C25, Malignant neoplasm of pancreas. That is what someone in Jerry's family had; therefore, Z80.0 is correct.

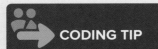

CODING TIP

Family is a description of a type of history.

Malignant is a description of a type of neoplasm.

Open is a description of a type of wound.

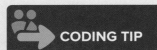

CODING TIP

Once you find the appropriate main key word from the notes in the Alphabetic Index, the next item you want to identify is the adjective, or descriptor, used by the provider.

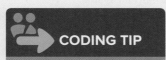

CODING TIP

When looking through these long lists with lots of indentations, you must be conscientious and go down the columns carefully. Use a ruler or your finger to keep things in line.

LO 2.3 The Tabular List

Volume 1 of the ICD-10-CM book lists all the codes and their descriptions. However, it lists all its information in alphanumeric order, starting at A00 and running all the way through to Z99.89 (see Figure 2-2). This section is called the *Tabular List.* Let's investigate the different types of codes shown in the list and discuss when you would use each kind.

CODING TIP

The Alphabetic Index will suggest a possible diagnosis code. Then you must find the code suggested by the Alphabetic Index in the Tabular List (Volume 1). This step is not a suggestion—it is mandatory. The Tabular List provides more detail for the code description, as well as additional notations such as *includes* and *excludes* notes and directives for the requirement of additional characters and codes. *NEVER, NEVER, NEVER code from the Alphabetic Index.*

B67 Echinococcosis
  Includes: hydatidosis
  B67.0 Echinococcus granulosus infection of liver
  B67.1 Echinococcus granulosus infection of lung
  B67.2 Echinococcus granulosus infection of bone
  B67.3 Echinococcus granulosus infection, other and multiple sites
    B67.31 Echinococcus granulosus infection, thyroid gland
    B67.32 Echinococcus granulosus infection, multiple sites
    B67.39 Echinococcus granulosus infection, other sites
  B67.4 Echinococcus granulosus infection, unspecified
    Dog tapeworm (infection)
  B67.5 Echinococcus multilocularis infection of liver
  B67.6 Echinococcus multilocularis infection, other and multiple sites
    B67.61 Echinococcus multilocularis infection, multiple sites
    B67.69 Echinococcus multilocularis infection, other sites
  B67.7 Echinococcus multilocularis infection, unspecified
  B67.8 Echinococcosis, unspecified, of liver
  B67.9 Echinococcosis, other and unspecified
    B67.90 Echinococcosis, unspecified
      Echinococcosis NOS
    B67.99 Other echinococcosis
  B68 Taeniasis
    Excludes1: cysticercosis (B69.-)
    B68.0 Taenia solium taeniasis
      Pork tapeworm (infection)
    B68.1 Taenia saginata taeniasis
      Beef tapeworm (infection)
      Infection due to adult tapeworm Taenia saginata
    B68.9 Taeniasis, unspecified
  B69 Cysticercosis
    Includes: cysticerciasis infection due to larval form of Taenia solium
    B69.0 Cysticercosis of central nervous system
    B69.1 Cysticercosis of eye
    B69.8 Cysticercosis of other sites
      B69.81 Myositis in cysticercosis
      B69.89 Cysticercosis of other sites
    B69.9 Cysticercosis, unspecified
  B70 Diphyllobothriasis and sparganosis
    B70.0 Diphyllobothriasis
      Diphyllobothrium (adult) (latum) (pacificum) infection
      Fish tapeworm (infection)
      Excludes2: larval diphyllobothriasis (B70.1)

FIGURE 2-2 Example of a Page from ICD-10-CM Tabular List

confirmed
Found to be true or definite.

outpatient services
Health care services provided to individuals without an overnight stay in the facility.

ICD-10-CM Codes As discussed previously in this chapter, the majority of the ICD-10-CM book contains codes that are from three to seven characters that identify specific, **confirmed** diagnoses of illness (disease) or injury and other valid reasons why a physician would provide care to a patient.

When coding **outpatient services,** you must be certain that the patient's file, including the physician's notes, verifies that the patient actually has the condition, disease, illness, or injury. The guideline (Section IV.H, Uncertain diagnosis) states that you are to use the code or codes that identify the condition to its highest level of certainty. This means that you code only what you know for a fact. You are *not permitted* to assign an ICD-10-CM diagnosis code for a condition that is described by the provider as *probably, suspected, possible, questionable,* or *to be ruled out.* If the health care professional has not been able to confirm a diagnosis, then you must code the signs, symptoms, abnormal test results, or other element stated as the reason for the visit.

EXAMPLE

Larry Glass, a 39-year-old male, came to see Dr. Walden, in his office, because of a sharp pain in his abdomen. After doing a thorough examination, Dr. Walden suspects that Larry may have enteritis due to the rotavirus, so he orders a blood test. If the blood test comes back *positive* to confirm enteritis due to the rotavirus (after the physician documents it in the file), you would use the following code:

R80.0 Rotaviral enteritis

If the blood test comes back *negative,* meaning Larry does *not* have enteritis due to the rotavirus (after the physician documents it in the file), then you would use code:

K52.9 Enteritis, NOS (not otherwise specified)

inpatient facility
An establishment that provides health care services to individuals who stay overnight on the premises.

The rules for coding uncertain diagnoses for patients of an **inpatient facility** are different from those for outpatients. As directed by the guideline (Section II.H, Uncertain diagnosis), when at the time of discharge the diagnosis is described as probable, possible, suspected, likely, or still to be ruled out, you must code that condition as if it did exist. This directive applies only when you are coding services provided in a short-term, acute, long-term care, or psychiatric hospital or facility. It is one of the few circumstances in which you will find the guidelines differ between coding for outpatient and inpatient services.

YOU CODE IT! CASE STUDY

Jenna Butler, a 59-year-old female, was admitted to the hospital for observation after she complained of having severe chest pain radiating to her left shoulder and down her arm. Dr. Halberton discharged her the next day with a diagnosis of probable variant angina pectoris.

You Code It!

As the hospital's coder, go through the steps of coding, and determine the diagnosis code that should be reported for this encounter between Dr. Halberton and Jenna Butler.

Step 1: Read the case completely.

Step 2: Abstract the notes: Which key words can you identify relating to why Dr. Halberton cared for Jenna?

_____

Step 3: Query the provider, if necessary.

Step 4: Code the diagnosis or diagnoses.

_____

Step 5: Code the procedure(s): One-night hospital stay for observation.

Step 6: Link the procedure codes to at least one diagnosis code to confirm medical necessity.

Step 7: Back code to double-check your choices.

Answer:

Did you determine the correct code?

I20.1 Angina pectoris with documented spasm (variant angina)

Good job!

LO 2.4 Z Codes

There are times when an individual comes to see a health care provider without having a particular illness or injury. In such cases, you might assign a Z code, which describes an encounter between a provider and an individual who does not have a current health condition.

1. A healthy person might go to see a physician for the following reasons:
   a. Preventive care such as a flu shot or vaccination: such as code Z23.
   b. Routine and administrative exams, such as an annual physical or a well-baby checkup: such as code category Z00.
   c. Monitoring care and screenings for someone:
      i. With a personal history of a condition: such as code category Z87.
      ii. With a family history: such as code category Z83.
      iii. In a population subgroup, such as mammograms for women over 40 or prostate examinations for men over 50: such as code category Z12.
   d. Counseling for the patient and/or family members relating to the circumstances involved with an illness or injury or to help with family problems or social concerns such as contraceptive or procreative management: such as code category Z63.
   e. Organ donation (to be a donor): such as code category Z52.

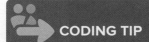

CODING TIP

A Z code is used for a patient who doesn't have a current disease or injury but comes to see the physician to validate his or her current healthy status—to prevent something from going wrong or to ensure continued health.

EXAMPLE

Kinley Washington finds out his brother has end-stage renal disease (ESRD). He comes in today to be tested to see if he can donate his kidney: code Z00.5.

2. A person might require continuous care for the following:
   a. Chronic illness or injury.
   b. Healing illness or injury requiring aftercare, such as follow-up after surgery: such as code category Z48.

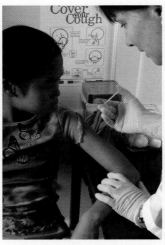

© McGraw-Hill Education/Jill Braaten, photographer

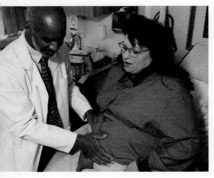
© Getty Images

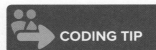

CODING TIP

When you identify why the physician cared for the patient, ask yourself, "Is the patient currently sick or injured?" If this is not a current, active issue, then there is a good chance the medical necessity for this encounter will be reported with a Z code. Another question you can ask yourself is, "Did the patient have signs or symptoms, or did the patient come to the encounter because the calendar said to?" The calendar tells patients to come in for an annual exam, seasonal flu vaccine, or 12-week prenatal exam. These are all reported with Z codes.

c. Status identification, which is a follow-up for someone who is a carrier of a disease, has residual effects of a past condition, or has a prosthetic or mechanical device: such as code categories Z14 and Z44.

d. Follow-up examinations for a condition that has already been treated or no longer exists: such as code category Z47.

EXAMPLE

Dr. Rosin sees Don Bowlin in the office 6 weeks after performing a carpal tunnel release before closing this case: code Z47.89.

3. A person without any signs or symptoms of a disease but who comes to the health care professional because he or she:

a. Was exposed to an infected individual: such as category Z20.

b. Might be a carrier or suspected carrier of a disease: such as category Z22.

c. Needs to be observed for a suspected condition that is ruled out: such as category Z03.

EXAMPLE

Robert Boatman, a 19-year-old male, discovers that his roommate has been diagnosed with tuberculosis. He visits his physician to find out what he should do: code Z20.1.

4. Obstetrics and neonatal evaluations and circumstances including regularly planned, periodic checkups, the outcome of delivery, birth status, and health supervision and observations of an infant or child may be reported with a Z code such as Z00.110 or Z37.1.

EXAMPLE

Tiffany Sherwood, a 29-year-old female, is 7 weeks pregnant with her first child. She has an appointment with Dr. Nelson today for her regularly scheduled prenatal checkup: code Z34.01.

5. When coding a visit for routine lab work or radiology services, when there are no current signs, symptoms, or related diagnosis, report the visit with a Z code such as a code from category Z13.

EXAMPLE

Rhonda Shultz comes in for a routine chest x-ray. She does not see Dr. Fahey or have any other services provided: code Z13.83.

6. When routine testing is performed during an encounter at which an unrelated sign, symptom, or diagnosis is evaluated, code both the Z code for the routine test and the reason for the evaluation.

EXAMPLE

Kallie Pasternak, a 25-year-old female, is here for her annual well-woman exam. She asks Dr. Walli to do a genetic disease test because she and her husband are discussing beginning a family: codes Z01.41 (routine gynecologic examination) and Z31.430, Encounter of female for testing for genetic disease carrier status for procreative management.

LET'S CODE IT! SCENARIO

Lewis Elliott brings his daughter Marissa to Dr. Cruse, her pediatrician, for a rubella vaccination. Marissa is 4 years old and will be going to preschool next month. The school requires just this one shot. Marissa chooses a sunflower sticker as her prize for being a good patient.

Let's Code It!

Marissa did not come to Dr. Cruse because she was ill or injured. She came so that he could *prevent* her from becoming ill. Dr. Cruse indicates that the reason why he saw Marissa today was to give her a *vaccination* to prevent her from getting rubella. Let's go to the Alphabetic Index.

Looking up the key word *vaccination,* you will see:

Vaccination (prophylactic)

> **complication or reaction**—*see* Complications, vaccination
>
> **delayed Z28.9**
>
> **encounter for Z23**
>
> **not done**—*see* Immunization, not done, because (of)

Which of these describes the reason why Dr. Cruse cared for Marissa?

> **Vaccination, encounter for Z23**

Let's turn to the Tabular List (remember to always begin reading at the three-character code category):

> **Z23 Encounter for immunization**

That's it? You, as the coder, are required to tell the whole story, yet this explains only that Marissa came to get a vaccine (also known as *immunization*). How do we explain that the specific immunization she received was for rubella? Read the note directly below code Z23:

> **Note: Procedure codes are required to identify the types of immunizations given**

That will work, because every physician-patient encounter requires at least one diagnosis code and at least one procedure code. This is how you will be able to explain the rest of this story.

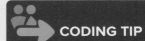

CODING TIP

Remember that a diagnostic code identifies the reason *why* the physician treated this patient during this encounter. In Marissa's case this is because she needed to have the vaccination. The diagnostic code is not the code for the actual provision of the injection. That will come from the procedure coding book. This is just the *why,* not the *what.*

Some Z codes cover a variety of miscellaneous issues: problems relating to lifestyle, such as codes in category Z57, or encounters for administrative purposes, such as codes in category Z02. There are even codes to report when a procedure was not performed, such as code category Z53. Take a few minutes to review the Z code category descriptions so you can get a sense of the wide variety of valid reasons why a physician may need to provide care for a patient who is not currently ill.

LET'S CODE IT! SCENARIO

After having surgery to remove a cancerous tumor, Caroline completed her planned sequence of chemotherapy treatments. She comes to see Dr. Masters for a follow-up.

Let's Code It!

Caroline has completed her treatments, so she is technically no longer ill. However, it would be remiss of Dr. Masters not to examine her to ensure that she is doing as well as expected and that the treatments worked. You cannot report the visit with a code for cancer, because Caroline no longer has cancer. This visit is a follow-up as a part of her completed treatment, so she actually does not yet qualify for a personal history code. Let's try the best key word we have: *follow-up.*

In the Alphabetic Index, you see:

Follow-up—*see* Examination, follow-up

Let's turn to the key term:

Examination (for)(following)(general)(of)(routine) Z00.00

And read down the indented list to:

Examination

    Follow-up (routine)(following) Z09

        Chemotherapy NEC Z09

        Malignant neoplasm Z08

Go back to the scenario. Caroline came to Dr. Masters after finishing her chemotherapy, but the scenario also states she had a malignant neoplasm ("cancerous tumor"). This means that Z08 is more accurate. So let's go to the Tabular List and read the entire code description:

Z08 Encounter for follow-up examination after completed treatment for malignant neoplasm

    Use additional code to identify any acquired absence of organs (Z90.-)

    Use additional code to identify the personal history of malignant neoplasm (Z85.-)

Good! Z08 reports why Dr. Masters is spending time caring for Caroline. Yet you are not done yet. Did you notice the two "Use additional code . . ." notations beneath code Z08? These are not suggestions; they are required. Now, we don't have the details in our short scenario. However, when you are on the job, you will need to look further into the physician's notes, or query the physician, to obtain the details about Caroline's "surgery to remove a cancerous tumor" so you can accurately report these additional codes.

Augustina Saciolo, a 26-year-old female who is approximately 15 weeks pregnant with her first baby, comes to see Dr. Apple for a routine pregnancy checkup. The sonogram shows no abnormalities with a fetus that appears to have appropriate size and growth for the approximated gestation.

You Code It!

Go through the steps of coding, and determine the diagnosis code that should be reported for this encounter between Dr. Apple and Augustina.

Step 1: Read the case completely.

Step 2: Abstract the notes: Which key words can you identify relating to why Dr. Apple cared for Augustina?

_____

Step 3: Query the provider, if necessary.

Step 4: Code the diagnosis or diagnoses.

_____

Step 5: Code the procedure(s): Regular pregnancy checkup; sonogram.

Step 6: Link the procedure codes to at least one diagnosis code to confirm medical necessity.

Step 7: Back code to double-check your choices.

Answer:

Did you determine the correct code?

Z34.02 Encounter for supervision of normal first pregnancy, second trimester

Good job!

LO 2.5 External Cause Codes V01–Y99

When an individual has an injury, has been poisoned, or has had an adverse effect, something had to cause it. You can't catch a broken leg or wake up with a case of poisoning. Something outside the body caused the problem. There has to be an **external cause. External cause codes** are used, along with other ICD-10-CM codes, to explain exactly what has happened.

external cause
An event, outside the body, that causes injury, poisoning, or an adverse reaction.

external cause codes
Codes that report *how* and/or *where* an injury or poisoning happened.

EXAMPLE

How did Jason get that wound? W61.33xA Pecked by chicken, initial encounter
What was Jason doing at this time? Y93.K9 Activity, other involving animal care
Where was Jason at this time? Y92.72 Chicken coop as the place of occurrence of the external cause
Why was Jason doing this at this time? Y99.2 Volunteer activity

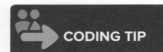

CODING TIP

External cause codes explain the *external* cause of the individual's injury, poisoning, or adverse reaction.

How did Helina get hurt? X36.1xxA Avalanche, landslide, or mudslide, initial encounter

What was Helina doing at this time? Y93.H3 Activity, building and construction

Where was Helina when this happened? Y92.017 Garden or yard in single-family (private) house as the place of occurrence of the external cause

Why was Helina at this location? Y99.0 Civilian activity done for income or pay

How did Bobby get his brain concussion? X52.xxxA Prolonged stay in weightless environment, initial encounter

Where was Bobby when this happened? Y92.138 Other place on military base as the place of occurrence of the external cause

Why was Bobby in a weightless environment? Y99.1 Military activity

LET'S CODE IT! SCENARIO

Ellen Depew was brought to Dr. Davis's office with a bad headache. She had been on a swing in the park and had fallen off the swing and hit her head fiercely against the ground. After x-rays have been taken, Dr. Davis determines that Ellen has a brain concussion.

Let's Code It!

Why do the claim forms and the reports need to identify *how* or *where* Ellen got hurt? The answer is that the situation responsible for Ellen's concussion affects which insurance carrier's policy pays the medical expenses. If Ellen hit her head:

At work, then *workers' compensation* insurance would pay the medical bills, not her health care plan.

While shopping at a store, the store's *liability insurance* might pay for the medical bills.

In an automobile accident, then her *automobile insurance* would probably be billed.

In her own home, then her own *health care policy* would be billed first.

Therefore, as a coding specialist, you must use codes to explain what happened so that it will be clear which insurance carrier is responsible for, and should receive, the medical bills. In addition, your state or federal agencies may need to know the circumstances for statistical analysis or other research purposes.

You will use external cause codes, *after* the diagnosis code(s), to provide this important information. Now let's look back at Ellen Depew's scenario and pick out the key words that will lead us to the correct codes. With our diagnosis codes and external cause codes, the entire story must be reported to explain *why* Ellen came to see Dr. Davis for this visit. As you learned, because Ellen has an injury, you must also report *how* and *where* she became injured.

Dr. Davis's notes tell us that Ellen had a headache that turned out to be a concussion: "Dr. Davis determines that Ellen has a *brain concussion*." In the Alphabetic Index, find:

Concussion (brain)(cerebral)(current) S06.0x-

Now turn to the tabular list, and find:

S06 Intracranial injury

Beneath this code you can see an *includes* note and some *excludes* notes. None of these relate to Ellen's diagnosis, so continue reading down the column looking at all of the fourth-character choices:

S06.0 Concussion

S06.0x Concussion

The notes do not mention anything about her losing consciousness after she hurt her head, so now review the choices for the sixth and seventh characters. Find:

S06.0x0A Concussion without loss of consciousness, initial encounter

Now you know that a concussion is an injury, so you will need to explain *how* and *where* she hurt her head. Go back to the notes, and find the documentation to explain how she injured herself: "*She had fallen off the swing and hit her head fiercely against the ground.*" For the correct code to report the *how* and *where* information about an injury, you will need to look this up in the Alphabetic Index to external causes in Volume 2, Section 3, and then confirm it in the Tabular List. Let's begin with the *how*. . . . In the Alphabetic Index to External Causes, find:

Fall, falling (accidental) W19

Read down the indented list under this key term, and find the item from which she fell:

Fall, falling (accidental) W19

> **from, off, out of**
>> **playground equipment W09.8**
>>> **swing W09.0**

Turn to the Tabular List and find:

W09 Fall on and from playground equipment

Continue to read down to determine the accurate fifth and sixth characters. Which one matches the notes?

W09.1xx- Fall from playground swing

Perfect! Now notice the hyphen to the right of the code. Remember that this means that a seventh character is required. There is nothing below this code, so read up and find the choices directly below W09:

The appropriate 7th character is to be added to each code from category W09

> **A initial encounter**
>
> **D subsequent encounter**
>
> **S sequela**

Let's go back to the scenario and check. Is this the first time Ellen is seeing Dr. Davis for this concussion? Yes. Terrific! So now you know that the correct code you need to report what Ellen was doing when she got her brain concussion is:

W09.1xxA Fall from playground swing, initial encounter

You still have some additional information to share. You need to explain *where* she was (known as *place of occurrence*) and *why* she was doing what she was doing when she got hurt. Take a look at:

Y92.830 Public park as the place of occurrence of the external cause

Y99.8 Other external cause status (leisure activity)

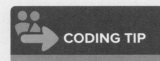

CODING TIP

An external cause code can *never* be a principal, or first-listed, code. In other words, it cannot be the first code on a claim form, and it can never be the only diagnosis code on a claim form.

Don't worry, you will learn more, and practice more, with external cause codes later on. For now, you are just laying a foundation. So you are now ready to report why Dr. Davis provided care to Ellen during this encounter:

S06.0x0A Concussion without loss of consciousness, initial encounter

W09.1xxA Fall from playground swing, initial encounter

Y92.830 Public park as the place of occurrence of the external cause

Y99.8 Other external cause status (leisure activity)

Good work!

You may have to ask the intake nurse, the attending physician, or the patient himself or herself to obtain all the information you need to code an injury properly. However, in some circumstances, additional information may not be available. If the patient is unconscious, for example, you may know the *how* with regard to the event (e.g., fell off a ladder, in an automobile accident, overdose of aspirin?) but not have a confirmation on the intent (e.g., was the injury or poisoning an accident, assault, or attempted suicide?). In such cases, you can use a code from the following:

Y21-Y33 Event of undetermined intent

Undetermined and unspecified codes should be used only as a last resort, when you have no way of getting additional information. Most insurers are wary of such codes and will typically pull claims using them for further investigation. This will delay payment.

Occasionally, the ICD-10-CM book will actually remind you to include an external cause code.

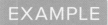

EXAMPLE

T75.3xx- Motion sickness
   Use additional external cause code to identify vehicle or type of motion (Y92.81-, Y93.5-)

Most of the time, however, you have to use your judgment as to whether an external cause code is necessary. These code descriptions are *not* included in the main Alphabetic Index. So once you have determined that an external cause code is necessary, you will begin the search for the most accurate code in Section 3 of Volume 2: the *Alphabetic Index to External Causes.*

Remember: The main purpose of the external cause code is to help guide you in your determination as to which insurance policy should be responsible for paying the bill. Therefore, be certain you know the whole story so that your codes can tell the whole story. While external cause codes are not required in all states or by all insurance carriers, including the codes on your health claim form will speed the process along and get your claim paid faster. And that's what this is all about!

LO 2.6 Sequelae (Late Effects)

When the patient has come to see the health care professional for the treatment of a **sequela** (also known as a **late effect**), you must code the particular problem as a sequela *only* in the following situations:

- Scarring.
- Nonunion or malunion of a fracture.
- When the connection is specifically documented by the physician or health care professional confirming the new condition as a sequela (a late effect) of a previous condition.

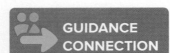

GUIDANCE CONNECTION

Review the ICD-10-CM Coding Guidelines, Section 1.B, General coding guidelines, Subsection 10, **Sequela (late effects).**

sequela (late effect)
Cause-and-effect relationship between an original condition, illness, or injury and an additional problem caused by the existence of that original condition. Time is not a requirement for a diagnosis as a late effect because the additional concern may be present at any time.

Coding a late effect requires at least two codes, in the following order:

1. The sequela condition, which is the condition that resulted and that is being treated.
2. The sequela (late effect) or original-condition code with the seventh character "S."

Seventh Character "S" for Sequela

When available, the seventh character "S" is used to report a condition that has directly resulted from another condition. A scar that has formed as an aftereffect of a burn, laceration, wound, or other injury is a perfect example of a sequela. When reporting a code with the seventh character "S," you must use both the original-injury code from which the sequela came and the code for the sequela condition itself. The "S" is added to the injury code only, not the sequela code. This is your way, as the coder, to explain the injury that was responsible for the resulting condition (the sequela). The sequela condition code is sequenced first, followed by the injury code with the seventh character "S."

> ## EXAMPLE
>
> Bruce Bucholz, a 27-year-old male, comes to see Dr. Walker for treatment of adherent scars on the back of his hand. Bruce is a firefighter and suffered third-degree burns on his left hand last year when he reached in to save a child from a burning house. Dr. Walker evaluates Bruce's scars and proceeds to plan out a series of plastic surgeries.
>
> L90.5 Scar conditions and fibrosis of skin (adherent scar)
> T23.362S Burn of third degree of back of left hand, sequela
> X00.0xxS Exposure to flames in uncontrolled fire in building or structure
> Y99.0 Civilian activity done for income or pay

Sequelae (Late Effects) of External Cause

A condition considered to be a late effect or sequela of an injury must be documented as such. Sequelae of external cause codes are used with a code reporting a sequela (late effect) of a previous (not current) injury. This is indicated using a seventh character of "S" for sequela with both the injury code and the external cause code.

Sequelae of Cerebrovascular Disease

When the physician identifies a condition, such as a neurologic deficit, as a late effect of cerebrovascular disease, a cardiovascular accident (CVA), or other diagnosis originally reported with a code from the I60–I67 range, report this sequela using a code from category I69, Sequelae of cerebrovascular disease, to connect the current problem (the late effect) with the original condition.

Sequelae of Complication of Pregnancy, Childbirth, and the Puerperium

Similar to the codes in category I69 for reporting the sequela of cardiovascular disease, there is a dedicated code for reporting the sequela of a complication with the pregnancy, the birth of the child, and/or the puerperium. When that complication creates a condition that requires treatment or services later on, after the postpartum period (within 6 weeks after delivery), and the condition is documented as a late effect of a pregnancy complication, you will use code O94, sequencing it after the code to report the complication or condition.

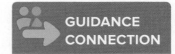

GUIDANCE CONNECTION

Review the ICD-10-CM Coding Guidelines, Section I.C.19, Chapter 19: **Injury, poisoning, and certain other consequences of external causes,** Subsection a, **Application of 7th characters in Chapter 19.**

GUIDANCE CONNECTION

Review the ICD-10-CM Coding Guidelines, Section I.C.20, Chapter 20: **External causes of morbidity,** Subsection i, **Sequelae (late effects) of external cause guidelines.**

GUIDANCE CONNECTION

Review the ICD-10-CM Coding Guidelines, Section I.C.9, Chapter 9: **Diseases of the circulatory system,** Subsection d, **Sequelae of cerebrovascular disease.**

GUIDANCE CONNECTION

Review the ICD-10-CM Coding Guidelines, Section I.C.15, Chapter 15: **Pregnancy, childbirth, and the puerperium,** Subsection p, **Code O94 sequelae of complication of pregnancy, childbirth, and the puerperium.**

Marion Rilea, a 71-year-old female, came to see Dr. Miller for continued treatment of the acute gastric ulcer in her stomach. The ulcer developed as a result of her taking aspirin for her arthritis, as instructed. Dr. Miller recommends surgery, and Marion agrees.

You Code It!

Go through the steps of coding, and determine the codes that should be reported for this encounter between Dr. Miller and Marion Rilea.

Step 1: Read the case completely.

Step 2: Abstract the notes: Which key words can you identify relating to why Dr. Miller cared for Marion?

_____

Step 3: Query the provider, if necessary.

Step 4: Code the diagnosis or diagnoses.

_____

Step 5: Code the procedure(s): Office visit

Step 6: Link the procedure codes to at least one diagnosis code to confirm medical necessity.

Step 7: Back code to double-check your choices.

Answer:

Did you determine the correct codes?

K25.3 Acute gastric ulcer without hemorrhage or perforation

T39.015D Adverse effect of aspirin, subsequent encounter

Chapter Summary

This chapter is just an overview of what the following chapters will be discussing, in detail, about coding diagnoses. As you look back over this chapter, you should notice one very important thing: The ICD-10-CM book will almost always guide you to the correct code. The Alphabetic Index will guide you to the correct page in the Tabular List (Volume 1), so you can read the notations and symbols, evaluate all the choices, and determine the best, most accurate code. If no codes seem to match the attending physician's notes, just go back and keep looking.

Two principles important to becoming a good coder:

1. Identify the key words in the physician's notes so that you can look up the best, most accurate code or codes.

2. In case of an injury, poisoning, or adverse effect, you will need to add an external cause code.

The ICD-10-CM book will guide you through the rest with its notations and instructions. The Official Coding Guidelines are always there, in the book for you to reference—no memorization! All the information can point you in the right direction toward the best, most accurate code. Just look and read. And when the time comes, you will have no problem transitioning from student to professional coding specialist.

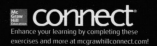

Using Terminology

Match each key term to the appropriate definition.

_____ **1.** LO 2.1 A separate condition or illness present in the same patient at the same time as another, unrelated condition or illness.

_____ **2.** LO 2.3 Health care services provided to individuals without an overnight stay in the facility.

_____ **3.** LO 2.6 Cause-and-effect relationship between an original condition, illness, or injury and an additional problem caused by the existence of that original condition.

_____ **4.** LO 2.1 A condition caused or developed from the existence of another condition.

_____ **5.** LO 2.1 A condition named after a person.

_____ **6.** LO 2.1 An unexpected, bad result; also known as an *adverse reaction*.

_____ **7.** LO 2.5 An event, outside the body, that causes injury, poisoning, or an adverse reaction.

_____ **8.** LO 2.2 A specific location or part of the human body.

_____ **9.** LO 2.3 Found to be true or definite.

_____ **10.** LO 2.1 A health-related situation.

_____ **11.** LO 2.3 An establishment that provides acute care services to individuals who stay overnight on the premises.

A. Adverse effect
B. Anatomical site
C. Co-morbidity
D. Condition
E. Confirmed
F. Eponym
G. External cause
H. Inpatient facility
I. Manifestation
J. Outpatient services
K. Sequela (late effect)

Checking Your Understanding

Choose the most appropriate answer for each of the following questions.

1. LO 2.1 An example of an *eponym* is

  a. fracture.
  b. wounds.
  c. Cushing's disease.
  d. mitral valve disease.

2. LO 2.1 An example of a *condition* is

  a. heart.
  b. acute.
  c. subcutaneous.
  d. infection.

3. LO 2.2 After abstracting the key terms, a coder will go next to the

  a. Tabular listings.
  b. Alphabetic Index.
  c. external cause codes.
  d. Appendix A.

4. LO 2.1 Diagnosis codes explain
   a. who the patient is.
   b. what the physician did for the patient.
   c. why the physician treated the patient.
   d. how the patient came to be ill.

5. LO 2.3 The Tabular List (Volume 1) shows diagnoses
   a. in alphanumeric order.
   b. in ledger format.
   c. in numeric order.
   d. in cost order, from least expensive to most expensive.

6. LO 2.3 When coding outpatient services, code any condition documented as
   a. suspected.
   b. possible.
   c. probable.
   d. confirmed.

7. LO 2.4 A Z code is used to report an encounter for
   a. applying a cast to a broken arm.
   b. an annual checkup.
   c. a stomach ache.
   d. a fall from a ladder.

8. LO 2.5 An external cause code can be used
   a. as a first-listed diagnosis code.
   b. as the only diagnosis code.
   c. with other ICD-10-CM codes.
   d. to report what the physician did for the patient.

9. LO 2.5 In case of an injury, poisoning, or adverse effect, you will need to add a(n)
   a. Z code.
   b. external cause code.
   c. sequela code.
   d. eponym.

10. LO 2.6 All of the following are sequelae *except*
    a. scarring.
    b. nonunion of a fracture.
    c. malunion of a fracture.
    d. influenza.

Applying Your Knowledge

1. LO 2.1 Explain what the principal or first-listed diagnosis is for a hospital admission. _____

_____

2. LO 2.1 What does *abstracting the physician's notes* mean? _____

_____

3. LO 2.1/2.6 Explain the difference between co-morbidities and manifestations. _____

_____

4. LO 2.5 What is an external cause code, and what part of the patient encounter does it tell? _____

_____

5. LO 2.6 What is the minimum number of codes required to code a sequela or late effect, and in what sequence or order are they listed? _____

_____

6. LO 2.4 What is a Z code, and when would it be assigned? _____

_____

7. LO 2.3 Explain the difference in the guidelines between coding for outpatient services and coding for inpatient services. _____

_____

8. LO 2.2 When is it appropriate to code from the Alphabetic Index? _____

_____

Using the techniques described in this chapter, carefully read through the case studies and determine the most accurate ICD-10-CM code(s) and external cause code(s), if appropriate, for each case.

1. Jonathan Masters, a 16-year-old male, goes to Dr. Principal for a medical examination required by his school so that he can play on the basketball team.

   _____

2. Marilyn Chase, a 57-year-old female, comes in today to see Dr. Jamison, her family physician. Dr. Jamison saw Marilyn 5 days ago and prescribed Amobarbital, a sleeping pill. Marilyn states she has been taking the medication as prescribed and now she is having generalized abdominal cramps. Dr. Jamison completes an examination and determines Marilyn is having an adverse reaction to the medication and orders her to discontinue use.

   _____

3. Harrison Richmond, a 27-year-old male, is seen in the emergency room for a sprained back (coccyx) suffered as a result of falling off a horse he was riding in the local public park.

   _____

4. Karyn Felder, a 31-year-old female, comes to Dr. Vistas complaining of pain in her left ear. Dr. Vistas diagnoses Karyn with acute otitis media.

   _____

5. Raul Boca, a 13-year-old male, was recently diagnosed with asthma. He comes in to Dr. Wilder's office for counseling on the correct use of his nebulizer.

   _____

6. Eleanor McKee, a 43-year-old female, comes to Dr. Geoffrey for her annual gynecologic exam with Pap smear.

   _____

7. Mary Chase, a 23-year-old female, comes to Dr. Hernandez for the evaluation of a pilonidal cyst.

   _____

8. Kim Wong, a 9-day-old female, is brought to Dr. Johannson for the evaluation of congenital skin tags that are on her outer ear and earlobe.

   _____

9. Millie Andujar, a 43-year-old female, comes to Seaside Diagnostic Imaging for another mammogram because her mother died of breast cancer.

   _____

10. Edward Madison, an 81-year-old male, is brought to Dr. Abbott for a follow-up on the progress of the malignant melanoma on his forehead.

_____

11. Lawrence Bowers, a 33-year-old male, comes to the emergency room for treatment of second-degree sunburn on his shoulder area.

_____

12. Salvatore Mulkey, a 2-year-old male, is brought to the ER by ambulance after his mother found him extremely drowsy. Her bottle of ampicillin was found half empty next to him.

_____

13. Debra Gilliam, a 19-year-old female, went camping with her boyfriend 10 days ago. While she was at the campsite, she was bitten by a tick. She began to feel sick this morning and came to see Dr. Chung. After a thorough examination, Debra is diagnosed with Lyme disease.

_____

14. Kathleen Wilcox, a 4-year-old female, is brought by her father to Dr. Bridges to remove a jellybean from Kathleen's nostril. The jellybean is making it difficult for Kathleen to breathe.

_____

15. Christopher Edison, a 1-year-old male, is brought in to Dr. Vasquez for Christopher's routine examination.

_____

YOU CODE IT! Application
Chapter 2: Introduction to ICD-10-CM

The following exercises provide practice in abstracting physicians' notes and learning to work with SOAP notes from our health care facility, _Taylor, Reader, & Associates_. These case studies (SOAP notes) are modeled on real patient encounters.

SOAP notes are a standardized documentation process used by health care providers to create a patient's file. The SOAP note has four parts; each part will differ in length and support the patient's encounter for that day.

So, what does the acronym _SOAP_ stand for?

S = subjective
O = objective
A = assessment
P = plan

What the **subjective** portion of the SOAP note includes:
A short statement in the patient's own words as to the reason for the encounter, the chief complaint.

What the **objective** portion of the SOAP note includes:
The results of the physical examination, any measurable result. A few examples are vital signs, height, weight, and lab and diagnostic results.

What the **assessment** portion of the SOAP note includes:
A concise summation of the physician's diagnosis.

What the **plan** portion of the SOAP note includes:
The physician's plan of care (treatment) for the patient's encounter.

Carefully read through the notes. Then, using the techniques you learned in the practice exercises, determine the most accurate ICD-10-CM code(s) and external cause code(s), if appropriate, for each case study.

TAYLOR, READER, & ASSOCIATES
A Complete Health Care Facility
975 CENTRAL AVENUE • SOMEWHERE, FL 32811 • 407-555-4321

PATIENT: VAN DYKE, OLIVIA
ACCOUNT/EHR #:   VANDOL001
DATE: 09/16/18

Attending Physician: Suzanne R. Taylor, MD

S: Pt is a 25-year-old female who has had a sore throat for the past week. She states that she has felt feverish for the last two days, and had a temperature of 100.5 degrees last night.

O: Ht 5′5″ Wt. 159 lb. R 16. T 99. BP 110/85 Pharynx is inspected, and there is obvious purulent material in the left posterior pharynx. Neck: supple, no nodes. Chest: clear. COR: RRR without murmur.

A: Acute pharyngitis

P: 1. Send pt for test to rule/out Strep
     2. Recommend patient gargle with warm salt water and use OTC lozenges to keep throat moist
     3. Will write Rx once results of Strep test come back
     4. Return in three weeks for follow-up

Suzanne R. Taylor, MD

SRT/pw   D: 9/16/18 09:50:16   T: 9/18/18 12:55:01

Determine the most accurate ICD-10-CM code(s).

_____

_____

_____

TAYLOR, READER, & ASSOCIATES
A Complete Health Care Facility
975 CENTRAL AVENUE • SOMEWHERE, FL 32811 • 407-555-4321

PATIENT: WILLIAMS, CONRAD
ACCOUNT/EHR #:   WILLCO001
DATE: 06/21/18

Attending Physician: Suzanne R. Taylor, MD

S: Pt is a 51-year-old male who I have not seen since his annual physical exam last September. He states that 5–6 weeks ago he noted some intermittent soft stool and decrease in the caliber of stools. He also noted some bleeding that discontinued four days ago. He denies any cramps or abdominal pain.

O: External examination of the anus revealed some external skin tags present in the left anterior position. Anal examination revealed an extremely tight anal sphincter. This was dilated manually to allow instrumentation with the anoscope, which was accomplished in a 360-degree orientation. There was some prominence of the crypts and some inflammation of the rectal mucosa, a portion of which was sent for biopsy. This was friable. In the left anterior position there was a fistula that was healing with some formation of a sentinel pile on the outside, which had been noticed on external examination.

A: Anal fissure, unusual position, nontraumatic

P: 1. Rule out inflammatory bowel disease with air contrast barium enema examination and reflux into terminal ileum.
     2. Patient to return for sigmoidoscopy after BE.

Suzanne R. Taylor, MD

SRT/pw   D: 06/21/18 09:50:16   T: 06/25/18 12:55:01

Determine the most accurate ICD-10-CM code(s).

_____

_____

_____

TAYLOR, READER, & ASSOCIATES
A Complete Health Care Facility
975 CENTRAL AVENUE • SOMEWHERE, FL 32811 • 407-555-4321

PATIENT: BEVINS, NANCY
ACCOUNT/EHR #:   BEVINA001
DATE: 08/11/18

Attending Physician: Willard B. Reader, MD

S: Pt is a 37-year-old female who comes in every six months for an abdominal scan. She had been diagnosed with bladder cancer three years ago. After a sequence of radiation and chemotherapy, she was pronounced malignant-free one year ago. Since that time, she comes in for a check every six months. Pt denies any signs or symptoms indicating a return of the malignancy.

O: Ht 5'3". Wt. 119 lb. R 18. T 98.6. BP 120/95. Abdomen appears to be normal upon manual examination. Results of CT scan indicated no abnormalities.

A: Personal history of bladder cancer

P: Pt to return PRN

_____

Willard B. Reader, MD

WBR/pw   D: 08/11/18 09:50:16   T: 08/13/18 12:55:01

Determine the most accurate ICD-10-CM code(s).

_____

_____

_____

TAYLOR, READER, & ASSOCIATES
A Complete Health Care Facility
975 CENTRAL AVENUE • SOMEWHERE, FL 32811 • 407-555-4321

PATIENT: ROMANO, JOSEPH
ACCOUNT/EHR #:   ROMAJO001
DATE: 07/11/18

Attending Physician: Suzanne R. Taylor, MD

S: Pt is a 25-year-old male who states that he cut the back of his right index finger while cutting up a chicken while at work. Pt works as a chef at a local restaurant. He cannot extend his finger since the accident, and he had some bleeding, which he stopped with pressure. Pt had a tetanus toxoid administered last year when he sustained a wound to the forearm while at work. He has no past history of serious illnesses, operations, or allergies. Social history and family history are noncontributory.

O: Examination reveals a 3-cm laceration, dorsum of right index finger, with laceration of extensor tendon, proximal to the interphalangeal joint. The patient cannot extend the finger; he can flex, adduct, and abduct the finger. Sensation at this time appears to be normal. Pt was prepped, and a digital nerve block using 1% Carbocaine was carried out. When the block was totally effective, the wound was explored. After thorough irrigation of the wound with normal saline, the joint capsule was repaired with two sutures of 5-0 Dexon. The tendon repair was then carried out using 4-0 nylon. Dressings were applied, and a splint was applied holding the interphalangeal joint in neutral position, in full extension but not hyperextension. The Pt tolerated the procedure well and left the surgical area in good condition.

A: 3-cm laceration, dorsum of right index finger, with laceration of extensor tendon

P: 1. Rx Percocet, q4h prn for pain
     2. Rx Augmentin, 250 mg tid
     3. Patient to return for follow-up in three days

Suzanne R. Taylor, MD

SRT/pw   D: 07/11/18 09:50:16   T: 07/13/18 12:55:01

Determine the most accurate ICD-10-CM code(s).

_____

_____

_____

TAYLOR, READER, & ASSOCIATES
A Complete Health Care Facility
975 CENTRAL AVENUE • SOMEWHERE, FL 32811 • 407-555-4321

PATIENT: HADLEY, HELEN
ACCOUNT/EHR #:   HADLHE001
DATE: 10/19/18

Attending Physician: Willard B. Reader, MD

S: Pt is a 37-year-old female who parachuted from a plane yesterday and landed in a tree. She banged her head against a tree limb and lost consciousness for approximately three minutes.

O: Ht 5′7″ Wt. 129 lb. R 17. T 98.6. BP 120/95. HEENT unremarkable. Pupils are equal and reactive. EEG shows indication of a mild head trauma. CT scan confirmed the brain concussion. Pt told to rest, with no physical activity for the next 72 hours.

A: Concussion with brief loss of consciousness

P: 1. Rx aspirin for pain prn
      2. Pt to return in one week

Willard B. Reader, MD

WBR/pw   D: 10/19/18 09:50:16   T: 10/23/18 12:55:01

Determine the most accurate ICD-10-CM code(s).

_____

_____

_____

GENERAL GUIDELINES AND NOTATIONS

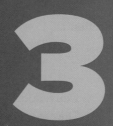

Learning Outcomes *After completing this chapter, the student should be able to:*

LO 3.1 Identify the manner in which to report codes with the greatest specificity.

LO 3.2 Apply the guidelines for properly using placeholder characters.

LO 3.3 Identify when a seventh character is required.

LO 3.4 Use the punctuation presented to clarify code choices.

LO 3.5 Abstract physicians' notes to pinpoint key terms related to the diagnoses.

LO 3.6 Determine the most accurate diagnosis code.

ICD-10-CM diagnosis codes are from three to seven characters in length. What's the difference?

Diagnoses, signs, and symptoms each need various levels of detail to completely explain them. Some are simple and straightforward, while others can be very complex. All of the specifics are needed for continuity of care and medical decision making, as well as the determination of reimbursement. The codes used to report the reason why a health care provider cared for and treated a patient must relate all of the available details because each and every specific element is important to the process. Therefore, various levels of details require various levels of codes.

The use of these codes is governed by the conventions and guidelines presented in *ICD-10-CM Official Guidelines for Coding and Reporting* (see Figure 3-1).

LO 3.1 Three-Character Codes Categories

Each type of illness or injury is divided into a separate category identified by a three-character code. Sometimes the three-character code is all that is needed to report the whole story about the patient's condition. Consider the following ICD-10-CM code:

J14 Pneumonia due to *Hemophilus influenzae*

The three-character code is complete and requires no further information or detail.

Key Terms

Acute

Chronic

Manifestation

Nonessential modifier

Not elsewhere classifiable (NEC)

Not otherwise specified (NOS)

Other specified

Principal diagnosis

Underlying condition

Unspecified

Section I.   Conventions, general coding guidelines and chapter specific guidelines

The conventions, general guidelines and chapter-specific guidelines are applicable to all health care settings unless otherwise indicated. The conventions and instructions of the classification take precedence over guidelines.

A. Conventions for the ICD-10-CM

The conventions for the ICD-10-CM are the general rules for use of the classification independent of the guidelines. These conventions are incorporated within the Alphabetic Index and Tabular List of the ICD-10-CM as instructional notes.

1. The Alphabetic Index and Tabular List

The ICD-10-CM is divided into the Alphabetic Index, an alphabetical list of terms and their corresponding code, and the Tabular List, a structured list of codes divided into chapters based on body system or condition. The Alphabetic Index consists of the following parts: the Index of Diseases and Injury, the Index of External Causes of Injury, the Table of Neoplasms and the Table of Drugs and Chemicals.

See Section I.C2.   General guidelines
See Section I.C.19.   Adverse effects, poisoning, underdosing and toxic effects

2. Format and Structure:

The ICD-10-CM Tabular List contains categories, subcategories and codes. Characters for categories, subcategories and codes may be either a letter or a number. All categories are 3 characters. A three-character category that has no further subdivision is equivalent to a code. Subcategories are either 4 or 5 characters. Codes may be 3, 4, 5, 6 or 7 characters. That is, each level of subdivision after a category is a subcategory. The final level of subdivision is a code. Codes that have applicable 7th characters are still referred to as codes, not subcategories. A code that has an applicable 7th character is considered invalid without the 7th character.

The ICD-10-CM uses an indented format for ease in reference.

3. Use of codes for reporting purposes

For reporting purposes only codes are permissible, not categories or subcategories, and any applicable 7th character is required.

4. Placeholder character

The ICD-10-CM utilizes a placeholder character "X". The "X" is used as a placeholder at certain codes to allow for future expansion. An example of this is at the poisoning, adverse effect and underdosing codes, categories T36–T50.

ICD-10-CM Official Guidelines for Coding and Reporting
FY 2015
Page 7 of 116

Figure 3-1 Example of a Page from ICD-10-CM Official Guidelines

LET'S CODE IT! SCENARIO

Bruce Morrison, a 56-year-old male, went to see his physician, Dr. Thurston, with complaints of chest congestion and a cough. After a thorough exam, Dr. Thurston diagnosed Bruce with bronchitis.

Let's Code It!

Read through the notes, and recognize the key words that identify *why* the patient came to see the physician. Bruce came because of the chest congestion and the cough. However, Dr. Thurston determined that these were signs of a condition called *bronchitis*. Dr. Thurston confirmed the diagnosis of *bronchitis*. Let's turn to *bronchitis* in the Alphabetic Index:

Bronchitis (diffuse) (fibrinous)(hypostatic)(infective) (membranous) J40

Dr. Thurston did not include any other specifications or descriptions of the bronchitis; therefore, none of the other descriptions in the indented list below *Bronchitis* applies.

Now let's turn to the Tabular List:

J40 Bronchitis, not specified as acute or chronic

   Bronchitis NOS

NOS is the acronym for *not otherwise specified*. This is true. Dr. Thurston did not provide any additional specifications. In the Tabular List, look at all the other codes and their descriptions as they relate to the diagnosis of bronchitis in general and particularly with regard to this encounter between Dr. Thurston and Bruce. The description for J40 is best and most clearly matches the physician's notes. Therefore, the three-character code J40 is correct because it relates the *whole story*.

Four-Character, Five-Character, and Six-Character Codes (Subcategories)

In some cases, additional characters are *required* to report a more specific description. If so, the ICD-10-CM Tabular List will tell you with an indented listing of all the available choices for these extended descriptions, shown below the code category.

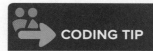

CODING TIP

Now is the time to begin good habits. When you turn to the Tabular List, begin reading at the three-character category to be certain that you review all the applicable notations and guidelines.

LET'S CODE IT! SCENARIO

Renee Klepp, a 61-year-old female, has been under the care of Dr. Ledbetter, a dentist. He recently diagnosed her with localized, chronic periodontitis.

Let's Code It!

Okay, this one is easy when it comes to finding the diagnostic key words. You can clearly see that the diagnosis is *localized, chronic periodontitis*.

Let's turn to the Alphabetic Index, and look up:

Periodontitis (chronic)(complex)(compound)(local)(simplex) K05.30

   Acute K05.20

   Apical K04.5

   Generalized K05.32

   Localized K05.31

That last one, K05.31, looks like a good match. But you know you are never permitted to report a code from the Alphabetic Index. You must confirm this is the correct code in the Tabular List. Turn to the Tabular List, and, as always, let's begin reading at the three-character code:

K05 Gingivitis and periodontal diseases

Directly below this code is a notation:

Use additional code to identify:

Alcohol abuse and dependence (F10.-)

. . .etc. . . .

Notations like this are terrific because they actually help us to determine the codes to report the whole story. This notation is directing you to go back to the physician's notes and determine if any of the listed circumstances are documented. If so, you will need to report it with a second code.

For now, let's continue on our journey for the accurate code to report Renee's periodontitis. Read down all the choices for a fourth character in this code category. Did you find:

K05.3 Chronic periodontitis

This matches what Dr. Ledbetter wrote in his notes. But this one code does not tell the whole story about Renee's condition, so let's continue reading the indented list below:

K05.31 Chronic periodontitis, localized

The differences between K05.30, K05.31, and K05.32 mean quite a lot to the patient, and to the health care professionals who are caring for Renee now and in the future. In addition, the third-party payer needs to know all the facts.

The details you will need in order to determine which code is correct should be found in the medical notes. Here, Dr. Ledbetter's notes state that Renee's chronic periodontitis is localized. This is how you know that K05.31 is correct. And thanks to the *use additional code* notation, you also know to go back to the complete documentation to determine if an additional code is necessary.

CODING TIP

If you had not read up to the three-character code description, you might have missed the *use additional code* notation. The notation and others like it are very important to your ability to code accurately. We will discuss more about notations in the next few pages.

EXAMPLE

L02 Cutaneous abscess, furnuncle and carbuncle
  L02.2 Cutaneous abscess, furuncle and carbuncle of trunk
    L02.21 Cutaneous abscess of trunk
      L02.214 Cutaneous abscess of groin

Remember! When codes with additional characters (and details) are available, you must use them. This is not optional—it is mandatory. And when a six-character code is available, the three-, four-, and five-character codes become invalid.

LET'S CODE IT! SCENARIO

Eileen Sucher, a 15-year-old female, is seen by Dr. Mazar. After a thorough examination and talking with Eileen, Dr. Mazar diagnoses her with bulimia nervosa.

Dr. Mazar has diagnosed Eileen with *bulimia nervosa*. In the Alphabetic Index, find:

Bulimia (nervosa) F50.2

　atypical F50.9

　normal weight F50.9

Great! Bulimia, nervosa F50.2, appears to match the notes perfectly. But you never, never, never code from the Alphabetic Index, so let's go to the Tabular List for code category F50:

F50 Eating disorders

　F50.2 Bulimia nervosa

There are no guidelines or notations that apply to Dr. Mazar's notes or Eileen's case to alter the code, so it still matches Dr. Mazar's notes exactly. Good work!

LO 3.2 Placeholder Character

There are times when a fourth, fifth, sixth, or seventh character is required, yet there are no previous characters. In these cases, ICD-10-CM uses a placeholder character, the letter "x," so the following characters will fall into their correct locations.

EXAMPLE

T15.01xA Foreign body in cornea, right eye, initial encounter

T47.5x2D Poisoning by digestants, intentional self-harm, subsequent encounter

T88.6xxS Anaphylactic reaction due to adverse effect of correct drug or medicament properly administered, sequela

Y26.xxxA Exposure to smoke, fire, and flames, undetermined intent, initial encounter

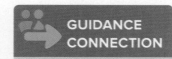

GUIDANCE CONNECTION

Refer to Official Guidelines: Section I.A.4, **Placeholder character.**

LO 3.3 Seventh Character

Some ICD-10-CM codes require a seventh character. Different subsections use this position—the seventh character—to add different types of information. Most often, these choices will be listed at the top of the code category and are used for all codes within that category. With this in mind, you must always check the top of the code category for this information.

EXAMPLE

In the **Diseases of the musculoskeletal system and connective tissue** chapter:
The appropriate 7th character is to be added to each code:

　A initial encounter for fracture

　D subsequent encounter for fracture with routine healing

　G subsequent encounter for fracture with delayed healing

　K subsequent encounter for fracture with nonunion

　P subsequent encounter for fracture with malunion

　S sequela

Within the **Pregnancy, childbirth, and the puerperium** chapter:
The appropriate 7th character is to be added to code:

> 0 not applicable or unspecified
> 1 fetus 1
> 2 fetus 2
> 3 fetus 3
> 4 fetus 4
> 5 fetus 5
> 9 other fetus

Within the **Injury, poisoning, and certain other consequences of external causes** chapter:
The appropriate 7th character is to be added to each code:

> A initial encounter
> D subsequent encounter
> S sequela

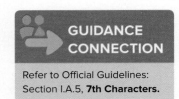

GUIDANCE CONNECTION

Refer to Official Guidelines: Section I.A.5, **7th Characters.**

The Tabular List contains all the details you need. All you have to do is read the choices and determine which is the most accurate, as per the physician's documentation.

LET'S CODE IT! SCENARIO

Oscar Tollson, a 73-year old male, went to see Dr. Auerback, an ophthalmologist, because of problems with his eyes. After taking a history and performing a physical exam, Dr. Auerback diagnosed Oscar with bilateral, mild-stage, chronic primary angle-closure glaucoma.

Let's Code It!

We see that Dr. Auerback diagnosed Oscar with *bilateral, mild-stage, chronic primary angle-closure glaucoma.* In the Alphabetic Index, find:

> **Glaucoma H40.9**

You know from the physician's notes that Oscar's glaucoma is "angle-closure," so read down the indented list beneath the key term *Glaucoma* and find:

> **Glaucoma H40.9**
> > **Angle-closure (primary) H40.20-**

Now, this term also has an indented list below it. Are there any more details available that match Dr. Auerback's notes?

> **Glaucoma H40.9**
> > **Angle-closure (primary) H40.20-**
> > > **Acute (attack)(crisis) H40.21-**
> > > **Chronic H40.22-**
> > > **Intermittent H40.23-**
> > > **Residual stage H40.24-**

Excellent! The notes also state that Oscar's glaucoma is chronic. Good job. Now let's turn to the Tabular list and begin reading at H40:

> **H40 Glaucoma**

Read through all of the fourth-character options, and determine which matches Dr. Auerback's notes:

H40.0 Glaucoma suspect

H40.1 Open-angle glaucoma

H40.2 Primary angle-closure glaucoma

H40.3 Glaucoma secondary to eye trauma

H40.4 Glaucoma secondary to eye inflammation

H40.5 Glaucoma secondary to other eye disorders

H40.6 Glaucoma secondary to drugs

H40.8 Other glaucoma

H40.9 Unspecified glaucoma

Did you notice that H40.2, Primary angle-closure glaucoma, matches Dr. Auerback's notes? Great! Now, you need to read through the fifth-character choices:

H40.20x Unspecified primary angle-closure glaucoma

H40.21 Acute angle-closure glaucoma

H40.22 Chronic angle-closure glaucoma

H40.23 Intermittent angle-closure glaucoma

H40.24 Residual stage of angle-closure glaucoma

Match these code descriptions to the documentation. Did you determine that H40.22, Chronic angle-closure glaucoma, matches Dr. Auerback's notes? Terrific! Now, this specific subcategory also provides sixth-character options:

H40.221 Chronic angle-closure glaucoma, right eye

H40.222 Chronic angle-closure glaucoma, left eye

H40.223 Chronic angle-closure glaucoma, bilateral

H40.229 Chronic angle-closure glaucoma, unspecified eye

Go back to Dr. Auerback's notes and see if she noted which of Oscar's eyes was affected by this condition. Then match that to the accurate code:

H40.223 Chronic angle-closure glaucoma, bilateral

You are really doing a great job! However, you are not done yet. Did you notice that symbol directing you to determine a seventh character for this code? The options are directly below code H40.22:

One of the following 7th characters is to be assigned to code H40.22 to designate the state of glaucoma

0 stage unspecified

1 mild stage

2 moderate stage

3 severe stage

4 indeterminate stage

What do the notes document about the stage of Oscar's glaucoma? Determine this and construct the correct code to report the reason why Dr. Auerback cared for Oscar:

H40.2231 Chronic angle-closure glaucoma, bilateral, mild stage

Good work!

Notations

Throughout the ICD-10-CM code book, directions, tips, symbols, and helpful notations are available to guide you to the accurate code for the patient encounter. Let's go through each, with examples, so you can develop a clear understanding of their meanings.

Includes, Excludes1, and Excludes2

Let's begin this explanation with an example. Turn, in the ICD-10-CM Tabular List, to code F31:

> **F31 Bipolar disorder**
> | INCLUDES | manic-depressive illness |
> | | manic-depressive psychosis |
> | | manic-depressive reaction |
> | EXCLUDES1 | bipolar disorder, single manic episode (F30.-) |
> | | major depressive disorder, single episode (F32.-) |
> | | major depressive disorder, recurrent (F33.-) |
> | EXCLUDES2 | cyclothymia (F34.0) |

These notations are there, in the Tabular List, to help you always determine the correct code. They provide you with additional terms and alternate codes that you might find better match what the physician wrote. This is all designed to make the coding process easier.

Includes This notation provides you with additional terms and diagnoses that are also reported with the above code or included in this code's description. They offer you variations to expand the opportunity for this code description to match what the physician wrote in the documentation. Looking at our example, this means that diagnoses of *bipolar disorder, manic-depressive illness, manic-depressive psychosis,* and *manic-depressive reaction* are all reported from code category F31.

Excludes1 There are times when two diagnostic statements may be close to each other, yet actually conflict. The *Excludes1* notation identifies codes that cannot be used on the same health claim form with the originally listed code. The notation signifies that the two codes:

- Are contradictory to each other.
- Cannot coexist in the same person at the same time.
- Are redundant.

Using our example above, this notation tells you that F32, Major-depressive disorder, single episode, is mutually exclusive to (cannot be reported with) F31, Bipolar disorder.

Excludes2 The *Excludes2* notation is the ICD-10-CM book's way of alerting you to a possible error. An *Excludes2* notation is a warning not to mistakenly use the code above when the code below is more accurate. It lists specific conditions that are *not* a part of the code and notify you that an alternate code or additional code may be needed. Using our example, you can see that this notation tells you that F34.0, Cyclothymia, is not the same as F31, Bipolar disorder. Now you can go back to the physician's notes, double-check the information, and determine which is the more accurate code to report.

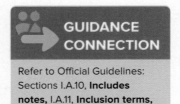

GUIDANCE CONNECTION

Refer to Official Guidelines: Sections I.A.10, **Includes notes,** I.A.11, **Inclusion terms,** and I.A.12, **Excludes notes.**

Code First

Certain conditions and diseases can cause additional problems in the body. Individuals with diabetes are known to have problems with their eyes or circulation, just to name a few, as a direct result of having diabetes. Patients found to be HIV-positive are prone to such conditions as pneumonia, again, directly linked to the fact that they have human immunodeficiency virus infection. This is known as an **underlying condition.** The resulting condition (e.g., pneumonia) is called a **manifestation.**

The *code first* notation is a reminder that you are going to need another code to identify the underlying disease that caused this condition. This notation is also telling you in what order to report the two codes: the underlying condition first, followed by the code for the manifestation (see Figure 3-2). Often, the notation will offer you a reference to the most common underlying diseases along with their codes! Cool!

EXAMPLE

C80.2 Malignant neoplasm associated with transplanted organ
Code first complication of transplanted organ (T86.-)

This notation tells you that:

1. You need to report both code C80.2 and a code from category T86 (as per the physician's notes).

2. You need to report the code from T86.- first, followed by C80.2.

13. **Etiology/manifestation convention ("code first", "use additional code" and "in diseases classified elsewhere" notes)**

Certain conditions have both an underlying etiology and multiple body system manifestations due to the underlying etiology. For such conditions, the ICD-10-CM has a coding convention that requires the underlying condition be sequenced first followed by the manifestation. Wherever such a combination exists, there is a "use additional code" note at the etiology code, and a "code first" note at the manifestation code. These instructional notes indicate the proper sequencing order of the codes, etiology followed by manifestation.

In most cases the manifestation codes will have in the code title, "in diseases classified elsewhere." Codes with this title are a component of the etiology/manifestation convention. The code title indicates that it is a manifestation code. "In diseases classified elsewhere" codes are never permitted to be used as first-listed or principal diagnosis codes. They must be used in conjunction with an underlying condition code and they must be listed following the underlying condition. See category F02, Dementia in other diseases classified elsewhere, for an example of this convention.

There are manifestation codes that do not have "in diseases classified elsewhere" in the title. For such codes, there is a "use additional code" note at the etiology code and a "code first" note at the manifestation code and the rules for sequencing apply.

In addition to the notes in the Tabular List, these conditions also have a specific Alphabetic Index entry structure. In the Alphabetic Index both conditions are listed together with the etiology code first followed by the manifestation codes in brackets. The code in brackets is always to be sequenced second.

FIGURE 3-2 ICD-10-CM Manifestation Convention

Use Additional Code

Similar to the *code first* notation, the *use additional code* notation is the ICD-10-CM's way of informing you that you may need to report another code as well as the code above to tell the whole story and that this extra code would be reported after the code above this notation.

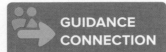

GUIDANCE CONNECTION

Refer to Official Guidelines: Section I.A.17, **"Code also note."**

EXAMPLE

> L58 Radiodermatitis
> *Use additional code* to identify the source of the radiation (W88, W90)

This notation tells you that:

1. You need to report both the code from category L58 and either W88 or W90 (as per the physician's notes).
2. You need to report the code from L58 first, followed by W88 or W90.

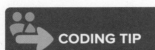

CODING TIP

Sometimes notations appear under the three-character code at the top of the category but are not repeated after each additional code in its section. This is another reason why it is important to read up to the three-character code, even when the Alphabetic Index directs you to the perfect code. You don't want to miss any important directives, such as *includes, excludes, code first,* or *use additional code* notations.

Code Also

A *code also* notation is similar to the *code first* and *use additional code* notations without the predetermination of sequencing. ICD-10-CM is alerting you that the physician's notes may contain some additional condition or issue that should be reported with a separate code, in addition to the code above this notation. This notation leaves it up to you to decide whether or not the additional code is needed to tell the whole story. If it is needed, you will need to use the Official Guidelines, Sections II and III, to determine in what order to report them.

EXAMPLE

> C7A Malignant neuroendocrine tumors
> *Code also* any associated multiple endocrine neoplasia (MEN) syndromes (E31.2-)

Category Notes

Occasionally, you may see informational notes under the description of a three-character code or at the top of a subsection in the Tabular List.

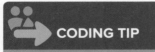

CODING TIP

Forgetting that, in ICD-10-CM, the word *and* really means "and/or" can throw a new coder off a correct code because the notes do not indicate both elements of the code description. Therefore, you need to make yourself a special note so you don't forget.

EXAMPLE

> I69 Sequelae of cerebrovascular disease
> Note: Category I69 is to be used to indicate conditions in I60–I67 as the cause of sequelae. The "sequelae" include conditions specified as such or as residuals which may occur at any time after the onset of the causal condition.

And

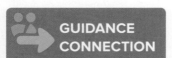

GUIDANCE CONNECTION

Refer to Official Guidelines: Section I.A.14, **"And."**

The guidelines for the accurate use of ICD-10-CM instruct you to interpret the use of the word *and* in a code description as "and/or." Therefore, if the physician's notes include only one part but not the other, the code may still be correct.

C41.0 Malignant neoplasm of bones of skull and face

You would be correct to report code C41.0 on the basis of physician's notes that confirm a diagnosis of a malignant neoplasm of the bones of the skull, a malignant neoplasm of the bones of the face, or a malignant neoplasm of the skull and face.

Other Notations

NEC **Not elsewhere classifiable (NEC),** or not elsewhere classified, indicates that the physician provided additional details of the condition but the ICD-10-CM book did not include those extra details in any of the other codes in the book.

M12.8 Other specific arthropathies, not elsewhere classified
Infection, coronavirus NEC B34.2

Other Specified The phrase **other specified** means the same thing as NEC: The physician specified additional information that the ICD-10-CM book doesn't have in any of the other codes in the category.

H80.81 Other otosclerosis, right ear
K03.8 Other specified diseases of hard tissues of teeth

NOS **Not otherwise specified (NOS)** means that the physician did not document any additional details that are identified in any of the other available code descriptions.

O03.9 Miscarriage NOS
K08.20 Unspecified atrophy of edentulous alveolar ridge (atrophy of the mandible NOS)

Unspecified **Unspecified** has the same meaning as NOS: The physician was not specific in his or her notes. Its notations are examples of how the ICD-10-CM diagnosis book will guide you to the correct code, if you pay attention.

H81.92 Unspecified disorder of vestibular function, left ear
Tumor, yolk sac, unspecified site, male C62.90

---

not elsewhere classifiable (NEC)
Specifics that are not described in any other code in the ICD-10-CM book; also known as *not elsewhere classified.*

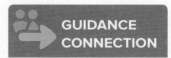

Refer to Official Guidelines: Section I.A.9.a, **"Other" codes.**

other specified
Additional information the physician specified that isn't included in any other code description.

not otherwise specified (NOS)
The absence of additional details documented in the notes.

unspecified
The absence of additional specifics in the physician's documentation.

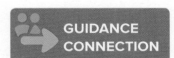

Refer to Official Guidelines: Section I.A.9.b, **"Unspecified" codes.**

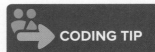

Before choosing any code with NOS or *unspecified* in the description, double-check the notes and patient record to be certain you cannot find a more specific code. If not, then query the provider and ask for the additional details you may need to determine a more accurate code. An unspecified or NOS code should always be a last resort.

See In the Alphabetic Index of ICD-10-CM, you may look up a term and notice that next to it, the book instructs you to *see* another term. This is an instruction in the index that the information you are looking for is listed under another term. In the example below, you can see that the Alphabetic Index is sending you to a different spelling of the diagnostic term.

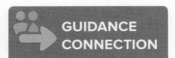
> ### EXAMPLE
>
> Ankylostoma—*see* Ancylostoma

See Also In other places in the Alphabetic Index, you may see that the instruction *see also* is next to the term you are investigating. Here, the ICD-10-CM index is explaining that additional details may be found under another term, as well as what you see here. In the example below, you can see that several suggested codes follow the main term. The index is providing you with an alternate term that may show terms more accurate to the physician's documentation.

> ### EXAMPLE
>
> Angiofibroma—*see also* Neoplasm, benign, by site
> Disease, diseased—*see also* Syndrome

See Condition The Alphabetic Index may also point you in a less detailed way when you look up a term and the notation tells you to *see condition*. This can be confusing. The index is not telling you to look up the term *condition*. What it is instructing you to do is to find the term that describes the health-related situation involved with this word and look up that term. You will see this most often next to the listing for an anatomical site.

> ### EXAMPLE
>
> Heart—*see condition*

This instruction comes back to the reason you are looking for a code in the first place. Remember, you are looking for a code to explain why the physician cared for the patient during the encounter. Using our example, having a heart is not a reason for a physician to meet with a patient. Everyone has a heart. Therefore, the index is telling you to look, instead, for the term that describes the condition of this patient's heart—the problem or concern about his or her heart that brought the patient together with the physician at this time. So, instead of *heart, cervix,* or *lung,* you need to look up *atrophy, fracture,* or *deformity.*

As you go through this material, you will learn more about determining the condition and the best way to look up terms in both the Alphabetic Index and the Tabular List of ICD-10-CM.

LO 3.4 Punctuation

Punctuation in ICD-10-CM adds information and helps you further in your quest for the best, most appropriate code.

[ ] Found in the Tabular List, *brackets* will show you alternate terms, alternate phrases, and/or synonyms to provide additional detail or explanation to the description. In our example below, the provider may have diagnosed the patient with foodborne intoxication

due to either *Clostridium perfringens* or *C. welchii*. In either case, A05.2 would be the correct code. The same for our second example: If the documentation reads either "third nerve palsy" or "palsy of the oculomotor nerve," code H49.02 is valid.

> ## EXAMPLE
>
> A05.2 Foodborne Clostridium perfringens [C. welchii] intoxication
> H49.02 Third [oculomotor] nerve palsy, left eye

[ ] *Italicized,* or *slanted, brackets,* used in the Alphabetic Index, will surround an additional code or codes (i.e., secondary codes) that *must* be included with the initial code. It is the Alphabetic Index's version of the *code first* and *use additional code* notations.

The italic brackets tell you that if the patient has been diagnosed with a muscle disorder due to leprosy, you have to use two codes: first, A30.9 for the underlying cause of the muscle disorder (the leprosy) and, second, M63.80 for the muscle disorder itself.

> ## EXAMPLE
>
> Leprosy A30.-
>   with muscle disorder A30.9 *[M63.80]*

( ) *Parentheses* show you additional descriptions, terms, or phrases that are also included in the description of the particular code. The additional terms are called **nonessential modifiers.** The modifiers can be used to provide additional definition but do not change the description of the condition. The additional terms are not required in the documentation, so if the provider did not use the additional term, the code description is still valid.

Take a look at the first example below. Whether the physician wrote the diagnosis as "malaria" or "malarial fever," code B54 would still apply.

In our second example, this code would be valid for a diagnosis written by the physician as "sarcoma of dendritic cells" or "sarcoma of accessory cells."

> ## EXAMPLE
>
> Malaria, malarial (fever) B54
> C96.4 Sarcoma of dendritic cells (accessory cells)

: A *colon* (two dots, one on top of the other), used in the Tabular List, will emphasize that one or more of the following descriptors are *required* to make the code valid for the diagnosis.

Combination Codes

If one code exists with a description that includes two or more diagnoses identified in one patient at the same time, you must choose the code that includes as many conditions as available. You may not code each separately.

When the physician's notes indicate that the patient suffered with both **acute** respiratory failure and **chronic** respiratory failure, you must use the code J96.2-. You are not allowed to use J96.0- and J96.1-, even though, technically, you are reporting the patient's conditions accurately. It is required that you use the combination code, as discussed in the Official Guidelines.

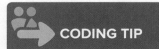

CODING TIP

If you ever forget what one of the symbols, abbreviations, or notations means, look for the pages in your ICD-10-CM book titled *ICD-10-CM Official Conventions.* On these pages, you will find the explanation for all of the footnotes, symbols, instructional notes, and conventions used.

In addition, most versions of ICD-10-CM include a legend across the bottom of the pages throughout Volume 1 with the symbols used and a brief description.

nonessential modifiers
Descriptors whose inclusion in the physician's notes is not absolutely necessary and that are provided simply to further clarify a code description; optional terms.

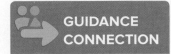

GUIDANCE CONNECTION

Refer to Official Guidelines: Sections I.B.8, **Acute and chronic conditions,** and I.B.9, **Combination code.**

acute
Severe; serious.

chronic
Long duration; continuing over a long period of time.

LO 3.5 Which Conditions to Code

As you abstract the provider's notes, you are looking for the information that will direct you to those codes that explain or describe the answer to the question, "Why did this health care provider care for and treat this individual during this encounter?" That is it. The codes do not report the individual's complete medical history.

> **GUIDANCE CONNECTION**
>
> Review the ICD-10-CM Coding Guidelines, Section I.B, **General coding guidelines,** specifically subsections **4, Signs and symptoms; 5, Conditions that are an integral part of a disease process;** and **6, Conditions that are not an integral part of a disease process.**

1. Identify only those symptoms, conditions, problems, or complaints that directly correlate to this encounter, that is, those that are directly addressed by the provider or influence the way treatments or services are presented at this encounter.

   The attending physician may include information in his or her notes that report a condition or diagnosis that is unrelated to this encounter. Remember that the physician does not write the notes just for you to code from. The notes have other, important purposes, such as documenting past history. You must learn to distinguish among notations. You will code only those diagnoses, signs, and/or symptoms related to procedures, services, treatments, and/or medical decision making occurring during this visit.

LET'S CODE IT! SCENARIO

Justine Cowen, a 33-year-old female, came to see Dr. Robinson complaining of severe pain in her shoulder. She stated that she was cleaning out her garage and a box fell off a shelf onto her left shoulder. Justine is 12 weeks pregnant. Normally, Dr. Robinson would have sent Justine for an x-ray. However, because she is pregnant, Dr. Robinson decided to examine her, diagnosed Justine with a sprained corahumeral shoulder, and strapped her shoulder and arm. The doctor also documented that Justine's pregnancy was incidental to the treatment for her shoulder.

Let's Code It!

Dr. Robinson diagnosed Justine with a *sprained shoulder.* Turn to the Alphabetic Index and look up *sprain, shoulder.*

Sprain, shoulder joint S43.40-

In the Tabular List, begin reading at code category S43 and read the *includes* and *excludes* notes carefully. There is nothing here that relates to this patient, so continue reading.

S43 Dislocation and sprain of joints and ligaments of shoulder girdle

You can see that you need additional characters, so continue reading down the column. Match the terms to the physician's notes. The fact is that Dr. Robinson did not provide any further specifics, so the most accurate code is:

S43.412A Sprain of left corahumeral (ligament), initial encounter

This is the only diagnosis confirmed by Dr. Robinson at this encounter. However, the notes clearly indicate that the fact that Justine is pregnant influenced the way the doctor needed to treat her. Therefore, the codes need to tell that part of the story. The code for the pregnancy must be included to accurately report this visit. The Alphabetic Index suggests:

Pregnancy incidental finding Z33.1

Let's go to the tabular list, and you will see:

Z33 Pregnant state

Keep reading to review the fourth-character choices. The most accurate is:

Z33.1 Pregnant state, incidental

This code explains the situation perfectly. Justine is pregnant, and that pregnancy was involved in the treatment of her shoulder injury, but it was not the principal reason she came to see Dr. Robinson. This code means that her pregnancy was incidental to the encounter. Perfect!

Of course, the claim form for the encounter between Justine and Dr. Robinson would also include three other codes—W20.8xxA, Other cause of strike by thrown, projected or falling object; Y93.E9, Activity, other interior property and clothing maintenance; and Y99.8, Other external cause status—because the injury was caused by a box falling on her while she was at her own home.

2. ICD-10-CM guidelines specifically direct you to exclude any diagnoses or conditions from a patient's history that have no impact on the current treatment or service.

LET'S CODE IT! SCENARIO

Kim Chen brought her son, Lee, to Dr. Killam, a pediatrician, because he was having a nosebleed that wouldn't stop. Lee is an otherwise healthy 3-year-old male with a history of allergic asthma. Dr. Killam examined his nasal passages and packed the nostrils. The doctor then discussed the situation with Kim and told her to bring Lee back the next day for a follow-up.

Let's Code It!

Lee came to see Dr. Killam because he had a *nosebleed*. Turn to the Alphabetic Index and look up the diagnosis.

Nosebleed R04.0

Surprised it was that easy? Well, sometimes it is. Check the code in the Tabular List, and you will see:

R04 Hemorrhage from respiratory passages

The nose is on the head, so you are in the correct category. Read the *excludes* notes and confirm that neither relates to this encounter. Neither do, so continue reading down the column to review your choices for the fourth-digit:

R04.0 Epistaxis
Hemorrhage from nose; nosebleed

Yes. I guess it was easy. Is that all you need to code? The notes state that Lee has a history of asthma. However, it has nothing to do with the reason Lee came to the doctor, and it did not affect the way Dr. Killam treated Lee. Therefore, you will not code it for this encounter because it had nothing to do with this visit.

3. Identify screening diagnosis codes when a screening test is performed with no signs, symptoms, or diagnosis of a condition. Many times, you can identify such instances because they are usually determined not by the patient's feelings or health but by the calendar.

EXAMPLE

Annual mammogram
Yearly physical
Well-baby visit

4. Remember, from Chapter 1, that in outpatient facilities you are not permitted to code diagnoses identified as *probable, suspected, rule out,* or *possible.* You may code only what you know for a fact: a confirmed diagnosis or signs and/or symptoms that form the basis for the encounter, additional testing, and/or procedures. That rule will also apply should tests be done and result in a normal, or negative, finding.

EXAMPLE

Kyana Parsons had pain in her abdomen. Dr. DeFacci did tests to rule out appendicitis. The tests were negative, and Dr. DeFacci diagnosed Kyana with abdominal pain RLQ (right lower quadrant). Report this with code R10.31, Abdominal pain, right lower quadrant.

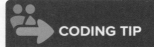

CODING TIP

When coding for a hospital (inpatient), you will be coding from discharge documents, so many of the answers will have already been found. In some hospitals, concurrent coding is done for patients who are in the facility for a long period of time. Chapter 22 of this textbook contains more detail on hospital (inpatient) coding.

GUIDANCE CONNECTION

Review the ICD-10-CM Coding Guidelines, Section 1.B, **General coding guidelines,** specifically subsection 7, **Multiple coding for a single condition.**

LO 3.6 Multiple and Additional Codes

If the patient has several conditions or concerns, the physician might possibly indicate more than one diagnosis. Sometimes, the doctor will list the diagnoses, making it easier for you to know which additional codes are needed.

How Many Codes Do You Need?

A professional coding specialist's job is to tell the *whole story* about the encounter between the health care provider and the patient. With diagnosis codes, we relate the whole story about WHY the physician provided the services, treatments, and procedures to the patient at this time. We must support *medical necessity* for all of these procedures.

Let's use a scenario as an example:

Kalem Wisceen, a 15-year-old male, came to see Dr. MacRhone because the side of his face and area around his ear was really hurting. He couldn't open his mouth. In addition, the area around his right eye was swollen and the conjunctiva in the eye was red. After examining him, Dr. MacRhone took a head x-ray which confirmed a closed fracture of the left mandible. Kalem admitted that he got into a fight at school with two other kids.

Dr. MacRhone wired Kalem's left jaw and ordered him NPO except liquids for the next 3 weeks. He also ordered cold, wet compresses for his eye, three times a day, and wrote a prescription for some eyedrops. Diagnosis was fracture of the left mandible, angle (closed), and black eye.

So, how many codes do you need?

You need as many codes as necessary to tell the *whole story* about WHY Kalem was cared for by Dr. MacRhone at this visit. Why did Dr. MacRhone examine Kalem, take the x-ray, and then wire his jaw shut? Because Kalem's jaw was fractured. The first code to use is S02.65xA to relate this part of the story.

S02.65xA Fracture of angle of mandible, initial encounter

That's one part of the story. Is there anything else to relate about this reason WHY Dr. MacRhone did all those services for Kalem? Ask yourself, *why* did Dr. MacRhone examine Kalem and order cold compresses and eyedrops for his eye? Because Kalem had a black eye. The second code to use is S00.11xA to relate more of the story.

S00.11xA Contusion of right eyelid and periocular area, initial encounter

Now, you also learned earlier that *when a patient is injured (or poisoned)*, you must also relate HOW and WHERE the injury occurred. This is used not only for statistical purposes but also to confirm which third-party payer will be responsible for paying the medical expenses. HOW and WHERE are reported with external cause codes. Ask yourself, how did Kalem's jaw get fractured and his eye injured? Code Y04.0xxA relates this part of the story.

Y04.0xxA Assault by unarmed brawl or fight, initial encounter

Where was Kalem when his jaw got fractured and his eye injured? Code Y92.213 explains this detail.

Y92.213 High school as the place of occurrence of the external cause

Y99.8 Other external cause status

Now you can see that, with these five codes, you and anyone reading these codes clearly can see that Dr. MacRhone cared for Kalem because he had a fractured jaw and a black eye and that the fractured jaw was the result of a fight at school. Without ALL FIVE codes, you don't have the *whole story.* So, for every case, every encounter, every scenario, you are responsible for telling *the WHOLE STORY about the encounter.*

Code Sequencing

When more than one diagnosis code is required to tell the whole story of the encounter accurately, you then must determine in which order the codes should be listed. The code reporting the most important reason for the encounter is called the **principal diagnosis.**

Sometimes the ICD-10-CM book will tell you which code should come first and which should come second with the *code first* and *use additional code* notations. Remember, an external cause code can never be the principal, or first-listed, diagnosis.

principal diagnosis
The condition that is the primary, or main, reason for the encounter.

EXAMPLE

Roman Fletcher was diagnosed with myocarditis due to *E. coli.* You will find notations directing you on how to sequence these two codes.

I41 Myocarditis in diseases classified elsewhere
   Code first underlying disease, such as: typhus (A75.0–A75.9)
I40.0 Infective myocarditis
   Use additional code (B95–B97) to identify infectious agent

In cases when there are multiple confirmed diagnoses identified, the guidelines instruct you to list the codes in order of severity from the most severe to the least severe. Take a look at the example below about Wade Padgett.

EXAMPLE

Wade Padgett came to see Dr. Stein after falling off his bicycle. After a thorough examination, Dr. Stein diagnosed Wade with a closed fracture of the fifth, left metacarpal shaft and an anterior dislocation of his left shoulder.

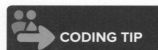

CODING TIP

Remember, an external cause code can never be the principal, or first-listed, diagnosis.

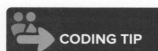

CODING TIP

If two (or more) diagnoses are of equal severity, then it will not matter in which order you list them.

For Wade's encounter, a fracture is more severe than a dislocation. Therefore, you would show the codes in the following order:

S62.357A Nondisplaced fracture of shaft of fifth metacarpal bone, left hand

M25.812 Other specified joint disorders, left shoulder

Acute and Chronic Conditions

If one patient has one health concern diagnosed by the physician as being both acute (severe) and chronic (ongoing) and the condition offers you separate codes for the two descriptors, you should report the code for the acute condition first, as directed by the guidelines. Remember, from your medical terminology lessons, acute is more serious than chronic.

YOU CODE IT! CASE STUDY

Varna Jackson has acute lymphoblastic leukemia and chronic lymphocytic leukemia of B-cell type, now in remission. She is seeing Dr. Roosevelt today for a checkup of this condition.

You Code It!

Can you determine the correct codes for Varna's visit with Dr. Roosevelt?

Step 1: Read the case completely.

Step 2: Abstract the notes: Which key words can you identify relating to why Dr. Roosevelt cared for Varna?

_____

Step 3: Query the provider, if necessary.

Step 4: Code the diagnosis or diagnoses.

_____

Step 5: Code the procedure(s): Office visit.

Step 6: Link the procedure codes to at least one diagnosis code to confirm medical necessity.

Step 7: Back code to double-check your choices.

Answer:

Did you determine the correct codes?

C91.01 Acute lymphoblastic leukemia, in remission

C91.11 Chronic lymphocytic leukemia of B-cell type in remission

Great job!

Two or More Conditions—Only One Confirmed Diagnosis

There may be cases where the physician documents treatment of two (or more) complaints and only one is identified by a confirmed diagnosis.

LET'S CODE IT! SCENARIO

Louise Jorgensen, a 61-year-old female, came to see Dr. Mulkey. Earlier in the day, she was lightheaded and a little dizzy. In addition, she complained that her heart was beating so wildly that she thought she may have had a heart attack. Due to her previous diagnosis of type 1 diabetes, Dr. Mulkey ordered a blood glucose test. He also performed an EKG to check her heart. After getting the results of the tests, Dr. Mulkey determined that Louise's lightheadedness and dizziness were a result of her glucose being too high. He spoke with Louise about how to bring her diabetes under control. He also told her that her EKG was negative and that there were no signs of a heart attack.

Let's Code It!

Dr. Mulkey confirmed that Louise's *type 1 diabetes mellitus* was *uncontrolled*. (This is indicated by his discussion with her on how to bring it under control.) Turn to the Alphabetic Index and find:

Diabetes

Turn to the Tabular List and see:

E10 Type 1 diabetes mellitus

   E10.9 Type 1 diabetes mellitus without complications

Uncontrolled type 1 diabetes mellitus seems to be the only confirmed diagnosis in Dr. Mulkey's notes. However, the doctor performed an EKG. A diagnosis for diabetes does not provide any medical rationale for doing an EKG. In addition, the test was negative and, therefore, provided no diagnosis. So you still need a diagnosis code to report the medical necessity for running the EKG. Why did Dr. Mulkey perform the EKG? Because Louise complained of a *rapid heartbeat*. The Alphabetic Index suggests:

Rapid, heart (beat) R00.0

The Tabular List confirms

R00 Abnormalities of heart beat

   R00.0 Tachycardia, unspecified

For the encounter, you have one confirmed diagnosis (the diabetes) and one symptom (rapid heartbeat). The guidelines state that a confirmed diagnosis should precede a sign or symptom, so you will list the diabetes code first and then the tachycardia.

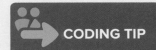

CODING TIP

Louise Jorgensen's case illustrates that sometimes asking yourself "*Why* did the physician provide a specific test, treatment, or service" can help you find the necessary diagnostic key words for an encounter.

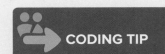

CODING TIP

An electrocardiogram may be referred to as either an ECG or an EKG. *Tachycardia* is the medical term for rapid heartbeat.

Differential Diagnoses

In the case where a provider indicates a differential diagnosis by using the word *versus* or *or* between two diagnostic statements, you need to code both as if they were confirmed, and either may be listed first.

YOU CODE IT! CASE STUDY

Colin Oliver, a 63-year-old male complaining of chest pain and shortness of breath, was seen by his family physician. Dr. Budman admitted him into the hospital with a differential diagnosis of congestive heart failure versus pleural effusion with respiratory distress.

You Code It!

Review the notes of the encounter between Dr. Budman and Colin Oliver, and determine the applicable diagnosis code(s).

Step 1: Read the case completely.

Step 2: Abstract the notes: Which key words can you identify relating to why Dr. Budman cared for Colin?

_____

Step 3: Query the provider, if necessary.

Step 4: Code the diagnosis or diagnoses.

_____

Step 5: Code the procedure(s): Admission to hospital for observation.

Step 6: Link the procedure codes to at least one diagnosis code to confirm medical necessity.

Step 7: Back code to double-check your choices.

Answer:

Did you determine the correct code?

I50.9 Congestive heart failure, NOS

J90 Pleural effusion, NOS

R06.00 Dyspnea, unspecified

Other Current Conditions

Another important issue that needs to be coded is a current condition that might be subtly addressed by the physician. It might be the writing of a prescription refill or a short discussion on the state of the patient's well-being as the result of ongoing therapy for a matter other than that which brought the patient to see the physician today.

YOU CODE IT! CASE STUDY

Leon Wilcox, a 47-year-old male, came to see Dr. Thackery for a follow-up on a previous diagnosis of paroxysmal atrial fibrillation. Dr. Thackery examined Leon and did a blood test to monitor the effectiveness of the prescription medication Coumadin, a blood thinner. Dr. Thackery told Leon he was very pleased with his progress and that he was doing well. Before he left, Leon asked Dr. Thackery for a refill of trinalin, his allergy medication. This time of year typically provoked his allergy to pollen, which caused a lot of inflammation and irritation in his nose (rhinitis). Dr. Thackery wrote the refill prescription.

You Code It!

Read Dr. Thackery's notes regarding this encounter with Leon, and determine the correct diagnostic code or codes.

Step 1: Read the case completely.

Step 2: Abstract the notes: Which key words can you identify relating to why Dr. Thackery cared for Leon?

_____

Step 3: Query the provider, if necessary.

Step 4: Code the diagnosis or diagnoses.

_____

Step 5: Code the procedure(s): Office visit and exam, blood test.

Step 6: Link the procedure codes to at least one diagnosis code to confirm medical necessity.

Step 7: Back code to double-check your choices.

Answer:

Did you determine the correct code?

I48.0 Paroxysmal atrial fibrillation

J30.1 Allergic rhinitis, due to pollen (hayfever)

Z79.01 Long-term (current) use of anticoagulants

The code for the atrial fibrillation supports the office visit and exam, the code for long-term use of the Coumadin (an anticoagulant) justifies the blood test, and the code for the allergic rhinitis supports the medical necessity for the trinalin prescription.

Test Results

Even though you didn't go to medical school, you still know the difference between a positive test result and a negative test result. However, you are not permitted to affirm a diagnosis from a test result without the physician's documentation. This refers to laboratory tests, x-rays and other imaging, pathology, and any other diagnostic testing done for a patient. In such cases, especially when the health care professional has ordered additional tests based on an abnormal finding, you should query, or ask, the physician whether or not you should document the results. Be certain to get your answer in writing in the patient's record. If it's not in writing, you can't code it!

In outpatient settings, if a physician, or other health care professional, interpreted the test results and the final report has been placed in the patient's file with a diagnostic statement, you should include the code.

Laboratory report in patient's file shows:

Glucose   155   Norm Range: 65–105 mg/dL

You can see that the patient's glucose is abnormally high. However, you cannot code it without a physician's written interpretation and diagnostic statement.

Report from radiology states: "X-ray shows an open fracture of the anatomical neck of the humerus, right arm. Signed: Frederick L. McCoy, MD, Chief of Radiology."

The report, signed by a physician, includes a specific diagnostic statement that should be coded. However, you should always check with the attending physician and permit him or her the opportunity to update the patient's chart with the confirmed diagnosis. It is a sign of respect.

Preoperative Evaluations

Whenever a patient is scheduled for a surgical procedure (on a non-emergency basis), there are typical tests that must be done to ensure that the patient is healthy enough to have the operation. Cardiovascular, respiratory, and other examinations are often done within a couple of days prior to the date of surgery. Often these tests do not necessarily relate directly to the diagnostic reason the surgery will be performed. Therefore, they will need a different diagnosis code to report medical necessity.

Coding those encounters carries a specific guideline. In such cases, the principal, or first-listed, diagnosis code will be from the following category:

Z01.8 Encounter for other specified special examinations

Follow that code with the code or codes that identify the condition(s) documented as the reason for the upcoming surgical procedure.

Tameka was diagnosed with carpal tunnel syndrome in her right wrist. Dr. Rothenstein recommended a surgical solution. Because of her history of atrial fibrillation, Tameka was required to get approval from her cardiologist before she could have the procedure.

G56.01, Carpal tunnel syndrome, right upper limb, is the code that will be used to report the medical necessity for the surgery on Tameka's wrist. However, it will not support the examination performed by her cardiologist. Think about it . . . who would agree to pay for a cardiologist to examine a patient with a diagnosis of carpal tunnel syndrome? The cardiologist is not qualified to do the job that is better suited for an orthopedist.

Z01.810, Encounter for preprocedural cardiovascular examination, will support the cardiologist's time and expertise to clear Tameka for the procedure on her wrist.

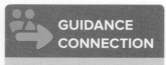

GUIDANCE CONNECTION

Review the ICD-10-CM Coding Guidelines, Section II, **Selection of Principal Diagnosis,** and Section III, **Reporting Additional Diagnoses.**

Preoperative/Postoperative Diagnoses

You may have already noticed that procedure and operative reporting usually include both a preoperative diagnosis and a postoperative diagnosis. For cases where the two statements differ, the guidelines state that you should code the postoperative diagnosis because it is expected that it is the more accurate of the two.

Chapter Summary

ICD-10-CM is formatted to guide you toward the best, most accurate code. Notations, symbols, and punctuation help you, the coder, follow guidelines and ensure that codes are complete in their descriptions of why the health care provider cared for the patient during this encounter. Three- to seven-character codes are offered so the coder can use the highest level of specificity to report the medically necessary rationale for the procedures, services, and treatments provided.

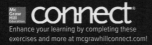

Using Terminology

Match each key term to the appropriate definition.

_____ **1.** LO 3.4 Descriptors whose inclusion in the physician's notes is not absolutely necessary and that are provided simply to further clarify a code description; optional terms.

_____ **2.** LO 3.3 Specifics that are not described in any other code in the ICD-10-CM book; also known as *not elsewhere classified.*

_____ **3.** LO 3.4 Long duration; continuing over a long period of time.

_____ **4.** LO 3.3 A condition caused or developed from the existence of another condition.

_____ **5.** LO 3.3 One disease that affects or encourages another condition.

_____ **6.** LO 3.3 The absence of additional specifics in the physician's documentation.

_____ **7.** LO 3.3 Additional information the physician specified that isn't included in any other code description.

_____ **8.** LO 3.6 The condition that is the primary, or main, reason for the encounter.

_____ **9.** LO 3.3 The absence of additional details documented in the notes.

_____ **10.** LO 3.4 Severe; serious.

A. Acute

B. Chronic

C. Manifestation

D. Nonessential modifiers

E. Not elsewhere classifiable (NEC)

F. Not otherwise specified (NOS)

G. Other specified

H. Principal diagnosis

I. Underlying condition

J. Unspecified

Checking Your Understanding

Choose the most appropriate answer for each of the following questions.

1. LO 3.1 When all are available, the code with the most specificity is the one with

   a. three characters.
   b. four characters.
   c. five characters.
   d. six characters.

2. LO 3.1/3.3 NOS means

   a. the hospital didn't provide more details.
   b. the physician didn't provide more details.
   c. the ICD-10-CM didn't provide a code with more details.
   d. the patient didn't provide more details.

3. LO 3.2 When a fourth, fifth, sixth or seventh character is required and there are no previous characters ICD-10-CM uses a placeholder character the letter _____.

   a. X.
   b. G.
   c. Z.
   d. B.

4. LO 3.4 A descriptor presented within parentheses is

   a. a mandatory part of the code description.
   b. an optional part of the code description.
   c. a previously deleted code description.
   d. a manifestation.

5. LO 3.3 NEC means

   a. the hospital didn't provide more details.
   b. the physician didn't provide more details.
   c. the ICD-10-CM didn't provide a code with more details.
   d. the patient didn't provide more details.

6. LO 3.3 An underlying condition

   a. encourages another condition.
   b. causes another condition.
   c. is the result of another condition.
   d. is a late effect of another condition.

7. LO 3.4 A nonessential modifier is a word or phrase that does all *except*

   a. further describe the condition.
   b. invalidate the code.
   c. provide alternate phrasing or terms.
   d. provide an optional description.

8. LO 3.4 When one code describes two concurrent conditions, it is known as

   a. preventive code.
   b. history code.
   c. combination code.
   d. procedure code.

9. LO 3.5 Diagnosis codes are important because they

   a. describe why the provider treated the patient.
   b. identify medical necessity for procedures and services.
   c. both describe why the provider treated the patient and identify medical necessity for procedures and services.
   d. none of these.

10. LO 3.1 When ICD-10-CM identifies that an additional character is available for a particular code,

    a. the additional character is required.
    b. the additional character is optional.
    c. the code with the smaller number of characters is invalid.
    d. the additional character is required, and the code with the smaller number of characters is invalid.

Applying Your Knowledge

1. LO 3.4 What is a nonessential modifier? _____

_____

2. LO 3.4 Explain the difference between acute and chronic. _____

_____

3. LO 3.2 What is the placeholder character, and why is it needed in ICD-10-CM? _____

_____

4. LO 3.3 Explain a *code first* notation. _____

_____

5. LO 3.3 How are you to interpret the word *and* in regard to ICD-10-CM? _____

_____

6. LO 3.3 What does the *use additional code* notation tell you? _____

_____

7. LO 3.3 What does *unspecified* mean? _____

_____

8. LO 3.4 How are slanted brackets *[ ]* used in ICD-10-CM? _____

_____

Using the techniques described in this chapter, carefully read through the case studies and determine the most accurate ICD-10-CM code(s) and external cause code(s), if appropriate, for each case.

1. Helen Whitworth, an 18-year-old female, came to see Dr. Hunter after falling off a ladder at home and twisting her left ankle. Dr. Hunter confirmed that her ankle was sprained and wrapped it with an Ace bandage.

   _____

2. Gary Beatty went to see Dr. Meredith with a complaint of shortness of breath and chest pain. Dr. Meredith diagnosed him with congestive heart failure.

   _____

3. Patrick Glass, a 59-year-old male, was seen by Dr. Grayson because Patrick was very upset and agitated. After a complete psychological evaluation, Dr. Grayson diagnosed Patrick with severe major depressive disorder with psychotic features.

   _____

4. Beatrice Hayward, a 29-year-old female, is a professional water skier and comes to see Dr. Maudi with a recurrent dislocation of her right shoulder.

   _____

5. Rudy Shaw, a 63-year-old male, comes to see Dr. Witsil for the results of his cervical lymph node biopsy. Dr. Witsil informs Rudy that the test confirmed Hodgkin's sarcoma disease.

   _____

6. Dennis Curran, a 35-year-old male, attended a beach party and barbecue where he had hot dogs and potato salad. Several hours later, he began vomiting and having severe diarrhea. The next morning, he went to see Dr. Haberstock, who diagnosed him with dehydration caused by *Salmonella* infection.

   _____

7. Charlene Goodwin, a 73-year-old female, is diagnosed with left arm paralysis (her dominant side), a late effect of poliomyelitis, which she had when she was a child.

   _____

8. Cecil Williams, a 7-year-old male, came in to see Dr. Beasley for a therapeutic bronchoscopy due to the doctor's diagnosis of cystic fibrosis.

   _____

9. Norman Siegel, a 3-year-old male, was brought into the clinic and seen by Dr. Norris. After a complete examination, Dr. Norris diagnosed Norman with severe malnutrition.

_____

10. Gayle Sentine, a 9-year-old female, is brought in to Dr. Matlock because she is having trouble in school. Dr. Matlock, after a thorough examination and testing, diagnoses her with attention deficit disorder with hyperactivity.

_____

11. Carlos Siplin, an 81-year-old male, was unable to speak. Dr. Permane performed a laryngoscopy and determined a diagnosis of complete bilateral paralysis of Carlos's vocal cords.

_____

12. Craig Liefer, a 49-year-old male, was diagnosed with Lou Gehrig's disease and came to the testing center for an EMG series.

_____

13. After having a grand mal seizure, Louise Garrett, a 39-year-old female, was taken to the emergency room by her husband, and Dr. Sherman diagnosed her with intractable epilepsy with status epilepticus.

_____

14. Eliot Cox, a 4-year-old male, was brought to his pediatrician, Dr. Germain, because of a cough and fever. After a complete examination, Dr. Germain confirmed Eliot had an upper respiratory infection with bilateral acute conjunctivitis.

_____

15. Roger Simpkin, a 43-year-old male, was diagnosed with an enlarged prostate without LUTS and came into the ambulatory surgery center (ASC) to have a prostatectomy performed.

_____

YOU CODE IT! Application

Chapter 3: General Guidelines and Notations

The following exercises provide practice in abstracting physicians' notes and learning to work with SOAP notes from our health care facility, *Taylor, Reader, & Associates*. These case studies (SOAP notes) are modeled on real patient encounters. Using the techniques described in this chapter, carefully read through the case studies and determine the most accurate ICD-10-CM code(s) for each case study.

TAYLOR, READER, & ASSOCIATES
A Complete Health Care Facility
975 CENTRAL AVENUE • SOMEWHERE, FL 32811 • 407-555-4321

PATIENT: FALLON, WILLA
ACCOUNT/EHR #:   FALLWI001
DATE: 07/16/18

Attending Physician: Suzanne R. Taylor, MD

S: This Pt is a 26-year-old female who I have not seen since last September when she came in for her annual physical. She presents today with burning upon urination, pink urine, and lower back pain. She stated that the symptoms began 2–3 days ago. She had been on vacation in Mexico and arrived back home yesterday.

O: Ht 5′ 7″ Wt. 169 lb. R 19. HEENT: unremarkable. Abdomen is tender. I ordered an automated urinalysis with microscopy, which was analyzed in our laboratory on the second floor. After the UA showed the presence of erythrocytes and leukocytes in the urine, I ordered a culture and sensitivity test, which was positive for *E. coli.*

A: Cystitis cystica due to *E. coli*

P: 1. Rx. Broad-spectrum antibiotics
     2. Return prn

Suzanne R. Taylor, MD

SRT/pw   D: 7/16/18 09:50:16   T: 7/18/18 12:55:01

Determine the most accurate ICD-10-CM code(s)

_____

_____

_____

TAYLOR, READER, & ASSOCIATES
A Complete Health Care Facility
975 CENTRAL AVENUE • SOMEWHERE, FL 32811 • 407-555-4321

PATIENT: MARSHALL, BARRY
ACCOUNT/EHR #:   MARSBA001
DATE: 11/09/18

Attending Physician: Willard B. Reader, MD

S: Pt is a 51-year-old male who comes in concerned about a sore he noticed on his left temple, directly at the hairline. He states that his mother died 6 years ago from melanoma, and his brother was diagnosed with precancerous cells of the epidermis. Pt states he is the captain of a beach volleyball team and volunteers at the local YMCA as a water aerobics instructor. He says that he tries to be diligent about sunscreen, but sometimes he forgets.

O: Ht 5′ 11″ Wt. 189 lb. R 20. T 98.6. BP 120/95 Cultures of lesion were taken and sent to our in-house lab. The pathology report confirms the lesion is malignant. I discussed options with the patient and recommended surgical removal of the lesion as soon as possible.

A: Malignant melanoma of skin of scalp

P: Pt to call to make appointment for surgical procedure.

_____

Willard B. Reader, MD

WBR/pw   D: 11/09/18 09:50:16   T: 11/13/18 12:55:01

Determine the most accurate ICD-10-CM code(s).

_____

_____

_____

TAYLOR, READER, & ASSOCIATES
A Complete Health Care Facility
975 CENTRAL AVENUE • SOMEWHERE, FL 32811 • 407-555-4321

PATIENT: GARISON, BENJAMIN
ACCOUNT/EHR #:   GARIBE001
DATE: 09/16/18

Attending Physician: Suzanne R. Taylor, MD

S: This Pt is a 5-month-old male brought in by his father because of severe rash on Benjamin's buttocks.

O: Ht 35″ Wt. 19 lb. T 98.6 Pt appears in minor distress; however, examination shows nothing out of the ordinary.

A: Diaper rash

P: 1. Rx A&D ointment to be applied after each diaper change
       2. Return prn

_____

Suzanne R. Taylor, MD

SRT/pw   D: 9/16/18 09:50:16   T: 9/18/18 12:55:01

Determine the most accurate ICD-10-CM code(s).

_____

_____

_____

TAYLOR, READER, & ASSOCIATES
A Complete Health Care Facility
975 CENTRAL AVENUE • SOMEWHERE, FL 32811 • 407-555-4321

PATIENT: BENTON, EARL
ACCOUNT/EHR #:   BENTEA001
DATE: 12/01/18

Attending Physician: Willard B. Reader, MD

S: Pt is a 44-year-old male who comes in with severe pain in the lower right quadrant of his abdomen. He states that the pain is sharp and shoots across his belly from right to left. Patient also states that he has been somewhat nauseated over the last 2 days.

O: Ht 5′ 9″ Wt. 177 lb. R 21. T 101.6. BP 130/95 Abdomen appears to be tender upon manual examination. Comprehensive metabolic blood test, general health panel blood workup, and an MRA, abdomen, angiography are taken. Results of all tests confirm diagnosis of appendicitis.

A: Acute appendicitis, w/o peritonitis

P: Pt to go to hospital immediately to be admitted for appendectomy

_____

Willard B. Reader, MD

WBR/pw   D: 12/01/18 09:50:16   T: 12/01/18 12:55:01

Determine the most accurate ICD-10-CM code(s).

_____

_____

_____

TAYLOR, READER, & ASSOCIATES
A Complete Health Care Facility
975 CENTRAL AVENUE • SOMEWHERE, FL 32811 • 407-555-4321

PATIENT: TESKE, KENDRA
ACCOUNT/EHR #:   TESKKE001
DATE: 09/25/18

Attending Physician: Willard B. Reader, MD

S: Pt is a 41-year-old female who presents today with complaints of malaise and fatigue. She states that she has lost weight without any change in her eating habits, and has had a fever recently. Her joints have been achy and sometimes painful, and she has suffered with a rash across her cheeks and nose.

O: Ht 5′ 7″ Wt. 181 lb. R 21. T 99.2. BP 125/85 Pt has butterfly rash over nose and cheeks. CBC with differential, platelet count, erythrocyte sedimentation rate, and serum electrophoresis. Antinuclear antibody, anti-DNA, and lupus erythematosus cell tests are all performed. Anti-DNA test is positive for SLE.

A: Systemic lupus erythematosus

P: 1. Rx 325 aspirin prn
     2. Rx flurandrenolide cream for topical treatment of skin lesions
     3. Rx prednisone, 60 mg, tapering dosage

Willard B. Reader, MD

WBR/pw   D: 09/25/18 09:50:16   T: 09/28/18 12:55:01

Determine the most accurate ICD-10-CM code(s).

_____

_____

_____

4 CODING INFECTIOUS DISEASES

Learning Objectives
After completing this chapter, the student should be able to:

LO 4.1 Explain the differences between bacterial, viral, and parasitic.

LO 4.2 Discuss the impact of communicable diseases.

LO 4.3 Identify the concerns related to reporting HIV infections.

LO 4.4 Distinguish between septicemia and SIRS.

LO 4.5 Interpret correctly documentation about MRSA.

LO 4.6 Code common other infectious and communicable conditions.

Key Terms

Acute
Asymptomatic
Bacteria
Chronic
Endemic
Epidemic
Fungi
Human immunodeficiency virus (HIV)
Infection
Infectious
Inflammation
Nosocomial
Pandemic
Parasites
Pathogen
Sepsis
Septic shock
Septicemia
Severe sepsis
Systemic
Systemic inflammatory response syndrome (SIRS)
Tuberculosis
Viruses

Many conditions and illnesses can be disseminated from one individual to another. **Infectious** diseases are spread by personal contact, such as a handshake or the exchange of bodily fluids; other diseases can be spread by the touch of a doorknob that has been handled by someone else. This chapter will discuss the essential factors of disease, as well as how diseases spread.

You have heard about some of these conditions, such as meningitis, hepatitis, **tuberculosis,** and **human immunodeficiency virus (HIV).**

As a coding specialist, your vulnerability to infectious diseases and conditions while on the job is limited. However, you should realize that protecting your health is the basis for certain safety protocols, such as wearing gloves and using special waste receptacles. As long as you follow important safety policies, there is no reason to be afraid.

LO 4.1 Pathogens

There are wars going on, constantly, throughout your body as **pathogens** (vehicles of disease) insert themselves into your cells and multiply. There are many types of pathogens, and each carries its own threat to your health. The most common are discussed below.

Bacteria

If you have watched enough yogurt commercials on television, you already know about good **bacteria** and bad bacteria. The good bacteria are situated in the walls of your small and large intestines and participate in the digestive process.

Bacteria are single-celled organisms named by their shape (see Figure 4-1). Rod-shaped bacteria, called *bacilli,* are responsible for the development of diphtheria, tetanus, and tuberculosis, among others. *Spirilla,* bacterial organisms shaped like a spiral, may cause cholera or syphilis,

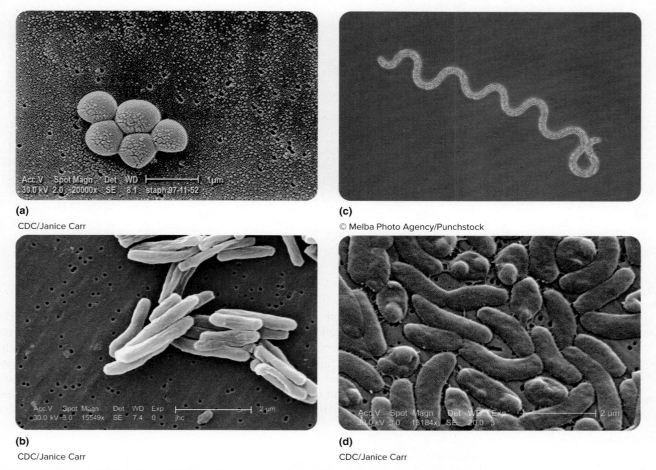

(a)
CDC/Janice Carr

(c)
© Melba Photo Agency/Punchstock

(b)
CDC/Janice Carr

(d)
CDC/Janice Carr

FIGURE 4-1 Types of Bacteria: (a) coccus, (b) bacillus, (c) spirillum, and (d) vibrio

while dot-shaped bacteria known as *cocci* cause gonorrhea, tonsillitis, scarlet fever, and bacterial meningitis.

EXAMPLE

A05.4 Foodborne <u>Bacillus</u> cereus intoxication

A27.9 Lepto<u>spiro</u>sis, unspecified

A49.1 Strepto<u>coccal</u> infection, unspecified site

Viruses

Viruses are tiny microorganisms that are not easily treated with medication because they embed themselves within the host cells and are, therefore, difficult to isolate (see Figure 4-2). These invaders can remain dormant (latent) for long periods of time. Examples include varicella (chickenpox), hepatitis, and viral pneumonia, as well as the common cold.

EXAMPLE

A85.0 Enteroviral encephalitis

B18.0 Chronic viral hepatitis B with delta-agent

B33.21 Viral endocarditis

infectious
A condition that can be transmitted from one person to another.

tuberculosis
An infectious condition that causes small rounded swellings on mucous membranes throughout the body.

human immunodeficiency virus (HIV)
A condition affecting the immune system.

pathogen
Any agent that causes disease; a microorganism such as a bacterium or virus.

bacteria
Single-celled microorganisms that cause disease.

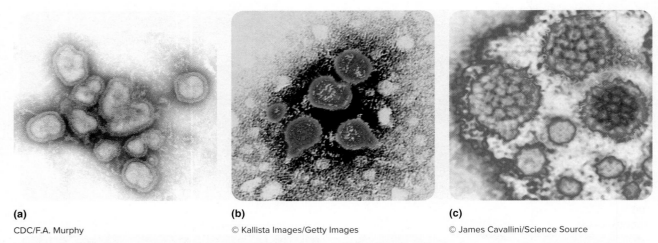

(a)
CDC/F.A. Murphy

(b)
© Kallista Images/Getty Images

(c)
© James Cavallini/Science Source

FIGURE 4-2 Types of Viruses: (a) influenza, (b) hepatitis, and (c) warts

virus
A microscopic particle that initiates disease, mimicking the characteristics of a particular cell; can reproduce only within the body of the cell which it has invaded.

parasites
Tiny living things that can invade and feed off other living things.

Parasites

Parasites are tiny living things that can invade and feed off other living things—like humans. They are one-celled organisms (protozoa), insects (lice and mites), worms (*Helminthiasis*), and others (see Figure 4-3) that can interfere with a healthy body. Tapeworms, hookworms, and pinworms are internal parasites. Parasites can be transmitted in food (e.g., protozoa like *Giardia intestinalis* and *Cyclospora cayetanensis*); spread by mosquitoes and other insects through the bloodstream (as in malaria and leishmaniasis); or ingested in contaminated water (as in amebiasis and schistosomiasis).

EXAMPLE

B86 Scabies (mites)
B71.9 Tapeworm (infection) NOS
B89 Parasitic infestation of the eyelid

fungi
Group of organisms, including mold, yeast, and mildew, that cause infection; fungus (singular).

Fungi

There are many versions of **fungi** (the plural form of *fungus*) in our lives. Mushrooms on your pizza or in your salad and yeast in your bread or beer are tasty. Mold, a form of fungus, can be delicious when it is called blue cheese or feta cheese, and it can be helpful when developed in a pill containing penicillin. Then there are fungi that cause illness, such as *aspergillus,* which may cause lower respiratory tract dysfunction, or *Candida albicans,* which causes infection in the oral mucosa and the walls of the vagina. *Onychomycosis* is the most common nail fungal infection.

EXAMPLE

P37.5 Neonatal candidiasis
B44.81 Allergic bronchopulmonary aspergillosis
B40.3 Cutaneous blastomycosis

infection
The invasion of pathogens into tissue cells.

systemic
Spread throughout the entire body.

Infection and Inflammation

Once a pathogen successfully invades the body and begins to replicate, this is known as an **infection.** This multiplication of the organism, known as *colonization,* causes damage to cell structures and can remain localized in one area (such as an infected toe), spread to a larger area (such as infection of the foot and leg), or become **systemic**

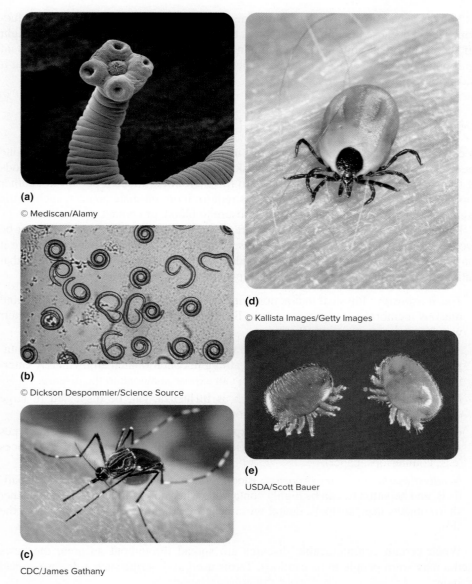

(a)

© Mediscan/Alamy

(b)

© Dickson Despommier/Science Source

(c)

CDC/James Gathany

(d)

© Kallista Images/Getty Images

(e)

USDA/Scott Bauer

FIGURE 4-3 Parasitic worms: (a) tapeworms and (b) *Trichinella.* Parasitic insects: (c) mosquitoes, (d) deer ticks, and (e) mites.

(spreading throughout the entire body). The body is designed to alert you, and your doctor, to the existence of infection by exhibiting specific signs and symptoms:

- Increased body temperature (commonly known as a *fever*)
- Increased white blood cell count
- Increase or decrease in heart rate (tachycardia or bradycardia)
- Increase or decrease in respiratory rate (hyperventilation or dyspnea)

In some cases, you might not be aware that there is an infection in your body. This is known as a *subclinical* or *asymptomatic* infection. In other cases, the condition can become **acute** (severe) and a specific area may show signs of **inflammation.** This can be visible when the inflammation is located in the epidermis; then it causes symptoms such as erythema (reddening), swelling, warmth to the touch, and often pain. When located internally, the inflammation can cause lack of function, especially when found within a joint.

When inflammation is left untreated, or if treatment is ineffective, the condition can become **chronic** (ongoing).

acute
Severe.

inflammation
The reaction of tissues to infection or injury; characterized by pain, swelling, and erythema.

chronic
Long-lasting; ongoing.

You may be aware that young children and the elderly are most susceptible to infection. This is because the immune system is the body's defense, the army that will fight off these pathogenic invaders. The immune system does not complete development until puberty, and by age 70, its effectiveness has diminished to about 25% of what it was prior to puberty.

LO 4.2 Communicable Disease

A cough or a sneeze may send pathogens into the air, and a doorknob or a telephone receiver easily transfers pathogens to the skin that touches it next—these are methods of transportation for bacteria or viruses to travel from an infected person to another soon-to-be-infected person. Some diseases require more intimate contact, such as the exchange of bodily fluids (during sex, exposure to blood, or contact with mucus).

People interact in society, and, therefore, the transmission of pathogens cannot be avoided. The level of interaction and the severity of the pathogen (how aggressive it may be) will impact how many individuals are infected. There are many ways that patients and health care workers can be exposed to an infection and become ill.

- *Touch exposure:* Physical interaction with blood, bodily fluids, nonintact skin, and mucous membranes can enable a long list of bloodborne pathogens to make their way from one person to another.
- *Airborne exposure:* Some pathogens travel in small particles that remain contagious in the air, such as chickenpox. Breathing in contaminated air by merely entering an examination room or patient area can expose someone to the disease.
- *Droplet exposure:* Some diseases, such as influenza, can be dispersed in large droplets, such as those transmitted by coughing, spitting, talking, and sneezing.
- *Contact exposure:* As with touch exposure, some infections, such as herpes simplex virus, are communicated by skin-to-skin contact or skin to other surfaces (e.g., countertops, paper).
- *Needlestick/sharps injury exposure:* Bloodborne pathogens, including HIV, hepatitis B, and hepatitis C, can be highly contagious when contaminated needles or other sharp objects (e.g., scalpels, dental wire) penetrate the protective outer layer of the skin.

When certain communicable diseases are spread throughout an area, the news media may warn people to be cautious. Terms used to describe such a disease spread include:

- **Epidemic:** The pathogen spreads quickly and easily, infecting even those with healthy immune systems.
- **Endemic:** The spread of the pathogen is contained within a small area. This may be a school with an outbreak of meningitis or a small geographic area such as a neighborhood.
- **Pandemic:** The pathogen has infected a large geographic area, possibly involving populations in multiple countries.

Health care–acquired infections (HAI), also known as **nosocomial** infections, are those conditions that are contracted solely due to interactions with a health care facility, during which exposure to various types of pathogens occurs. Take note that HAIs are infections that occur in hospitals, outpatient clinics, nursing homes, and other health care provider locations. This is not just the concern of inpatient acute care facilities. Of course, the entire concept of health care–acquired infection is contradictory to the reasons health care professionals and facilities exist. Health care is the business of keeping patients healthy and working to make them healthy when they are ill. From physicians' offices to acute care hospitals to nursing homes, everyone must take the steps necessary to ensure the provision of care does not actually cause harm.

epidemic
The pathogen spreads quickly and easily.

endemic
The spread of the pathogen is contained within a small area.

pandemic
The pathogen has infected a large geographic area.

nosocomial
A hospital-acquired condition; a condition that develops as a result of being in a health care facility.

LO 4.3 Human Immunodeficiency Virus Infections

Human immunodeficiency virus (HIV) infection not only is a serious illness but also carries with it a huge societal stigma. Therefore, whether you are coding for an inpatient facility (an exception to the guideline discussed earlier) or an outpatient facility, you will code that condition *only* when it has been *clearly specified in the physician's notes* that the patient is HIV-positive.

Testing for Human Immunodeficiency Virus

Anyone possibly exposed to HIV should be tested. Similar to so many other conditions, like malignancies, the earlier a diagnosis is made, the sooner treatment can begin. Early treatment translates into a longer, better-quality life for the patient.

Of course, when an individual with no symptoms comes to a health care facility to be tested for a condition, you will need a diagnosis code to provide medical necessity for the test. As with other preventive health care encounters, you will use a Z code. For the first office visit, to discuss possible exposure to HIV, you will use code:

> **Z20.6 Contact with and (suspected) exposure to human immunodeficiency virus [HIV]**

For the diagnosis code used to support the actual test, generally, you will use code:

> **Z11.4 Encounter for screening for human immunodeficiency virus [HIV]**

However, if the patient is documented by the physician as a member of a known high-risk group, you may use:

> **Z72.5- High-risk sexual behavior**
>
> **Z72.8- Other problems related to lifestyle**

Remember, until there is a specific diagnostic statement in the physician's notes, you are not to report anything connected to HIV. If the patient is tested because of specific signs and/or symptoms, you will code those signs and symptoms, rather than any of the above.

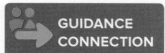

GUIDANCE CONNECTION

Review the ICD-10-CM Coding Guidelines, Section I.C.1, Chapter 1: **Certain Infectious and parasitic diseases,** Subsections a, **Human immunodeficiency virus (HIV) infections,** and a(2)(h), **Encounters for testing for HIV.**

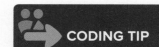

CODING TIP

In some states, information in the patient's record relating to HIV testing (positive or negative result), HIV AIDS status, sexually transmitted diseases, genetic information (such as the results of any genetic testing), mental health conditions, and substance abuse is categorized as *superconfidential* information. This information has additional legal protection, above the requirements of HIPAA, with regard to disclosure and use. Be certain to find out if your state has this additional protection for patients as well as the requirements for compliance.

LET'S CODE IT! SCENARIO

Kenneth Armstrong got drunk and had unprotected intercourse last night. He comes to Dr. Frank's office to discuss his concerns about possible exposure to HIV.

Let's Code It!

Kenneth went to see Dr. Frank because he was concerned that he had been *exposed to HIV.* Let's turn to the Alphabetic Index and look up *exposure:*

> **Exposure to HIV Z20.6**

Confirm the complete code description in the Tabular List; start reading at the top of the chapter subsection titled:

> **Persons with potential health hazards related to communicable diseases (Z20-Z28)**

Be certain to read the *Excludes1* and *Excludes2* notes. While these excluded diagnoses do not relate to our current case of Kenneth's visit to Dr. Frank, this is a critical habit that you need to build—to always read up and down and around the code that was suggested by the Alphabetic Index. This time, the notes do not apply, but next time, they might. Continue reading down the column.

Z20 Contact with or (suspected) exposure to communicable diseases

This fits the documentation which notes that Kenneth is concerned that he has been "exposed." Keep reading down the column to find that required fourth digit. You will realize that HIV is not specifically mentioned. Instead, it is included in the code:

Z20.6 Contact with and (suspected) exposure to human immunodeficiency virus [HIV]

Directly beneath this code is another *Excludes1* notation:

Asymptomatic human immunodeficiency virus [HIV] infection status (Z21)

This reminds you that contact or exposure is not the same as a positive status asymptomatic HIV diagnosis.

Test Negative

There are rapid HIV tests that use oral swabs or finger sticks and can provide results in minutes. Other HIV tests may take several days to provide an answer. Therefore, a return visit to the health care provider will sometimes be required.

The entire experience of being tested and then having to wait for the results can be psychologically difficult, even when the news is good. In addition, it is the health care professional's responsibility to counsel the patient on how to prevent being at risk in the future. Therefore, when an individual returns to get the results of an HIV test and the results are negative, counseling should be provided. For that reason, when documented, use:

Z71.7 Human immunodeficiency virus [HIV] counseling

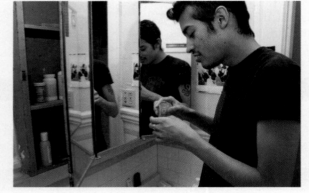

© McGraw-Hill Education/Christopher Kerrigan, photographer

Test Inconclusive

It can happen that the serology (pathology testing) comes back inconclusive for HIV. There can be no specific diagnosis for HIV or any direct manifestations of the illness, because there is nothing to confirm or deny HIV-positive status. In such cases, you have to use code:

R75 Inconclusive laboratory evidence of human immunodeficiency virus [HIV]

Test Positive but Asymptomatic

Thanks to research and the development of new drug therapies, patients who have HIV are living longer and with a better quality of life. Therefore, testing positive for HIV is not quite as devastating as it was years ago. When a patient comes to receive the HIV test results that are positive but the patient has no signs, symptoms, or manifestations, the patient is **asymptomatic.** You will assign code:

Z21 Asymptomatic human immunodeficiency virus [HIV] infection status

When the physician provides counseling for the patient, discusses therapeutic treatments, and/or any other elements of dealing with the disease, you should report the counseling code as well.

Test Positive with Symptoms or Manifestations

Once the individual has been diagnosed and exhibits any manifestations associated with this disease, the code to report the condition will change from Z21 to:

B20 Human immunodeficiency virus [HIV] disease

Code B20 includes a diagnosis of acquired immune deficiency syndrome (AIDS), which is essentially HIV with manifestations. When you use code B20, you have to follow it with a code or codes to identify the specific manifestations, such as pneumonia, or HIV-2 infection. There is a notation in the ICD-10-CM book, below code B20's description in the Tabular List, reminding you to do that. If the patient is seen for a condition or illness directly related to his or her HIV-positive status, list code B20 first, followed by the code or codes for the conditions.

asymptomatic
No symptoms or manifestations.

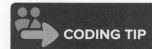

Once a patient has been diagnosed with manifestations of HIV-positive status, you are no longer permitted to use code Z21, even when the manifestations are no longer present.

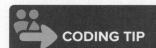

NEVER report a code for HIV infection or illness without a specific physician diagnostic statement—a confirmed diagnosis. This is an exception to hospital inpatient guidelines Section II, Subsection H, **Uncertain diagnosis.**

LET'S CODE IT! SCENARIO

Tyler Fairchild has been HIV-positive for 10 years. He comes to see Dr. Jeppahpi because of severe headaches and vision problems. After a complete physical examination (PE) and appropriate tests, Dr. Jeppahpi diagnoses Tyler with noninfectious acute disseminated encephalomyelitis, secondary to HIV.

Let's Code It!

Tyler has been diagnosed with *noninfectious acute disseminated encephalomyelitis, secondary to HIV.* Do you know whether the noninfectious acute disseminated encephalomyelitis is an HIV-related manifestation? There are two ways to tell. First, the physician's notes state that the condition is *secondary to HIV.* That means that not only are the two conditions related to each other but the HIV is the underlying condition (it came first). The second way to tell is shown in the Tabular List. Let's first go to the Alphabetic Index to find encephalomyelitis. The indented descriptions of encephalomyelitis include terms used by the physician in her notes.

Encephalomyelitis
acute disseminated (ADEM) (postinfectious) G04.01

Notice that this description, however, also includes the term *postinfectious.* Tyler was diagnosed with noninfectious encephalomyelitis. Keep reading down and find:

Encephalomyelitis, acute disseminated, noninfectious G04.81

That seems to match the doctor's notes, so now, let's turn to the Tabular List and read the complete descriptions. Start reading at:

G04 Encephalitis, myelitis, and encephalomyelitis

This code category contains both *includes* and *Excludes1* and *Excludes2* notes, which you need to read carefully. Is there anything that leads you away from this code category? No, there isn't, so you need to read down the column to find the most accurate, required fourth digit:

G04.8 Other causes of encephalitis, myelitis, and encephalomyelitis

None of the other descriptions match, or work with Dr. Jeppahpi's notes, so this looks like the best option. Take a look at your choices for the required fifth digit:

G04.81 Other encephalitis and encephalomyelitis
G04.89 Other myelitis

Check the notes and you will see that Tyler was diagnosed with encephalomyelitis, leading you directly to code:

G04.81 Other encephalitis and encephalomyelitis; noninfectious acute disseminated encephalomyelitis (ADEM)

That matches Dr. Jeppahpi's notes exactly.

Now you need the code for Tyler's HIV-positive status. Now that you know that the encephalomyelitis is a manifestation of that status, you should be clear as to what the code should be. In the Alphabetic Index, find:

Human immunodeficiency virus (disease) (infection) B20

asymptomatic status Z21

Which one should you follow? You know from the notes that Tyler does have symptoms and has manifested a secondary illness. Therefore, turn to the Tabular List to confirm:

B20 Human immunodeficiency virus [HIV] disease

You now have two codes to report the reasons Dr. Jeppahpi cared for Tyler at this encounter. Which gets listed first? The notation below the description reminds you to "use additional code(s) to identify all manifestations of HIV." This tells you that B20 is listed first. So your report for Dr. Jeppahpi's encounter with Tyler will show:

B20 Human immunodeficiency virus [HIV] disease
G04.81 Other causes of encephalitis, noninfectious acute disseminated encephalomyelitis

Good job!

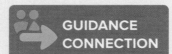

GUIDANCE CONNECTION

Review the ICD-10-CM Coding Guidelines, Section I.C.1, Chapter 1: **Certain infectious and parasitic diseases,** Subsection 2.f, **Previously diagnosed HIV-related illness.**

HIV Status with Unrelated Conditions

An individual who is HIV-positive can still be affected by conditions, illnesses, or injuries that have nothing to do with the HIV status. As you have learned, the first-listed code should answer the question, "Why did the health care provider care for the patient at this encounter?" Therefore, the code for the condition that caused the patient to visit the physician should come first. Because HIV is a systemic disease, affecting the entire body, you have to include a code for that condition as well, even if it has nothing to do with the services or treatment provided by the physician, because it will have an impact on the physician's decision making.

EXAMPLE

Roseanne Estes came to see Dr. Noonan because she slipped on the ice and hurt her ankle. Dr. Noonan examined her and took x-rays that confirmed a sprain of the deltoid ligament of the right ankle. Roseanne was diagnosed with HIV 2 years ago and is asymptomatic.

    S93.421A Sprain, of deltoid ligament of right ankle, initial encounter

    Z21 Asymptomatic human immunodeficiency virus [HIV]

EXAMPLE

Bernard Harris fell off a ladder and hurt his lower back. Dr. Kelly determined that Bernard had a fractured coccyx. Bernard was hospitalized last year with HIV-related pneumonia.

    S32.2xxA Fracture of coccyx, initial encounter

    B20 Human immunodeficiency virus [HIV] disease

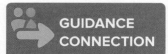

GUIDANCE CONNECTION

ICD-10-CM guideline Section I.C.1.a(2)(b): *"If a patient with HIV disease is admitted for an unrelated condition (such as a traumatic injury), the code for the unrelated condition (e.g., the nature of injury code) should be the principal diagnosis. Other diagnoses would be B20 followed by additional diagnosis codes for all reported HIV-related conditions."*

HIV Status in Obstetrics

When a woman with HIV-positive status is pregnant, giving childbirth, or in the post-partum period, the systemic disease must be a consideration in determining her care. Therefore, whether or not she has symptoms or manifestations of the HIV condition, the first-listed code must be:

O98.7- Human immunodeficiency virus [HIV] disease complicating pregnancy, childbirth, or the puerperium

This should be followed by the appropriate HIV positive status code: Z21 or B20.

YOU CODE IT! CASE STUDY

Lisa LaGuardia, a 27-year-old female, 19 weeks pregnant, was playing tennis when she felt a pain in her right knee. She went to see her physician, Dr. Jackman, who diagnosed her problem as a derangement of the posterior horn of the lateral cystic meniscus. Lisa has been HIV-positive and asymptomatic for 5 years.

You Code It!

Go through the steps of coding, and determine the diagnosis code(s) to be reported for this encounter between Dr. Jackman and Lisa LaGuardia.

    Step 1:   Read the case completely.

    Step 2:   Abstract the notes: Which key words can you identify relating to why Dr. Jackman cared for Lisa?

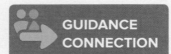

GUIDANCE CONNECTION

Are you wondering why the knee condition is listed first, when the guideline for HIV infection in pregnancy states the O98.7- code category should be listed first? In this case, you have two guidelines that need to be followed:

Section I.C.1.a(2)(b), **Patient with HIV disease admitted for unrelated condition**

Section I.C.1.a(2)(g), **HIV infection in pregnancy, childbirth, and the puerperium**

To break the tie, let's look at one more guideline, either:

Section II, **Selection of Principal Diagnosis (for inpatient admission)**

or

Section IV, **Diagnostic Coding and Reporting Guidelines for Outpatient Services, Subsection H (for outpatient)**

---

septicemia
Generalized infection spread through the body via the bloodstream; blood infection.

systemic inflammatory response syndrome (SIRS)
A definite physical reaction, such as fever, chills, etc., to an unspecified pathogen.

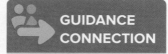

GUIDANCE CONNECTION

Review the ICD-10-CM Coding Guidelines, Section I.C.1, Chapter 1: **Certain infectious and parasitic diseases,** Subsection d, **Sepsis, severe sepsis, and septic shock.**

Step 3:   Query the provider, if necessary.

Step 4:   Code the diagnosis or diagnoses.

Step 5:   Code the procedure(s): Office visit.

Step 6:   Link the procedure codes to at least one diagnosis code to confirm medical necessity.

Step 7:   Back code to double-check your choices.

Answer:

Did you determine the correct codes?

M23.051 Internal derangement, cystic meniscus, posterior horn of lateral meniscus, right knee

O98.712 Human immunodeficiency virus [HIV] disease complicating pregnancy, childbirth, or the puerperium, antepartum condition, second trimester

Z21 Asymptomatic human immunodeficiency virus [HIV] infection status

Good job!

Whether you are coding for outpatient or inpatient services, the guidelines agree that the principal or first-listed diagnosis code should be the condition "chiefly responsible" for the encounter. In Lisa's case, the reason she went to the doctor for care was the pain in her knee—not the pregnancy and not the HIV. Then why code them at all? Because Dr. Jackman must take Lisa's pregnant status and her HIV status into consideration in his medical decision-making process to determine the best way to treat her knee.

LO 4.4 Septicemia and Other Blood Infections

Blood infections are very dangerous, as you might imagine, because of their potential effect on the entire body. Blood circulates through the body and touches all the cells and organs in some fashion. So you can understand that if the blood circulating through the body is carrying a disease, it can have the potential to cause real problems. There are several types of blood infections, and each needs to be coded differently.

Essentially, **septicemia** is identified as the presence of a microorganism or toxin in the bloodstream. The organism might be a virus, a fungus, a bacterium, or another pathologic substance. Septicemia is very serious. A physician may refer to this condition as *bacteremia;* however, they are really not the same. Bacteremia may not be clinically significant, but septicemia is always significant.

The code used for a diagnosis of septicemia may be taken from category:

A41.9 Sepsis, unspecified sepsis (Septicemia NOS)

You will need to determine a more accurate code by the pathogen or toxin found in the blood, such as streptococcus or staphylococcus.

A diagnosis of **systemic inflammatory response syndrome (SIRS)** is used when the basic cause, or *pathogen,* is unknown. The human body is amazing and is designed to fight any and all intruders (disease or infection). The system's response to infection may be:

- Increased body temperature.
- Change in heart rate.
- Change in respiratory rate.
- Increased white blood cell count.

> **Systemic inflammatory response syndrome (SIRS) of non-infectious origin R65.10**
>
> **Systemic inflammatory response syndrome (SIRS) of non-infectious origin with acute organ dysfunction R65.11**

YOU CODE IT! CASE STUDY

Caroline Culpepper, 15 years old, was brought by her mother to see Dr. Trevianni. Caroline was coughing, wheezing, and listless. After running some tests, Dr. Trevianni diagnosed Caroline with sepsis due to pseudomonas.

You Code It!

Go through the steps of coding, and determine the diagnosis code or codes that should be reported for this encounter between Dr. Trevianni and Caroline Culpepper.

Step 1: Read the case completely.

Step 2: Abstract the notes: Which key words can you identify relating to why Dr. Trevianni cared for Caroline?

_____

Step 3: Query the provider, if necessary.

Step 4: Code the diagnosis or diagnoses.

_____

Step 5: Code the procedure(s): Office visit, blood test.

Step 6: Link the procedure codes to at least one diagnosis code to confirm medical necessity.

Step 7: Back code to double-check your choices.

Answer:

Did you determine the correct codes?

A41.52 Sepsis due to pseudomonas

Terrific!

Sepsis

When one individual exhibits two or more systemic responses or when the presence of a specific pathogen has been identified in the bloodstream, the diagnosis is typically **sepsis.**

Reporting a diagnosis of sepsis will begin with the identification of the underlying systemic infection—the pathogen that initiated the septic condition. This code will

sepsis
Condition typified by two or more systemic responses to infection; a specified pathogen.

come from category A40.- or A41.-. You may find this detail in the physician's documentation or the pathology report.

On occasion, a physician might diagnose a patient with *urosepsis*. This is not a synonym for sepsis and cannot be coded as sepsis. Should you find this term used in the documentation, you will need to query the physician for clarification.

A patient may be diagnosed with sepsis and acute organ failure during the same encounter, without a relationship (or cause and effect) between the two. In these situations, the organ failure is a co-morbidity and is reported separately from the sepsis.

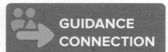

GUIDANCE CONNECTION

The Official Guidelines, Section I.C.1.d(3), warn you that a code from subcategory R65.2, **Severe sepsis,** is *never* permitted to be the first-listed or principal diagnosis code reported.

EXAMPLE

Timothy Roberts was in the hospital and diagnosed with group A streptococcus sepsis.

A40.0 Sepsis due to streptococcus, group A

Severe Sepsis

When left untreated, sepsis may become severe and cause an organ to fail—a life-threatening condition. In some cases, this can occur when treatment is provided but is ineffective. A diagnosis of sepsis in combination with acute organ failure due to the septic condition is reported as **severe sepsis.** The physician's notes that contain a diagnosis of severe sepsis will be reported with:

severe sepsis
Sepsis with signs of acute organ dysfunction.

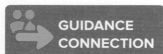

GUIDANCE CONNECTION

Review the ICD-10-CM Coding Guidelines, Section I.C.1, Chapter 1: **Certain infectious and parasitic diseases,** Subsection d(1)(b), **Severe sepsis.**

- *First:* the code for the underlying systemic infection, such as streptococcus or other bacteria (e.g., a code from A40.- or A41.-). If the organism is not known, you may report A41.9, Sepsis, unspecified organism
- *Followed by:* a code from subcategory R65.2, Severe sepsis. An additional character is required to report whether or not the physician has documented that the patient is in "septic shock."
- *Followed by:* a code to report the specific organ failure caused by the septic condition. To remind you, code subcategory R65 has a *use additional code* notation.

LET'S CODE IT! SCENARIO

Dr. Kahanni admitted Burton Chapel with acute renal failure due to severe sepsis resulting from pneumonia.

Let's Code It!

Dr. Kahanni diagnosed Burton with "acute renal failure due to severe sepsis resulting from pneumonia." Remember the Official Guideline at Section l.c.1.d(1)(b): The coding of severe sepsis requires first a code for the underlying systemic infection, followed by a code from R65.2-, and then the code for the acute organ dysfunction. Turn to the Alphabetic Index and find:

Sepsis

Pneumococcal A40.3

Turn to the Tabular list to confirm this code:

A40 Steptococcal sepsis

Read the fourth-character choices and find:

A40.3 Sepsis due to streptococcus pneumoniae (Pneumococcal sepsis)

Next, let's turn to R65.2- and see what will accurately report Dr. Kahanni's diagnosis for Burton.

R65.2 Severe sepsis

Read the fifth-character descriptions, and determine which one matches:

R65.20 Severe sepsis without septic shock

The notations above this code help you further. They remind you to "code first underlying infection," which you have done already with the pneumococcal sepsis code. The second notation directs you to:

Use additional code to specify acute organ dysfunction, such as: acute kidney failure (N17.-)

Next, confirm the code for the acute renal (kidney) failure:

N17 Acute kidney failure

Carefully read the *code also* and *Excludes1* notes. There is no relevance here to Burton's diagnosis at this encounter, so read down the column to review all of your choices for the required fourth character. With no documentation of any lesions on Burton's kidneys, the best choice is:

N17.9 Acute renal failure, unspecified

You will report these codes in the order specified by the guidelines: A40.3, R65.20, N17.9 . . .

Good job!

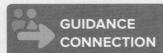

CODING TIP

The code for septic shock may not be the principal or first-listed diagnosis.

GUIDANCE CONNECTION

Review the ICD-10-CM Coding Guidelines, Section I.C.1, Chapter 1: **Certain infectious and parasitic diseases,** Subsection d.2, **Septic shock.**

Septic Shock

Should a patient also develop hypotension (low blood pressure) in addition to having severe sepsis, the diagnosis becomes **septic shock.** Septic shock cannot be present without the existence of severe sepsis—and it all must be documented. When coding septic shock, report the codes in the following order:

1. The code for the systemic infection (e.g., A40.-.)
2. The code for the severe sepsis with septic shock (e.g., R65.21.)
3. The code for the organ dysfunction.

septic shock
Severe sepsis with hypotension; unresponsive to fluid resuscitation.

Sepsis and Septic Shock Relating to Pregnancy or Newborns

Sepsis during Labor During the process of giving birth, a woman might develop a septic infection. In this case, code O75.3, Other infection during labor (Sepsis during labor), is reported. A code from B95–B97, Bacterial and viral infectious agents, should follow to specify the pathogen causing the infection.

Puerperal Sepsis Puerperal sepsis, also known as *postpartum sepsis, puerperal peritonitis,* or *puerperal pyemia,* results from an infection that develops in a woman's reproductive organs and was initiated during, or following, miscarriage or childbirth. This diagnosis is reported with code O85, Puerperal sepsis.

In addition, a code from B95–B97, Bacterial and viral infectious agents, is required to specify the pathogen causing the infection. If severe sepsis is documented, a code from R65.2- should also be reported.

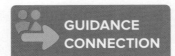

GUIDANCE CONNECTION

Review the ICD-10-CM Coding Guidelines, Section I.C.15, Chapter 15: **Pregnancy, Childbirth, and the Puerperium,** Subsection s j, **Sepsis and septic shock complicating abortion and pregnancy,** and k, **Puerperal sepsis,** and Section I.C.16.f, **Bacterial sepsis of newborn, sepsis.**

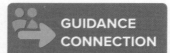

GUIDANCE CONNECTION

Review the ICD-10-CM Coding Guidelines, Section I.C.I, Chapter 1: **Certain infectious and parasitic diseases,** Subsection d(5), **Sepsis due to a postprocedural infection.**

Neonatal Sepsis A fetus may contract an infection in utero, during the birth process (delivery), or during the first 28 days after birth. In these cases, when a neonate is diagnosed with sepsis, the code will be reported from category P36, Bacterial sepsis of newborn. An additional character is required to identify the pathogen that caused the infection. If severe sepsis is documented, a code from R65.2- should also be reported.

Septic Condition Resulting from Surgery

Should a patient develop sepsis from an infection as a complication of a surgical procedure, you will list a code for that situation first. In the Alphabetic Index, find:

> Sepsis, postprocedural T81.4

In the Tabular List, find:

> T81.4xx- Infection following a procedure

Read the *Excludes1* notes. You will see that there are three diagnoses that would be easy to code incorrectly from this subcategory:

> Obstetric surgical wound infection (O86.0)
>
> postprocedural fever NOS (R50.82)
>
> postprocedural retroperitoneal abscess (K68.11)

This is a great example of why it is so important to read carefully. Don't forget the notation below this code:

> Use additional code to identify infection

Then continue with the usual coding sequence for sepsis, as reviewed earlier in this chapter. Remember to refer to the physician's documentation and the pathology report to gather all of the details you need to code accurately.

YOU CODE IT! CASE STUDY

Gregory Parrale, a 31-year-old male, had his appendix taken out last week. He comes to Dr. Gorman's office for his postsurgical follow-up visit, and Dr. Gorman finds the surgical wound is erythematous, swollen, and painful to the touch. He takes a swab of the fluid oozing from the site. The lab confirms a postoperative staph infection.

You Code It!

Go through the steps of coding, and determine the diagnosis code(s) to be reported for this encounter between Dr. Gorman and Gregory Parrale.

Step 1: Read the case completely.

Step 2: Abstract the notes: Which key words can you identify relating to why Dr. Gorman cared for Gregory?

_____

Step 3: Query the provider, if necessary.

Step 4: Code the diagnosis or diagnoses.

_____

Step 5: Code the procedure(s): Office visit, blood tests.

Step 6: Link the procedure codes to at least one diagnosis code to confirm medical necessity.

Step 7: Back code to double-check your choices.

Answer:

Did you determine the correct codes?

T81.4xxA Infection following a procedure, initial encounter

B95.8 Unspecified staphylococcus as the cause of diseases classified elsewhere

Good job!

Systemic Inflammatory Response Syndrome Without Infection

Systemic inflammatory response syndrome (SIRS) can develop in patients who have not developed an infection. Instead the reaction may occur due to the presence of a burn or other trauma, a malignant neoplasm, or the presence of pancreatitis. In such cases, coding the condition will change slightly. You will code the following sequence:

1. The code for the underlying condition (e.g., T22.311-, Third-degree burn of right forearm).
2. The code for SIRS from the subcategory R65.1-, Systemic inflammatory response syndrome.
3. The code for the acute organ dysfunction, when applicable.

If the documentation indicates that the patient later developed an infection, you will code the diagnosis for the infection as shown earlier in the chapter, along with the additional code for the underlying trauma or condition.

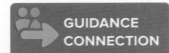

GUIDANCE CONNECTION

Review the ICD-10-CM Coding Guidelines, Section I.C.18, Chapter 18: **Symptoms, signs, and abnormal clinical laboratory findings, not elsewhere classified,** Subsection g, **SIRS due to non-infectious process.**

LO 4.5 Methicillin-Resistant *Staphylococcus Aureus*

Methicillin-resistant *Staphylococcus aureus* (MRSA) is a bacterial (staph) infection that is essentially unaffected by certain antibiotics. MRSA is spread from one person to another by direct contact with the infection, such as touching a skin bump or infection that is draining pus. MRSA can be spread directly, for example, by touching an infected person's rash, or it can be spread indirectly, such as by touching a used bandage contaminated with MRSA or by sharing a towel or razor that has come in contact with infected skin. One of the most frequent anatomical sites of MRSA colonization is the nose; bacteria can be found in nasal secretions.

Methicillin-Resistant *Staphylococcus Aureus* Colonization

When the patient is documented as having a MRSA screening or nasal swab test that is positive, yet there is no current illness, this is called colonization. Colonization indicates that the patient is a carrier. When this is the case, report either:

Z22.321 Carrier or suspected carrier, Methicillin susceptible Staphylococcus aureus (MSSA)

or

Z22.322 Carrier or suspected carrier, Methicillin resistant Staphylococcus aureus (MRSA)

The coding guidelines state that it is possible for one patient to be a MRSA carrier *and* have a current MRSA infection at the same encounter. When this is the case, you are permitted to report code Z22.322 and a code for the MRSA infection.

Methicillin-Resistant *Staphylococcus Aureus* Infection

There are some infections commonly known to be caused by the patient's current MRSA status. In these cases, ICD-10-CM provides a combination code that can be used—the one code instead of two different codes. Two examples of these combination codes are:

A41.02 Sepsis due to Methicillin resistant Staphylococcus aureus

J15.212 Pneumonia due to Methicillin resistant Staphylococcus aureus

Notice that the code descriptions include both the MRSA and another infection: septicemia in the first code and pneumonia in the second.

Not all infections occurring at the same time a patient has a MRSA infection will have a combination code available. To properly report these diagnoses, code the current infection due to MRSA and the MRSA infection separately with code:

A49.02 Methicillin resistant Staphylococcus aureus infection, unspecified site

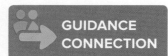

GUIDANCE CONNECTION

Review the ICD-10-CM Coding Guidelines, Section I.C.1, Chapter 1: **Certain infectious and parasitic diseases**, Subsection e, **Methicillin resistant Staphylococcus aureus (MRSA) conditions.**

EXAMPLE

Taneshia Novack was diagnosed with acute cystitis due to MRSA.

    N30.00 Acute cystitis

    B95.62 Methicillin resistant Staphylococcus aureus infections as the causes of diseases classified elsewhere

Tuberculosis

Tuberculosis (TB) is a threat to the community because it is highly contagious. You may have been required to take a TB skin test as a part of your entry into the health care field. *Mycobacterium tuberculosis,* the causative agent of TB, is a bacterial infection that is transmitted through the air. It means that someone can become infected by being coughed on by someone who has TB. One version of TB is called *latent tuberculosis infection (LTBI),* because it is dormant and may not show symptoms right away. That is why individuals must take a TB test, because not everyone who has been infected is symptomatic. Most types of TB and LTBI are successfully treated with medication.

There is a specific cultural group of people who will get a positive result to the skin test but not actually have the disease. A simple chest x-ray confirms that situation. Should you have a patient in such a circumstance, you will use code:

R76.11 Nonspecific reaction to tuberculin skin test without active tuberculosis

In cases where a patient tests positive for TB and actually does have the disease, you will choose the best, most appropriate code from the range A15–A19, Tuberculosis. As you look through the section, you will notice that TB is a disseminated disease. While most people think of TB as a pulmonary infection, infiltrating only the lungs, it can actually leach throughout the body and be identified in many different anatomical sites. You have to know which anatomical site is infected with the TB bacterium so that you can find the most accurate code.

Henry Kensington was brought into the emergency department (ED) by ambulance because he was having pain in his abdomen. Dr. Stanton diagnosed Henry with renal tuberculosis, confirmed histologically, with pyelonephritis.

You Code It!

Go through the steps of coding, and determine the diagnosis code or codes that should be reported for this encounter between Dr. Stanton and Henry Kensington.

Step 1: Read the case completely.

Step 2: Abstract the notes: Which key words can you identify relating to why Dr. Stanton cared for Henry?

_____

Step 3: Query the provider, if necessary.

Step 4: Code the diagnosis or diagnoses.

_____

Step 5: Code the procedure(s): ED visit

Step 6: Link the procedure codes to at least one diagnosis code to confirm medical necessity.

Step 7: Back code to double-check your choices.

Answer:

Did you determine the correct code?

A18.11 Tuberculosis of kidney and ureter (Pyelitis tuberculous)

Terrific!

Bacterial Infections

Some bacterial infections that you will encounter in a typical health care facility are those that are foodborne, commonly called *food poisoning.* According to the Centers for Disease Control (CDC), approximately 76 million cases of foodborne illness and 5,000 associated deaths occur in the United States annually. Do not let this fool you: These diagnoses are not poisonings (as far as coding goes); they are infections. Therefore, the diagnosis codes will not include external cause codes. Some of the most frequently seen bacterial infections, and their sources, are as follows:

- *Campylobacter:* From foods including raw poultry; raw meat; untreated milk: code A04.5.
- *Listeria:* Untreated milk; dairy products; raw salads and vegetables: code A32.-.
- *Salmonella:* Raw poultry; eggs; raw meat; untreated milk and dairy products: code A02.9.
- *Shigella:* Untreated water; milk and dairy products; raw vegetables and salads; shellfish; turkey; apple cider: codes A03.-.
- *Vibrio:* Raw and lightly cooked fish and shellfish: code A00.-.
- *Clostridium perfringens:* Animal and human excreta; soil; dust; insects; raw meat: code B96.7.

- *Escherichia coli (E. coli 0157):* Human and animal gut; sewage; water; raw meat: code A49.8.

Almost all the above infections induce symptoms of diarrhea, abdominal pain, nausea, fever, and vomiting. Other serious effects include dehydration, headache, and kidney damage or failure. Therefore, you must be careful not to report unnecessary codes for signs and symptoms that are actually included in a definitive diagnosis that has been made.

LET'S CODE IT! SCENARIO

Robyn Julianni, a 23-year-old female, came to see Dr. Chou due to severe abdominal pain. She had a fever and stated that she has had bloody diarrhea for the past 2 days. Dr. Chou's examination revealed that she was dehydrated as well. Robyn stated she ate at a new restaurant at the beach where she had a salad and a vegetable plate. After taking some tests, he diagnosed Robyn with Shigella dysenteriae *(bacillary dysentery).*

Let's Code It!

Dr. Chou found Robyn to be suffering from *Shigella.* Turn to the Alphabetic Index and find

Shigella (dysentery) (see Dysentery, bacillary)
Dysentery, bacillary A03.9

Turn to the Tabular List, and check the code's complete description:

A03 Shigellosis

There are no notations or directives, so read down the column to review all of the choices for the required fourth character. The code suggested by the Alphabetic Index:

A03.9 Shigellosis, unspecified

Is this the most accurate code? You will note that the other fourth-character code choices want specifics on which group (A, B, C, or D) of the *Shigella* infection is present. Do you know? Dr. Chou did specify in the notes—*Shigella dysenteriae,* which matches the description for:

A03.0 Shigellosis due to Shigella dysenteriae

Therefore, A03.0 is the most accurate code available. Excellent!

LO 4.6 Other Infections

There are a large number of infectious diseases that you may have to code, depending upon the type of facility that employs you, combined with geographic and other factors. Let's review some of the most common infections, their descriptions, and their code ranges.

Viral Hepatitis

Hepatitis (*hepat* = liver; *-itis* = inflammation) actually refers to several different viral infections. According to the Centers for Disease Control (CDC), viral hepatitis is the most prevalent cause of malignant neoplasms of the liver. Millions of people are living with one of these conditions in the United States. As you know, prevention is a much better path than treatment. For those coming to your facility to get a hepatitis vaccine, you will report one of these codes:

Z20.5 Contact with or (suspected) exposure to other viral diseases

Z22.5- Carrier of viral hepatitis

Z23 Encounter for immunization

Viral Hepatitis, Type A The CDC estimates that an additional 25,000 people each year become infected with viral hepatitis, type A, a viral infection of the liver caused by the hepatitis A virus (HAV). The virus can travel from person to person by personal contact, as with other infections. However, in addition, one can become infected by being exposed to contaminated water or ice. Shellfish harvested from sewage-contaminated water, as well as fruits, vegetables, and other foods that have been contaminated and eaten uncooked, may also carry the hepatitis A virus. Viral hepatitis A is reported with either:

B15.0 Hepatitis A with hepatic coma

or

B15.9 Hepatitis A without hepatic coma

Viral Hepatitis, Type B Caused by the hepatitis B virus (HBV), viral hepatitis, type B, is transmitted through contact with infected bodily fluids, such as blood or semen. The infection can also be spread by the use of equipment that has been contaminated with the virus, which is why when getting a tattoo, body piercing, or even fingernail application, one must be careful that the needles and files have been sterilized properly. The CDC estimates 43,000 new cases of hepatitis B are diagnosed each year. Viral hepatitis B is reported with:

B16.0 Acute hepatitis B with delta-agent with hepatic coma

B16.1 Acute hepatitis B with delta-agent without hepatic coma

B16.2 Acute hepatitis B without delta-agent with hepatic coma

B16.9 Acute hepatitis B without delta-agent and without hepatic coma

To choose the most accurate code, you have to know if the patient has a hepatic coma, whether or not the condition is identified as acute or chronic, and whether or not hepatitis D (delta) is involved.

Viral Hepatitis, Type C The hepatitis C virus (HCV) infection is estimated by the Centers for Disease Control (CDC) to chronically affect 3.2 million people in the United States. It is considered to be the most widespread chronic bloodborne infection. Those individuals at the highest risk for infection are those using injected drugs. Each year, it is believed that an additional 17,000 individuals become hepatitis C positive. Report this diagnosis with one of these codes:

B17.11 Acute hepatitis C with hepatic coma

B18.2 Chronic hepatitis C

B17.10 Acute hepatitis C without hepatic coma

B19.2 Unspecified viral hepatitis C

Viral Hepatitis, Type D Also known as *hepatitis delta,* this is a serious liver disease that requires the HBV (hepatitis B virus) to replicate itself. This condition is not seen often in the United States. Hepatitis D is transmitted through direct contact with infected blood, similar to how hepatitis B is passed from one person to another. Currently, there is no vaccine for hepatitis D. Hepatitis D is referred to as *hepatitis delta* in the code descriptions, and reported with code:

B17.0 Acute delta-(super) infection of hepatitis B carrier

Viral Hepatitis, Type E Occurrences of hepatitis E in the United States are rare; it is known to be common in countries with poor sanitation and contaminated water supplies. This liver disease, caused by the hepatitis E virus (HEV), does not lead to chronic infection. There is no vaccine currently approved by the FDA for hepatitis E. Report this diagnosis with:

B17.2 Acute Hepatitis E

Meningitis

Meningitis is the inflammation of the meningeal membranes of the brain and/or the spinal cord. Meningitis can be bacterial; however, it is more often the result of a viral infection. When meningitis is caught early, the prognosis is good and the complications are rare.

In order to code a diagnosis of meningitis, you have to know which virus or bacterium is at the core of the inflammation.

EXAMPLE

Meningococcal meningitis A39.0

In some cases, ICD-10-CM will identify the requirement of a second code.

EXAMPLE

Meningitis due to poliovirus A80.9 *[G02]*

Tetanus (Lockjaw)

You are probably more familiar with the tetanus vaccine than you are with the disease. Tetanus is an infection of the nervous system and is caused by the entry of bacteria into the body through a break in the skin. It causes death in about 11% of all cases. The illness can be prevented by the administration of the tetanus toxoid, included in the DTaP, DT, and Td vaccines.

When the patient has come for inoculation with the tetanus toxoid only, you will use Z23. However, read the notes carefully. If the development of tetanus is a complication arising from the vaccination, use code T88.1. If it is a result of an incident, such as stepping on a rusty nail, report it with code A35 plus an external cause code. Should this disease occur with or following an abortion or ectopic pregnancy, then you will report it as a complication of pregnancy, using A34 or O08.89. And in cases where the tetanus is affecting a neonate, it will be reported with code A33.

Influenza

There is a reason why so much commotion is made annually about individuals getting their flu shots. A seemingly ordinary infection, influenza (commonly called the *flu*) can be deadly. It is caused by the influenza A or B virus and can be transmitted by casual contact, such as a handshake, or touching a contaminated doorknob. It is estimated that as many as 36,000 people die in the United States each year from influenza.

The diagnosis of influenza will be reported with code J09.-, J10.-, or J11.-, depending upon the accompanying complications and coexisting conditions.

Sexually Transmitted Diseases

There are more than 25 infectious organisms that are passed from one person to another during sexual activity of any kind that involves the exchange of bodily fluids. Herpes, gonorrhea, syphilis, and HIV are the most common sexually transmitted diseases (STDs). When not caught early, STDs can frequently result in serious long-term complications, including pelvic inflammatory disease (PID), genital cancer, infertility, and even mental illness.

You will find some STDs coded from the subsection titled: Infections with a predominantly sexual mode of transmission (A50–A64). However, that is not all inclusive; STDs such as HIV (code Z21 or B20) and herpes simplex (code B00.-) are listed elsewhere.

Another serious group of STDs are types of human papilloma virus (HPV). There are more than 70 types of HPV diagnoses, including condylomata acuminata, penile warts, venereal warts, and condyloma (genital warts).

Varicella

Varicella, commonly known as *chickenpox,* is generally not perceived to be serious, most particularly for children. Complications from varicella, however, may include pneumonia in adults and bacterial infections of the skin and soft tissue in affected children. The infections can be severe and lead to septicemia, toxic shock syndrome, necrotizing fasciitis, osteomyelitis, bacterial pneumonia, and septic arthritis. There may also be a connection between varicella and development of herpes zoster, also known as *shingles,* later in life. The availability of the varicella vaccine has made contracting the infection almost nil.

Code varicella from B01.- if the patient has been diagnosed. If the patient has come to receive a varicella vaccine, then use code Z23. However, if the patient has been exposed to varicella, the code will change to Z20.820.

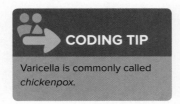

CODING TIP

Varicella is commonly called *chickenpox.*

Rubeola

Commonly referred to as measles, the risk of catching the childhood illness of rubeola is very low because of the success of the measles vaccine. Your coding experience relating to measles should be limited to office visits for administering the vaccine.

When an individual has come to get vaccinated against rubeola only, code the encounter using Z23. However, a patient who is seeing a health care professional because of having been exposed to rubeola will be reported with Z20.828. A diagnosis of rubeola (measles) should be reported with code B05.-

Rubella

An acute viral disease that can affect anyone of any age, rubella is thought of by many to be a children's disease known as the *German measles.* While the symptoms are most often not more than a mild rash, the health danger of rubella can be serious to a pregnant woman in her first trimester. When contracted during the early months of pregnancy, rubella can be associated with a condition known as *congenital rubella syndrome (CRS).* CRS may cause any of a large number of birth defects, including deafness and, possibly, fetal death. The vaccine has almost eliminated CRS.

Rubella is coded with B06.- when it has been diagnosed. For those cases in which a patient is being vaccinated against rubella alone, you will use Z23, and if the patient has been exposed to rubella, report this with code Z20.4.

Mumps

Another childhood viral infection, the mumps has been virtually eliminated with the licensure of the vaccine in 1967. Report the encounter for administering a mumps vaccine alone with code Z23. If the diagnosis is confirmed, the encounter should be reported with code B26.-

Parasitic Infestations

Many parasites can affect the health of both children and adults. The spread of lice is one of the most commonly seen. Children share head lice during sports or on the playground, while pubic or body lice are more often seen in sexually active adults. Parasitic infestations are coded from the B35–B89 categories, using additional characters to specify the particular vermin, as documented by the physician.

YOU CODE IT! CASE STUDY

Meredith Frasier brought her 5-year-old daughter Megan to see Dr. Washington, complaining that her daughter keeps scratching her head. After a thorough exam, Dr. Washington explains that Megan has a case of head lice. He instructs her to buy Nix, an over-the-counter permethrin, and gives her an instruction sheet on how to rid her child and her household of the parasites.

You Code It!

Go through the steps of coding, and determine the diagnosis code or codes that should be reported for this encounter between Dr. Washington and Megan Frasier.

Step 1: Read the case completely.

Step 2: Abstract the notes: Which key words can you identify relating to why Dr. Washington cared for Megan?

_____

Step 3: Query the provider, if necessary.

Step 4: Code the diagnosis or diagnoses.

_____

Step 5: Code the procedure(s): Office visit.

Step 6: Link the procedure codes to at least one diagnosis code to confirm medical necessity.

Step 7: Back code to double-check your choices.

Answer:

Did you determine the correct codes?

B85.0 Pediculus capitis [head louse]

Great work!

Chapter Summary

The contagious nature of infectious diseases makes them very serious. The coding of such conditions and their treatment has statistical significance, in addition to the importance of reimbursement.

Ordinary day-to-day activities, such as sneezing, coughing, having sex, or playing baseball, may pass an infectious disease from one person to another. Health care advancements have enabled the use of vaccines to prevent such conditions as measles, mumps, varicella, or human papilloma virus (HPV). Other conditions require behavioral or lifestyle changes to prevent their spread.

In any case, the health care industry is charged with helping patients, and it is, or will be, your job to code all of these infectious diseases correctly.

CHAPTER **4** REVIEW
Coding Infectious Diseases

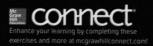
Enhance your learning by completing these
exercises and more at mcgrawhillconnect.com!

Using Terminology

Match each key term to the appropriate definition.

_____ **1.** LO 4.1 Group of organisms, including mold, yeast, and mildew, that cause infection.

_____ **2.** LO 4.4 Condition typified by two or more systemic responses to infection; a specified pathogen.

_____ **3.** LO 4.1/4.5 An infectious condition that causes small, rounded swellings on mucous membranes throughout the body.

_____ **4.** LO 4.1 Any agent that causes disease; a microorganism such as a bacterium or virus.

_____ **5.** LO 4.1 Spread throughout the entire body.

_____ **6.** LO 4.1 A single-celled microorganism that causes disease.

_____ **7.** LO 4.2 The pathogen has infected a large geographic area.

_____ **8.** LO 4.1 Severe.

_____ **9.** LO 4.1 A microscopic particle that initiates disease, mimicking the characteristics of a particular cell, and that can reproduce only within the body of the cell which it has invaded.

_____ **10.** LO 4.2 The spread of the pathogen is contained within a small area.

_____ **11.** LO 4.1 Tiny living things that can invade and feed off other living things.

_____ **12.** LO 4.1/4.3 A condition affecting the immune system.

_____ **13.** LO 4.3 No symptoms or manifestations.

_____ **14.** LO 4.2 The pathogen spreads quickly and easily.

_____ **15.** LO 4.1 A condition that can be transmitted from one person to another.

_____ **16.** LO 4.1 Long lasting; ongoing.

_____ **17.** LO 4.4 A definite physical reaction, such as fever or chills, to an unspecified pathogen.

_____ **18.** LO 4.2 A hospital-acquired condition.

A. Acute

B. Asymptomatic

C. Bacteria

D. Chronic

E. Endemic

F. Epidemic

G. Fungi

H. Human immunodeficiency virus (HIV)

I. Infectious

J. Nosocomial

K. Pandemic

L. Parasites

M. Pathogen

N. Sepsis

O. Systemic

P. Systemic inflammatory response syndrome (SIRS)

Q. Tuberculosis

R. Virus

Checking Your Understanding

Choose the most appropriate answer for each of the following questions.

1. LO 4.1/4.2 An infection can be spread by

  a. physical contact.

  b. exchange of bodily fluids.

  c. touching a surface, such as a counter or doorknob.

  d. all of these.

2. LO 4.3 HIV can be spread by

 a. physical contact.
 b. exchange of bodily fluids.
 c. touching a surface, such as a counter or doorknob.
 d. all of these.

3. LO 4.3 A test for HIV will be coded if

 a. the test is positive.
 b. the test is negative.
 c. the test is inconclusive.
 d. all of these.

4. LO 4.3 A patient who is HIV-positive is coded with an HIV code

 a. at all encounters.
 b. only at encounters for the HIV and/or related conditions.
 c. never, to protect the patient's privacy.
 d. only when a manifestation is diagnosed.

5. LO 4.1 The body's response to an infection may include the sign or symptom of

 a. rash.
 b. blurred vision.
 c. increased body temperature.
 d. reduced body temperature.

6. LO 4.4 When coding for SIRS in a patient who has *not* developed an infection, you would code in which sequence?

 a. the code for the acute organ dysfunction, the code for SIRS, the code for the underlying condition.
 b. the code for SIRS, the code for the acute organ dysfunction, the code for the underlying condition.
 c. the code for the underlying condition, the code for SIRS, the code for the acute organ dysfunction.
 d. none of these.

7. LO 4.4 The diagnosis of severe sepsis must include identification of

 a. the organ that is dysfunctional.
 b. the specific pathogen.
 c. the type of medication prescribed.
 d. the patient's age.

8. LO 4.4 The code for septic shock may be all of the following *except*

 a. the first-listed diagnosis code.
 b. an additional code.
 c. used to identify the inclusion of hypotension.
 d. added to the codes required for severe sepsis.

9. LO 4.5 Tuberculosis can occur

    a. in the lungs only.

    b. almost anywhere in the body.

    c. as a positive skin test only when active TB is present.

    d. only outside the United States.

10. LO 4.5 Foodborne bacterial infections can be contracted from

    a. red meat.

    b. dairy products.

    c. vegetables.

    d. all of these.

Applying Your Knowledge

1. LO 4.1 Explain the difference between a bacterial infection and a viral infection, and give examples of each. _____

_____

2. LO 4.2 List three ways you can be exposed to an infection and become ill. _____

_____

3. LO 4.2 What is a nosocomial infection, and where do such infections occur? _____

_____

4. LO 4.4 Discuss the difference between septicemia and SIRS. _____

_____

5. LO 4.5 What is MRSA? _____

_____

YOU CODE IT! Practice

Chapter 4: Coding Infectious Diseases

Using the techniques described in this chapter, carefully read through the case studies and determine the most accurate ICD-10-CM code(s) and external cause code(s), if appropriate, for each case.

1. Dr. Tully diagnosed Margaret Tulane with tuberculosis peritonitis, confirmed histologically.

   _____

2. Marion Norris came back from a trip overseas and wasn't feeling well. Dr. Delbert diagnosed her with typhoid fever.

   _____

3. Brian Townsend came home from active military duty with an intestinal problem. Dr. Vanderhooten diagnosed him with hemorrhagic dysentery.

   _____

4. Cheryl Laurens woke up with itchy spots all over her body. Dr. Malaga diagnosed her with chickenpox.

   _____

5. Arthur Lang comes to see Dr. Fahey because of his chronic viral hepatitis C.

   _____

6. Leanne Kinnerson went hiking with friends in the woods. Dr. Gaitlin diagnosed her with Rocky Mountain spotted fever.

   _____

7. Sheila Brennan has difficulty breathing. She is 19 weeks pregnant and was diagnosed with AIDS 2 years ago. Dr. Workman diagnoses her with *Pneumocystis carinii* pneumonia.

   _____

8. Greg Wooten had an eruption of molluscum contagiosum on his penis.

   _____

9. Faith Hardy had severe abdominal cramps. Dr. Stevenson diagnosed her with acute amebiasis.

   _____

10. Martin Kinsey was admitted to the hospital with severe sepsis due to anaerobic streptococci. Martin developed acute respiratory failure.

_____

11. Dr. Heinek diagnosed William Anderson with bacteremia due to *H. pylori*.

_____

12. Jesse Berman tested HIV positive 8 years ago. She is admitted with herpes zoster with meningitis.

_____

13. Irving Durran was diagnosed with aseptic meningitis due to ECHO virus.

_____

14. Dr. Lovell diagnosed Emily Norman with American histoplasmosis with pericarditis. Emily was diagnosed with AIDS 1 year ago.

_____

15. Sidney Lukenstrom was admitted into the hospital with food poisoning due to *Clostridium botulinum*.

_____

The following exercises provide practice in abstracting physicians' notes and learning to work with SOAP notes from our textbook's health care facility, *Taylor, Reader, & Associates*. These case studies (SOAP notes) are modeled on real patient encounters. Using the techniques described in this chapter, carefully read through the case studies and determine the most accurate ICD-10-CM code(s) and external cause code(s), if appropriate, for each case study.

TAYLOR, READER, & ASSOCIATES
A Complete Health Care Facility
975 CENTRAL AVENUE • SOMEWHERE, FL 32811 • 407-555-4321

PATIENT: ACCOLINO, JEANETTE
ACCOUNT/EHR #:   ACCOJE001
DATE: 09/16/18

Attending Physician: Suzanne R. Taylor, MD

This 55-year-old female was admitted for a high fever and obtundation. She had been treated with oral antibiotics for a left ear fullness (clogged up) and decreased hearing for 1 week. Three days ago, I saw the patient in the office, and her left ear spontaneously drained.

On PE, the Pt appears confused and febrile. Her left ear continues to drain. Spinal fluid is turbid and showed 6250 WBC, 33 g/L protein, and 21 mg/dL glucose.

Two blood cultures indicate arbovirus. She responded to antimicrobial therapy and except for the reduction of hearing on the left, there are no neurologic sequelae.

DX. Meningitis due to arbovirus, urban; acute suppurative otitis media

---

Suzanne R. Taylor, MD

SRT/pw   D: 09/16/18 09:50:16   T: 09/18/18 12:55:01

Determine the most accurate ICD-10-CM code(s).

TAYLOR, READER, & ASSOCIATES
A Complete Health Care Facility
975 CENTRAL AVENUE • SOMEWHERE, FL 32811 • 407-555-4321

PATIENT: RYAN, MAYLENE
ACCOUNT/EHR #:   RYANMA001
DATE: 08/11/18

Attending Physician: Willard B. Reader, MD

Pt is admitted with a chief complaint of shortness of breath of approximately 1-week duration. Pt was found to be HIV-positive in March 2000, and diagnosed with AIDS in August 2003.

Patient reports that she has lost approximately 12 lb within the last 4 weeks.

T 102.58. Wt 115 lb. Ht 5'7". Red and blue skin lesions are noted in her mouth, specifically the upper palate.

DX. Kaposi's sarcoma of the palate, secondary to AIDS

Willard B. Reader, MD

WBR/pw   D: 08/11/18 09:50:16   T: 08/13/18 12:55:01

Determine the most accurate ICD-10-CM code(s).

_____

_____

_____

TAYLOR, READER, & ASSOCIATES
A Complete Health Care Facility
975 CENTRAL AVENUE • SOMEWHERE, FL 32811 • 407-555-4321

PATIENT: COLLIER, LINDA
ACCOUNT/EHR #:   COLLLI001
DATE: 09/16/18

Attending Physician: Suzanne R. Taylor, MD

Pt presented to the urgent care center with a laceration to the left elbow that occurred 2 weeks ago and was left untreated. She states that she fell off a barstool at her local tavern.

An infected gaping wound was found, with resulting cellulitis to the forearm and upper arm. Extensive irrigation and debridement using sterile water were performed, but closure was not attempted pending resolution of the infection. Culture of the wound revealed streptococcus D.

1,200 units of Bicillin CR IM was given.
Rx for oral antibiotics was given to Pt.
Pt to return in 3 days for follow-up.

Suzanne R. Taylor, MD

SRT/pw   D: 09/16/18 09:50:16   T: 09/18/18 12:55:01

Determine the most accurate ICD-10-CM code(s).

_____

_____

_____

TAYLOR, READER, & ASSOCIATES
A Complete Health Care Facility
975 CENTRAL AVENUE • SOMEWHERE, FL 32811 • 407-555-4321

PATIENT: FEENEY, WANDA
ACCOUNT/EHR #:   FEENWA01
DATE: 08/11/18

Attending Physician: Willard B. Reader, MD

Pt is a 21-year-old female, who came today with complaints of a sore throat. She stated that her throat was scratchy 1 week ago. The scratchiness progressed into a sharp pain in the last day or two.
    PE reveals acute tonsillitis. Quick strep test confirms the presence of streptococcal infection.
    Rx. Antibiotics.
    Recommendation for bed rest, lots of fluids. Pt to return prn.

Willard B. Reader, MD

WBR/pw   D: 08/11/18 09:50:16   T: 08/13/18 12:55:01

Determine the most accurate ICD-10-CM code(s).

_____

_____

_____

TAYLOR, READER, & ASSOCIATES
A Complete Health Care Facility
975 CENTRAL AVENUE • SOMEWHERE, FL 32811 • 407-555-4321

PATIENT: LOCKSEN, MICHELLE
ACCOUNT/EHR #:   LOCKMI001
DATE: 09/16/18

Attending Physician: Suzanne R. Taylor, MD

This 83-year-old female was admitted to the hospital with acute influenza. She also exhibited an apparent altered mental status.

The following day, her condition deteriorated with distinct signs of septic shock, pneumonia, and hypotension. She later suffered acute renal failure.

DX. Influenza with pneumonia due to *E. coli;* septic shock, acute renal failure

---

Suzanne R. Taylor, MD

SRT/pw   D: 09/16/18 09:50:16   T: 09/18/18 12:55:01

Determine the most accurate ICD-10-CM code(s).

_____

_____

_____

CODING NEOPLASMS

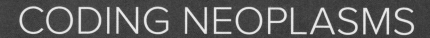

Learning Outcomes
After completing this chapter, the student should be able to:

LO 5.1 Explain the difference between screenings and diagnostic testing.

LO 5.2 Identify the various types of neoplasms: benign and malignant.

LO 5.3 Distinguish between primary and secondary malignancies.

LO 5.4 Determine the proper sequencing of coding multiple neoplasms.

LO 5.5 Apply the guidelines for reporting admissions for chemotherapy and radiation therapies.

LO 5.6 Code and sequence complications associated with malignancies.

When normal cells mutate, they may create a **neoplasm,** also known as a *tumor.* A tumor is an overgrowth or abnormal mass of tissue, and it may be either benign or malignant (cancerous). In all cases, a physician should check the abnormality and determine a course of action.

LO 5.1 Testing

Screenings

You may already know about preventive care and screenings. *Preventive care* consists of health care services designed to help a body stay healthy and not be affected by disease or injury. Examples of this include a flu shot administered so the individual will not get sick with influenza and a helmet worn to prevent traumatic brain injury.

Screenings, on the other hand, are a bit different. Screenings are provided with the intention of identifying a disease or abnormality as early as possible. When a neoplasm is detected and treated early in its formation, the treatment is less intense, making the process easier on the patient and less costly. Also important is the proven fact that the earlier a malignancy is dealt with, the better the chances of recovery and survival. Patients with no signs or symptoms are typically scheduled for various screenings based on guidelines related to age, family history, or personal history.

When you are coding for a patient encounter for a screening for a possible malignant neoplasm, such as a mammogram or a colonoscopy, you will report a code from category:

Z12 Encounter for screening for malignant neoplasms

Key Terms

Benign

Carcinoma

Functional activity

Gross

Histology

Malignant

Mass

Metastasize

Microscopic

Morphology

Neoplasm

Overlapping boundaries

Read the notation directly below this code category:

> **Screening is the testing for disease or disease precursors in asymptomatic individuals so that early detection and treatment can be provided for those who test positive for the disease.**

Also, pay attention to the notation:

> **Use additional code to identify any family history of malignant neoplasm (Z80.-)**

ICD-10-CM reminds you that an additional code should be reported when the prompting factor for the screening is not age but family history. A personal history code (Z85.-) should be reported for those patients who may receive screening tests more frequently than others. For example, a woman with a history of breast cancer may get mammograms every 6 months rather than annually. The personal history of breast cancer code will support medical necessity for this increase in testing.

This code category also carries an *Excludes1* notation to remind you of the difference between a diagnostic test, which is performed when a patient does exhibit signs or symptoms, and a screening test, which is performed with the intention of early detection of disease without signs or symptoms.

> **EXCLUDES1 encounter for diagnostic examination — code to sign or symptom**

Confirming a Diagnosis

Once the patient exhibits signs, such as a lump found during a physical examination or an abnormality identified during a screening test, a pathologist must determine the context of the neoplasm. This is the only way to factually distinguish between benign cells and malignant cells.

There are two types of tissue examination used:

gross
Inspection of the specimen by the naked eye.

microscopic
Inspection of the specimen using a microscope.

- **Gross:** inspection of the specimen by the naked eye.
- **Microscopic:** inspection of the specimen using a microscope.

Generally, specimens may be provided to the laboratory in various forms: blood (capillary or vein), urine, semen, sputum, swabs (that carry tissue cells, pus, or other excretion), or tissue specimens (surgical samples taken during a biopsy). Most often with neoplasms, this will require a biopsy to provide actual specimens of the tissue to be studied. You will need to ensure that an accurate ICD-10-CM diagnosis code is presented with the specimen to confirm medical necessity for the diagnostic testing, such as signs and symptoms.

EXAMPLE

> N63 Unspecified lump in breast
> R94.02 Abnormal brain scan

Blood tests can also provide important information with regard to malignancies in the body. For example, an increased white blood cell (WBC) count, also known as *leukocytosis,* may be a sign of neoplastic cells that have been produced in the bone marrow and released into the bloodstream—common in conditions such as leukemic neoplasia and other myeloproliferative disorders. Many types of pathologic and imaging tests can provide critical information to the physician seeking to confirm, or deny, a diagnosis of a malignancy, depending upon the anatomical site and the type of malignancy (see Table 5-1).

TABLE 5-1 Some Common Tests Performed for Various Types of Malignancies

Malignant Neoplasm of the Cervix

- Abdominal ultrasound
- Cervical biopsy
- Colposcopy
- CT scan of the abdomen and pelvis

Malignant Neoplasm of the Colon and Rectum

- Barium enema
- Carcinoembryonic antigen (CEA)
- Colonoscopy
- Stool for occult blood

Leukemia/Lymphoma

- Blood smear
- Bone marrow biopsy
- Cell surface immunophenotyping
- Cryoglobulins

Malignant Neoplasm of the Lung

- Alpha-1 antitrypsin
- Bone scan
- Bronchoscopy
- Chest x-ray
- Lung biopsy

Malignant Neoplasm of the Ovary

- CA-125
- Laparoscopy
- Paracentesis
- Pyelography

Malignant Neoplasm of the Prostate

- Acid phosphatase
- CT scan of the pelvis
- Cystoscopy
- MRI of the prostate
- Prostate specific antigen (PSA)

You will see pathology reports in the patient's chart, whether you work in a hospital or a physician's office. Some examples are:

- "Histopathology: A punch biopsy of the overlying skin reveals an adenocarcinoma with diffuse involvement of the dermis and extensive invasion of the dermal lymphatics. The adenocarcinoma is composed of irregular nests with some areas forming tubercles. Mitotic figures, including atypical forms, are seen. The tumor was ER −, PR −, Her2 +, CK7 +, and CK 20 −."

- "Tissue biopsy culture: Negative for any growth

  Blood culture: 2/2 positive for *Neisseria meningitidis*

  Lumbar puncture: negative for organisms"

- "Labs: WBC: 8.6, Hgb/Hct: 9.4/26.3, Platelets: 222, BUN: 71, Creatinine: 6.8, U/A: 2+ protein, 3+ blood, ANA: negative, Hepatitis B surface antigen: negative, Hepatitis C antibody: negative, Serum cryoglobulins: negative, HIV: negative, cANCA: positive (1:1280), Tissue culture: negative, Initial blood cultures: negative, CXR: bilateral opacities."

mass
Abnormal collection of tissue.

carcinoma
A malignant neoplasm or cancerous tumor.

malignant
Invasive and destructive characteristic of a neoplasm; possibly causing damage or death.

benign
Nonmalignant characteristic of a neoplasm; not infectious or spreading.

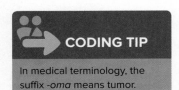
CODING TIP

In medical terminology, the suffix -oma means tumor.

LO 5.2 Neoplasms

Once a diagnosis is confirmed, you will need to accurately report it with the specific code or codes. Begin by ensuring you understand the details.

In some cases, you will see the term **mass** used to describe a patient's condition. Mass is *not* the same as a neoplasm. More often, mass is used to identify a cyst or other thickening of tissue.

While many people think that *neoplasm* and *cancer* are synonymous, they are not. Cancer is the common term for **carcinoma** (see Figure 5-1).

Neoplasms might be **malignant** or **benign** or have aspects of both characteristics. In diagnoses, neoplasms are also defined by individual name. The physician's notes may state one of the following:

- Adenoma
- Melanoma
- Leukemia
- Papilloma

When you see terms like those in the previous list, it is better to look for that specific term in the Alphabetic Index first, before looking under the term *neoplasm*. One of the most important reasons for doing so is to find additional information to help you code more accurately.

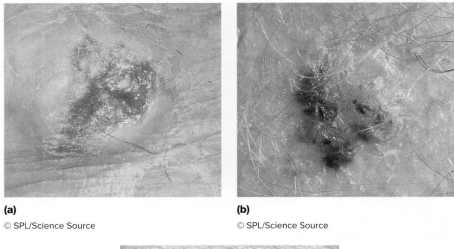

(a)
© SPL/Science Source

(b)
© SPL/Science Source

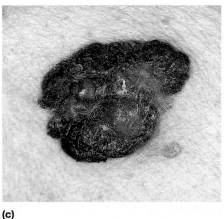

(c)
© SPL/Science Source

FIGURE 5-1 Types of Skin Cancer: (a) squamous cell carcinoma; (b) basal cell carcinoma; (c) malignant melanoma

Earl Show, a 46-year-old male, comes to see Dr. Lee to get the results of his biopsy. Dr. Lee explains that Earl has an alpha cell adenoma of the pancreas. Dr. Lee spends 30 minutes discussing treatment options.

Let's Code It!

Dr. Lee has diagnosed Earl with an *alpha cell adenoma of the pancreas.* You have been working with Dr. Lee as his coder for a while, so you know that an adenoma is a neoplasm, but what kind of neoplasm is it—benign or malignant? To help you determine this, instead of going to *neoplasm,* let's see if there is a listing in the Alphabetic Index under *adenoma.* When you find *adenoma,* the book refers you to:

> *see also* Neoplasm, benign, by site

This tells you an adenoma is a benign tumor. Or you can continue down this list to the indented term, and find:

> Adenoma, alpha-cell, pancreas D13.7

Turn to the Tabular List and read the complete description of code category D13:

> **D13 Benign neoplasm of other and ill-defined parts of digestive system**
>
> **D13.7 Benign neoplasm of endocrine pancreas**

That matches Dr. Lee's diagnosis. Good job!

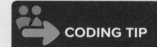

CODING TIP

Always begin with the terms the physician writes in his or her notes. Then, only when that does not bring you to an accurate code, you can look up alternate terms. This rule of thumb will save you a lot of time.

The Neoplasm Table

Another way to look up a diagnosis of a tumor in the ICD-10-CM book is to follow the Alphabetic Index's notation to turn to *neoplasm* in the Alphabetic Index. Here, you see a table.

In the first column of this table, neoplasms are listed by anatomical site (the part of the body where the tumor is located) in alphabetic order. To the right of the first column, you see six columns across: Malignant Primary, Malignant Secondary, Ca in situ, Benign, Uncertain, and Unspecified Behavior. Let's review each of these titles (see Figure 5-2).

LO 5.3 Malignant Primary

The term *primary* indicates the anatomical site (the place in the body) where the malignant neoplasm was first seen and identified. If the physician's notes do not specify primary or secondary, then the site mentioned is primary.

Malignant Secondary

The term *secondary* identifies the anatomical site to which the malignancy **metastasized.** One very strange thing about cancerous cells is that they travel through the body and do not necessarily spread to adjoining body parts. Cancer can be identified in the breast as the primary site and metastasize to the liver without actually interacting with anything in between. Notes will state that a site is "secondary to" *(primary site),* "metastasized from" *(primary site),* or *(primary site)* "metastasized to" *(secondary site).*

The terms *disseminated cancer, generalized cancer,* or *widely metastatic* would indicate that the malignancy has infiltrated the body throughout and affects all or most

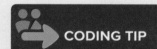

CODING TIP

To determine the code to report a neoplasm, you need to know:

- Where in the body (specifically, which anatomical site) is the neoplasm located?
- Is the neoplasm benign, malignant, in situ, or uncertain? Uncertain is a pathologic determination and is *not* the same as unspecified.
- If the neoplasm is malignant, is this the first diagnosis of malignancy for this patient? If so, this is the primary site. If not, this is a secondary malignancy because it metastasized from the primary.

metastasize
To proliferate, reproduce, or spread.

ICD-10-CM TABLE of NEOPLASMS

The list below gives the code numbers for neoplasms by anatomical site. For each site there are six possible code numbers according to whether the neoplasm in question is malignant, benign, in situ, of uncertain behavior, or of unspecified nature. The description of the neoplasm will often indicate which of the six columns is appropriate; e.g., malignant melanoma of skin, benign fibroadenoma of breast, carcinoma in situ of cervix uteri.

Where such descriptors are not present, the remainder of the Index should be consulted where guidance is given to the appropriate column for each morphological (histological) variety listed; e.g., Mesonephroma—see Neoplasm, malignant; Embryoma—see also Neoplasm, uncertain behavior; Disease, Bowen's—see Neoplasm, skin, in situ. However, the guidance in the Index can be overridden if one of the descriptors mentioned above is present; e.g., malignant adenoma of colon is coded to C18.9 and not to D12.6 as the adjective "malignant" overrides the Index entry "Adenoma—see also Neoplasm, benign."

Codes listed with a dash—following the code have a required additional character for laterality. The tabular must be reviewed for the complete code.

	Malignant Primary	Malignant Secondary	Ca in situ	Benign	Uncertain Behavior	Unspecified Behavior
Neoplasm, neoplastic	C80.1	C79.9	D09.9	D36.9	D48.9	D49.9
abdomen, abdominal	C76.2	C79.8—	D09.8	D36.7	D48.7	D49.89
cavity	C76.2	C79.8—	D09.8	D36.7	D48.7	D49.89
organ	C76.2	C79.8—	D09.8	D36.7	D48.7	D49.89
viscera	C76.2	C79.8—	D09.8	D36.7	D48.7	D49.89
wall—*see also Neoplasm, abdomen, wall, skin*	C44.509	C79.2—	D04.5	D23.5	D48.5	D49.2
connective tissue	C49.4	C79.8—	—	D21.4	D48.1	D49.2
skin	C44.509					
basal cell carcinoma	C44.519	—	—	—	—	—
specified type NEC	C44.599	—	—	—	—	—
squamous cell carcinoma	C44.529	—	—	—	—	—
abdominopelvic	C76.8	C79.8—	—	D36.7	D48.7	D49.89
accessory sinus—*see Neoplasm, sinus*						
acoustic nerve	C72.4—	C79.49	—	D33.3	D43.3	D49.7
adenoid (pharynx) (tissue)	C11.1	C79.89	D00.08	D10.6	D37.05	D49.0
adipose tissue—*see also Neoplasm, connective tissue*	C49.4	C79.89	—	D21.9	D48.1	D49.2
adnexa (uterine)	C57.4	C79.89	D07.39	D28.7	D39.8	D49.5
adrenal	C74.9—	C79.7—	D09.3	D35.0—	D44.1—	D49.7
capsule	C74.9—	C79.7—	D09.3	D35.0—	D44.1—	D49.7
cortex	C74.0—	C79.7—	D09.3	D35.0—	D44.1—	D49.7
gland	C74.9—	C79.7—	D09.3	D35.0—	D44.1—	D49.7
medulla	C74.1—	C79.7—	D09.3	D35.0—	D44.1—	D49.7
ala nasi (external)—*see also Neoplasm, skin, nose*	C44.301	C79.2	D04.39	D23.39	D48.5	D49.2
alimentary canal or tract NEC	C26.9	C78.80	D01.9	D13.9	D37.9	D49.0
alveolar	C03.9	C79.89	D00.03	D10.39	D37.09	D49.0
mucosa	C03.9	C79.89	D00.03	D10.39	D37.09	D49.0
lower	C03.1	C79.89	D00.03	D10.39	D37.09	D49.0
upper	C03.0	C79.89	D00.03	D10.39	D37.09	D49.0
ridge or process	C41.1	C79.51	—	D16.5—	D48.0	D49.2
carcinoma	C03.9	C79.8—	—	—	—	—
lower	C03.1	C79.8—	—	—	—	—
upper	C03.0	C79.8—	—	—	—	—

Page 1

FIGURE 5-2 The Neoplasm Table, in Part

of the patient's anatomy. That would be coded as a malignant neoplasm without specification of site (code C80.0). In such cases, it is not that the physician forgot to specify the site. It is that there are too many sites to list.

Ca in Situ

The term *Ca in situ* indicates that the tumor has undergone malignant changes but is still limited to the site where it originated (i.e., it has not spread). *Ca* is short for carcinoma, and you can remember *situ* as in the word *situated*. So think of it as a cancerous tumor that is staying in place.

Benign

As you learned earlier, the term *benign* means there is no indication of invasion of adjacent cells. Generally, benign means not cancerous.

Uncertain

The classification *uncertain* indicates that the pathologist is not able to specifically determine whether a tumor is benign or malignant because indicators of both are present.

Unspecified Behavior

Choose codes in the "Unspecified Behavior" column when the physician's notes do not include any specific information regarding the nature of the tumor. Before choosing a code from the column, please query the physician and make certain that a laboratory report is not available or on its way with the information you need.

LET'S CODE IT! SCENARIO

Stephen Mathis is a 44-year-old male who is seen by his regular primary care physician, Dr. Fornari. After the imaging and laboratory test results come back, Stephen is diagnosed with a benign neoplasm of the ascending colon.

Let's Code It!

Dr. Fornari diagnosed Stephen with *a benign neoplasm of the ascending colon.* Turn to the Neoplasm Table in the Alphabetic Index. Go down the list of anatomical sites until you reach *colon.* There is a notation that directs you to "*see also* Neoplasm, intestine, large." The ascending colon is actually the portion of the large intestine that goes from the cecum to the transverse colon. Indented under *colon* are the words *and rectum.* Go back to Dr. Fornari's notes. His diagnosis does not include the rectum, so follow the book's advice and turn to the listing for *intestine, large,* and find out what is shown there.

Continue through the list until you get to *intestine, intestinal.* Beneath the term *intestine,* you will find the word *large* indented. Indented under *large* is *colon.* Indented under *colon,* you see *ascending.* This matches Dr. Fornari's diagnosis of Stephen's neoplasm exactly! Now, go across the table to the right to the "Benign" column. Here, the code D12.2 is suggested. Remember the rule: Never, never code from the Alphabetic Index, and that includes the Neoplasm Table, so turn to the Tabular List to confirm this suggested code. Start reading at the three-character code category:

D12 Benign neoplasm of colon, rectum, anus, and anal canal

The *excludes* note does not relate to this patient's diagnosis for this encounter, so continue reading down the column to review all of the choices for the required fourth character.

D12.2 Benign neoplasm of ascending colon

Good coding!

Functional Activity

functional activity
Glandular secretion in abnormal quantity.

Certain neoplasms require an additional code to report **functional activity.** Take a look at the beginning of the Tabular List, Neoplasms (directly above code C00). There are several notes here to help you find the most accurate neoplasm code. Take a look at number 2, Functional activity. This note states, "An additional code from chapter 4 may be used to identify such functional activity associated with any neoplasm." Chapter 4 of the ICD-10-CM Tabular List is titled: Endocrine, nutritional, and metabolic diseases (E00–E89). The note beneath the heading for Chapter 4 (directly above code E00) reminds you of this detail:

> **Note: All neoplasms, whether functionally active or not, are classified in Chapter 2. Appropriate codes in this chapter (i.e. E05.8, E07.0, E16—E31.—) may be used as additional codes to indicate either functional activity by neoplasms and ectopic endocrine tissue or hyperfunction and hypofunction of endocrine glands associated with neoplasms and other conditions classified elsewhere.**

What the note means is that if a patient has been diagnosed with a neoplasm affecting the individual's glandular function, you have to identify the functional activity (of the gland) with an additional code.

For example, take a look beneath code category C56, Malignant neoplasm of ovary. There is a notation that says:

> **Use additional code to identify any functional activity**

This note regarding functional activity also appears under the following terms:

Benign neoplasm of ovary

Malignant neoplasm of endocrine glands

Benign neoplasm of endocrine glands

Malignant neoplasm of islets of Langerhans

Benign neoplasm of islets of Langerhans

Malignant neoplasm of the testis

Benign neoplasm of the testis

Malignant neoplasm of thyroid glands

Benign neoplasm of thyroid glands

EXAMPLE

Catecholamine-producing malignant pheochromocytoma of thyroid

C73 Malignant neoplasm of thyroid gland

E27.5 Adrenomedullary hyperfunction

Ovarian carcinoma, right side, with hyperestrogenism

C56.1 Malignant neoplasm of right ovary

E28.0 Hyperestrogenism (estrogen excess)

Basophil adenoma of pituitary with Cushing's disease

C75.1 Benign neoplasm of pituitary gland

E24.0 Cushing's syndrome

LET'S CODE IT! SCENARIO

Taylor Chattman, a 37-year-old male, came to see Dr. Bornstein for a checkup. He was diagnosed with functioning thyroid carcinoma. Dr. Bornstein reviews with Taylor the results of his latest thyroid scan, TSH and TRH stimulation tests and an ultrasonogram and inform him that Taylor has developed hyperthyroidism.

Let's Code It!

Dr. Bornstein has diagnosed Taylor with *functioning thyroid carcinoma* and *hyperthyroidism*. The hyperthyroidism is the functional activity of the thyroid carcinoma. Turn to the Alphabetic Index and look for:

Carcinoma—*see also* Neoplasm, by site, malignant

Look down the list. Neither the term *functioning* nor the term *thyroid* is shown here, so you will need to turn to the Neoplasm Table and find:

Neoplasm, thyroid, malignant, primary C73

Let's go to the Tabular List, to confirm:

C73 Malignant neoplasm of thyroid gland
Use additional code to identify any functional activity

This code is correct, and the ICD-10-CM book is telling you that you need an additional code to report the functional activity. The only other detail Dr. Bornstein included in her diagnostic statement is hyperthyroidism. Turn back to the Alphabetic Index, and look up hyperthyroidism:

Hyperthyroidism (latent) (preadult) (recurrent) E05.90

Turn to the Tabular List to confirm this suggested code.

E05 Thyrotoxicosis [hyperthyroidism]

The *excludes* note mentions nothing that relates to this encounter for our patient, so read down the column to review the choices for the required fourth character.

E05.9 Thyrotoxicosis unspecified

This matches the notes, so you are in the correct place. The symbol to the left of the code tells you that an additional character is required. There is nothing beneath this code, so you will need to read up the column until you find the box, directly below code E05.9, that provides your choices.

E05.90 Thyrotoxicosis unspecified without mention of thyrotoxic crisis or storm

Did you notice that this code is located in chapter 4 and is describing the functional activity of the neoplasm? Great! The two diagnosis codes for Taylor's claim are C73 and E05.90.

Overlapping Boundaries

The nature of a malignant neoplasm includes its potential to spread to adjoining tissue. As you learned earlier in this chapter, you code malignancies by their anatomical site in the order in which the malignancy developed: primary and secondary. However, there are cases where the condition of the patient involves more than one code subcategory. Neoplasms with **overlapping boundaries,** also known as *contiguous,* may blur the anatomical descriptors.

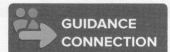

See the ICD-10-CM Official Coding Guidelines: Section I.C.2, Chapter 2: **Neoplasms,** under **General Guidelines:** "Primary malignant neoplasms overlapping site boundaries."

> ## EXAMPLE
>
> C60.8 Malignant neoplasm of overlapping sites of penis
> C76.8 Malignant neoplasm of other specified ill-defined sites (Malignant neoplasm of overlapping ill-defined sites)
> C83.78 Burkitt lymphoma, lymph nodes of multiple sites

For cases in which the physician cannot identify a specific site, usually because the malignancy has metastasized so dramatically, the code category C76 enables you to report the malignancy identifying only the section of the patient's body, such as head, abdomen, or lower limb.

> ## EXAMPLE
>
> C76.0 Malignant neoplasm of head, face, and neck
> C76.51 Malignant neoplasm of right lower limb

Neoplasms and Morphology Codes (M Codes)

In addition to the code for a neoplasm, you may be required to include an M code. The *M* stands for **morphology,** and the M code identifies the behavior and **histology** of the neoplasm.

"Morphology of Neoplasms" is available as a separate book, the *International Classification of Diseases for Oncology* (ICD-O). Morphology codes are not structured like the other diagnosis codes. The codes always begin with the letter "M," which is followed by four characters, a slash (/), and a single character. The neoplasm's histology is described by the first four characters of the M code.

> ## EXAMPLE
>
> Craniopharyngioma M9350/1

Some of the M code categories include:

M800 Neoplasms NOS
M809–M811 Basal cell neoplasms
M880 Soft tissue tumors and sarcomas NOS

> ## EXAMPLE
>
> Craniopharyngioma M9350/**1**

The single number, shown after the slash of the M code, describes the behavior of the neoplasm. The numbers represent:

/0 Benign

/1 Uncertain behavior whether benign or malignant; borderline malignancy

/2 Carcinoma in situ; intraepithelial; noninfiltrating; noninvasive

/3 Malignant, primary site

/6 Malignant, metastatic site; secondary site

/9 Malignant, uncertain whether primary or metastatic site

In our example, the behavior of this neoplasm is *uncertain behavior,* as indicated by the number 1 after the slash.

M codes are used for providing specific data about the site (topography) and the histology (morphology) of the affected tissue to tumor and cancer registries. Pathologists may also use the codes to provide more detail about a particular tissue sample. Normally, M codes are not used for reimbursement and are not placed on insurance claim forms.

LO 5.4 Coding Sequences

When you are coding encounters with a patient diagnosed with a neoplasm, our basic rule still applies. The principal diagnosis code should answer the question, "Why did the health care professional care for this patient today?"

When multiple issues are addressed during the visit, you report the primary site of malignancy first, followed by any secondary sites, in order of severity, and then anatomy (most severe first, top of the body first). As you know, however, every rule has an exception. When only the secondary site and not the primary site of a neoplasm is treated, you should list the secondary neoplasm first, followed by the code for the primary site.

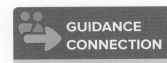

GUIDANCE CONNECTION

Review the ICD-10-CM Coding Guidelines, Section I.C.2, Chapter 2: **Neoplasms,** Subsection I, **Sequencing of neoplasm codes.**

LET'S CODE IT! SCENARIO

Sean O'Boyle, a 30-year-old male, presents today with concerns of a recurrent incident of cancer. He was diagnosed with osteogenic sarcoma of the left femur 3 years ago and went through a treatment sequence of surgery and chemotherapy. After reviewing his symptoms and running a battery of tests, Dr. Hostetler confirms the presence of chondrosarcoma of the ribs, secondary to osteogenic sarcoma. Dr. Hostetler discusses his recommendation of a surgical resection of the ribs, to be followed by radiation and chemotherapy treatments. Dr. Hostetler paid no attention to the previous diagnosis of osteogenic sarcoma.

Let's Code It!

Dr. Hostetler diagnosed Sean with *chondrosarcoma of the ribs, secondary to osteogenic sarcoma.* As you learned earlier in this chapter, this means that the primary site of the neoplasm is the osteogenic sarcoma, a malignant bone cancer most often in the ends of the long bones. Dr. Hostetler's notes specify the femur—a long bone in the thigh. In addition, the secondary site is documented as a chondrosarcoma of the ribs. A chondrosarcoma is a malignancy that forms in cartilage cells. Let's find the codes.

In the Alphabetic Index, next to the list for *osteosarcoma* (the combined form of osteogenic sarcoma), the notation states, "*See* Neoplasm, bone, malignant." Now turn to the Neoplasm Table in the Alphabetic Index and find *neoplasm, bone*. Beneath it, indented, find the anatomical site of Sean's osteosarcoma—his left *femur*. Look across the line to the "Malignant Primary" column. The code C40.2 is suggested. Let's turn to the Tabular List to confirm the code:

C40 Malignant neoplasm of bone and articular cartilage of limbs

This time, you have *excludes* notes above and below this code to read. None of these diagnoses relate to this case, so read down the column to review the choices for the required additional characters.

C40.22 Malignant neoplasm of long bones of left lower limb

Now you need to find the code for the second issue. Under *chondrosarcoma,* in the Alphabetic Index, the notation states, "*See also* Neoplasm, cartilage, malignant." At the Neoplasm Table, find *cartilage,* and then look for the anatomical part in which Sean was found to have chondrosarcoma—his ribs. Move across the line to the "Malignant Secondary" column this time, and find the suggested code C79.51. Confirm the code by looking at the complete code description in the Tabular List:

C79 Secondary malignant neoplasm of other and unspecified sites

There are a couple of *excludes* notes but they don't relate to this case, so read down the column and review all of the choices for the required additional characters.

C79.51 Secondary malignant neoplasm, bone

Good work! You have determined both diagnostic codes for Sean's encounter with Dr. Hostetler. However, you still must determine the order in which to list the two codes. When you go back to the notes for the visit, you read that Dr. Hostetler specifically mentions that *no attention to the previous diagnosis of osteogenic sarcoma* was provided. Our rule is that the first-listed code should identify the main reason why Sean came to see Dr. Hostetler. This rule is in sync with the exception to the neoplasm rule that tells you to code the condition that was the focus of treatment first. So the correct order of the codes is C79.51 followed by C40.22. You are doing a great job!

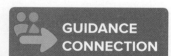

GUIDANCE CONNECTION

Review the ICD-10-CM Coding Guidelines, Section I.C.2, Chapter 2: **Neoplasms,** Subsection d, **Primary malignancy previously excised.**

Excised Malignancies

Thanks to modern medical science and technology, health care professionals are more successful than ever at getting rid of certain neoplasms (tumors), often by excising them, or cutting them out. When that happens, the patient no longer has the site of the malignancy and, therefore, can no longer have that condition. At that time, the code will change from a malignancy code (C00–C96) to a personal history of a malignancy code (category Z85).

EXAMPLE

Mary Alice Arkin was diagnosed with a malignant neoplasm of the central portion of the left breast. The diagnosis code was:

C50.112 Malignant neoplasm of central portion of left female breast

She underwent a mastectomy, a surgical procedure to remove her breast. Once the anatomical site (her breast) that contained the malignant neoplasm was removed, she no longer had the disease. From this point on, the diagnosis code is:

Z85.3 Personal history of malignant neoplasm, breast

Suppose a patient has a primary site of malignancy and the disease has already metastasized to a second location; if the primary site is removed, the secondary malignancy is still coded as secondary but listed first. Confusing? Let's look at an example.

EXAMPLE

Joshua Miller was diagnosed with prostate cancer. It spread to his liver before he was able to have surgery. The diagnosis codes, in this sequence, are:

C61 Malignant neoplasm of the prostate

C78.7 Secondary malignant neoplasm of liver, and intrahepatic bile duct

Dr. Farina removes Joshua's prostate successfully. The new codes are:

C78.7 Secondary malignant neoplasm of liver, and intrahepatic bile duct

Z85.46 Personal history of malignant neoplasm, prostate

Once Joshua has the site of his primary malignancy removed, his prostate condition becomes "history." His secondary malignancy in the liver moves up in order, but it will always be the *second* site at which Joshua developed a malignancy.

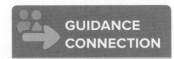

GUIDANCE CONNECTION

Review the ICD-10-CM Coding Guidelines, Section I.C.2.b, **Treatment of secondary site.**

YOU CODE IT! CASE STUDY

Randolph Holloway, a 47-year-old male, came to see Dr. Johnson, his dermatologist, for an annual checkup. Two years ago, Dr. Johnson removed a malignant melanoma from Randolph's left forearm. The malignancy was totally removed, but he comes to see his physician for a checkup once a year.

You Code It!

Go through the steps of coding, and determine the diagnosis code or codes that should be reported for this encounter between Dr. Johnson and Randolph Holloway.

Step 1: Read the case completely.

Step 2: Abstract the notes: Which key words can you identify relating to why Dr. Johnson cared for Randolph?

_____

Step 3: Query the provider, if necessary.

Step 4: Code the diagnosis or diagnoses.

_____

Step 5: Code the procedure(s): Annual dermatologic evaluation.

Step 6: Link the procedure codes to at least one diagnosis code to confirm medical necessity.

Step 7: Back code to double-check your choices.

Answer:

Did you determine the following diagnosis code?

Z85.820 Personal history of malignant melanoma of skin

Good job!

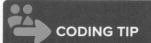

CODING TIP

Professional coding specialists must be cautious when determining the difference between a patient in remission and a patient with a personal history of a condition, such as leukemia. If the documentation is not absolutely clear on this, the physician must be queried. There is a big difference between these two diagnostic identifications.

Prophylactic Organ Removal

Advances in science have given us genetic predisposition testing and other identification exams. The information, along with personal and family histories, enables patients and health care professionals to predict an individual's risk for cancer and other diseases more accurately. Studies show, for example, that a woman who has inherited a mutation in the BRCA1 or BRCA2 gene faces a dramatically higher risk for developing breast cancer by age 65. A strong family history of colon cancer may lead an individual to be tested for a variant in the APC gene. There are many others that can now be tested.

Prophylactic, or preventive, surgery can reduce the risk by as much as 90%. In the case of breast cancer, it would mean having a double mastectomy (the surgical removal of both breasts) while they are still healthy and without any signs or symptoms of carcinoma.

As a coder, the question becomes, How do you code a diagnosis for a surgical procedure on a healthy anatomical site? Of course, you will use:

Z40.0 Encounter for prophylactic surgery for risk factors related to malignant neoplasms (Admission for prophylactic organ removal) *Use additional code to identify risk factor*

For those patients who have had genetic testing with a confirmed abnormal gene, you will also use a second code from category Z15, Genetic susceptibility to disease.

If the reason for the preventive surgery is due to a family history of cancer, you will add another code from the Z80, Family history of primary malignant neoplasm, category.

YOU CODE IT! CASE STUDY

Janis Olivette, a 29-year-old female, was admitted today for the prophylactic removal of her breasts. Her grandmother, mother, and sister have all had breast cancer, so she had genetic testing performed, indicating that she did have a genetic susceptibility to breast cancer. She elected to have the surgery instead of taking chances with her health.

You Code It!

Go through the steps of coding, and determine the diagnosis code or codes that should be reported for Janis Olivette's surgery.

Step 1: Read the case completely.

Step 2: Abstract the notes: Which key words can you identify relating to why Janis was admitted into the hospital?

Step 3: Query the provider, if necessary.

Step 4: Code the diagnosis or diagnoses.

Step 5: Code the procedure(s): Double mastectomy.

Step 6: Link the procedure codes to at least one diagnosis code to confirm medical necessity.

Step 7: Back code to double-check your choices.

Answer:

Did you determine the following diagnosis codes?

Z40.01 Prophylactic removal of breast

Z15.01 Genetic susceptibility to malignant neoplasm of breast

Z80.3 Family history of malignant neoplasm, breast

Good job!

LO 5.5 Chemotherapy and Radiation Therapy

Patients diagnosed with a malignancy often undergo chemotherapy and/or radiation therapy. During the course of treatment, the patient may be admitted into the hospital for the treatment and then discharged. When the only treatment or service provided for the patient during this stay at the hospital is the administration of the chemotherapy or radiation, you will code the chemotherapy or radiotherapy first and then the malignancy or malignancies being treated.

GUIDANCE CONNECTION

Review the ICD-10-CM Coding Guidelines, Section I.C.2, Chapter 2: **Neoplasms,** subsection e, **Admissions/ encounters involving chemotherapy, immunotherapy and radiation therapy.**

EXAMPLE

Douglas Brunner is admitted into the hospital for administration of chemotherapy for malignant neoplasm of the pharynx.

Z51.11 Encounter for antineoplastic chemotherapy

C14.0 Malignant neoplasm of pharynx, unspecified

In some cases, a patient is admitted into the hospital for surgical treatment of a malignancy with the plan to have chemotherapy or radiation follow immediately (during the same admission). In such cases, the standard coding rule will hold true. Why did the patient come to the hospital? To have a malignancy treated. How was this treated? First, surgery and then chemotherapy or radiation. Therefore, the code for the malignancy will be listed first, followed by the code for the chemotherapy or radiation.

EXAMPLE

Glynnis Gallimore is admitted to the hospital for the surgical removal of the navicular of her right ankle. Dr. Faison scheduled Glynnis to begin radiation treatments after the surgery has been successfully completed.

C40.31 Malignant neoplasm of short bones of right lower limb

Z51.0 Encounter for antineoplastic radiation therapy

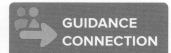

GUIDANCE CONNECTION

Review the ICD-10-CM Official Coding Guidelines: Section I.C.2.c, **Coding and sequencing of complications.**

Should the patient develop complications as a result of the chemotherapy or radiotherapy while still in the hospital and getting treatment, you will still code the Z51 code first and follow that with the appropriate code or codes for the symptoms, such as uncontrolled nausea and vomiting or dehydration. The code for the malignancy being treated by the radiation or chemotherapy should be listed after that.

LO 5.6 Admissions for Treatment of Complications

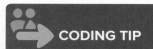

CODING TIP

To determine the correct code for an admission of a patient with a complication and a malignancy, you must identify whether both conditions were treated or only the complication. This will affect the sequencing of the codes.

Treatment for malignancies can wreak havoc on a patient's body. Complications of either the malignancy itself, surgical treatment of the malignancy, or chemotherapy/radiation treatments may need attention. In those cases, when the patient is treated for the complication, such as anemia or dehydration, the code for the complication should be listed first, followed by the code for the malignancy.

However, if the admission is for treatment of the malignancy and complications are *also* treated, then you must code the malignancy first, followed by the code or codes for the complications.

EXAMPLE

Lorina Lardner was admitted to the hospital for surgical treatment of a melanoma on her upper lip. While Lorina was there, Dr. Bowen treated her anemia, which she developed as a result of the chemotherapy.

C44.09 Other specified malignant neoplasm of skin of lip
D64.81 Anemia due to antineoplastic chemotherapy

YOU CODE IT! CASE STUDY

Kirby Graham has been receiving chemotherapy treatments for the last 6 weeks. He was diagnosed with malignant neoplasm of the pyloric canal 3 months ago. After Kirby began showing signs of dehydration, Dr. Rodriguez admitted him into the hospital for intravenous rehydration. He was discharged the next day.

You Code It!

Read Dr. Rodriguez's notes on his encounter with Kirby Graham, and find the best, most appropriate diagnosis code or codes.

Step 1: Read the case completely.

Step 2: Abstract the notes: Which key words can you identify relating to why Dr. Rodriguez cared for Kirby?

_____

Step 3: Query the provider, if necessary.

Step 4: Code the diagnosis or diagnoses.

_____

Step 5: Code the procedure(s): Intravenous rehydration.

Step 6: Link the procedure codes to at least one diagnosis code to confirm medical necessity.

Step 7: Back code to double-check your choices.

Answer:

Did you determine the following diagnosis codes?

E86.0 Volume depletion, dehydration

C16.4 Malignant neoplasm of pylorus

Good job!

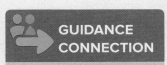

GUIDANCE CONNECTION

Review the ICD-10-CM Official Coding Guidelines: Section I.C.2.c(3), **Management of dehydration due to the malignancy.**

Chapter Summary

In this chapter, you learned how to identify the key words in physicians' notes and lab reports that can guide you toward the most accurate code. You learned the differences in the types of neoplasms, the proper sequencing of codes, and how to use morphology codes. In addition, you reviewed the correct way to code a patient's admission for various treatments and the services rendered for complications of those treatments.

There have been, and continue to be, incredible advancements made in the treatments of all types of neoplasms, as well as modifications to sociological behaviors to help prevent the development of those insidious health concerns. As a professional coding specialist, your ability to properly code the diagnostic tests and procedures used in the care of individuals can open many job opportunities for you.

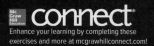

Using Terminology

Match each key term to the appropriate definition.

_____ **1.** LO 5.2 Invasive and destructive characteristic of a neoplasm; possibly causing damage or death.

_____ **2.** LO 5.3 Glandular secretion in abnormal quantity.

_____ **3.** LO 5.2 Nonmalignant characteristic of a neoplasm; not infectious or spreading.

_____ **4.** LO 5.1 Inspection of the specimen by the naked eye.

_____ **5.** LO 5.2 A malignant neoplasm or cancerous tumor.

_____ **6.** LO 5.1 Abnormal tissue growth; tumor.

_____ **7.** LO 5.3 To proliferate, reproduce, or spread.

_____ **8.** LO 5.3 The study of the microscopic composition of tissues.

_____ **9.** LO 5.1 Inspection of the specimen using a microscope.

_____ **10.** LO 5.3 Multiple sites of carcinoma without identifiable borders.

_____ **11.** LO 5.2 Abnormal collection of tissue.

_____ **12.** LO 5.3 The study of the configuration or structure of living organisms.

A. Benign

B. Carcinoma

C. Functional activity

D. Gross

E. Histology

F. Malignant

G. Mass

H. Metastasize

I. Microscopic

J. Morphology

K. Neoplasm

L. Overlapping boundaries

Checking Your Understanding

Choose the most appropriate answer for each of the following questions.

1. LO 5.1/5.2 A neoplasm is the same as a

　a. tumor.

　b. cancer.

　c. malignancy.

　d. metastasis.

2. LO 5.2 Different types of neoplasms include all of the following *except*

　a. adenoma.

　b. melanoma.

　c. carcinoma.

　d. chemotherapy.

3. LO 5.2/5.3 The column title of the Neoplasm Table that does *not* identify a malignancy is

　a. primary.

　b. benign.

　c. Ca in situ.

　d. secondary.

4. LO 5.3 Morphology codes are used

   a. for reimbursement.
   b. to describe treatment.
   c. to describe the behavior and histology of the neoplasm.
   d. for identification of manifestations.

5. LO 5.4 At subsequent encounters after the surgical removal of a neoplasm, the diagnosis code changes to a

   a. personal history of malignancy code.
   b. malignancy code.
   c. late effects code.
   d. co-morbidity code.

6. LO 5.5 When a patient is admitted for chemotherapy to treat a malignant neoplasm and that is the extent of treatment, the first code listed is the code for

   a. the primary malignancy.
   b. the secondary malignancy.
   c. the chemotherapy.
   d. observation in a hospital.

7. LO 5.6 When a patient is treated for a complication, such as anemia or dehydration, the code for this complication should be listed

   a. after the primary malignancy.
   b. first.
   c. after the chemotherapy or radiation code.
   d. as a Z code.

8. LO 5.3 Metastasized means

   a. spread.
   b. noncancerous.
   c. malignant.
   d. measured.

9. LO 5.3 The term *disseminated cancer* has the same meaning as

   a. widely metastatic.
   b. Ca in situ.
   c. uncertain behavior.
   d. unspecified.

10. LO 5.2/5.3 When coding a neoplasm, you must know

    a. the anatomical site.
    b. whether it is primary or secondary.
    c. whether it is benign or malignant.
    d. all of these.

Applying Your Knowledge

1. LO 5.2 Explain the difference between benign and malignant. _____

_____

2. LO 5.2 What three questions should you ask when reporting a neoplasm? _____

_____

3. LO 5.3 Explain the difference between primary, secondary, and Ca in situ. _____

_____

4. LO 5.3 Explain what overlapping boundaries are, and give another term for overlapping boundaries. _____

_____

5. LO 5.3 What is morphology, and why is it important? _____

_____

YOU CODE IT! Practice

Chapter 5: Coding Neoplasms

Using the techniques described in this chapter, carefully read through the case studies and determine the most accurate ICD-10-CM code(s) and external cause code(s), if appropriate, for each case study.

1. Scott Mercado was diagnosed with a malignancy of his pancreatic duct.

   _____

2. Dorinna Ziegler was diagnosed with bronchial adenoma.

   _____

3. Jonathan Jones, a 47-year-old male, was diagnosed with a malignant neoplasm of cerebral meninges metastasized from the left breast; both sites are being addressed in today's encounter.

   _____

4. Tina Baker was diagnosed with carcinoma in situ of the left eye.

   _____

5. Glenn Shutts was diagnosed with lymphoid leukemia now in remission.

   _____

6. Dr. Shaughnessy diagnosed Harriet Hubbell with a nonspecific tumor of the hilus lung.

   _____

7. Jeffrey Sharp was diagnosed with a malignant lymphosarcoma B-precursor.

   _____

8. Susan Kasbeer was told she had a carcinoma in situ of the vermilion border of her lower lip.

   _____

9. Thomas Kelly was diagnosed with a subcutaneous lipoma of the face.

   _____

10. Marissa Kirby was diagnosed with malignant ovarian cancer, left ovary.

   _____

11. Greg Phillips was told he had a benign neoplasm of the occipital bone.

_____

12. Davida Phillips developed a malignant tumor in her left lung that metastasized from the cancer she has in her upper-inner quadrant of her right breast. The lung tumor is being addressed in today's encounter.

_____

13. Marcelo Allen was diagnosed with an oat cell carcinoma in the upper lobe of his left lung.

_____

14. Barbara Shires was diagnosed with carcinoma of the right ovary with extensive metastasis to the omentum. Both sites are being addressed in today's encounter.

_____

15. Arlene Addenson was diagnosed with carcinoma in situ of the endocervix.

_____

YOU CODE IT! Application

Chapter 5: Coding Neoplasms

The following exercises provide practice in abstracting physicians' notes and learning to work with SOAP notes from our health care facility, *Taylor, Reader, & Associates*. These case studies (SOAP notes) are modeled on real patient encounters. Using the techniques described in this chapter, carefully read through the case studies and determine the most accurate ICD-10-CM code(s) and external cause code(s), if appropriate, for each case study.

TAYLOR, READER, & ASSOCIATES
A Complete Health Care Facility
975 CENTRAL AVENUE • SOMEWHERE, FL 32811 • 407-555-4321

PATIENT: MERCHANE, REBECCA
ACCOUNT/EHR #:   MERCRE001
DATE: 09/16/18

Attending Physician: Suzanne R. Taylor, MD

HPI: This patient will present to McGraw Medical Center for wide excision of a melanoma which is reported verbally as level 2, of the right side of the face. She comes here through the courtesy of Dr. Patton for its evaluation. Apparently she has had this lesion for what she describes as her whole life, but Dr. Patton felt rather uneasy about it and biopsied it and discovered it was a level 2 melanoma.

    This lesion is located just anterior to the ear on the right zygomatic region, and under the circumstances this will limit how wide we can resect this, but we should get a reasonably good margin from this lesion.

PAST MEDICAL HISTORY: The patient denies all major medical illnesses; however, she is hypothyroid and takes thyroid replacement medication.

PAST SURGICAL HISTORY: The patient had carcinoma of the breast and underwent a left mastectomy in 2003. She had a hysterectomy for benign ovarian tumors in 2009.
ALLERGIES: NKA
SOCIAL HISTORY: She quit smoking in 1998. She uses alcohol rarely.
FAMILY HISTORY: The patient's sister is diabetic.
ROS: Negative.

PHYSICAL EXAMINATION: BP 170/70. HEENT: Head is atraumatic, normocephalic: there is a pigmented lesion just anterior to the right ear over the zygomatic region, which is slightly irregular in shape and different shades of brown. It appears that there is a biopsy site that is healing.
NECK: Negative, there is no adenopathy.
CHEST: Clear and symmetrical
HEART: Regular rhythm, no murmurs or gallops
ABDOMEN: Soft, nontender, no masses or organomegaly
EXTREMITIES: No cyanosis, clubbing, or edema
NEUROLOGIC: Grossly intact

IMPRESSION: Melanoma of the right cheek, level 2

PLAN: Wide excision with flap advancement closure

SRT/pw   D: 9/16/18 09:50:16   T: 9/18/18 12:55:01

Determine the most accurate ICD-10-CM codes.

_____

_____

_____

TAYLOR, READER, & ASSOCIATES
A Complete Health Care Facility
975 CENTRAL AVENUE • SOMEWHERE, FL 32811 • 407-555-4321

PATIENT: CANNELLO, MORGAN
ACCOUNT/EHR #: CANNMO001
DATE: 08/11/18

Attending Physician: Willard B. Reader, MD

Pt is a 45-year-old female with terminal carcinoma of the breast, metastatic to the liver and the brain. She was admitted today with dehydration, due to the program of chemotherapy she has been on. Rehydrated 3 hours with IV infusion and discharged with no treatment given to the cancer.

Willard B. Reader, MD

WBR/pw   D: 08/11/18 09:50:16   T: 08/13/18 12:55:01

Determine the most accurate ICD-10-CM codes.

_____

_____

_____

TAYLOR, READER, & ASSOCIATES
A Complete Health Care Facility
975 CENTRAL AVENUE • SOMEWHERE, FL 32811 • 407-555-4321

PATIENT: BONHEUR, MORRIS
ACCOUNT/EHR #:   BONHMO001
DATE: 09/16/18

Attending Physician: Suzanne R. Taylor, MD

Pt is a 61-year-old male who has been having increasing amounts of pain. He was diagnosed with prostate cancer 5 years ago and had prostectomy 24 months ago. He was then found to have bone metastasis. Eight months ago, the CT scan showed extensive liver mets, as well.

     He is admitted today to have a central port-a-cath VAD (venous access device) tunneled centrally inserted with a sub q port because of problematic pain from his liver cancer.

_____

Suzanne R. Taylor, MD

SRT/pw   D: 9/16/18 09:50:16   T: 9/18/18 12:55:01

Determine the most accurate ICD-10-CM codes.

_____

_____

_____

TAYLOR, READER, & ASSOCIATES
A Complete Health Care Facility
975 CENTRAL AVENUE • SOMEWHERE, FL 32811 • 407-555-4321

PATIENT: RODRIQUEZ, KATRINA
ACCOUNT/EHR #:   RODRKA001
DATE: 08/11/18

Attending Physician: Willard B. Reader, MD

Pt is a 35-year-old female and is 3 days status post an exploratory laparotomy, lysis of adhesions; total abdominal hysterectomy; bilateral salpingo-oophorectomy; partial omentectomy; excision of small and large bowel implants; pelvic-abdominal peritoneal stripping; and placement of intraperitoneal port-a-cath; enterolyses. She has come to see me in my office today to discuss the results of the pathology of the material removed at that procedure.

    The specimen from the omentum was found to be metastatic adenocarcinoma consistent with ovarian origin.

    The ovaries were found to be poorly differentiated; serous carcinoma extended to the left fallopian tube. The right fallopian tube was found to have serosal fibrosis consistent with tubo-ovarian adhesion.

    The specimen from her cervix showed chronic cervicitis.

    A broad-based endometrial polyp was found in the endometrium while the myometrium showed leiomyomata, adenomyosis, multifocal serosal implants of poorly differentiated ovarian serous carcinoma.

    Lastly, the specimens from both the small and large bowel were positive for metastatic, poorly differentiated ovarian serous carcinoma.

The histomorphologic features of poorly differentiated ovarian serous carcinoma closely resemble that of a poorly differentiated fallopian tube primary adenocarcinoma. The bilateral ovarian involvement supports the primary ovarian origin of the neoplasm.

ASSESSMENT: Metastatic adenocarcinoma of the omentum; metastatic carcinoma of the small and large intestine.

Willard B. Reader, MD

WBR/pw   D: 08/11/18 09:50:16   T: 08/13/18 12:55:01

Determine the most accurate ICD-10-CM codes.

TAYLOR, READER, & ASSOCIATES
A Complete Health Care Facility
975 CENTRAL AVENUE • SOMEWHERE, FL 32811 • 407-555-4321

PATIENT: LIPSITZ, ELIOT
ACCOUNT/EHR #:   LIPSEL001
DATE: 09/16/18

Attending Physician: Oscar Hersh, MD

PREOP DIAGNOSIS: Lower extremity ischemia with rest pain and gangrene of the right third toe, probable atheroembolic disease to the right lower extremity
POSTOP DIAGNOSIS: Atheroembolic disease to the right lower extremity
PROCEDURE: Right, axillary femoral-femoral bypass utilizing an 8.0-mm ringed Gore-Tex axillary-to-femoral graft and a 6.0-mm ringed Gore-Tex femoral cross-over graft, right third toe amputation.

OPERATIVE INDICATIONS: This is a 67-year-old male, presenting with local recurrence of rectal carcinoma, with military metastases found on the liver surface.

PATHOLOGICAL FINDINGS: Specimen: Third right toe found to be consistent with ischemic necrosis

PLAN/RECOMMENDATIONS: At this time, given known early liver metastases and extensive local regional recurrence in the pelvis, I do not feel that further antineoplastic therapy will be of great benefit.
   Specifically, the patient has had previous full radiotherapy to the pelvis by history. In addition, he has had chemotherapy up until August of this year and this disease has recurred despite this.
   Secondly, secondline chemotherapy has not been shown to be of value in recurrent colorectal cancer and would certainly not be palliative in this otherwise frail and depressed man.
   With regard to pain management, I would recommend continuing his Duragesic patch. At this time, I would suggest the addition of Elavil at a low dose in the hopes of improving his neurogenic pain. Efforts will be made to improve his home situation and to increase his mobility. I will continue to follow the patient with you.

Oscar Hersh, MD

OH/pw   D: 9/16/18 09:50:16   T: 9/18/18 12:55:01

Determine the most accurate ICD-10-CM codes.

_____

_____

_____

6

CODING DISEASES OF THE BLOOD AND IMMUNE MECHANISM

Learning Outcomes *After completing this chapter, the student should be able to:*

LO 6.1 Identify the components of the blood and blood-forming organs.

LO 6.2 Express the function of antigens on red blood cells.

LO 6.3 Relate the role of blood in the human body.

LO 6.4 Explain the purpose of various blood tests.

LO 6.5 Describe the impact of diseases affecting the blood.

LO 6.6 Classify disorders involving the immune mechanism.

Key Terms

Agglutination

Antigen

Blood

Blood type

Coagulation

Hematopoiesis

Hemoglobin (hgb or Hgb)

Hemolysis

Hemostasis

Plasma

Platelets (Plat)

Red blood cells (RBCs)

Rh (rhesus) factor

Transfusion

White blood cells (WBCs)

Blood is a type of connective tissue consisting of **red blood cells (RBCs), white blood cells (WBCs),** and **platelets (Plats)**—all contained within liquid **plasma.** It is a transportation system for oxygen (nourishment for cells throughout the body) and for carbon dioxide (cell waste products). The average adult has between 5 and 6 liters of blood constantly circulating throughout the body.

LO 6.1 The Formation of Blood

Blood is created in the red bone marrow (see Figure 6-1) during a series of steps called **hematopoiesis.** During gestation, blood cells originate in the yolk sac from the mesenchyme (the section of the embryo in which blood, lymphatic vessels, bones, cartilage, and connective tissues form). As the fetus continues to develop, the liver, spleen, and thymus produce blood cells. At about the 20th week of gestation, the red bone marrow also begins to produce blood cells. Once the baby is born, blood cell formation is primarily the responsibility of the red bone marrow only, specifically in the sternum, ribs, and vertebrae. Red bone marrow produces red blood cells (erythrocytes) through a process called *erythropoiesis,* and the red bone marrow produces white blood cells (leukocytes) through a process called *leukopoiesis.*

How many blood cells does a healthy body need? Normal counts (per microliter of blood) are:

- *Red blood cell count:* 4 to 6 million cells.
- *White blood cell count:* 4,000 to 11,000 cells.
- *Platelet count:* 150,000 to 400,000 platelets.

Too many cells or too few cells may indicate a problem. This is why one of the first diagnostic tests run when a physician is trying to figure out what is wrong with the patient is a complete blood count (CBC).

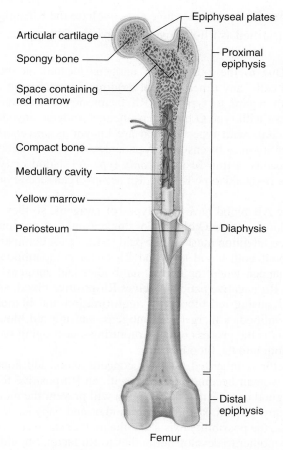

FIGURE 6-1 Bone Marrow

Source: David Shier et al., HOLE'S HUMAN ANATOMY & PHYSIOLOGY, 12/e. © 2010 MHE. Figure 7.2, p. 194

Labels on figure:
- Epiphyseal plates
- Articular cartilage
- Spongy bone
- Space containing red marrow
- Compact bone
- Medullary cavity
- Yellow marrow
- Periosteum
- Proximal epiphysis
- Diaphysis
- Distal epiphysis
- Femur

blood
Fluid pumped throughout the body, carrying oxygen and nutrients to the cells and wastes away from the cells.

red blood cells (RBCs)
Cells within the blood that contain hemoglobin responsible for carrying oxygen to tissues; also known as *erythrocytes.*

white blood cells (WBCs)
Cells within the blood that help to protect the body from pathogens; also known as *leukocytes.*

platelets (Plats)
Large cell fragments in the bone marrow that function in clotting; also known as *thrombocytes.*

plasma
The fluid part of the blood.

hematopoiesis
The formation of blood cells.

EXAMPLE

D72.818 Other decreased white blood cell count (plasmacytopenia)
R71.8 Abnormal red-cell volume

LO 6.2 Antigens on Red Blood Cells

Antigens sit on the surface of red blood cells, while antibodies are located in the blood plasma. Antigens are proteins that cause antibodies to form, and each antibody can connect with only one specific type of antigen. Antigens that are located on RBCs are categorized in two ways: blood type and Rh factor.

Blood Type You may know what **blood type** you have: type A, type B, type AB, or type O. This is something that is inherited from your parents.

- An individual with type A blood has only antigen A on his or her red blood cells.
- An individual with type B blood has only antigen B on his or her red blood cells.
- An individual with type AB blood has both antigens—A and B.
- An individual with type O blood has neither antigen—not A nor B.

Rh Factor Another antigen that may or may not be present on the surface of a red blood cell is called **Rh (Rhesus) factor.** This is also an inherited situation.

antigen
A substance that promotes the production of antibodies.

blood type
A system of classifying blood based on the antigens present on the surface of the individual's red blood cells; also known as *blood group.*

Rh (Rhesus) factor
An antigen located on the red blood cell that produces immunogenic responses in those individuals without it.

- An individual identified as Rh-negative does *not* have the Rh antigen.
- An individual identified as Rh-positive *does* have the Rh antigen.

transfusion
The provision of one person's blood or plasma to another individual.

Transfusions Due to the existence of antigens located on the surface of the patient's red blood cells, any time a patient requires a **transfusion** of blood, it must be compatible with regard to type and Rh factor or serious consequences could occur. Because those with type O blood have neither antigen, anyone can accept this blood type. Individuals with type O blood are known as *universal donors*. Again, Rh factor compatibility must be ensured. A patient with type A+ blood (type A blood, Rh positive) can receive a transfusion of *only* type A+ blood or type O blood. An individual with type B− blood (type B blood, Rh negative) can receive *only* type B− blood or type O blood.

Those with type AB blood have both types of antigens, so they can receive type A blood, type B blood, or type O blood. For this reason, they are known as *universal recipients*. However, attention must still be paid to Rh factor compatibility.

agglutination
The process of red blood cells combining together in a mass or lump.

The concern about both blood type and Rh factor compatibility arises from the dangers that can happen when the correct antibodies and antigens are not in place. For example, if an Rh-negative patient receives Rh-positive blood, anti-Rh antibodies would be created, causing red blood cell **agglutination** and **hemolysis.** Agglutination occurs when antibodies merge with antigens, causing red blood cells to clump together. Hemolysis is the process of cells rupturing—destroying red blood cells and releasing hemoglobin into the bloodstream.

hemolysis
The destruction of red blood cells, resulting in the release of hemoglobin into the bloodstream.

Because Rh factor is inherited, there is concern about additional complications if an Rh-negative woman becomes pregnant with an Rh-positive fetus (the father is Rh-positive). The good news is that the placenta will prevent the mother's blood from mixing with the baby's blood, keeping both mother and baby safe. However, during the birthing process, the possibility exists that the mother can be exposed to the baby's blood, causing the mother to develop antibodies to Rh factor. Should this occur and if the woman becomes pregnant again, the antibodies can transfer through the placenta and destroy RBCs.

EXAMPLE

O36.012 Maternal care for anti-D (Rh) antibodies, second trimester

Z31.82 Encounter for Rh incompatibility status

LET'S CODE IT! SCENARIO

Neonate female was born vaginally without incident, Apgar scores: 10/10. Three hours later, extensive purpura became visible on her abdomen, arms, and legs. No jaundice was observed. Her 29-year-old mother had a blood transfusion for a postpartum hemorrhage after her first pregnancy 2 years earlier. The mother's serum was found to contain IgG antibodies to father's platelets and to some of a panel of platelets from normal, unrelated donors. These antibodies were typed as specific anti-HPA-1A antibodies and had been incited by the previous pregnancy and transfusion. These antibodies crossed the placenta to cause alloimmune thrombocytopenia in the neonate. In addition, she had a red cell incompatibility. An exchange transfusion was performed to compensate for hemolysis. It is unusual for an ABO incompatibility to require an exchange transfusion, but it worked. Her platelet count returned to normal quickly due to free reactant antibody to platelets having been removed by the exchange.

The baby was born and diagnosed with *alloimmune thrombocytopenia.* In the Alphabetic Index, let's find our key term:

> ### Thrombocytopenia

As you read down the indented list, there are two choices that may pop out at you:

> ### Thrombocytopenia
> #### Congenital D69.42
> #### Neonatal, transitory P61.0
> ##### Due to
> ###### Exchange maternal thrombocytopenia P61.0

Congenital means "present at birth," and this condition was. However, the patient is a neonate, and the documentation states that this condition is due to the exchange with her mother. One thing to always remember: You can always look up both terms in the Tabular List. So let's do just that—take a look at them both:

> ### D69.42 Congenital and hereditary thrombocytopenia purpura
> ### P61.0 Transient neonatal thrombocytopenia

Let's go back to the documentation. The physician notes that the baby contracted this condition as a result of the transfusion her mother received previously. So this is not actually inherited because it is not the result of genetics; it is the result of circumstances. In addition, the treatment worked, so the baby no longer has the blood problem, meaning the thrombocytopenia was temporary (transient). This points us toward the accurate code of:

> ### P61.0 Transient neonatal thrombocytopenia

Good work!

LO 6.3 Blood Roles

As mentioned at the beginning of this chapter, blood's primary job is transporting oxygen from the lungs and delivering it to tissue cells throughout the body. As the oxygen passes from the lungs to the blood, it binds to the red blood cells and the **hemoglobin (hgb or Hgb)** inside those RBCs (see Figure 6-2), so it can travel through the heart and out through the body via the arteries. After delivering the oxygen (O_2) to the cells, the blood picks up carbon dioxide (CO_2) and carries it back to the lungs for expulsion from the body.

However, this is not blood's only job. In addition to transporting oxygen, blood transports regulatory hormones and nutrients to the tissues. In addition to carrying CO_2 to the lungs, blood carries metabolic wastes to the kidneys and skin. Blood also controls **hemostasis** (stopping the bleeding process) via **coagulation** (clotting). White blood cells (the production of antibodies) increase in response to infections and other antigens. Sensitized lymphocytes establish the body's immunity to viruses and cancer cells.

hemoglobin (hgb or Hgb)
The part of the red blood cell that carries oxygen.

hemostasis
The interruption of bleeding.

coagulation
Clotting; the change from a liquid into a thickened substance.

EXAMPLE

> D68.4 Acquired coagulation factor deficiency
> R79.1 Abnormal coagulation profile

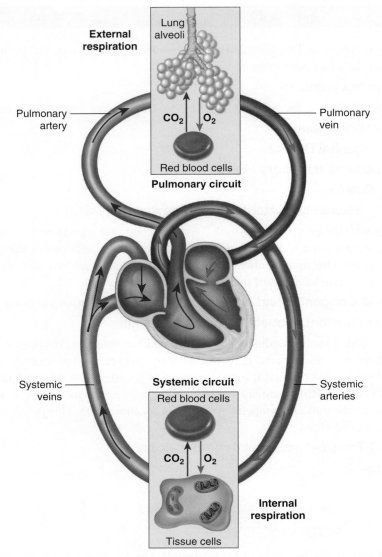

FIGURE 6-2 Oxygen and Carbon Dioxide Exchanging in Blood

LET'S CODE IT! SCENARIO

Dr. Longwood ordered a coagulation profile, including a partial thromboplastin time (PTT) and prothrombin time (PT), to be done on Oscar Nepolitano prior to scheduling his surgery. The pathology report showed an abnormally prolonged PTT. The surgery will be delayed until Dr. Longwood can confirm the cause.

Let's Code It!

The lab report identified an abnormal coagulation profile, and Dr. Longwood did not provide any confirmed diagnosis. Therefore, this is all you know for a fact, and this is what must be reported. Turn to the Alphabetic Index and find:

Abnormal

This is going to take some analysis. There is no listing under *Abnormal* for *Test* or *Coagulation*. Think about this. What is the body's reason for coagulation? To stop bleeding. Look for *Blood* or *Bleeding*. Did you find:

Abnormal

    Bleeding time R79.1

Now let's go into the Tabular List to check this out. Remember, always begin reading at the three-character category.

R79 Other abnormal findings of blood chemistry

Read down the fourth-character choices, and find:

R79.1 Abnormal coagulation profile (abnormal or prolonged partial thromboplastin time [PTT])

Good job!

LO 6.4 Blood Tests

Sending a patient for a blood test might sound like a simple thing. A vial or two of blood, taken by venipuncture, results in descriptive lab test data (see Figure 6-3) that can provide important clues about a patient's health. In addition to an RBC count and a WBC count, common blood tests performed include:

- *Bicarbonate:* Kidneys and lungs keep bicarbonate balanced to maintain homeostatic pH levels (ensure a balance of acid and alkali levels). Abnormal levels can indicate dysfunction of these organs (kidneys and lungs).
- *Blood culture:* This test measures the presence of bacteria or yeast in the blood, which is used to confirm (or deny) a suspected infection or sepsis.
- *Blood differential (Diff):* This test measures numbers of WBCs, which are used to identify presence of infection. Normal is less than 20%.
- *Blood urea nitrogen (BUN):* This test measures kidney function. A low count might indicate malnutrition, while a high count may identify the presence of heart failure, kidney disease, or liver disease. Normal range: 7–20 milligrams per deciliter (mg/dL).
- *Creatinine:* This test measures levels of this chemical excreted by the kidneys. It is used to determine muscle damage, dehydration, and/or kidney dysfunction. Normal range: 0.8–1.4 mg/dL.
- *Glucose:* This test measures the levels of sugar in the blood. Low levels may indicate hypoglycemia or liver disease, whereas high levels may indicate hyperglycemia (diabetes) or hyperthyroidism. Normal range: 70–99 mg/dL.
- *Erythrocyte sedimentation rate (ESR):* This test measures the speed with which red blood cells cling together, fall, and settle in the bottom of a glass tube within 60 minutes. It is used to detect inflammatory, neoplastic, infectious, and necrotic processes. When inflammation is present, the higher the rate, the greater the amount of inflammation. Normal range: male = up to 15 millimeters per hour (mm/h); female = up to 20 mm/h.
- *Hematocrit (HCT):* This test identifies the percentage of RBCs, which is used to identify anemia. Low counts may indicate bone marrow damage or vitamin deficiency, while high counts may indicate congenital heart disease, renal problems, or pulmonary disease. Normal range: 34%–45%.
- *Hemoglobin (Hgb):* This test measures oxygen being carried by the RBCs. Low counts may indicate bone marrow damage or vitamin deficiency, while high counts may indicate congenital heart disease, renal problems, or pulmonary disease. Normal range: 11.5–15.5 grams per deciliter (g/dL).

LABORATORIES

	Augusta, GA.	Oriando,	Tampa, FL
	Tel:	Tel:	Tel:
	Fax:	Fax:	Fax:

Patient:
DOB:　　　　Age: Yrs　Sex:
PID:
Phone:
Episode:
Notes:
Copy to:

Collecting Time: 03/26/20　08:27　　PHYSICIAN　　　　P96
Log in DT/TM:　03/27/20　00:57　　550
Report DT/TM:　03/27/20　05:02
Reprint DT/TM:　03/31/20　10:07
FASTING: Y　Priority: R　　Physician:

TEST NAME		RESULT	UNITS	REF RANGE	LAB
COMPREHENSIVE METABOLIC PANEL WITH eGFR					ORL
Sodium		139	mEq/L	(133–146)	
Potassium		3.9	mEq/L	(3.5–5.4)	
Chloride		101	mEq/L	(97–110)	
Carbon Dioxide		31	mEq/L	(21–33)	
Anion Gap		7.0	mEq/L	(5.0-–15.0)	
Glucose		96	mg/dL	(65–100)	
BUN		11	mg/dL	(8–25)	
Creatinine		0.64	mg/dL	(0.6–1.4)	
eGFR African American		113	mL/min	(>60)	
eGFR Non-African Am.		98	mL/min	(>60)	
BUN/Creatinine Ratio		17		(6–28)	
Calcium		9.3	mg/dL	(8.2–10.6)	
Total Protein		7.2	g/dL	(6.0–8.3)	
Albumin		4.5	g/dL	(3.5–5.7)	
Globulin		2.7	g/dL	(1.6–4.2)	
A/G Ratio		1.7		(0.9–2.5)	
Bilirubin Total		0.5	mg/dL	(0.1–1.30)	
Alkaline Phosphatase		87	U/L	(35–126)	
AST (SGOT)		17	U/L	(5–43)	
ALT (SGPT)		11	U/L	(7–56)	
TSH		4.199	ulU/mL	(0.550–4.780)	ORL
Free T4		1.16	ng/dL	(0.89–1.76)	ORL
LIPID PANEL					
Cholesterol	H	243	mg/dL	(80–199)	
Triglycerides		188	mg/dL	(30–150)	
HDL Cholesterol		55	mg/dL	(40–110)	
LDL Cholesterol Calc		141	mg/dL	(30–130)	
VLDL Cholesterol Calc		28	mg/dL	(10–60)	
Risk Ratio (CHOL/HDL)		3.6	Ratio	(0.0–5.0)	
Non-HDL Cholesterol		145	mg/dL		

Cholesterol/HDL　　Ratio　　Interpretation:
　　Gender　　CVD　Risk　Category
　　Female

　　　Average　Risk　　　4.4
　　　Twice　Average　Risk　　71

Printed at:03/31/20　10:07　　　　　"CONTINUED REPORT"

FIGURE 6-3　Pathology Report—Blood Tests

- *Mean corpuscular hemoglobin (MCH):* This test measures the amount of hemoglobin in RBCs. A low number may indicate an iron deficiency, whereas a high number may indicate a vitamin deficiency. Normal range: 27–34 picograms (pg).

- *Mean corpuscular volume (MCV):* This test identifies the average size of the RBCs. Small size may indicate an iron deficiency, whereas a large reading may indicate a vitamin deficiency. Normal range: 80–100 femtoliters (fL).

- *Partial thromboplastin time (PTT):* This test measures factors I (fibrinogen), II (prothrombin), V, VIII, IX, X, XI, and XII. Inadequate quantities of these factors cause the PTT to be prolonged, a delay in the clotting of the blood that increases the opportunity for the patient to hemorrhage. Normal PTT: 60–70 seconds.

- *Platelet count:* Low platelet counts can indicate a clotting disorder, putting the patient at risk for hemorrhage. Low levels may indicate pernicious anemia, lupus, or a viral infection, while high levels may identify leukemia. Normal range: 150–400 thousand per microliter (K/mcL).

- *Potassium:* This test measures levels of potassium in the blood. Low potassium levels can cause muscle cramps and/or weakness; abnormal levels (too high or low) can result in an abnormal heartbeat. Low levels can identify use of corticosteroids or diuretics, while high levels may signify kidney failure, diabetes, or Addison's disease. Normal range: 3.7–5.2 milliequivalents per liter (mEq/L).

- *Prothrombin time (PT):* This test evaluates the clotting ability of factors I (fibrinogen), II (prothrombin), V, VII, and X. Low quantities of these clotting factors result in a prolonged PT. PT results include the use of the international normalized ratio (INR) value as well as absolute numbers. Normal PT result: 85%–100% in 11–12.5 seconds and an INR of 0.8–1.1.

- *Sodium:* This test determines if the balance between sodium and liquid in the blood is at the correct proportion. Low levels of sodium can identify the use of diuretics or adrenal insufficiency, while high levels may indicate dehydration or kidney dysfunction. High levels of sodium can lead to hypertension. Normal range: 136–144 mEq/L.

LO 6.5 Blood Conditions

As with any other part of the body, malfunction of the blood or one of its components can result in problems. Some of the more common conditions include the following.

Anemia

While many believe anemia is the result of an iron deficiency, this is only one cause of an abnormally low count of hemoglobin, hematocrit, and/or RBCs. The low volume of RBCs reduces the amount of oxygen being transported, causing tissue hypoxia (low levels of oxygen). Classic signs and symptoms include tachycardia, dyspnea, and sometimes fatigue. *Nutritional anemia,* reported with codes from the D50–D53 range, is caused by an insufficient intake or absorption into the body of certain key nutrients. For example, pernicious anemia is a genetic condition that causes dysfunction of the ileum so it cannot properly absorb vitamin B_{12}; iron deficiency anemia may be caused by a diet lacking iron-rich foods. *Hemolytic anemia* (codes D55–D59) results from an insufficient number of healthy red blood cells due to abnormal or premature destruction, thereby retarding the delivery of oxygen to the tissues throughout the body. This premature destruction of the red blood cells may be caused by a genetic defect, an infection, or exposure to certain toxins. Hemolytic anemia can also be caused by a mismatched blood transfusion. *Aplastic anemia* (code category D61) is the inability of the bone marrow to manufacture enough new blood cells required by the body for proper function. *Hemorrhagic anemia,* also called *blood loss anemia* or *posthemorrhagic anemia* (code D62), can occur after the patient has lost a great deal of blood. This can be after a traumatic injury or internal bleeding, such as an untreated gastric ulcer.

D52.0 Dietary folate deficiency anemia
D57.1 Sickle-cell disease without crisis (Sickle-cell anemia NOS)
D62 Acute post-hemorrhagic (blood loss) anemia
P61.2 Anemia of prematurity

LET'S CODE IT! SCENARIO

Demetri Kosmopolus, an 18-month-old male, was brought to Dr. Katzman, a pediatrician specializing in blood disorders, by his mother. Dr. Katzman noted jaundice, an enlarged spleen on palpation, and other signs of failure to thrive. Dr. Katzman recognized these signs and symptoms and confirmed with blood tests a diagnosis of Cooley's anemia.

Let's Code It!

Dr. Katzman diagnosed Demetri with *Cooley's anemia.* Turn to the Alphabetic Index and find:

Anemia

Are you surprised by the long indented list of different types of anemia? Read down the list and find:

Anemia

Cooley's (erythroblastic) D56.1

Now let's go to the Tabular List to confirm this code. Remember, always begin reading at the three-character category.

D56 Thalassemia

Thalassemia is an inherited group of hemolytic anemias (*hemo* = blood + *-lytic* = involving lysis, the decomposition of a cell). Cooley's anemia, also known as *thalassemia major,* is one type of beta thalassemia, the most common form of this condition.

Read down the fourth-character choices, and find:

D56.1 *Beta thalassemia (Cooley's anemia)*

Good job!

Clotting Disorders

Essentially, there are two types of clotting disorders: hemostatic and thrombotic. A *hemostatic disorder* is a failure in the system to repair a damaged blood vessel. Because there is no clot to stop it, the vessel continues to bleed. These coagulation deficiencies—where clotting does not occur as it should (see Figure 6-4)—may be seen with bleeding into the muscles, joints, and viscera or with the appearance of purpura (dysfunction of blood vessels). Hemophilia is a common hemostatic condition, reported with code D66, Hereditary factor VIII deficiency (Classical hemophilia). *Thrombotic disorders* are the opposite: The blood clots without purpose, forming thrombi (blood clots) within the vessels, causing a blockage. Beyond the dangers from the thrombi themselves, should a clot dislodge (embolus) and travel through the blood vessels, it might get caught going through the lungs or heart, causing a blockage that could be deadly. Thrombophilia is an example of a thrombotic condition, reported with, for example, ICD-10-CM code D68.59, Other primary thrombophilia (Hypercoagulable state NOS).

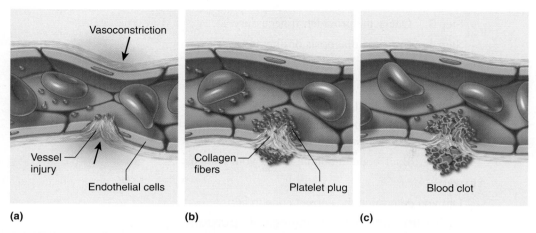

(a)   **(b)**   **(c)**

FIGURE 6-4 Hemostasis: (a) blood vessel spasm, (b) platelet plug formation, and (c) blood coagulation

Source: Deborah Roiger, ANATOMY & PHYSIOLOGY: FOUNDATIONS FOR THE HEALTH PROFESSIONS, 1/e. © 2013 MHE. Figure 9.8, p. 345

Thrombocytopenia This is a low platelet count most often due to increased platelet destruction, decreased platelet production, or malfunctioning platelets. Underlying conditions might include splenomegaly (enlarged spleen); destruction of bone marrow by medication, chemotherapy, or radiation therapy; or aplastic anemia. The condition will be reported most often with a code from ICD-10-CM code category D69, Purpura and other hemorrhagic conditions, although not exclusively. For example, postpartum puerperal thrombocytopenia is reported with code O72.3, Postpartum coagulation defects, and neonatal, transitory thrombocytopenia is reported with code P61.0, Transient neonatal thrombocytopenia.

YOU CODE IT! CASE STUDY

Arlene Tomlinson, a 27-year-old female, came to see Dr. Landau with complaints of spontaneous bruising on her arms and legs. She states she had two recent episodes of epistaxes but no other bleeding. She denied taking any drugs or smoking, and had no risk factors for HIV. Physical examination revealed the spleen was not palpable. Petechiae are noted scattered on her legs bilaterally. Lab tests showed: normal hemoglobin (138 g/L); normal white cell count; low platelet count of 10×10^9/L (normal $>150 \times 10^9$/L); erythrocyte sedimentation rate was 6 mm/h; direct Coombs' test was negative; antinuclear absent; DNA-binding antibodies absent; rheumatoid factor absent. Bone marrow aspiration showed high number of normal megakaryocytes but was otherwise normal. A diagnosis of immune thrombocytopenia purpura was confirmed. She is placed on a short course of prednisolone.

You Code It!

Go through the steps of coding, and determine the code or codes that should be reported for this encounter between Dr. Landau and Arlene.

    Step 1:   Read the case completely.

    Step 2:   Abstract the notes: Which key words can you identify relating to why Dr. Landau cared for Arlene?

Step 3: Query the provider, if necessary.

Step 4: Code the diagnosis or diagnoses.

Step 5: Code the procedure(s): Office visit.

Step 6: Link the procedure codes to at least one diagnosis code to confirm medical necessity.

Step 7: Back code to double-check your choices.

Answer:

Did you determine the correct code to be:

D69.3 Immune thrombocytopenic purpura

Hematologic Malignancies Both lymphomas and leukemias are included in this category. Leukemia is the presence of malignant cells within the bone marrow that produces blood cells (hematopoietic tissues), causing a reduction in the production of RBCs, WBCs, and platelets. This anemic state makes the patient very susceptible to infections and hemorrhaging. There are several types of leukemia reported from several ICD-10-CM code categories, including C92, Myeloid leukemia; C93, Monocytic leukemia; C94, Other leukemias of specified cell type; and C95, Leukemia of unspecified cell type.

LO 6.6 Disorders of the Immune Mechanism

Sarcoidosis The specific etiology of sarcoidosis is still unknown; however, most researchers believe it is a combination of a genetic susceptibility with a certain exposure to something that triggers the immune system to release chemicals that are ineffective at combating inflammation. Instead, the cells clump together and become granulomas (tumors that result from an ulcerated infection) situated within certain organs throughout the body, such as the lungs, liver, or skin. This diagnosis is reported with a code from category D86, Sarcoidosis.

Wiskott-Aldrich Syndrome When a patient suffers from Wiskott-Aldrich syndrome, this genetic mutation causes white blood cells to malfunction, increasing the body's susceptibility to inflammatory diseases and other immunodeficiency disorders. Eczema, thrombocytopenia, and pyogenic infections often develop and put the patient at a higher than normal risk of autoimmune diseases. This condition is reported with code D82.0, Wiskott-Aldrich syndrome.

YOU CODE IT! CASE STUDY

Marlena Robinson, a 33-year-old female, came in complaining of discomfort and tenderness under her arms and in her neck. Dr. Gorren performed a physical exam revealing swollen lymph nodes. Lab work showed she was suffering with sarcoidosis of her lymph nodes.

Go through the steps of coding, and determine the code or codes that should be reported for this encounter between Dr. Gorren and Marlena.

Step 1: Read the case completely.

Step 2: Abstract the notes: Which key words can you identify relating to why Dr. Gorren cared for Marlena?

_____

Step 3: Query the provider, if necessary.

Step 4: Code the diagnosis or diagnoses.

_____

Step 5: Code the procedure(s): Office visit.

Step 6: Link the procedure codes to at least one diagnosis code to confirm medical necessity.

Step 7: Back code to double-check your choices.

Answer:

Did you determine the correct code to be:

D86.1 Sarcoidosis of lymph nodes

Chapter Summary

Blood flows through your arteries and veins, transporting oxygen (O_2) to nourish tissues and carrying away the waste (CO_2) from those cells. Production of the components of the blood, including red blood cells, white blood cells, and platelets, occurs within the red bone marrow, specifically, within the sternum, ribs, and vertebrae in the adult. Since blood is systemic (traveling throughout the entire body), blood tests are an excellent diagnostic tool because the minor invasiveness of venipuncture can yield massive amounts of information about the health of the body. When the blood system malfunctions, serious health consequences result.

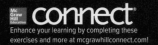

Using Terminology

Match each key term to the appropriate definition.

_____ **1.** LO 6.2 A system of classifying blood based on the antigens present on the surface of the individual's red blood cells.

_____ **2.** LO 6.1 Cells within the blood that help to protect the body from pathogens.

_____ **3.** LO 6.2 The process of red blood cells combining together in a mass or lump.

_____ **4.** LO 6.3 Clotting; the change from a liquid into a thickened substance.

_____ **5.** LO 6.3 The interruption of bleeding.

_____ **6.** LO 6.2 An antigen located on the red blood cell that produces immunogenic responses in those individuals without it.

_____ **7.** LO 6.2 The provision of one person's blood or plasma to another individual.

_____ **8.** LO 6.1 Fluid pumped throughout the body, carrying oxygen and nutrients to the cells and wastes away from the cells.

_____ **9.** LO 6.1 The fluid part of the blood.

_____ **10.** LO 6.1 Cells within the blood that contain hemoglobin responsible for carrying oxygen to tissues.

_____ **11.** LO 6.3 The part of the red blood cell that carries oxygen.

_____ **12.** LO 6.2 The destruction of red blood cells resulting in the release of hemoglobin into the bloodstream.

_____ **13.** LO 6.1 Large cell fragments in the bone marrow that function in clotting.

_____ **14.** LO 6.1 The formation of blood.

A. Agglutination
B. Blood
C. Blood type
D. Coagulation
E. Hematopoiesis
F. Hemoglobin
G. Hemolysis
H. Hemostasis
I. Plasma
J. Platelets (Plat)
K. Red blood cells (RBCs)
L. Rh factor
M. Transfusions
N. White blood cells (WBCs)

Checking Your Understanding

Choose the most appropriate answer for each of the following questions.

1. LO 6.1 Blood is composed of all of the following *except*

a. RBCs.
b. WBCs.
c. Plats.
d. HCT.

2. LO 6.1 Hematopoiesis means

a. formation of bone marrow.
b. formation of blood.
c. formation of nutrients.
d. formation of carbon dioxide.

3. LO 6.1 Which cells within the blood help protect the body from pathogens?

a. erythrocytes.
b. thrombocytes.
c. leukocytes.
d. lymphocytes.

4. LO 6.2 An individual with blood type _____ is known as a *universal donor.*

　　a. O.
　　b. A.
　　c. B.
　　d. AB.

5. LO 6.2 Blood type _____ has only A antigens on the red blood cells.

　　a. O.
　　b. A.
　　c. AB.
　　d. B.

6. LO 6.2 An individual with blood type B– can receive only which type of blood in a transfusion?

　　a. type B–.
　　b. type B+.
　　c. type O.
　　d. type B– or type O.

7. LO 6.4 The test that measures kidney function is

　　a. blood culture.
　　b. creatinine.
　　c. blood urea nitrogen.
　　d. hematocrit.

8. LO 6.5 Which type of anemia indicates the inability of the bone marrow to manufacture enough new blood cells required by the body to function properly?

　　a. hemolytic anemia.
　　b. aplastic anemia.
　　c. nutritional anemia.
　　d. hemorrhagic anemia.

9. LO 6.5 Which clotting disorder may be seen as bleeding into the muscles, joints, and viscera?

　　a. hemostatic disorder.
　　b. choroid disorder.
　　c. thrombotic disorder.
　　d. hypoglossal disorder.

10. LO 6.6 The genetic mutation causing white blood cells to malfunction, increasing the body's susceptibility to inflammatory diseases and other immunodeficiency disorders, is known as

　　a. Clarke-Hadfield syndrome.
　　b. Heubner-Herter syndrome.
　　c. Wiskott-Aldrich syndrome.
　　d. Lennox-Gastaut syndrome.

Applying Your Knowledge

1. LO 6.1 How many blood cells does a healthy body need? Why is this important? _____

   _____

2. LO 6.2 What are the blood types, and what differentiates each type? _____

   _____

3. LO 6.2 What is Rh factor, and why is it important? _____

   _____

4. LO 6.2 Who is a universal donor, and who can receive this donor's type of blood in a transfusion? Why? _____

   _____

5. LO 6.2 Who is a universal recipient, and what type of blood can this recipient receive? _____

   _____

6. LO 6.4 List six types of blood tests. _____

   _____

7. LO 6.5 What is anemia, and what are its common signs and symptoms? Include three examples of different types
   of anemia. _____

   _____

8. LO 6.5 How many types of clotting disorders are there? What are they, and how do they differ? _____

   _____

Using the techniques described in this chapter, carefully read through the case studies and determine the most accurate ICD-10-CM code(s) and external cause code(s), if appropriate, for each case study.

1. Pauline Meadows, a 33-year-old female, comes to see Dr. Morris because of bruising on her right leg. She states she does not remember hitting anything that would have caused the bruise. Blood work showed that Pauline has a vitamin K deficiency. She is diagnosed with hemostatic disorder due to vitamin K deficiency.

   _____

2. Jason Peak, an 11-month-old male, is brought in by his mother to see Dr. Watson. Jason is learning to walk and is showing a few large bruises and some swelling. After testing, Jason is diagnosed with classic hemophilia.

   _____

3. Joyce Allyson, a 56-year-old female, began heparin therapy 14 days ago. She comes to see Dr. Livingston for a heparin check. After blood work, Dr. Livingston finds Joyce's platelet level low. Joyce is diagnosed with heparin-induced thrombocytopenia (HIT).

   _____

4. April Sundell, an 18-year-old female, comes to the emergency room for treatment of a minor cut that will not stop bleeding. April states she was fixing a snack and cut her finger and cannot get the bleeding to stop. The ER physician notes the bleeding is heavy for this type of superficial laceration and can only be stopped for short periods of time. After blood work, April is diagnosed with Christmas disease.

   _____

5. Richard Sullivan, a 26-year-old male, comes in today to see Dr. Brighten, complaining of a dry cough he has had for almost 3 weeks that just won't go away and some shortness of breath. He admits to night sweats and low-grade fever. After a thorough exam and blood work, Dr. Brighten diagnoses Richard with sarcoidosis of lung.

   _____

6. Leigh Summers, a 67-year-old female, comes in today complaining of fever, chills, and night sweats. She also states that she has lost weight and feels tired. CBC shows hemoglobin of 7.9, and tissue biopsy is positive for extrapulmonary tuberculosis. Leigh is diagnosed with anemia due to tuberculosis.

   _____

7. Diana Gamble, an 8-month-old female, was brought in last week by her mother for blood work and a bone marrow biopsy. Diana's mother is here today to discuss the results of her daughter's tests. Dr. Hinson explains that Diana's white blood cells and platelets are normal, but her red blood cell count is low. The bone marrow biopsy confirms a diagnosis of Diamond-Blackfan anemia.

_____

8. James Bucklew, a 64-year-old male with chronic kidney disease, stage 3, comes to see Dr. Britton complaining of extreme tiredness and weakness. After complete blood work, Dr. Britton diagnoses James with anemia due to chronic kidney disease.

_____

9. Anna Haggins has been diagnosed with an acute Rh blood transfusion incompatibility less than 24 hours after transfusion.

_____

10. Albert Hoffmayer, an 8-year-old male, spent the summer on his uncle's farm. His father brings Albert to see Dr. Anderson due to weakness, a cough, and fever. After a physical examination and blood work, Dr. Anderson diagnoses Albert with hookworm anemia.

_____

11. Keith Guest, a 68-year-old male, comes to see Dr. Rabon, complaining of joint pain. After a thorough examination and blood work, Dr. Rabon diagnoses Keith with anemic thalassemia.

_____

12. Henry Haffner, a 7-year-old male, comes to see Dr. Causey for his 6-month checkup. Henry has no complaints. During Dr. Causey's physical exam, he notes a slightly enlarged spleen. After blood work, Dr. Causey diagnoses Henry with splenic anemia.

_____

13. Meagan Norris, a 28-year-old female, comes to see Dr. Dunkin with the complaint of flu-like symptoms, headaches, and unintentional weight loss. Dr. Dunkin does a complete physical examination and blood work and diagnoses Meagan with acute leukemia.

_____

14. John Newman, a 42-year-old male, comes to see Dr. Grover complaining of tiredness and weakness. After blood work and a bone marrow biopsy, Dr. Grover diagnoses John with chronic lymphocytic, B-cell-type leukemia.

_____

15. Chris Griffin, a 9-year-old female, is brought in by her mother to see Dr. Clarke with the complaint of paleness, fever, and a rash. Dr. Clarke does a complete physical exam and blood work and diagnoses Chris with juvenile myelomonocytic leukemia.

_____

YOU CODE IT! Application

Chapter 6: Coding Diseases of the Blood
and Immune Mechanism

The following exercises provide practice in abstracting physicians' notes and learning to work with SOAP notes from our health care facility, *Taylor, Reader, & Associates.* These case studies (SOAP notes) are modeled on real patient encounters. Using the techniques described in this chapter, carefully read through the case studies and determine the most accurate ICD-10-CM code(s) and external cause code(s), if appropriate, for each case study.

TAYLOR, READER, & ASSOCIATES
A Complete Health Care Facility
975 CENTRAL AVENUE • SOMEWHERE, FL 32811 • 407-555-4321

PATIENT: RABON, ROBYN
ACCOUNT/EHR #:   RABORO001
DATE: 09/23/18

Attending Physician: Willard B. Reader, MD

Robyn Rabon, a 41-year-old female, comes in to see her physician, Dr. Reader, with complaints of fatigue of about 3–4 weeks duration. She states mild shortness of breath with exertion such as walking up a flight of stairs, and she denies chest pain with exertion or at rest. She notes no bright red blood per rectum or melena, but she has had heavy menstrual periods for about a year.

PAST MEDICAL HISTORY: She was treated for anemia following her second pregnancy 9 years ago. She denies taking any prescribed medications.

FAMILY HISTORY: Her parents were born in Greece and passed away when she was 12 years old. She does not know their medical history.

     When asked if she takes any over-the-counter medication or herbal supplements, she notes that she has been taking aspirin 81 mg daily for several months.

     When asked about her diet, she notes that she is a vegetarian who eats a lot of cereal.

     She denies eating any nonfood substances, such as starch or talc, or any craving for ice.

PHYSICAL EXAM:
General appearance: Pale female in no acute distress.
Vital signs: Blood pressure 125/90, heart rate 88 regular, respirations 12/min. There were no significant changes in the blood pressure and heart rate between the supine and upright positions.

     The remainder of the physical examination was remarkable for pale conjunctiva. Mucous membranes were moist and without lesions. There was no adenopathy appreciated. The chest was clear to auscultation, and the heart had a regular rate and rhythm with a grade I/VI systolic ejection murmur. The abdomen was soft, nontender, and nondistended. There was no hepatosplenomegaly. Rectal examination revealed no masses and heme-negative brown stool was present.

     Hemoglobin levels are 7 g/dL. There is evidence of marked microcytosis and hypochromia with a markedly decreased hemoglobin level.

DIAGNOSIS: Anemia due to iron deficiency

_____

Willard B. Reader, MD

WBR/pw   D: 09/25/18 09:50:16   T: 09/25/18 12:55:01

Determine the most accurate ICD-10-CM code(s).

_____

_____

_____

TAYLOR, READER, & ASSOCIATES
A Complete Health Care Facility
975 CENTRAL AVENUE • SOMEWHERE, FL 32811 • 407-555-4321

PATIENT: PUTNAM, EDNA
ACCOUNT/EHR #:   PUTNED001
DATE: 09/25/18

Attending Physician: Suzanne R. Taylor, MD

Edna Putnam, a 31-year-old woman, comes in to the ED, referred by her dentist, Dr. Titah. She had gone to see him because her gums were bleeding. The bleeding started on the day prior to evaluation and seems to be getting steadily worse with time. After briefly evaluating her, Dr. Titah noted diffuse bleeding from the mucosal surfaces around multiple teeth and referred her for further evaluation to us.

The patient states that she has never had an episode of anything similar in the past. Her past medical history is remarkable only for a tonsillectomy at age 11 that was uncomplicated. There is no family history of a bleeding disorder. She denies taking any medication regularly, only acetaminophen occasionally for headaches. She denies smoking or drinking alcohol.

On a review of systems, patient states that over the past month she has been feeling gradually more fatigued, which she attributes to working overtime at her job as a teacher. She denies fevers or chills but states that she may have lost a few pounds due to decreased appetite. She states that on her way to the emergency department, she noticed some small bruises on her forearms and thighs and that her ankles and feet seem to have numerous small red dots on them. She denies any chest pain, shortness of breath, abdominal pain, edema, headaches, dizziness, or other neurologic symptoms.

PHYSICAL EXAMINATION:
General: Pale-appearing woman in no acute distress. T 98.9°F, P 105, BP 94/64, RR 16.
Skin: Notable for several 2–3-cm ecchymoses on the forearms and thighs bilaterally; in addition, there is a petechial rash over the ankles and feet bilaterally.
HEENT: The oropharynx is notable for a small amount of fresh blood at the gum line around the base of multiple upper and lower incisors and molars.
CV: Normal S1, S2, regular, with a grade I/VI systolic murmur appreciated at the left sternal border.
Pulm: Unlabored respiration, clear to auscultation and percussion bilaterally.
Abd: Soft, nontender, nondistended, without organomegaly or mass.
Extr: Warm, well perfused, no edema, but with the ecchymoses and petechiae noted above.
Neuro: Alert and oriented to person, place, and time. No motor or sensory defects.
Lab: Review of the peripheral blood smear reveals decreased platelets, 3 to 4 schistocytes per high-powered field. The bone marrow aspirate and biopsy findings, along with the flow cytometric analysis, both document acute promyelocytic leukemia (APL).

DIAGNOSIS: Acute promyelocytic leukemia (APL)

PLAN: Patient is referred to oncology.

Suzanne R. Taylor, MD

SRT/pw   D: 09/27/18 09:50:16   T: 09/27/18 12:55:01

Determine the most accurate ICD-10-CM code(s).

_____

_____

_____

TAYLOR, READER, & ASSOCIATES
A Complete Health Care Facility
975 CENTRAL AVENUE • SOMEWHERE, FL 32811 • 407-555-4321

PATIENT: KLUMP, DUSTIN
ACCOUNT/EHR #:   KLUMDU001
DATE: 09/28/18

Attending Physician: Willard B. Reader, MD

S: Dustin presents to the emergency room today with rapid and painful breathing. Patient states he was exercising and has not drunk an appreciable amount of fluid today.

O: Ht 5′ 6″ Wt. 155 lb. R 28. T 101.4. BP 100/70. Dustin was diagnosed with sickle cell disease 2 years ago. Patient appears to be in crisis. Chest x-ray confirms pulmonary infiltration.

A: Sickle cell/Hb-C crisis with acute chest syndrome (ACS)

P: Admit to inpatient

_____

Willard B. Reader, MD

WBR/pw   D: 09/30/18 09:50:16   T: 09/30/18 12:55:01

Determine the most accurate ICD-10-CM code(s).

_____

_____

_____

TAYLOR, READER, & ASSOCIATES
A Complete Health Care Facility
975 CENTRAL AVENUE • SOMEWHERE, FL 32811 • 407-555-4321

PATIENT: LAMB, JEFF
ACCOUNT/EHR #:   LAMBJE001
DATE: 10/03/18

Attending Physician: Suzanne R. Taylor, MD

Jeff Lamb, a 23-year-old male aeronautical engineer, came to see me with complaints of a rash on his ankles and shins. He also noticed that he has been bruising easily for 10 days. The rash is not itchy or painful. He denies recent contact with new soaps or detergents. The bruises occur on his arms and sides, unrelated to trauma.

 On further questioning, he reports having had nosebleeds and gum bleeding when he flosses. He states he had an upper respiratory infection about 3 weeks ago, which has now resolved. On physical exam, he has no lymphadenopathy or hepatosplenomegaly. Stool sample testing is guaiac-positive.

LABORATORY FINDINGS:
The patient is thrombocytopenic. This is very apparent on both CBC and peripheral smear. There are no abnormalities of other cell lines. Platelet function analyzer and bleeding time cannot be used to assess platelet function due to the low platelet count. There is no evidence of a disorder of coagulation.

DIAGNOSIS: Autoimmune thrombocytopenia (ITP)

Suzanne R. Taylor, MD

SRT/pw D: 10/05/18 09:50:16 T: 10/05/18 12:55:01

Determine the most accurate ICD-10-CM code(s).

_____

_____

_____

TAYLOR, READER, & ASSOCIATES
A Complete Health Care Facility
975 CENTRAL AVENUE • SOMEWHERE, FL 32811 • 407-555-4321

PATIENT: KULP, RACHEL
ACCOUNT/EHR #:   KULPRA001
DATE: 10/10/18

Attending Physician: Willard B. Reader, MD

Rachel Kulp, a 49-year-old woman, comes in to see Dr. Reader with complaints of abdominal cramping and diarrhea. She states she has seen a lot of blood in her stools. She has a past history of a peptic ulcer and hypertension. The referring physician states he wants us to rule out a coagulopathy.

The patient states that her visible gastrointestinal bleeding began 10 days ago, but symptoms of colitis have been present for 3–4 weeks. She has a previous history of menorrhagia and excessive surgical bleeding but no family history of bleeding.

Although the patient has taken medication for the colitis, she has not been exposed to drugs that might have provoked or aggravated bleeding (i.e., aspirin), and her diet has been adequate.

A preliminary laboratory evaluation reveals hemoglobin of 7.6 g/dL (normal values for women range from 11.5 to 14 g/dL). The mean corpuscular volume (MCV) is 75 fL (normal: 80–100 fL). The patient had a normal prothrombin time (PT) and a prolonged activated partial thromboplastin time (aPTT).

A von Willebrand factor antigen assay, a von Willebrand factor activity assay, and factor VIII measurement were ordered and confirmed the diagnosis.

DIAGNOSIS: von Willebrand disease

Willard B. Reader, MD

WBR/pw   D: 10/12/18 09:50:16   T: 10/12/18 12:55:01

Determine the most accurate ICD-10-CM code(s).

CODING CONDITIONS OF THE ENDOCRINE AND METABOLIC SYSTEMS

7

Learning Outcomes *After completing this chapter, the student should be able to:*

LO 7.1 Identify the organs included in the endocrine system.

LO 7.2 Discern between type 1, type 2, secondary, and gestational diabetes mellitus.

LO 7.3 Apply the guidelines for coding diabetic manifestations and co-morbidities.

LO 7.4 Correctly code the use of insulin and insulin pumps.

LO 7.5 Abstract encounter notes to determine the involvement of hormones in certain malignancies.

LO 7.6 Determine the impact of an individual's weight on his or her health.

The endocrine system of glands and secretions does not typically come to mind as easily as the musculoskeletal system or even the nervous system. Yet the hormones and glandular activity of the endocrine system are also important to a healthy, active life.

Certainly, there are functions of the endocrine system with which you are familiar. You may know about adrenaline, a chemical that is pumped through the body when a person is frightened and that can sometimes provide an energy boost. Adrenaline is secreted through the adrenal gland, and when this gland is not working properly, it can result in a patient feeling weak and experiencing gastrointestinal disturbances.

In this chapter, you will review what coders need to know about accurately reporting conditions affecting the endocrine system.

LO 7.1 The Endocrine System

The endocrine system (see Figure 7-1) consists of glands located throughout the body, from the head to the genitals. Each organ performs a different purpose, releasing hormones and other chemicals required for proper function of the body. The glands included are the hypothalamus, pituitary gland, pineal gland, thyroid gland, parathyroid glands, thymus gland, adrenal glands, and pancreas, as well as the testes in men and the ovaries in women.

Endocrine Glands

Endocrine glands are the primary locations for hormone production. Hormones are chemical agents that interact with specific *target* cells. They travel via the bloodstream, and their effects vary, based on the specific type of cell they are targeting.

Key Terms
Adrenal glands
Cushing's syndrome
Diabetes mellitus
Dyslipidemia
Gestational diabetes mellitus (GDM)
Hyperglycemia
Hypoglycemia
Hypothalamus
Hypothyroidism
Pancreas
Parathyroid glands
Pineal gland
Pituitary gland
Polydipsia
Polyuria
Secondary
Thymus gland
Thyroid gland
Type 1
Type 2

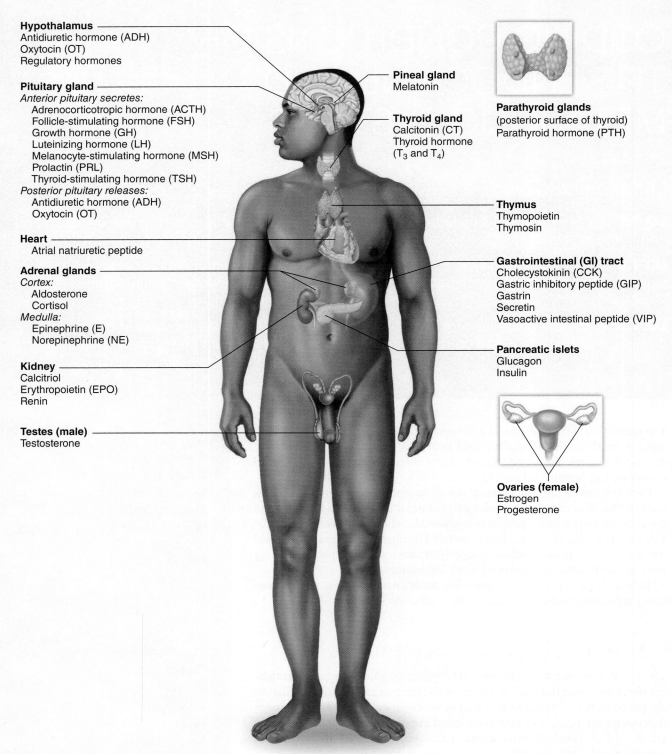

Hypothalamus
Antidiuretic hormone (ADH)
Oxytocin (OT)
Regulatory hormones

Pituitary gland
Anterior pituitary secretes:
  Adrenocorticotropic hormone (ACTH)
  Follicle-stimulating hormone (FSH)
  Growth hormone (GH)
  Luteinizing hormone (LH)
  Melanocyte-stimulating hormone (MSH)
  Prolactin (PRL)
  Thyroid-stimulating hormone (TSH)
Posterior pituitary releases:
  Antidiuretic hormone (ADH)
  Oxytocin (OT)

Heart
  Atrial natriuretic peptide

Adrenal glands
Cortex:
  Aldosterone
  Cortisol
Medulla:
  Epinephrine (E)
  Norepinephrine (NE)

Kidney
Calcitriol
Erythropoietin (EPO)
Renin

Testes (male)
Testosterone

Pineal gland
Melatonin

Thyroid gland
Calcitonin (CT)
Thyroid hormone
(T_3 and T_4)

Parathyroid glands
(posterior surface of thyroid)
Parathyroid hormone (PTH)

Thymus
Thymopoietin
Thymosin

Gastrointestinal (GI) tract
Cholecystokinin (CCK)
Gastric inhibitory peptide (GIP)
Gastrin
Secretin
Vasoactive intestinal peptide (VIP)

Pancreatic islets
Glucagon
Insulin

Ovaries (female)
Estrogen
Progesterone

FIGURE 7-1 The Endocrine System

Source: Booth et al., MA, 5e. Copyright © 2013 by McGraw-Hill. Figure 34-1, p. 659

hypothalamus

The part of the brain responsible for controlling body temperature and the autonomic nervous system.

Hypothalamus The **hypothalamus** is located within the third ventricle of the brain (see Figure 7-2) and is responsible for the creation of eight different hormones. Oxytocin and antidiuretic hormone (ADH) are stored in the posterior pituitary gland and are released as needed. In addition, the hypothalamus makes releasing hormones (RHs) that prompt the anterior pituitary gland to release hormones, as needed.

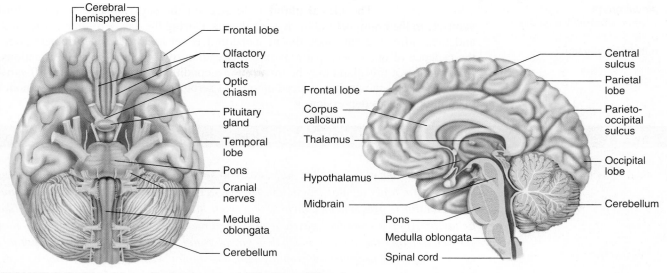

FIGURE 7-2 The Hypothalamus and Pituitary Gland

Source: Booth et al., MA, 5e. Copyright © 2013 by McGraw-Hill. Figure 30-6, p. 599

Pituitary Gland The **pituitary gland** (hypophysis) (see Figure 7-2) consists of two lobes: the *adenohypophysis,* the larger lobe sitting anteriorly, and the *neurohypophysis,* which is smaller and toward the posterior.

The adenohypophysis produces and releases hormones when prompted by the hypothalamus:

- *Adrenocorticotropic hormone (ACTH),* also known as *corticotropin,* is released to the adrenal glands to stimulate the production of corticosteroids.
- *Follicle-stimulating hormone (FSH)* is released to the ovaries to stimulate egg production in the female and is released to the testes to stimulate sperm production in the male.
- *Growth hormone (GH),* also known as *somatotropin,* is typically released to the liver as well as the bone, fat, and muscle tissues to encourage cells to enlarge and divide.
- *Luteinizing hormone (LH)* is used in the male, specifically the testes, to produce testosterone and is used in the female, specifically the ovaries, to stimulate ovulation as well as the secretion of estrogen and progesterone.
- *Prolactin (PRL)* is released to the mammary glands in women postpregnancy to stimulate milk production.
- *Thyroid-stimulating hormone (TSH),* also known as *thyrotropin,* is released to the thyroid gland to encourage the growth of the thyroid itself, as well as to stimulate the production of thyroxine.

The neurohypophysis is responsible for storing two types of hormones that, as you will remember from earlier in this chapter, come from the hypothalamus:

- *Oxytocin (OT)* is released during sexual intercourse to enhance the emotional bonding and feelings of satisfaction in both genders. In the female, during labor and delivery, OT encourages contractions of the uterus to expel the fetus. Postdelivery, OT promotes lactation to move the milk through the ducts into the nipple.
- *Antidiuretic hormone (ADH),* also known as *vasopressin,* reduces the amount of urine created by the kidneys.

pituitary gland
A two-lobed gland that creates and secretes hormones.

EXAMPLE

E23.0 Hypopituitarism (pituitary insufficiency NOS)
E24.3 Ectopic ACTH syndrome

Pineal Gland

The **pineal gland** is located on the superior aspect of the third ventricle in the brain, behind the hypothalamus. During the day, serotonin is secreted, and then, after the sun goes down, melatonin is released. These hormones affect the cadence of one's sleep patterns in the circadian rhythms and seasonal functions. Malfunction of this gland may be involved in a condition known as *seasonal affective disorder (SAD)*, in which a reduced amount of serotonin (due to a diminished amount of sunlight) causes depression.

LET'S CODE IT! SCENARIO

Clyde Bronsoner, a 53-year-old male, came to see Dr. Daniels, an endocrinologist, on a referral from his regular physician. He has been having visual disturbances (some hallucinations), frequent headaches, and what has been described as dementia-like behavior. After a complete physical examination, Dr. Daniels ordered an MRI that showed a neoplasm (tumor) on Clyde's pineal gland. Surgery and subsequent pathology revealed the neoplasm was malignant. The tumor was successfully excised and, ultimately, Clyde made a full recovery.

Let's Code It!

Dr. Daniels diagnosed Clyde with *a malignant neoplasm of the pineal gland.* When you turn to the Alphabetic Index (actually the Neoplasm Table within the index), you see:

Neoplasm, neoplastic

Pineal (body)(gland) C75.3 [Malignant primary]

Turn to the Tabular List and read:

C75 Malignant neoplasm of other endocrine glands and related structures

Read the *Excludes1* notation carefully. Several other endocrine organs are listed here, but not the pineal gland. Good! So keep reading down to evaluate the fourth-character choices for C75 to determine which code description matches Dr. Daniels's notes:

C75.3 Malignant neoplasm of pineal gland

Good job!

Thyroid Gland

The **thyroid gland** is located in the neck. Each of its two lobes reaches around the trachea laterally, and they connect anteriorly by an isthmus (see Figure 7-3).

The anterior pituitary gland transmits thyroid-stimulating hormone (TSH) to the thyroid, which then extracts iodine from the blood system to create two hormones. The two hormones secreted by this gland—triiodothyronine (T_3) and thyroxine (T_4)—are collectively known as *thyroid hormone (TH)*. Thyroid hormone is responsible for stimulating the production of proteins in virtually every tissue in the body, controlling the body's metabolic rate, and increasing the quantity of oxygen used by each cell. In addition, calcitonin is produced here from the C cells located in the follicles. This hormone, secreted in response to hypercalcemia (too much calcium in the blood), promotes the deposit of calcium and works in the formation of bone.

EXAMPLE

E03.1 Congenital hypothyroidism without goiter
E07.0 Hypersecretion of calcitonin

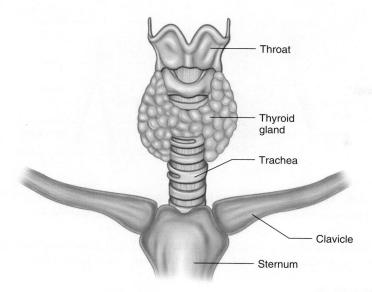

FIGURE 7-3 The Thyroid Gland

Parathyroid Glands   In the posterior aspect of the thyroid gland are four partially embedded **parathyroid glands.** When stimulated by hypocalcemia (too little calcium in the blood), they produce parathyroid hormone (PTH). PTH works in the opposite way of how calcitonin (produced by the thyroid) works.

parathyroid glands
Four small glands situated on the back of the thyroid gland that secrete parathyroid hormone.

> EXAMPLE
>
> E20.0 Idiopathic hypoparathyroidism
> E21.0 Primary hyperparathyroidism

Thymus Gland   Behind the sternum, medial to the two lobes of the lung and superior to the heart, lies the **thymus gland.** This gland, made of fibrous tissue, produces several hormones that encourage T-lymphocyte production.

thymus gland
A gland that assists in the development of the immune system prior to puberty.

> EXAMPLE
>
> E32.0 Persistent hyperplasia of thymus
> E32.1 Abscess of thymus

Adrenal Glands   Located on the superior aspect of each kidney (see Figure 7-4) are the **adrenal glands** (also known as the *suprarenal glands*). These glands produce more than 25 adrenocortical hormones (also known as *corticoids* or *corticosteroids*). Each of these hormones is categorized within one of the following groups:

adrenal glands
Glands situated on the superior aspect of each kidney that secrete critical hormones, including epinephrine; also known as *suprarenal glands.*

- *Mineralocorticoids* encourage the kidneys to retain sodium (salt) and excrete potassium. The primary hormone in this group is aldosterone.
- *Glucocorticoids* assist in the regulation of glucose levels in the blood as well as the catabolism of fats and proteins. The primary hormone in this group is hydrocortisone (also known as *cortisol*), which functions as an anti-inflammatory.
- *Androgens* are secreted to other tissues and converted into testosterone. This group includes dehydroepiandrosterone (DHEA).
- *Estrogens,* most particularly estradiol, are produced in the adrenal gland. They are also produced in the ovaries, but in smaller amounts.

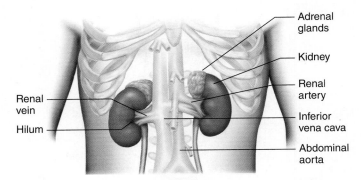

FIGURE 7-4 The Adrenal Glands (Golden Area) on Top of Each Kidney

Source: David Shier et al., HOLE'S HUMAN ANATOMY & PHYSIOLOGY, 12/e. © 2010 MHE. Figure 20.1, p. 776

The adrenal medulla (the interior aspect of the adrenal gland) produces epinephrine (also known as *adrenaline*) as well as norepinephrine, both known as *catecholamines*.

> ## EXAMPLE
>
> E26.02 Glucocorticoid-remediable aldosteronism
> E27.1 Primary adrenocortical insufficiency

Pancreas As a part of the digestive system, the **pancreas** functions in the processing of nourishment to the body. Its primary responsibility is to contribute digestive juices via a duct into the duodenum to assist in digestion. However, also included in the pancreas are clusters of endocrine cells known as the *islets of Langerhans,* or *pancreatic islets* (see Figure 7-5). These cells have their own responsibilities:

- Production of glucagon, via the alpha cells, that encourages the liver to release glucose into the blood to countermand low blood glucose.
- Production of insulin, via the beta cells, to reduce the amount of glucose in the blood—the opposite of the process of glucagon—by encouraging absorption of glucose into the muscle and fat cells.
- Production of somatostatin, via delta cells, which is a controlling hormone that discourages the secretion of both insulin and glucagon within the pancreas itself.

> ## EXAMPLE
>
> E16.3 Increased secretion of glucagon
> E16.9 Disorder of pancreatic internal secretion (Islet-cell hyperplasia)

Disorders of the Endocrine System

When any part of the complex endocrine system malfunctions, health problems arise. Let's review some of the most common concerns.

LO 7.2 Diabetes Mellitus

Diabetes mellitus (DM) is a chronic disease and a result of insulin deficiency or resistance due to a malfunction of the pancreatic beta cells (Figure 7-5). The body has a difficult time metabolizing carbohydrates, proteins, and fats. It is estimated that 16 million people have DM; however, many (possibly as many as 50%) do not know it yet.

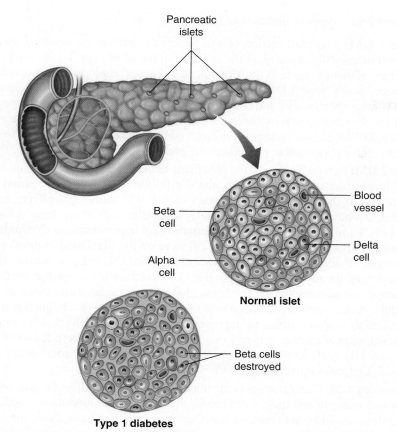

Pancreatic islets

Beta cell

Alpha cell

Blood vessel

Delta cell

Normal islet

Beta cells destroyed

Type 1 diabetes

FIGURE 7-5 The Pancreatic Islets

A physician can diagnose diabetes with a glucose lab test and the presence of the following signs and symptoms:

- Excessive thirst (**polydipsia**)
- Excessive appetite
- Increased urination (**polyuria**)
- Unusual weight change (loss or gain)
- Fatigue
- Nausea, vomiting
- Blurred vision
- Frequent vaginal infections (females)
- Yeast infections (both males and females)
- Dry mouth
- Slow-healing sores or cuts
- Itchy skin, especially in the groin or vaginal area

Measures for detecting diabetes include a glucose tolerance test (GTT) and evaluation of the results. Diabetes may be indicated by:

- A casual plasma glucose value greater than or equal to 200 mg/dL.
- A fasting plasma glucose level greater than or equal to 126 mg/dL.
- A plasma glucose value in the 2-hour sample of the oral glucose tolerance test greater than or equal to 200 mg/dL.

(*Note:* Normal blood glucose levels are less than 110 mg/dL.)

polydipsia
Excessive thirst.

polyuria
Excessive urination.

There are four types of diabetes mellitus:

- **Type 1 DM:** The malfunction of the pancreatic beta cells, resulting in no production of insulin naturally, is the underlying cause of type 1 (juvenile) diabetes mellitus, although there is no documented known etiology for idiopathic DM. Therapeutically, type 1 DM patients must administer insulin every day in addition to following specific diet and exercise programs. Implanted insulin pumps may be used for those requiring multiple dose regimens. This diagnosis will be reported from ICD-10-CM code category E10 with additional characters required to identify specific information about complications (manifestations).

- **Type 2 DM:** In type 2 patients, the pancreatic beta cells do produce insulin; however, the glucose transport is ineffective, thereby failing to deliver the required amount to the rest of the body. Type 2 diabetics often suffer pathologic effects, including increased body fat (obesity), especially when the individual does not exercise regularly. Family history of DM, co-morbidities of hypertension or **dyslipidemia,** or a personal history of gestational DM will increase the likelihood of developing this condition. In addition, patients of African-American, Latino, or Native American heritage are found to have a high risk. Diet and exercise are the first level of treatment and may resolve the condition. However, oral antidiabetic medications, such as sulfonylureas, may be prescribed to stimulate pancreatic beta cell function if diet and exercise fail to show sufficient improvement. Some type 2 DM patients require the administration of insulin. A type 2 diagnosis will be reported from ICD-10-CM code category E11 with additional characters required to identify specific information about complications (manifestations).

- **Secondary DM:** Certain drugs or chemicals can negatively affect the pancreatic beta cells and may prevent them from producing the required amount of insulin. Also, other diseases and conditions, such as Cushing's syndrome, can cause the patient to develop diabetes mellitus. This diagnosis is reported from code category E08, Diabetes mellitus due to underlying condition; E09, Drug or chemical induced diabetes mellitus; or E13, Other specified diabetes mellitus; additional characters are required to provide specific information about complications. The underlying condition, drug, or chemical causing the secondary DM will be reported first, and any codes required to identify specific manifestations will be reported following the E08, E09, or E13 code.

- **Gestational DM:** When a woman is pregnant, the weight gain, along with the higher levels of estrogen and the increase of placental hormones, may retard the production of insulin. This is considered a temporary type of DM due to the fact that, typically, the problem with the pancreatic beta cells resolves itself after the baby is delivered. Report this with a code from the ICD-10-CM code subcategory O24.4, Gestational diabetes mellitus, with an additional character to report additional details.

LO 7.3 Diabetic Manifestations

Due to its involvement with the blood system as well as muscle and fat tissue, there can be serious manifestations—the development of other illnesses and conditions—caused by suffering with DM long-term, especially when the condition goes untreated.

Ophthalmic Manifestations The problems that diabetics frequently experience with their eyes are actually related to vascular concerns. Diabetic retinopathy, one of the leading causes of irreversible blindness, may be one of several types:

- *Background retinopathy:* blood vessel damage with no current vision problems.
- *Maculopathy:* damage to the macula part of the eye, resulting in a considerable loss of vision.
- *Proliferative retinopathy:* a microvascular complication of diabetes in which the small vessels of the eye become diseased as a result of diminishing oxygen.
- *Other eye problems often suffered by diabetics:* diabetic cataracts and macular edema.

GUIDANCE CONNECTION

Review the ICD-10-CM Coding Guidelines, Sections I.C.4, Chapter 4: **Endocrine, nutritional, and metabolic diseases (E00–E90),** Subsection a, **Diabetes mellitus,** and I.C.15, Chapter 15: **Pregnancy, childbirth, and the puerperium,** Subsections g, **Diabetes mellitus in pregnancy,** and i, **Gestational (pregnancy induced) diabetes.**

Diabetic retinopathy is evidenced by microcirculatory changes in the eye that interfere with the blood supply and therefore the health of the eye. Nonproliferative diabetic retinopathy is seen in the blood vessels of the retina leaking plasma or fatty substances, resulting in diminished blood flow. Proliferative diabetic retinopathy encourages neovascularization (the growth of new blood vessels) in the vitreous of the eye; these vessels then rupture, causing a hemorrhage and sudden loss of vision. Without treatment, this can cause blindness. A diagnosis of type 1 diabetic retinopathy would be reported with a code from ICD-10-CM code subcategory E10.3, Type I diabetes mellitus with ophthalmic complications, with the required additional characters determined by the specifics (proliferative/nonproliferative, with/without macular edema, mild/moderate/severe).

Neurologic Manifestations Uncontrolled diabetes can cause damage to the patient's nerves, causing diabetic neuropathy—in particular, sensory diabetic neuropathy, or a lack of feeling. Sensory diabetic neuropathy can be dangerous because the damaged nerves do not transmit feelings of heat, cold, or pain. Such a patient might be burned or cut and not know it. The injuries might become infected, causing additional health problems. In addition, the nerve damage can retard healing, making additional complications more viable.

Renal Manifestations *Diabetic nephropathy* develops due to the reduced control of blood sugar. Almost 30% of diabetics develop diabetic nephropathy (kidney disease) or other kidney-related problems, such as bladder infections and nerve damage to the bladder. The nephrons within the kidneys thicken, and the scarring that forms results in leakage of albumin (protein) into the urine. Quantitative lab tests examine the levels of albumin in the patient's urine (microalbuminuria), as well as other levels such as blood urea nitrogen (BUN) and serum creatinine. Diabetic kidney disease can cause severe illness and possibly death. Therefore, early diagnosis and treatment to prevent the progression of the condition is important. Angiotensin-converting enzyme (ACE) inhibitors as well as angiotensin receptor blockers (ARB) are considered the best medications in these cases. A diagnosis of type 2 diabetic nephropathy is reported from ICD-10-CM subcategory E11.2, Type 2 diabetes mellitus with kidney complications, with an additional character to report a chronic or other condition.

You may need a second code to identify the exact nature of the renal complication, such as the stage of the chronic kidney failure. Type 2 diabetes–related chronic kidney disease may be reported with E11.22, Type 2 diabetes mellitus with diabetic chronic kidney disease; diabetic nephropathy may be reported with E10.21, Type 1 diabetes mellitus with diabetic nephropathy.

Circulatory Manifestations Peripheral vascular disease is another likely complication because diabetes mellitus disturbs the blood flow, increasing the development of ulcers. It is estimated that as many as 10% of diabetics develop foot ulcers. Gangrene, a condition by which necrosis (tissue death) occurs as a result of lack of blood, is another relatively common manifestation. When gangrene is not caught early enough, the resulting treatment to stop the spread of the necrosis is often amputation. You might report one of these diagnoses with code E09.52, Drug or chemical induced diabetes mellitus with diabetic peripheral angiopathy with gangrene, or E11.51, Type 2 diabetes mellitus with diabetic peripheral angiopathy without gangrene.

LET'S CODE IT! SCENARIO

Andrew Claussen, a 50-year-old male, came to see Dr. Scout for his annual checkup. He is a type 1 insulin-dependent diabetic. He has been feeling fine and has no diabetic-related manifestations.

Dr. Scout's notes state that Andrew has *type 1 diabetes mellitus* with *no complications*. When you turn to the Alphabetic Index, you see:

Diabetes, diabetic (mellitus)(sugar) E11.9

When you turn to the Tabular List, you confirm:

E11 Type 2 diabetes mellitus

Oh, wait a minute. This code category is for type 2 diabetes. Dr. Scout's notes document that Andrew has type 1 diabetes. Turn the pages and review this whole section to see if you can find a more accurate code category. Did you find:

E10 Type 1 diabetes mellitus

There is an *includes* note as well as an *Excludes1* notation listing several diagnoses. Take a minute to review them and determine if any apply to Andrew's condition. No, none of them do, so continue down and review all of the fourth-character choices. Which matches Dr. Scout's notes?

E10.9 Type 1 diabetes mellitus without complications

Perfect!

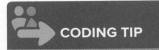

CODING TIP

The code for long-term insulin use is not used for patients with type 1 diabetes mellitus. Remember, type 1 DM is known as insulin-dependent diabetes making Z79.4 unnecessary.

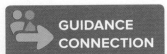

GUIDANCE CONNECTION

Review the ICD-10-CM Coding Guidelines, Section I.C.4, Chapter 4: **Endocrine, nutritional, and metabolic diseases (E00–E90)**, Subsection a(3), **Diabetes mellitus and the use of insulin**.

LO 7.4 Long-Term Insulin Use

In cases where a patient diagnosed with type 2 diabetes has been using insulin on a regular basis, you have to include a code stating that fact:

Z79.4 Long-term (current) use of insulin

You can see the notation at the beginning of the E11, Type 2 diabetes mellitus, code category:

Use additional code to identify any insulin use (Z79.4)

The additional code will accurately report that:

- A patient with non-insulin-dependent diabetes mellitus has been using insulin steadily.
- The insulin use is not a one-time or temporary treatment.

YOU CODE IT! CASE STUDY

Renyatta Tackler, a 43-year-old female, was diagnosed with type 2 diabetes a year ago. Dr. Eng had prescribed tolbutamide to stimulate her pancreatic insulin release. However, 6 months ago, he became concerned that the medication was not working and started her on a regime of insulin injections. She is here today for Dr. Eng to check her insulin levels.

You Code It!

Go through the steps of coding, and determine the code or codes that should be reported for this encounter between Dr. Eng and Renyatta Tackler.

Step 1: Read the case completely.

Step 2: Abstract the notes: Which key words can you identify relating to why Dr. Eng cared for Renyatta?

_____

Step 3: Query the provider, if necessary.

Step 4: Code the diagnosis or diagnoses.

_____

Step 5: Code the procedure(s): Office visit for long-term insulin use.

Step 6: Link the procedure codes to at least one diagnosis code to confirm medical necessity.

Step 7: Back code to double-check your choices.

Answer:

Did you determine the correct codes to be:

E11.9 Type 2 diabetes mellitus without complications

Z79.4 Long-term (current) use of insulin

Hyperglycemia

A patient with **hyperglycemia** is *not* diagnosed with diabetes. Hyperglycemia, just like **hypoglycemia,** is a separate condition.

Chronic hyperglycemia may impair one's resistance to infection, resulting in diabetic skin problems and urinary tract infections. A diabetic patient that has hypoglycemia may have administered too much insulin or antidiabetic medication.

hyperglycemia
Abnormally high levels of glucose.

hypoglycemia
Abnormally low glucose levels.

Hypothyroidism (Adults)

Hypothyroidism is caused by an insufficient production of thyroid hormone (TH). This might be the result of irradiation therapy, infection, Hashimoto's disease (chronic autoimmune thyroiditis), or pituitary failure to produce the required amount of thyroid-stimulating hormone (TSH). Fatigue, hypercholesterolemia, unexplained increase in weight, forgetfulness, or even unusual sensitivity to colder temperatures are early signs of this condition.

To confirm this diagnosis, radioimmunoassay and/or lab tests are performed to look at the levels of TSH. Lab tests can identify the patient's TSH levels; however, reference ranges may fluctuate depending upon the patient's age and family history. Treatment for hypothyroidism includes medication, such as levothyroxine, to replace TH. Disorders of the thyroid gland, including hypothyroidism, are reported from code categories E00–E07, Disorders of thyroid gland.

hypothyroidism
A condition in which the thyroid converts energy more slowly than normal, resulting in an otherwise unexplained weight gain and fatigue.

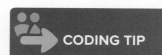

CODING TIP

If you recognize a patient's condition from a lab report, but the physician did not document a confirmed diagnosis, you must *query* the physician. You may *not* code from the lab report.

Cushing's Syndrome

Cushing's syndrome is caused by excessive production of corticotropin (ACTH) in the hypothalamus and too much secretion from the adenohypophysis (pituitary gland). This may be caused by a tumor in another organ affecting this process—possibly a bronchogenic tumor or a malignant neoplasm of the pancreas. Approximately 30% of such cases are the result of a benign neoplasm of the adrenal gland.

Cushing's syndrome may cause diabetes mellitus, hypokalemia (low potassium in the blood), pathologic fractures, slow wound healing, hypertension, irritability, and other conditions. Lab tests for plasma steroid levels measured by 24-hour urine samples can

Cushing's syndrome
A condition resulting from the hyperproduction of corticosteroids, most often caused by an adrenal cortex tumor or a tumor of the pituitary gland.

be used to confirm a diagnosis of Cushing's syndrome. An adrenal tumor can be seen on an ultrasound, CT scan, or angiography, while MRI and CT scans can illuminate the presence of a pituitary tumor.

Administration of radiation therapy, drug therapy with a medication such as aminoglutethimide, or surgery to remove the tumor can be successful to control or reverse the effects of Cushing's syndrome. ICD-10-CM code category E24, Cushing's syndrome, requires an additional character to provide more specific information about the condition.

LO 7.5 Functional Activity of Hormones in Neoplasms

When a gland has been found to have a neoplasm (tumor), whether it is benign or malignant, an additional code may be necessary to identify the *functional activity* of the affected gland. Functional activity identifies that the gland is secreting hormones in abnormal quantities.

For example, in the Tabular List of ICD-10-CM, beneath code D13.7, Benign neoplasm of endocrine pancreas (benign neoplasm of islets of Langerhans), is a notation:

Use additional code to identify any functional activity

Correspondingly, at the beginning of ICD-10-CM Chapter 4, Endocrine, nutritional, and metabolic diseases (E00–E89), within the Tabular List, you will see this note:

All neoplasms, whether functionally active or not, are classified in Chapter 2 [Neoplasms]. Appropriate codes in this chapter (i.e. E05.8, E07.0, E16–E31, E34-) may be used as additional codes to indicate either functional activity by neoplasms and ectopic endocrine tissue or hyperfunction and hypofunction of endocrine glands associated with neoplasms and other conditions classified elsewhere.

If you follow our example of D13.7, Benign neoplasm of islets of Langerhans, the documentation may also state the patient is experiencing increased secretion of somatostatin. In this case, you would report D13.7 followed by E16.8, Other specified disorders of pancreatic internal secretion.

LET'S CODE IT! SCENARIO

Barry Swanzer, a 55-year-old male, has been feeling excessively tired and irritable. He tells Dr. Brickman that he has felt edgy and nervous while experiencing cold sweats and trembling. Dr. Brickman performs a glucose-screening test using a reagent strip with a reading of less than 45 mg/dL. He orders a lab test to confirm a diagnosis of reactive hypoglycemia and provides Barry with a diet to follow and a referral to a nutritionist.

Let's Code It!

Barry has been diagnosed with *reactive hypoglycemia*. Let's turn to the Alphabetic Index and look it up:

Hypoglycemia (spontaneous) E16.2

Read all the way down the indented list to find:

Reactive (not drug-induced) E16.1

The Tabular List describes the code as:

E16 Other disorders of pancreatic internal secretion

There are no notations or directives, so keep reading down the column.

E16.1 Other hypoglycemia

E16.2 Hypoglycemia, unspecified

How do you decide between these two codes? Let's think about this. Dr. Brickman *did* specify the type of hypoglycemia that Barry has, so you cannot report that this detail was "unspecified." This eliminates E16.2 and confirms that E16.1, Other hypoglycemia, is accurate.

Notice that the *Excludes1* note under code E16.1 states that neither hypoglycemia in infant of diabetic mother (P70.1) nor neonatal hypoglycemia is to be reported with this code. Does it apply to Barry's case? Dr. Brickman indicated that Barry is an adult; therefore, it does not apply.

The correct diagnosis code for the encounter between Dr. Brickman and Barry is:

E16.1 Other Hypoglycemia

Excellent!

Insulin Pumps

Technology has provided patients with an easier and more controlled manner by which to get their insulin: an insulin pump. However, nothing is perfect, so there may be a concern with the patient as a result of the insulin pump not working correctly.

Underdose of Insulin It can be very dangerous for a patient to receive less than the proper amount of insulin, as prescribed by the physician, on schedule. If that occurs and is the reason the physician is caring for the patient at the encounter, your first-listed code should be:

T85.614* Breakdown (mechanical) of insulin pump

(*This T code requires a seventh character to identify the encounter as initial, subsequent, or for sequela of this breakdown.)

Follow that code with the proper diabetes mellitus code and any other appropriate codes, including codes for any effects, or conditions, caused by the insulin underdose.

If the patient's ill health is caused by an underdose of insulin that the patient injects by hand (not using a pump), meaning that the patient is not taking the correct amount as often as it was prescribed, you might use the following code:

Z91.1* Patient's noncompliance with medical treatment and regimen

(*This Z code requires a fifth character to identify the intent of the noncompliance, such as intentional, unintentional, etc.)

Also note that beneath code Z91.12 and Z91.13 is a notation:

Code first underdosing of medication (T36–T50) with fifth or sixth character 6

This T code will enable you to report which specific medication was underdosed. So, in this example, you would also report:

T38.3x6* Underdosing of insulin and oral hypoglycemic (antidiabetic) drugs

(*This T code requires a seventh character to identify the encounter as initial, subsequent, or for sequela of this breakdown.)

Blossom Glascow, an 18-year-old female, was diagnosed with type 1 diabetes 2 years ago. Starting college, Blossom kept forgetting to take her insulin as prescribed. She comes into the University Health Center because she feels dizzy, weak, and confused. Dr. Primo, the on-call physician, finds her to have poor skin turgor and dry mucous membranes. He diagnoses her with dehydration caused by insulin deficiency and diabetes mellitus, type 1, uncontrolled.

You Code It!

Go through the steps of coding, and determine the code or codes that should be reported for this encounter between Dr. Primo and Blossom Glascow.

Step 1: Read the case completely.

Step 2: Abstract the notes: Which key words can you identify relating to why Dr. Primo cared for Blossom?

_____

Step 3: Query the provider, if necessary.

Step 4: Code the diagnosis or diagnoses.

_____

Step 5: Code the procedure(s): Office visit.

Step 6: Link the procedure codes to at least one diagnosis code to confirm medical necessity.

Step 7: Back code to double-check your choices.

Answer:

Did you determine the correct codes to be:

E86.0 Dehydration

E10.9 Type 1 diabetes mellitus without mention of complications

T38.3x6* Underdosing of insulin and oral hypoglycemic (antidiabetic) drugs

Z91.138 Patient's unintentional underdosing of medication regimen for other reason

(*This T code requires a seventh character to identify the encounter as initial, subsequent, or for sequela of this issue.)

Overdose of Insulin Patients with an insulin pump that malfunctions can dose with a higher quantity of insulin than prescribed by the attending physician. For such a case, you will use the following code (which is the same as the code for an underdose):

T85.614* Breakdown (mechanical) of insulin pump

(*This T code requires a seventh character to identify the encounter as initial, subsequent, or for sequela of this breakdown.)

Follow that code with a poisoning code:

T38.3x Poisoning by insulin and oral hypoglycemia (antidiabetic) drugs**

(*This T code requires a sixth character to identify the motivation [intentional, accidental, undetermined] and a seventh character to identify the encounter as initial, subsequent, or for sequela of this breakdown.)

Follow that code with the appropriate diabetes mellitus code and any other appropriate codes, including the codes identifying the reaction or conditions caused by the overdose.

If the patient delivers a dose of insulin manually and suffers an overdose, you will code it the same way you do any other poisoning, including the determination of the cause of the overdose (such as accident, attempted suicide, or assault). Unless the health concern with the patient is an adverse reaction to the insulin and not related to the actual dosage, you will not use the code reporting therapeutic usage.

GUIDANCE CONNECTION

Review the ICD-10-CM Coding Guidelines, Section I.C.4, Chapter 4: **Endocrine, nutritional, and metabolic diseases (E00–E90)**, Subsection a(5), **Complications due to insulin pump malfunction.**

Diabetes Insipidus

Another type of diabetes that few people have heard of is *diabetes insipidus (DI)*. DI is a disorder of water metabolism that is the result of an antidiuretic hormone (ADH) deficiency. Intracranial neoplastic or metastatic lesions, hypophysectomy or other neurosurgery, or skull fractures or other head trauma that damages the neurohypophyseal structures can all incite DI. The condition can also result from infection. Diabetes insipidus is also known as *pituitary diabetes insipidus* and is coded using E23.2 from the subsection for disorders of the pituitary gland.

Nephrogenic diabetes insipidus, another form of DI, is a very rare congenital disturbance of water metabolism resulting from a renal tubular resistance to vasopressin. Interestingly, it is not coded from the congenital anomalies, but is reported using code N25.1, Disorders resulting from impaired renal function.

YOU CODE IT! CASE STUDY

Chet McKeen, a 19-year-old male, comes to see Dr. Turner with complaints of extreme thirst and muscle weakness. During examination, Dr. Turner identifies that Chet has poor tissue turgor, dry mucous membranes, and hypotension. UA results show urine of low osmolality at 75 mOsm/kg. Dr. Turner diagnoses Chet with diabetes insipidus and prescribes vasopressin IM qid.

You Code It!

Go through the steps of coding, and determine the code or codes that should be reported for this encounter between Dr. Turner and Chet McKeen.

Step 1:   Read the case completely.

Step 2:   Abstract the notes: Which key words can you identify relating to why Dr. Turner cared for Chet?

_____

Step 3:   Query the provider, if necessary.

Step 4:   Code the diagnosis or diagnoses.

_____

Step 5: Code the procedure(s): Office visit, urinalysis.

Step 6: Link the procedure codes to at least one diagnosis code to confirm medical necessity.

Step 7: Back code to double-check your choices.

Answer:

Did you determine the correct code to be:

E23.2 Diabetes insipidus

Good job!

LO 7.6 Weight Factors

Obesity

The definitions of *overweight, obese,* and *morbidly obese* can get lost in societal norms and self-perception. Of course, the health care industry has its own official determinations of these conditions, further specified by reporting the patient's body mass index (BMI).

Overweight merely means weighing too much. This can be a reference to the individual's muscles, bones, fat, or fluid retention when calculated along with the person's height. This condition is calculated as a BMI of 25 to 29.9.

Obesity is a condition calculated as a body mass index of 30 to 38.9. Typically, a person becomes obese when more calories are consumed than expended. While some critics believe extra pounds are caused only by eating too much and not exercising enough, the facts are that one's genetics and current medications (including herbal supplements) can also influence this condition.

Being diagnosed as obese is a true health condition that not only can result in self-esteem problems and social anxiety but also may increase the risk of developing diabetes, heart disease, arthritis, stroke, and even certain malignancies.

Morbid obesity is diagnosed when a patient's current overweight status increases to the extent that it actually interferes with normal, daily activities. This condition is calculated as a BMI over 39.

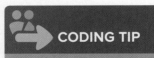

CODING TIP

Several different types of health care professionals, such as a dietician or a nutritionist, may be involved in the care of a patient determined to be overweight, obese, or morbidly obese. However, the first time this diagnosis code is reported it may be coded only from physician documentation.

EXAMPLE

E66 Overweight and obesity
Use additional code to identify Body Mass Index (BMI) if known (Z68.-)
E66.01 Morbid (severe) obesity due to excess calories
E66.09 Other obesity due to excess calories
E66.1 Drug-induced obesity
E66.2 Morbid (severe) obesity with alveolar hypoventilation
E66.3 Overweight
E66.8 Other obesity
E66.9 Obesity, unspecified

As you can see, ICD-10-CM reminds you to use an additional code to specify the patient's BMI.

Body Mass Index

It is important for health care professionals to determine specifically what is a healthy amount of body fat and what falls or rises to an unhealthy level. Body mass index (BMI) is a calculation using an individual's actual weight and current height to determine a workable measure of body fat. However, some people, such as athletes, may have a BMI that indicates he or she is overweight even though there is no excess body fat. This can occur because BMI does not actually measure body fat but instead determines a ratio with which to work. BMI is just an indicator of potential health risks related to an individual's being outside the normal weight range.

BMI ranges are listed differently for adults than they are for children and teens. The pediatric ranges, used for individuals aged 2 to 20 years, are based on the growth charts of the Centers for Disease Control and take into account the normal differences in body fat for various ages as well as differences between boys and girls.

Z68 Body Mass Index [BMI]

Adult BMI codes range from Z68.1–Z68.45. The Pediatric BMI code is:

Z68.5* Body Mass Index [BMI] pediatric

(*An additional character is required to identify the percentile for the patient's age.)

Underweight

With all the discussion regarding how many people in the United States are overweight or clinically obese, the opposite—being underweight—can also cause health concerns. Unlike the codes for overweight conditions, codes for reporting an abnormal weight loss or underweight condition are listed in the Symptoms, signs, and ill-defined conditions section of ICD-10-CM. In certain cases, the BMI will also need to be reported.

EXAMPLE

R63.4 Abnormal weight loss
R63.6 Underweight
Use additional code to identify Body Mass Index (BMI) if known (Z68.-)

When a patient is diagnosed with anorexia, you may need more information from the physician before determining the correct code.

R63.0 Anorexia

(This is used when the cause of the anorexia has not been determined as organic [physiological)] or nonorganic [psychological].)

F50.0* Anorexia nervosa

F50.2 Bulimia nervosa

F50.8* Loss of appetite of non-organic origin

Other Metabolic Disorders

When you eat, it is your metabolism that processes nutrition into energy. The chemicals in the digestive system portion out glucoses and acids from the carbohydrates, fats, and proteins in the food. This process is known as *metabolization*. The energy created by this process can be used right away—for example, when someone eats before taking a test or running a race. If the body doesn't need the energy at this time, the tissues in the liver and the muscular system, as well as the adipose (body fat), can store it for future use.

Dysfunction of the metabolic processes can interfere with the various systems of the body getting what they need to work properly. This may be realized as too little of a

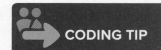

CODING TIP

While you may see issues of overweight status accompanying diagnoses such as diabetes mellitus or hypertension, in cases of underweight patients, be alert to initial or additional diagnoses of malnutrition.

chemical needed, such as when the pancreas cannot create enough insulin (a condition known as *diabetes mellitus*). You have already learned about what havoc can be caused in the other organs and systems when this disorder continues. Metabolic disorders can also result in too much of a chemical being present in the body. For example, hyperchloremia is an excessive level of chloride anion in the blood and can cause tachycardia (rapid heartbeat), hypertension, dyspnea (shortness of breath), and agitation.

The long list of metabolic diagnoses includes:

- Acid lipase disease
- Amyloidosis
- Barth's syndrome
- Central pontine myelinolysis
- Metabolic diseases of muscle
- Farber's disease
- G6PD deficiency
- Gangliosidoses
- Hunter's syndrome
- Trimethylaminuria
- Lesch-Nyhan syndrome
- Lipid storage diseases
- Metabolic myopathies
- Mitochondrial myopathies
- Mucopolysaccharidoses (MPS)
- Mucolipidoses
- Mucopolysaccharidoses
- Type I glycogen storage disease
- Pompe's disease
- Urea cycle disorder
- Hyperoxaluria
- Oxalosis

YOU CODE IT! CASE STUDY

Marilyn brought her 4-year-old son, Elian, to his pediatrician, Dr. Willows. She was very distressed because Elian had eruptions on his arms, legs, and face that appeared after he had spent the day at the beach. She had also noticed that his urine appeared to be reddish in color. Dr. Willows examined Elian and discovered that he had splenomegaly (enlargement of the spleen). The blood test came back positive for hemolytic anemia. Both of these conditions are signs of erythropoietic porphyria, also known as Gunther's disease. Dr. Willows diagnosed Elian with this condition.

You Code It!

Go through the steps of coding, and determine the code or codes that should be reported for this encounter between Dr. Willows and Elian.

Step 1: Read the case completely.

Step 2: Abstract the notes: Which key words can you identify relating to why Dr. Willows cared for Elian?

Step 3: Query the provider, if necessary.

Step 4: Code the diagnosis or diagnoses.

Step 5: Code the procedure(s): Office visit, blood work.

Step 6: Link the procedure codes to at least one diagnosis code to confirm medical necessity.

Step 7: Back code to double-check your choices.

Answer:

Did you determine the correct code to be:

E80.0 Hereditary erythropoietic porphyria

Good job!

Thyroid Disorders

Above your collarbone, in your neck, is the thyroid gland. This gland secretes hormones as a part of the metabolic system of the body.

Hypothyroidism is a condition in which the thyroid converts energy more slowly than normal, resulting in an otherwise unexplained weight gain and fatigue. In addition, individuals with hypothyroidism may often feel cold or have greater sensitivity to cold temperatures.

Hyperthyroidism, also known as *overactive thyroid,* is a condition in which the thyroid secretes too many hormones, more than the body needs to function properly. Signs and symptoms include unexplained weight loss, rapid heart rate, and sensitivity to heat.

Additional disorders of the thyroid include:

- Goiter
- Graves' disease
- Hashimoto's disease
- Thyroid nodules
- Thyroiditis
- Myxedema

Conditions and diseases that are related to or involve the thyroid and its function include:

- Celiac disease
- Iodine deficiency
- Thyroid eye disease (protruding, irritated eyes)
- Thyrotoxic myopathy

YOU CODE IT! CASE STUDY

Gretel Hanson, a 63-day-old female, was having dyspnea and her cry sounded hoarse. In addition, Dr. Grissom noticed her skin color was jaundiced. Her mother stated that she is a good baby and sleeps all the time. After running a TSH blood test and performing a thyroid scan, he diagnosed Gretel with infantile cretinism, also known as congenital hypothyroidism. Dr. Grissom also noted mild cognitive impairment, which is associated with the cretinism. He explained to Gretel's mother that the mental impairment is likely to be progressive.

Go through the steps of coding, and determine the code or codes that should be reported for this encounter between Dr. Grissom and Gretel.

Step 1: Read the case completely.

Step 2: Abstract the notes: Which key words can you identify relating to why Dr. Grissom cared for Gretel?

_____

Step 3: Query the provider, if necessary.

Step 4: Code the diagnosis or diagnoses.

_____

Step 5: Code the procedure(s): Office visit, blood work.

Step 6: Link the procedure codes to at least one diagnosis code to confirm medical necessity.

Step 7: Back code to double-check your choices.

Answer:

Did you determine the correct codes to be:

E03.1 Congenital hypothyroidism without goiter

G31.84 Mild cognitive impairment, so stated

Good for you!

Chapter Summary

The glands of the endocrine system produce and release various types of hormones that are used by numerous organs throughout the body—all a part of the function of a healthy body. When a component of this system does not function properly, the harm can cascade and reveal itself as signs and symptoms evident with other body systems, such as the urinary system or reproductive system. Diabetes mellitus is probably the most common of the conditions and diseases affecting the endocrine system. From the hypothalamus of the brain to the genitals, every part of this system, like all of the others that make up the human body, can malfunction or become diseased.

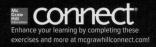

Using Terminology

Match each key term to the appropriate definition.

Part One

_____ **1.** LO 7.2 A form of diabetes mellitus with a gradual onset.

_____ **2.** LO 7.2 A chronic disease, a result of insulin deficiency or resistance.

_____ **3.** LO 7.2 A temporary diabetes mellitus occurring during pregnancy.

_____ **4.** LO 7.4 Abnormally high levels of glucose.

_____ **5.** LO 7.2 Excessive thirst.

_____ **6.** LO 7.2 Diabetes caused by medication or another condition or disease.

_____ **7.** LO 7.2 Excessive urination.

_____ **8.** LO 7.2 Abnormal lipoprotein metabolism.

_____ **9.** LO 7.4 Abnormally low glucose levels.

_____ **10.** LO 7.4 A condition in which the thyroid converts energy more slowly than normal, resulting in an otherwise unexplained weight gain and fatigue.

_____ **11.** LO 7.2 A sudden onset of insulin deficiency.

A. Diabetes mellitus

B. Dyslipidemia

C. Gestational diabetes mellitus (GDM)

D. Hyperglycemia

E. Hypoglycemia

F. Hypothyroidism

G. Polydipsia

H. Polyuria

I. Secondary DM

J. Type 1 DM

K. Type 2 DM

Part Two

_____ **1.** LO 7.1 Consists of the hypothalamus, pituitary gland, pineal gland, thyroid gland, parathyroid glands, thymus gland, adrenal glands, and pancreas, as well as the testes in men and the ovaries in women.

_____ **2.** LO 7.1 Consists of two lobes: the adenohypophysis, the larger lobe sitting anteriorly, and the neurohypophysis, which is smaller and toward the posterior.

_____ **3.** LO 7.1 A gland that secretes insulin and other hormones from the islet cells into the bloodstream and manufactures digestive enzymes that are secreted into the duodenum.

_____ **4.** LO 7.1 Two lobes located in the neck that reach around the trachea laterally and connect anteriorly by an isthmus.

_____ **5.** LO 7.1 The part of the brain responsible for controlling body temperature and the autonomic nervous system.

_____ **6.** LO 7.1 Four partially embedded glands in the posterior aspect of the thyroid gland.

_____ **7.** LO 7.1 Located on the superior aspect of each kidney and also known as the *suprarenal glands.*

_____ **8.** LO 7.1 A gland that assists in the development of the immune system prior to puberty.

_____ **9.** LO 7.1 A gland situated within the brain and responsible for the release of melatonin.

A. Adrenal glands

B. Endocrine system

C. Hypothalamus

D. Pancreas

E. Parathyroid glands

F. Pineal gland

G. Pituitary gland

H. Thymus gland

I. Thyroid gland

Checking Your Understanding

Choose the most appropriate answer for each of the following questions.

1. LO 7.4 Joe Jackson is seen at his doctor's office with a previous lab test result of positive for hyperglycemia. Dr. Ansewa writes in his chart that his diagnosis is suspected diabetes mellitus. The correct diagnosis code would report

   a. diabetes mellitus with unspecified complication.
   b. hyperglycemia; diabetes mellitus uncomplicated.
   c. hyperglycemia.
   d. diabetes mellitus with specified complication.

2. LO 7.2 Which of these is *not* a type of diabetes?

   a. hypertension.
   b. gestational.
   c. type 1.
   d. type 2.

3. LO 7.1 Which of the following is included in the endocrine system?

   a. liver.
   b. stomach.
   c. pituitary.
   d. kidney.

4. LO 7.2 Karin is diagnosed with type 2 diabetic hyperosmolarity. The hyperosmolarity should

   a. be coded first.
   b. be coded after the diabetes code.
   c. be coded after the effect code.
   d. not be coded—it is included in the diabetes code.

5. LO 7.3 Diabetic retinopathy may be manifested in all of the following *except*

   a. background.
   b. maculopathy.
   c. proliferative.
   d. neurologic.

6. LO 7.3 Diabetes mellitus is a condition that affects an individual's

   a. heart.
   b. lungs.
   c. liver.
   d. entire system.

7. LO 7.3 An individual with type 2 diabetes

   a. may use insulin.
   b. never uses insulin.
   c. always uses insulin.
   d. has temporary diabetes that will go away with treatment.

8. LO 7.4 An underdose of insulin may be caused by

    a. an incorrect dosage.

    b. a malfunctioning insulin pump.

    c. patient noncompliance.

    d. all of these.

9. LO 7.4 Hypoglycemia is

    a. another term for diabetes.

    b. an abnormally low level of glucose.

    c. an abnormally high level of glucose.

    d. caused by eating too much salt.

10. LO 7.2 Gestational diabetes is a condition that can affect only an individual

    a. over the age of 65.

    b. under the age of 4.

    c. who is pregnant.

    d. with hypertension.

Applying Your Knowledge

1. LO 7.1 List five of the glands in the endocrine system. _____

_____

2. LO 7.1 Where is the adenohypophysis located, and what hormones does it produce? _____

_____

3. LO 7.1 Where are the islets of Langerhans located, and what are their responsibilities? _____

_____

4. LO 7.2 Physicians can diagnose diabetes with a glucose lab test and certain signs and symptoms. List six of the signs and symptoms. _____

_____

5. LO 7.2 Explain the difference between type 1 diabetes mellitus and type 2 diabetes mellitus. _____

_____

6. LO 7.2 What is gestational diabetes mellitus? _____

_____

7. LO 7.2 What is secondary diabetes mellitus? _____

_____

8. LO 7.5 What is diabetes insipidus, and how does it differ from diabetes mellitus? _____

_____

Using the techniques described in this chapter, carefully read through the case studies and determine the most accurate ICD-10-CM code(s) and external cause code(s), if appropriate, for each case study.

1. Debra-Anne Jenner, a 37-year-old female, has type 2 diabetes and is admitted into the hospital in a diabetic hypoglycemic coma.

   _____

2. Juan Merced, a 69-year-old male with severe congestive heart failure, was admitted with a DX of nocturnal dyspnea and orthopnea. He has type 2 diabetes mellitus, insulin-dependent. During his stay in the hospital, insulin was administered to control his blood sugar, and he was treated with medication for his hypertension as well.

   _____

3. Herman Rivers, a 55-year-old male, has atherosclerosis and gangrene of the right lower extremity due to type 1 diabetes mellitus.

   _____

4. Robyn Winger, a 41-year-old female, is seen by Dr. Terrace for her quarterly evaluation of her type 1 diabetes mellitus. Patient states she is in good control with the continued insulin therapy but is having some problems with her eyes. After examination and testing, Dr. Terrace determines she has confirmed mild nonproliferative diabetic retinopathy.

   _____

5. Uma Thacher, a 29-year-old female, is seen in a clinic and has wheezing and a productive cough. Dr. Chintaz writes the DX as "probably bronchitis—pending CXR results." The chest x-ray confirms bronchitis. A glucose test is also taken to confirm that the patient's previously diagnosed diabetes (non-insulin-dependent) remains under control. Uma tells the doctor that her previous problems with arthritis and insomnia are not currently an issue.

   _____

6. Gene Reynolds, a 61-year-old male, is seen by his regular physician, Dr. Garrison. Gene complains of having headaches, a dry mouth, and excessive thirst; he also states he is urinating frequently. Gene is diagnosed with diabetes insipidus.

   _____

7. James Emmerson, a 59-year-old male, requires dialysis due to his diagnosis of insulin-dependent (type 1) diabetic nephropathy and chronic renal failure, stage 2.

   _____

8. Alma Taylor, a 31-year-old female, 38 weeks gestation, comes into the ED and complains that she has not felt the baby move all day. It is her first pregnancy, and her type 2 diabetes (which she has had for 5 years) has been relatively under control.

   _____

9. Russell Gaitlin, an 18-year-old male, was diagnosed with Addison's disease 2 years ago and then developed diabetic ketoacidosis and then type 1 diabetes mellitus.

   _____

10. June Haberstock, a 27-year-old female, G2 P0 at 40 weeks gestation, comes in today for induction secondary to gestational DM, insulin-dependent, to keep it under control. She is given an insulin drip and sent home without labor beginning.

   _____

11. Dr. Tomas diagnosed Luther Irvin with proliferative diabetic retinopathy due to type 1 diabetes mellitus.

   _____

12. Leanne Beasley, a 43-year-old female, was diagnosed with insulin-dependent (type 1) diabetes mellitus with polyneuropathy and peripheral angiopathy.

   _____

13. Melinda Carswell was diagnosed with type 2 diabetes with left midfoot ulcer.

   _____

14. Arthur Garrett is treated for mild malnutrition. He was diagnosed with uncontrolled type 2 DM 2 years ago.

   _____

15. Joan Kelhoffer came to see Dr. Peterman to check on her hypoglycemia in type 1 diabetes.

   _____

The following exercises provide practice in abstracting physicians' notes and learning to work with SOAP notes from our health care facility, *Taylor, Reader, & Associates*. These case studies (SOAP notes) are modeled on real patient encounters. Using the techniques described in this chapter, carefully read through the case studies and determine the most accurate ICD-10-CM code(s) and external cause code(s), if appropriate, for each case study.

TAYLOR, READER, & ASSOCIATES
A Complete Health Care Facility
975 CENTRAL AVENUE • SOMEWHERE, FL 32811 • 407-555-4321

PATIENT: GALINDA, GABRIEL
ACCOUNT/EHR #:   GALIGA001
DATE: 09/16/18

Attending Physician: Suzanne R. Taylor, MD

This 53-year-old male came to see me today to review the results of his blood tests, ordered last week. Patient had come in with complaints of hyperactive deep tendon reflexes, muscle cramps, and carpopedal spasm.

Pathology report shows abnormally decreased blood calcium levels. I discussed the details of this condition and reviewed treatment options. He wants to discuss this with his wife, and he will call within the next few days.

DX: Hypocalcemia

Suzanne R. Taylor, MD

SRT/pw   D: 09/16/18 09:50:16   T: 09/18/18 12:55:01

Determine the most accurate ICD-10-CM code(s).

_____

_____

_____

TAYLOR, READER, & ASSOCIATES
A Complete Health Care Facility
975 CENTRAL AVENUE • SOMEWHERE, FL 32811 • 407-555-4321

PATIENT: EMERALD, PEARL
ACCOUNT/EHR #:   EMERPE001
DATE: 08/11/18

Attending Physician: Willard B. Reader, MD

S: Pt is a 37-year-old female, comes in for a 10-week follow-up since her diagnosis with secondary diabetes mellitus due to hyperthyroidism. Patient states she has been taking her methimazole, as I had prescribed at that last visit. She says that she has been experiencing occasional tachycardia and this worries her.

O: W 110, T 98.6, BP 130/70; HEENT: unremarkable. She is exhibiting a wide pulse pressure. Lung sounds are also normal. EKG indicates paroxysmal supraventricular tachycardia.
    The importance of drug and diet compliance was emphasized with the patient. I reviewed the plan to control the secondary diabetes with diet and exercise initially, and explained that vigilant care was needed to monitor her heart rate, blood pressure, and pulse rate.

A: Hyperthyroidism with secondary diabetes mellitus

P: 1. Rx propranolol to manage tachycardia. Methimazole continued.
     2. Rx TSH blood test. Patient to go to lab for test within the week.
     3. Patient to return in 10 days to 2 weeks.

_____

Willard B. Reader, MD

WBR/pw   D: 08/11/18 09:50:16   T: 08/13/18 12:55:01

Determine the most accurate ICD-10-CM code(s).

_____

_____

_____

TAYLOR, READER, & ASSOCIATES
A Complete Health Care Facility
975 CENTRAL AVENUE • SOMEWHERE, FL 32811 • 407-555-4321

PATIENT: HEALLEY, GRAYSON
ACCOUNT/EHR #:   HEALGR001
DATE: 09/16/18

Attending Physician: Suzanne R. Taylor, MD

Procedure: Vitrectomy followed by laser panretinal photocoagulation. An ocutome is used to go behind the right iris and cut and suction the vitreous mechanically. After the vitreous removal, an endolaser is used to treat the remaining retinal disorders in all four retinal quadrants and prevent further retinal hemorrhage.

DX: Juvenile diabetes, insulin-dependent; severe retinal hemorrhage; proliferative diabetic retinopathy.

Suzanne R. Taylor, MD

SRT/pw   D: 09/16/18 09:50:16   T: 09/18/18 12:55:01

Determine the most accurate ICD-10-CM code(s).

_____

_____

_____

TAYLOR, READER, & ASSOCIATES
A Complete Health Care Facility
975 CENTRAL AVENUE • SOMEWHERE, FL 32811 • 407-555-4321

PATIENT: OCCASSIO, SANDY
ACCOUNT/EHR #: OCCASA001
DATE: 08/11/18

Attending Physician: Willard B. Reader, MD

S: Pt is a 33-year-old male complaining of an unhealed sore on his left foot. He states the sore is of 3 weeks' duration with no evidence of healing despite multiple home remedies and over-the-counter treatments. Pt has been a type 2 diabetic for 6 years.

O: Wt 195 lb, Ht 5′7″, T 99, BP 150/90; HEENT: unremarkable. Left extremity shows a diabetes-related ulcer directly above the third phalange. Ulcer is debrided (skin and subcutaneous tissue), ointment applied, and a bandage placed. Patient is given wound care instructions.

A: Type 2 diabetes; pressure ulcer, stage II, of midfoot.

P: Pt to return in 2 weeks for follow-up.

_____

Willard B. Reader, MD

WBR/pw   D: 08/11/18 09:50:16   T: 08/13/18 12:55:01

Determine the most accurate ICD-10-CM code(s).

_____

_____

_____

TAYLOR, READER, & ASSOCIATES
A Complete Health Care Facility
975 CENTRAL AVENUE • SOMEWHERE, FL 32811 • 407-555-4321

PATIENT: CONIG, DEMETRI
ACCOUNT/EHR #:   CONIDE001
DATE: 08/11/18

Attending Physician: Willard B. Reader, MD

Surgeon: Colleen Infanti, MD

Patient is a 27-year old male with insulin-dependent (type 1) diabetic nephropathy and chronic renal failure, stage 5. He presents today for an arteriovenous shunt for dialysis.

   A Cimino-type direct arteriovenous anastomosis is performed by incising the skin of the left antecubital fossa. Vessel clamps are placed on the vein and adjacent artery. The vein is dissected free, and the downstream portion of the vein is sutured to an opening in the artery using an end-to-side technique. The skin incision is closed in layers.

_____

Colleen Infanti, MD

CI/pw   D: 08/11/18 09:50:16   T: 08/13/18 12:55:01

Determine the most accurate ICD-10-CM code(s).

_____

_____

_____

8

CODING MENTAL AND BEHAVIORAL DISORDERS

Learning Outcomes *After completing this chapter, the student should be able to:*

LO 8.1 Identify underlying physiological conditions manifesting mental disorders.

LO 8.2 Distinguish substance use, abuse, and dependence.

LO 8.3 Classify nonmood disorders and psychotic disorders.

LO 8.4 Distinguish signs and symptoms of mood (affective) disorders.

LO 8.5 Understand the types of anxiety and nonpsychotic disorders.

LO 8.6 Apply the official guidelines for reporting stress-related disorders.

Key Terms

Abuse

Anxiety

Behavioral disturbance

Dependence

Depressive

Manic

Phobia

Posttraumatic stress disorder (PTSD)

Schizophrenia

Somatoform disorder

Use

Mental and behavioral disorders have long been a mystery to the average person, and the lack of understanding has fed fear of patients with these disorders. The dysfunction of a person's brain is often the result of many of the same things that cause other bodily health concerns, including genetics, congenital anomalies, traumatic injury, or the invasion of a pathogen. Any of these, along with other conditions and circumstances, have the ability to impact the health and function of the brain. Scientific research has evidenced shared signs and symptoms between psychiatric illness and neurologic illness.

The accepted understanding of mental illness is a condition that negatively affects an individual's thoughts, emotions, behaviors, ability to maintain effective social interactions, and ability to appropriately carry out the activities of daily living.

Brain Neurons

The control center of the human body is the brain. Within the brain, neurons (nerve cells) and other structures enable us to think, make decisions and plans, react to our surroundings, and take actions. Supported by the nervous system, the autonomic processes necessary for life, such as breathing and heart contractions, activate vital functions. Other aspects of the brain are responsible for memory, learning, sensory perceptions, and emotions.

The neurons communicate with each other, aided by neurotransmitters (brain chemicals), using electrical impulses (synapses) millions of times per second. This is how the brain processes information and directs certain actions and behaviors throughout the body. These actions and behaviors include conscious actions, such as reaching out your hand to pick up a pen, as well as subconscious actions, such as breathing. There has been quite a lot of scientific research performed seeking information about the brain's involvement in psychiatric illnesses. Evidence indicates that neurotransmitter imbalances have caused faulty communications between neurons, resulting in improper information being sent to various parts of the body, which, at times, may lead to some of the signs and symptoms of known mental illnesses. In addition, researchers have observed changes in the size and shape of certain structures within the brain, which may also result in psychiatric disorders.

LO 8.1 Mental Disorders due to Known Physiological Conditions

In some cases, a mental disorder is caused by another condition in the body. The physiological condition may be any of various diagnoses, including an infarction of the brain, hypertensive cerebrovascular disease, or a disease such as Creutzfeldt-Jakob disease, Parkinson's disease, or trypanosomiasis (a condition commonly known as *sleeping sickness*). Moreover, some endocrine disorders, exogenous hormones, and toxic substances can cause cognitive and/or intellectual malfunction, including signs and symptoms of problematic memory, impaired judgment, and diminished intellect.

Dementia is included in this subsection of the chapter on mental and behavioral disorders in ICD-10-CM. This diagnosis can be identified by evidence of both neurologic and psychological signs and symptoms, such as differences in personality, altered thoughts and feelings, and behavioral changes.

When it comes to reporting diagnoses for mental disorders that are manifestations of physiological conditions, you need to identify from the documentation the specific known etiology in cerebral disease, brain injury, or other insult leading to this cerebral dysfunction.

Vascular Dementia

A patient may develop vascular dementia after having experienced an infarction of the brain that is known to be a manifestation of a previously existing vascular disease. In ICD-10-CM, code category F01 also includes a diagnosis of hypertensive cerebrovascular disease as well as arteriosclerotic dementia. Vascular dementia is often defined as a "disease with a cognitive impairment resulting from cerebrovascular disease and ischemic or hemorrhagic brain injury" (*Source:* Iemolo et al, Pathophysiology of vascular dementia, *Immunity & Ageing* 2009, 6:13. doi:10.1186/1742-4933-6-13).

Therefore, the notation to "code first the underlying physiological conditions or sequelae of cerebrovascular disease" logically supports your correct sequencing of codes that may be involved in the reporting of this diagnosis.

EXAMPLE

F01.50 Vascular dementia without behavioral disturbance
F01.51 Vascular dementia with behavior disturbance
Use additional code, if applicable, to identify wandering in vascular dementia (Z91.83)

In addition to identifying the underlying physiological condition, you will also need to identify whether or not the patient is documented as having behavioral disturbance. If so, has the patient also been documented as having episodes of "wandering"? These details will guide you toward the correct code or codes to accurately report this patient's condition.

Amnestic Disorder due to Known Physiological Condition

Reporting amnestic disorder due to known physiological condition will take you to code category F04, Amnestic disorder, with the additional descriptions of Korsakov's psychosis and Syndrome, nonalcoholic. You can see that the *code first underlying condition* notation requires that the underlying condition be physiological, thereby eliminating any psychological underlying conditions from qualifying for this code.

Note that ICD-10-CM reporting of this diagnosis has an *Excludes1* notation. An *Excludes1* notation identifies other diagnoses that are mutually exclusive to the diagnosis above the notation (in this case, F04). This is the absolute statement that the excluded code can never be used at the same time because the two conditions cannot occur together in one patient at one time.

EXCLUDES1   amnesia NOS (R41.3)

anterograde amnesia (R41.1)

dissociative amnesia (F44.0)

retrograde amnesia (R41.2)

F04 also carries an *Excludes2* notation identifying several amnestic disorders that are not included in F04, therefore requiring either a different code or an additional code:

EXCLUDES2   alcohol-induced or unspecified Korsakov's syndrome (F10.26, F10.96)

Korsakov's syndrome induced by other psychoactive substances (F13.26, F13.96, F19.16, F19.26, F19.96)

Mood Disorder due to Known Physiological Condition

A mood disorder is a daily issue of dealing with one's emotional state. This category of mental illnesses includes major depressive disorder, dysthymic disorder, and bipolar disorder. Code subcategory F06.3* differentiates itself from other diagnoses under "Mood [affective] disorders," which includes bipolar disorder (F30–F39), because this diagnosis (reported with F06.3*) includes a documented physiological underlying cause.

EXAMPLE

F06.30 Mood disorder due to known physiological condition, unspecified
F06.31 Mood disorder due to known physiological condition, with depressive features
F06.32 Mood disorder due to known physiological condition, with major depressive-like episode
F06.33 Mood disorder due to known physiological condition, with manic features
F06.34 Mood disorder due to known physiological condition, with mixed features

Beneath F06.3 is an *Excludes2* notation, indicating specific diagnoses that are not included in this subcategory:

EXCLUDES2   mood disorders due to alcohol and other psychoactive substances (F10–F19 with .14, .24, .94)

mood disorders, not due to known physiological condition or unspecified (F30–F39)

Personality and Behavioral Disorders due to Known Physiological Condition

There have been known physiological conditions that manifest personality changes or behavioral disorders. Traumatic brain injury—specifically, damage to the patient's frontal lobe—can be evidenced by apathy, a lack of ability to formulate plans, emotional bluntness, and inability to perform abstract thinking. In this code category, you will find a *code first the underlying physiological condition* notation applicable to all codes within.

EXAMPLE

> F07.0 Personality change due to known physiological condition (Frontal lobe syndrome) (Organic pseudopsychopathic personality)(Postleucotomy syndrome) Code first underlying physiological condition

Beneath F07.0 are two *excludes* notations, which further clarify which diagnoses are reported with this code and which require the coder to look elsewhere in the code set:

EXCLUDES1	mild cognitive impairment (G31.84)
	postconcussional syndrome (F07.81)
	postencephalitic syndrome (F07.89)
	signs and symptoms involving emotional state (R45.-)
EXCLUDES2	specific personality disorder (F60.-)

EXAMPLE

> F07.81 Postconcussion syndrome (Postcontusion syndrome or encephalopathy) (Posttraumatic brain syndrome, nonpsychotic)
> *Use additional code to identify associated post-traumatic headache, if applicable (G44.3-)*

EXCLUDES1	Current concussion (brain)(S06.0-)
	Postencephalitic syndrome (F07.89)

Remember that an *Excludes1* notation in ICD-10-CM identifies diagnoses that are mutually exclusive—that cannot be reported for the same patient at the same time.

LET'S CODE IT! SCENARIO

Amelia Rasmussen, a 33-year-old female, came with her husband Ralph to see Dr. Blackman, a psychiatrist, on a referral from her regular physician. She complains about unusual fatigue and problems remembering things. Her husband has complained that she has been unusually irritable. Ralph stated that he has found Amelia wandering the neighborhood several times over the last few weeks. Amelia admitted to being on a new dairy-free, animal product–free diet. After a complete physical examination, Dr. Blackman performed a complete psychology exam and ordered blood work that confirmed his diagnosis of dementia caused by vitamin B_{12} deficiency.

Dr. Blackman diagnosed Amelia with *dementia caused by vitamin B₁₂ deficiency*. You also read that she did have incidents of *wandering*. When you turn to the Alphabetic Index, you see:

Dementia

> **In (due to)**
>> **Vitamin B12 deficiency E53.8 *[F02.80]***
>>> **With behavioral disturbance E53.8 *[F02.81]***

You should remember from Chapter 3 that the second code, in italicized brackets, tells you that you will need two codes for this diagnosis and in which order to report these two codes. Turn to the Tabular List to read the first suggested code:

E53 Deficiency of other B group vitamins

Read down and review all of the fourth-character choices to determine the most accurate code:

E53.8 Deficiency of other specified B group vitamins

Next, you know that you will need to follow this code with a code from F02—either F02.80 or F02.81. Let's take a look at both codes and see what exactly is meant by **behavioral disturbance:**

behavioral disturbance
A type of common behavior that includes mood disorders (such as depression, apathy, and euphoria); sleep disorders (such as insomnia and hypersomnia); psychotic symptoms (such as delusions and hallucinations); and agitation (such as pacing, wandering, and aggression).

F02.80 Dementia in other diseases classified elsewhere without behavioral disturbance

F02.81 Dementia in other diseases classified elsewhere with behavioral disturbance

Did you notice the notation beneath F02.81?

Use additional code, if applicable, to identify wandering in dementia in conditions classified elsewhere (Z91.83)

Aha! This tells you that "wandering" is considered a behavioral disturbance. Dr. Blackman documented that Amelia had been wandering, so you will need one more code:

Z91.83 Wandering in conditions classified elsewhere

Good job! You determined the three codes required to accurately report Dr. Blackman's encounter with Amelia:

E53.8 Deficiency of other specified B group vitamins

F02.81 Dementia in other diseases classified elsewhere with behavioral disturbance

Z91.83 Wandering in conditions classified elsewhere

LO 8.2 Mental and Behavioral Disorders due to Psychoactive Substance Use

Reporting Alcohol- and Drug-Related Disorders

When a patient is diagnosed with an alcohol- or drug-related disorder, the diagnosis is often more complex, as such conditions are susceptible to both psychological and physiological signs, symptoms, manifestations, and co-morbidities. Alcohol use doesn't damage the actual brain cells, but it does damage the ends of neurons, which are called *dendrites*. This results in problems conveying messages between the neurons.

EXAMPLE

NOTE: All codes in this example require additional characters.

F10.1 Alcohol abuse
F10.2 Alcohol dependence
F10.9 Alcohol use, unspecified
F11.1 Opioid abuse
F11.2 Opioid dependence
F11.9 Opioid use, unspecified
F12.1 Cannabis abuse
F12.2 Cannabis dependence
F12.9 Cannabis use, unspecified
F13.1 Sedative, hypnotic or anxiolytic-related abuse
F13.2 Sedative, hypnotic or anxiolytic-related dependence
F13.9 Sedative, hypnotic or anxiolytic-related use, unspecified
F14.1 Cocaine abuse
F14.2 Cocaine dependence
F14.9 Cocaine use, unspecified

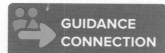

GUIDANCE CONNECTION

Review the ICD-10-CM Coding Guidelines, Section I.C.5, Chapter 5: **Mental, behavioral, and neurodevelopmental disorders (F01–F99),** Subsection b, **Mental and behavioral disorders due to psychoactive substance use,** (2) **Psychoactive substance use, abuse and dependence** and (3) **Psychoactive substance use.**

The first thing you might notice about these codes is that details are required from the documentation to identify *abuse* of or *dependence* on the psychoactive substance. Also, there are codes for specifically reporting the *use* of alcohol and drugs that enable the tracking of the patient's behavior, which often will ultimately have a negative impact on his or her health. These details can give providers and researchers a great deal of useful information as they look for better ways to care for patients and their maladies.

What is the clinical difference between these terms?

Use: Consumption of a substance without significant clinical manifestations.

Abuse: Ongoing, regular consumption of a substance with resulting clinical manifestations.

Dependence: Ongoing, regular consumption of a substance with resulting significant clinical manifestations and a dramatic decrease in the effect of the substance with continued use, therefore requiring an increased quantity of the substance to achieve intoxication. In addition, the patient will require continued consumption of the substance to avoid withdrawal symptoms and other serious behavioral effects, occurring at any time in the same 12-month period.

All of these codes require additional characters to identify details from the documentation about manifestations and co-morbidities. Let's take *alcohol abuse* as an example of what details you may need to abstract from the clinical documentation.

use
Occasional consumption of a substance.

abuse
Regular consumption of a substance with manifestations.

dependence
Ongoing consumption with significant manifestations.

EXAMPLE

F10.1 Alcohol abuse
F10.10 Alcohol abuse, uncomplicated
F10.120 Alcohol abuse with intoxication, uncomplicated
F10.121 Alcohol abuse with intoxication delirium
F10.14 Alcohol abuse with alcohol-induced mood disorder
F10.150 Alcohol abuse with alcohol-induced psychotic disorder with delusions
F10.180 Alcohol abuse with alcohol-induced anxiety disorder
F10.181 Alcohol abuse with alcohol-induced sexual dysfunction
F10.182 Alcohol abuse with alcohol-induced sleep disorder
F10.188 Alcohol abuse with other alcohol-induced disorder

As you can see, ICD-10-CM requires an understanding of the psychological and behavioral impacts of the use, abuse, or dependence. Signs, symptoms, manifestations, and co-morbidities such as delirium, mood disorder, and hallucinations will be reported with one combination code from this subsection.

In the subcategories for alcohol use and dependence, you will also find codes including a state of withdrawal, again providing one combination code to report this condition.

EXAMPLE

F10.231 Alcohol dependence with withdrawal delirium

The extended descriptions and combination-code choices include those codes used to report the use of other nontherapeutic substances as well. Take, for example, hallucinogens, caffeine, and inhalant use.

EXAMPLE

F15.120 Other stimulant abuse with intoxication, uncomplicated (caffeine) (amphetamine-related disorders)

F15.920 Other stimulant use with intoxication, uncomplicated (caffeine) (amphetamine-related disorders)

F16.1 Hallucinogen abuse

F16.2 Hallucinogen dependence

F16.9 Hallucinogen use, unspecified

F18.1 Inhalant abuse

F18.9 Inhalant use, unspecified

ICD-10-CM code descriptions separate inhalant abuse and dependence into its own specific code category (F18), and caffeine (yes, this is considered a substance) is included in the "Other" code category, now combined with amphetamine-related disorders.

As with the previous code categories in this subsection, the additional characters required for these ICD-10-CM codes include abstracting documentation for details on accompanying intoxication, delirium, perceptual disturbance, mood disorder, psychotic disorder with delusions or hallucinations, **anxiety** disorder, flashbacks, and other manifestations.

One more addition to this subsection of Chapter 5, Mental, behavioral, and neurodevelopmental disorders, in ICD-10-CM is code category F17, Nicotine dependence. The *Excludes1* note reminds you that nicotine dependence is not the same diagnosis as tobacco use (Z72.0) or history of tobacco dependence (Z87.891). Therefore, the documentation will need to specifically discern between tobacco use and nicotine dependence.

anxiety
The feelings of apprehension and fear, sometimes manifested with physical manifestations such as sweating and palpitations.

EXAMPLE

F17.210 Nicotine dependence, cigarettes, uncomplicated

F17.211 Nicotine dependence, cigarettes, in remission

F17.213 Nicotine dependence, cigarettes, with withdrawal

F17.218 Nicotine dependence, cigarettes, with other nicotine-induced disorders

F17.220 Nicotine dependence, chewing tobacco, uncomplicated

F17.221 Nicotine dependence, chewing tobacco, in remission

F17.223 Nicotine dependence, chewing tobacco, with withdrawal

F17.228 Nicotine dependence, chewing tobacco, with other nicotine-induced disorders

F17.290 Nicotine dependence, other tobacco product, uncomplicated

F17.291 Nicotine dependence, other tobacco product, in remission

F17.293 Nicotine dependence, other tobacco product, with withdrawal

F17.298 Nicotine dependence, other tobacco product, with other nicotine-induced disorders

The bottom line is that ICD-10-CM has organized these codes in a logical and efficient order and provided you with many combination codes.

LET'S CODE IT! SCENARIO

Herbert DeLauder, a 57-year-old male, has been a salesman for the last 30 years. He travels throughout the Midwest and has had a less than stellar career. Very often, he has come close to being fired for not making quota, but his supervisor takes pity on him because he has been with the company for so long. He is at the medical office today by court order after being arrested for his third DUI in the last 6 months. Seeking treatment is part of his plea deal, so he doesn't lose his driver's license. He needs to be able to drive to see his customers.

Herbert states he has tried to stop drinking but can't because it is part of his job. He must take customers out for a drink. And when he is back at his office, all the guys go out for drinks after work. When he is on the road, he finds nothing to do in the motel at night, so he drinks away the loneliness. The one time he tried to quit drinking, he got really sick. The only thing that helped him feel better was a little "hair of the dog."

He states that at times he is very sad and hopeless, while other times, especially when he is with clients, he is the life of the party and knows some of the best jokes. He pleads for help and begins to cry.

Dr. Jullienne diagnoses Herbert with alcohol dependence with alcohol-induced mood disorder.

Let's Code It!

Dr. Jullienne diagnosed Herbert with *alcohol dependence with alcohol-induced mood disorder.* Turn in the Alphabetic Index to find:

Dependence (on)(syndrome) F19.20

    Alcohol (ethyl)(methyl)(without remission) F10.20

        With

            Mood disorder F10.24

Now let's turn to find this suggested code in the Tabular List:

F10 Alcohol related disorder

Use additional code for blood alcohol level, if applicable (Y90.-)

This is not applicable in Herbert's case, so continue reading to review all of the options for the required fourth character. Did you choose:

F10.2 Alcohol dependence

Don't skip over the *Excludes1* or *Excludes2* notations. You must read them all carefully, and then determine whether they apply to the specific case you are coding. In this case, they do not. Keep reading all of the fifth-character choices to determine the most accurate code. You can see the code that matches Dr. Jullienne's notes perfectly!

F10.24 Alcohol dependence with alcohol-induced mood disorder

Good work!

LO 8.3 Schizophrenia, Schizotypal, Delusional, and Other Nonmood Psychotic Disorders

Schizophrenia

schizophrenia
A psychotic disorder with no known cause.

There is no known cause of **schizophrenia** (a psychotic disorder); however, evidence does exist that it may have an etiology of genetic, biological, cultural, and/or psychological foundations. The belief of a genetic predisposition is supported with statistical research showing that the close relatives of a schizophrenic are 50 times more likely to develop the condition. There is also a widely held belief of a biochemical imbalance, specifically excessive activity of dopaminergic synapses, encouraging the signs and symptoms of schizophrenia. Five types of schizophrenia are recognized by psychiatric professionals:

- *Paranoid,* also known as *paraphrenic schizophrenia* [F20.0]
- *Disorganized,* also known as *hebephrenic schizophrenia* or *hebephrenia* [F20.1]
- *Catatonic,* also known as *schizophrenic catalepsy, catatonia,* or *flexibilitas cerea* [F20.2]
- *Undifferentiated,* also known as *atypical schizophrenia* [F20.3]
- *Residual,* also known as *restzustand* [F20.5]

The signs and symptoms of schizophrenia are generally categorized into three groups: positive symptoms, negative symptoms, and cognitive symptoms. The specific behaviors related to this diagnosis will vary depending upon the type and phase of the disorder.

EXAMPLE

F20.0 Paranoid schizophrenia
F20.1 Disorganized schizophrenia
F20.2 Catatonic schizophrenia
F20.3 Undifferentiated schizophrenia (Atypical schizophrenia)
F20.5 Residual schizophrenia
F20.81 Schizophreniform disorder
F20.89 Other schizophrenia (Simple schizophrenia)
F21 Schizotypal disorder (Latent schizophrenia)
F25.0 Schizoaffective disorder, bipolar type
F25.1 Schizoaffective disorder, depressive type
F25.8 Other schizoaffective disorders

Coders working with health care professionals caring for patients diagnosed with schizophrenia should be aware of the known adverse effects of the antipsychotic drugs most often used to treat this condition. Also known as *neuroleptic drugs,* antipsychotics (such as haloperidol) are known to result in a high incident rate of extrapyramidal effects, including:

- Drug-induced parkinsonism [G21.11] with signs of propulsive gait, stooped posture, muscle rigidity, tremors
- Drug-induced dystonia [G24.02] showing signs of severe muscle contractions
- Drug-induced akathisia [G25.71] showing signs of restlessness and pacing

Some low-potency drugs in this category have been known to cause orthostatic hypotension [I95.2]—a sudden drop in blood pressure when the patient changes position quickly, such as standing up. A development of neuroleptic malignant syndrome [G21.0] has been reported in as many as 1 percent of patients taking antipsychotics.

Remember that when these adverse effects have been diagnosed, you will need to include an external cause code to identify the "drug taken for therapeutic purposes" as the reason for this condition. You would choose a code from category E939, Psychotropic agents causing adverse effects in therapeutic use, or category T43, Poisoning by, adverse effect of and underdosing of psychotropic drugs, not elsewhere classified, in ICD-10-CM.

Schizoid Personality Disorder (F60.1)

There may appear to be some overlap in the signs and symptoms of schizophrenia (a psychotic disorder) and schizoid personality disorder; however, they are very different conditions.

Patients diagnosed with schizoid personality disorder exhibit a limited range of emotions and an aversion to social relationships and personal interactions. These patients have little to no interest in sex and are indifferent to both praise and criticism. Overall, these patients have a flat affect.

YOU CODE IT! CASE STUDY

Elliot M., a 19-year-old male, is a junior at a state university. Over the past month, his parents have noticed that his behavior has become quite peculiar. Several times, his mother has overheard him speaking in a quiet yet angry tone, even though no one was in the room with him. Over the past 7 to 10 days, Elliot has refused to answer or make calls on his cell phone, stating that he knows if he uses the phone, it will activate a deadly chip that has been implanted in his brain by evil men from space.

Elliot's parents, as well as his brother and his best friend, have attempted to convince him to join them at an appointment with a psychiatrist for an evaluation, but he adamantly refused, until today. Several times, Elliot has accused his parents of conspiring with the aliens to steal his brain. He no longer attends classes and will soon flunk out unless he can get some help.

Other than a few beers with his friends, Elliot denies abusing alcohol or drugs. There is a family history of psychiatric illness; an estranged aunt has been in and out of psychiatric hospitals over the years due to erratic and bizarre behavior.

Dr. Leiber diagnosed Elliot with paranoid schizophrenia.

You Code It!

Go through the steps of coding, and determine the code or codes that should be reported for this encounter between Dr. Leiber and Elliot.

Step 1: Read the case completely.

Step 2: Abstract the notes: Which key words can you identify relating to why Dr. Leiber cared for Elliot?

_____

Step 3: Query the provider, if necessary.

Step 4: Code the diagnosis or diagnoses.

_____

Step 5: Code the procedure(s): Psychiatric evaluation.

Step 6: Link the procedure codes to at least one diagnosis code to confirm medical necessity.

Step 7: Back code to double-check your choices.

Answer:

Did you determine the correct code to be:

F20.0 Paranoid schizophrenia

LO 8.4 Mood (Affective) Disorders

Bipolar Disorders

The etiology of bipolar disorders is uncertain and complex. The strongest evidence leads to the belief that many factors act together to activate the signs and symptoms. While some evidence exists that the condition tends to have familial connections, there have been studies of identical twins in which only one twin is affected.

Bipolar disorder is categorized as a "mood disorder" identified by acute swings exhibited by the patient, ranging from euphoria and hyperactivity to depression and lethargy. An overly elated or overexcited state is called a **manic** episode, and an acute sad or hopeless state is known as a **depressive** episode. Bipolar disorder may also be present in a *mixed* state, during which the patient experiences both mania and depression simultaneously.

Bipolar disorder is a chronic illness, therefore requiring long-term, continuous treatment to control symptoms. Mood stabilizers (e.g., lithium carbonate), atypical antipsychotics (e.g., clozapine), and antidepressants are most commonly prescribed in combination.

This diagnosis is categorized into two types: Type I bipolar disorder is identified as alternating between manic episodes and depressive episodes, while type II bipolar patients deal with recurring depressive episodes with occasional mania.

manic
An emotional state that includes elation, excitement, and exuberance.

depressive
An emotional state that includes sadness, hopelessness, and gloom.

EXAMPLE

F31 Bipolar disorder

F31.0 Bipolar disorder, current episode hypomanic

F31.11 Bipolar disorder, current episode, manic without psychotic features, mild

F31.12 Bipolar disorder, current episode, manic without psychotic features, moderate

F31.13 Bipolar disorder, current episode, manic without psychotic features, severe

F31.2 Bipolar disorder, current episode, manic, severe, with psychotic features

F31.31 Bipolar disorder, current episode, depressed, mild

F31.32 Bipolar disorder, current episode, depressed, moderate

F31.4 Bipolar disorder, current episode, depressed, severe, without psychotic features

F31.5 Bipolar disorder, current episode, depressed, severe, with psychotic feature

F31.6* Bipolar disorder, current episode, mixed

F31.81 Bipolar II disorder

F31.89 Other bipolar disorder (recurrent manic episodes NOS)

The categorization of those patients in partial or full remission is also available, so you will need to check the documentation for this detail or query the physician.

EXAMPLE

F31.7 Bipolar disorder, currently in remission

F31.71 Bipolar disorder, in partial remission, most recent episode hypomanic

F31.72 Bipolar disorder, in full remission, most recent episode hypomanic

F31.73 Bipolar disorder, in partial remission, most recent episode manic

F31.74 Bipolar disorder, in full remission, most recent episode manic

F31.75 Bipolar disorder, in partial remission, most recent episode depressed

F31.76 Bipolar disorder, in full remission, most recent episode depressed

F31.77 Bipolar disorder, in partial remission, most recent episode mixed

F31.78 Bipolar disorder, in full remission, most recent episode mixed

Major Depressive Disorder

Everyone feels sad or depressed at times. It is part of life. However, major depressive disorder causes patients to feel hopeless, guilty, and worthless. The typical activities of life (work, study, sleep, and fun) become difficult and, for some, nearly impossible. Some patients may experience ongoing (recurrent) episodes, while others suffer only a one-time (single) episode. Additional diagnostic terms used by some psychiatrists include *agitated depression, depressive reaction, major depression, psychogenic depression, reactive depression,* and *vital depression.*

Major depressive disorder may be mild, moderate, or severe and may be described as with or without psychotic features. Patients diagnosed with this illness may also experience partial or full remission. As the professional coding specialist, it is your job to ensure that your physician documents all of these details.

EXAMPLE

F32.* Major depressive disorder, single episode

F33.* Major depressive disorder, recurrent

YOU CODE IT! CASE STUDY

Olivia C., a 27-year-old female, came in to see Dr. Paulter, a psychiatrist. She has a very demanding and high-stress life, being a second-year law student. In addition, she is clerking for a judge, and she is planning her wedding for this coming summer.

She states that she has always been highly motivated to achieve her goals. After graduating with top honors from college, she went on to achieve a 3.95 GPA in her first year in law school. She admits that she can be very self-critical when she is not able to achieve perfection, even though, intellectually, she knows that perfection is not necessary for success. Recently, she has been struggling with considerable feelings of worthlessness and shame due to her inability to perform as well as she has in the past.

For the past few weeks, Olivia has noticed that she is constantly feeling fatigued, no matter how much she has slept. She also states that it has been increasingly difficult to concentrate at work and pay attention in class. Her best friend, Bethany, who works with her at the courthouse, stated that, recently, Olivia is irritable and withdrawn, not at all her typical upbeat and friendly disposition. While she has always prided herself on perfect attendance at school and at work, Olivia has called in sick on several occasions. On those days she stayed in bed all day, watching TV and sleeping.

At home, Olivia's fiancé has noticed changes in her as well. He states that, in the last 6 months, it seems that she has lost interest in sex despite a very healthy sex life during the previous 2 years they had been together. He also has noticed that she has had difficulties falling asleep at night. Her tossing and turning for an hour or two after they go to bed has been keeping him awake. He confesses that he overheard her having tearful phone conversations with Bethany and her sister that have worried him. When he tries to get her to open up, she denies anything is wrong, emphatically stating "I'm fine" and walking away.

Olivia states that she has found herself increasingly dissatisfied with her life. She admits to having frequent thoughts of wishing she was dead, yet denies ever considering suicide. She gets frustrated with herself because she feels that she has every reason to be happy yet can't seem to shake the sense of a heavy dark cloud enshrouding her. Dr. Paulter diagnosed Olivia with major depressive disorder, single episode, moderate severity.

You Code It!

Go through the steps of coding, and determine the code or codes that should be reported for this encounter between Dr. Paulter and Olivia.

Step 1: Read the case completely.

Step 2: Abstract the notes: Which key words can you identify relating to why Dr. Paulter cared for Olivia?

_____

Step 3: Query the provider, if necessary.

Step 4: Code the diagnosis or diagnoses.

_____

Step 5: Code the procedure(s): Psychiatric evaluation.

Step 6: Link the procedure codes to at least one diagnosis code to confirm medical necessity.

Step 7: Back code to double-check your choices.

Answer:

Did you determine the correct code to be:

F32.1 Major depressive disorder, single episode, moderate

LO 8.5 Anxiety, Dissociative, Stress-Related, Somatoform, and Other Nonpsychotic Mental Disorders

Phobias

Are you terrified of something, with no real rationale? The definition of a **phobia** is the excessive and irrational fear of an object, activity, or situation. Of course, a slight fear of a spider or of flying would not typically result in a physician encounter or documented diagnosis. Therefore, for the most part, the code categories for phobias will be used to report the condition in which this fear has risen to the level at which it actually interferes with daily life and, therefore, requires treatment.

phobia
Irrational and excessive fear of an object, activity, or situation.

EXAMPLE

F40.0 Agoraphobia
F40.1 Social phobia
F40.23 Blood, injection, injury type phobia
F41.0 Panic disorder [episodic paroxysmal anxiety] with agoraphobia
F41.1 Generalized anxiety disorder

Somatoform Disorders

The term **somatoform disorders** may be new to you; however, you have probably heard of one type, *hypochondria (hypochondriacal disorder),* in which patients have an ongoing belief that they have an illness that they do not have. This group of psychological disorders causes the patient to exhibit, or believe he or she exhibits, physical signs and symptoms.

somatoform disorder
The sincere belief that one is suffering an illness that is not present.

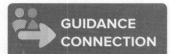

GUIDANCE CONNECTION

Review the ICD-10-CM Coding Guidelines, Section I.C.5, Chapter 5: **Mental, behavioral, and neurodevelopmental disorders (F01–F99),** Subsection a, **Pain disorders related to psychological factors.**

EXAMPLE

F45.0 Somatization disorder (Multiple psychosomatic disorder)
F45.22 Body dysmorphic disorder
F45.41 Pain disorder exclusively related to psychological factors
F45.42 Pain disorder with related psychological factors
Code also associated acute or chronic pain (G89.-)

YOU CODE IT! CASE STUDY

Aaron K., a 41-year-old divorced father of two teenagers, states he has a successful, financially rewarding career. He has been with this company for the last 9 years, the last 3 as vice president of his division. Even though his job performance evaluations are good and he has been lauded by his boss, he worries constantly about losing his job and being unable to provide for his children. This worry has been troubling him for about the last 8 or 9 months. Despite really trying, he can't seem to shake the negative thoughts.

Over these last months, he noticed that he feels restless, tired, and stressed out. He often paces in his office when he's alone, especially when not deeply engaged in tasks.

He's found difficulty in expressing himself and has been humiliated in a few meetings when this has occurred. At night, when attempting to go to sleep, he often finds that his brain won't shut off. Instead of resting, he finds himself obsessing over all the worst-case scenarios, including losing his job and ending up homeless.

Dr. Sheppard diagnoses Aaron with generalized anxiety disorder and discusses a treatment plan with him.

You Code It!

Go through the steps of coding, and determine the code or codes that should be reported for this encounter between Dr. Sheppard and Aaron.

Step 1: Read the case completely.

Step 2: Abstract the notes: Which key words can you identify relating to why Dr. Sheppard cared for Aaron?

_____

Step 3: Query the provider, if necessary.

Step 4: Code the diagnosis or diagnoses.

_____

Step 5: Code the procedure(s): Psychiatric evaluation.

Step 6: Link the procedure codes to at least one diagnosis code to confirm medical necessity.

Step 7: Back code to double-check your choices.

Answer:

Did you determine the correct code to be:

F41.1 Generalized anxiety disorder

LO 8.6 Stress-Related Disorders

posttraumatic stress disorder (PTSD)

An ongoing sense of fear after the danger has gone.

Posttraumatic stress disorder (PTSD) is a condition in which a horrible experience leaves a lasting imprint on the patient's sense of danger. Normally, when an individual senses danger, a "fight or flight" response initiates feelings of worry and fear. For those suffering from PTSD, the harmful or dangerous situation is gone, yet the sensation of fear continues.

Most people associate PTSD with our brave servicemen and servicewomen coming home from combat duty. However, there are other types of incidents that may affect someone very deeply, such as having been abused, having been in a plane crash, or having witnessed a car accident with injuries. Living though natural disasters—such as hurricanes, earthquakes, or tornadoes—may also invoke ongoing fear. PTSD affects an estimated 7.5 million adults in the United States.

Signs and symptoms of PTSD include bad dreams (nightmares), flashbacks, and pathophysical reactions triggered by everyday objects, words, or experiences. These reactions may include diaphoresis (sweating) and tachycardia (rapid heart rate) and are known as *reexperiencing symptoms*. Some patients may experience *avoidance symptoms* and become depressed, avoid locations that are reminiscent of the event, or just feel emotionally numb. At times, patients may feel edgy, easily startled, or overly nervous; these feelings are known as *hyperarousal symptoms*.

When diagnosing PTSD, the psychiatrist or psychologist will look for the patient's having experienced at least three avoidance symptoms, two hyperarousal symptoms, and at least one reexperiencing symptom over the previous 30 days. These symptoms can make it very difficult for the patient to go to school or work, enjoy time with friends, or be involved in his or her typical daily life.

ICD-10-CM provides three code options for reporting this diagnosis:

F43.10 Post-traumatic stress disorder, unspecific

F43.11 Post-traumatic stress disorder, acute

F43.12 Post-traumatic stress disorder, chronic

Chapter Summary

Due to an increase in available care, more patients are receiving treatment for mental and behavioral disorders. Therefore, it is important for professional coding specialists to understand both psychological and physiological concerns. Through education and understanding, these patients can receive treatment and their providers can receive accurate reimbursement.

CHAPTER **8** REVIEW
Mental and Behavioral Disorders

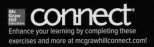

Enhance your learning by completing these
exercises and more at mcgrawhillconnect.com!

Using Terminology

Match each key term to the appropriate definition.

_____ **1.** LO 8.4 An emotional state that includes sadness, hopelessness, and gloom.

_____ **2.** LO 8.2 Consumption of a substance without significant clinical manifestations.

_____ **3.** LO 8.1 A type of common behavior that includes mood disorders, sleep disorders, psychotic symptoms, and agitation.

_____ **4.** LO 8.4 An emotional state that includes elation, excitement, and exuberance.

_____ **5.** LO 8.2 Ongoing, regular consumption of a substance with resulting significant clinical manifestations and a dramatic decrease in the effect of the substance with continued use, therefore requiring an increased quantity of the substance to achieve intoxication.

_____ **6.** LO 8.2 Ongoing, regular consumption of a substance with resulting clinical manifestations.

_____ **7.** LO 8.5 Irrational and excessive fear of an object, activity, or situation.

_____ **8.** LO 8.3 A psychotic disorder with no known cause.

_____ **9.** LO 8.5 The sincere belief that one is suffering an illness that is not present.

A. Abuse
B. Behavioral disturbance
C. Dependence
D. Depressive
E. Manic
F. Phobia
G. Schizophrenia
H. Somatoform disorder
 I. Use

Checking Your Understanding

Choose the most appropriate answer for each of the following questions.

1. LO 8.1 The control center of the human body is the

   a. dendrites.
   b. neurons.
   c. brain.
   d. synapses.

2. LO 8.2/8.3/8.4 All of the following are mood disorders *except*

   a. depression.
   b. apathy.
   c. euphoria.
   d. hallucinations.

3. LO 8.2 An ongoing, regular consumption of a substance with resulting clinical manifestations is

   a. use.
   b. abuse.
   c. dependence.
   d. depressive.

4. LO 8.3 _____ schizophrenia is also known as *hebephrenic schizophrenia* or *hebephrenia.*

    a. paranoid.

    b. catatonic.

    c. disorganized.

    d. undifferentiated.

5. LO 8.3 Atypical schizophrenia is also known as which type of schizophrenia?

    a. paranoid.

    b. disorganized.

    c. catatonic.

    d. undifferentiated.

6. LO 8.3 What is the appropriate code to assign for drug-induced dystonia?

    a. G21.11.

    b. G24.02.

    c. G25.71.

    d. G21.0.

7. LO 8.4 The feelings of hopelessness, guilt, and worthlessness are signs of which disorder?

    a. major depressive disorder.

    b. bipolar disorder.

    c. phobia disorder.

    d. somatoform disorder.

8. LO 8.5 Which of the following is a somatoform disorder?

    a. panic disorder.

    b. bipolar disorder.

    c. body dysmorphic disorder.

    d. schizophreniform disorder.

9. LO 8.2 The patient has been diagnosed with nicotine dependence, chewing tobacco in remission. What is the appropriate code to assign?

    a. F17.221.

    b. F17.223.

    c. F17.218.

    d. F17.291.

10. LO 8.1 It is important for professional coding specialists to understand

    a. psychological concerns.

    b. physiological concerns.

    c. psychological and physiological concerns.

    d. none of these.

Applying Your Knowledge

1. LO 8.2 What is the clinical difference between use, abuse, and dependence? _____

   _____

2. LO 8.4 What is a mood disorder? Give an example. _____

   _____

3. LO 8.3 List five types of schizophrenia. _____

   _____

4. LO 8.3 Explain schizoid personality disorder. _____

   _____

5. LO 8.4 Explain the difference between a bipolar manic episode and a bipolar depressive episode. _____

   _____

6. LO 8.5 What is a phobia? _____

   _____

Using the techniques described in this chapter, carefully read through the case studies and determine the most accurate ICD-10-CM code(s) and external cause code(s), if appropriate, for each case study.

1. Joe Burns, a 17-year-old male, was brought in by his mother to see Dr. Anderson. Mrs. Burns is concerned because her son is getting forgetful and loses interest in things quickly. Dr. Anderson examines Joe, and blood work reveals an alcohol level of 18 mg. Dr. Anderson diagnoses Joe with Korsakoff's syndrome.

_____

2. Anne Keels, a 27-year-old female, comes in today to see Dr. Goldbloom. Anne states that she has a constant anxious feeling without an obvious reason. Dr. Goldbloom diagnoses Anne with generalized anxiety disorder.

_____

3. Jimmy Henderson, a 4-year-old male, is brought in today by his father. Jimmy has started kindergarten, and when it is time for his mother to drop him off at school, Jimmy clings to his mother, refuses to let go, and cries. Dr. Stevenson diagnoses Jimmy with separation anxiety disorder (SAD).

_____

4. Sally Josephson, a 32-year-old female, comes in to see Dr. Elder. Sally has a history of depression, and today she states that she feels sad and hopeless and gets angry easily. She also says she does not feel like eating and is having difficulty sleeping. Dr. Elder diagnoses Sally with bipolar depressive disorder (current episode) without psychotic features, moderate level.

_____

5. Sam Coins, a 25-year-old male, comes in today for a follow-up appointment concerning his bipolar episode. Sam states he is doing well, without any negative feelings. Dr. Clarke diagnoses Sam's bipolar disorder as currently in remission.

_____

6. Susan Hills, a 43-year-old female, has a previous history of mood disorders. Susan is seeing Dr. Dunn today due to feeling increased energy, impulsiveness, and also sadness. Dr. Dunn diagnoses Susan's current episode as bipolar disorder, mixed state, mild level.

_____

7. Thomas Reynolds, a 37-year-old male, went on a mountain retreat last weekend. Tom comes in today to see Dr. Edwards because he experienced what he described as a panic attack during the retreat when he climbed a mountain and looked down. After a thorough examination, Dr. Edwards diagnosed Tom with acrophobia.

_____

8. Karin Griffith, an 18-year-old female, is scared to death of spiders and is diagnosed with arachnophobia.

   _____

9. Allen Ray, a 56-year-old male, is brought in by his wife to see Dr. Holder. Mrs. Ray states she is concerned because her husband has stated on several occasions that everyone is out to get him, and today he came home from work at noon because he said a coworker tried to poison his lunch. After a thorough examination, Dr. Holder diagnoses Allen with paranoid schizophrenia.

   _____

10. Judy Witt, a 16-year-old female, is brought in today by her mother after being found drinking alcohol and singing very loudly. After Dr. Daily's examination and blood work, which showed a blood alcohol level of 22 mg/100 mL, Judy is diagnosed with alcoholic intoxication.

    _____

11. Hal Pierson, a 45-year-old male, has been smoking cigarettes since he was 16 years old and has been trying to stop smoking on his own. Hal comes to see Dr. Tyler today with the complaint of irritability, inability to sleep, restlessness, and constant hunger. Dr. Tyler diagnoses Hal with nicotine dependence withdrawal.

    _____

12. Connie Franklin, a 20-year-old female, comes to see Dr. Dingle. Connie is a single female with a neat, attractive appearance. Connie states she feels deformed and would like to have the deformity fixed. After a thorough examination, Dr. Dingle found no physical deformity and diagnoses Connie with body dysmorphic disorder.

    _____

13. Billie Williams, a 32-year-old female, gave birth to a healthy baby boy 2 months ago. Billie comes in today complaining of feeling empty and numb, overwhelmed, and scared. Dr. Gaines diagnoses Billie with postpartum depression.

    _____

14. Robert Foley, a 67-year-old male, comes in today with the complaint that he's having trouble eating and swallowing and has been somewhat anxious. He also says he is concerned about his memory. Dr. Thomas examines Robert and diagnoses him with dementia.

    _____

15. Angela Cummings, a 51-year-old female, has a previous diagnosis of parkinsonism. She presents today complaining of speech and cognition difficulties. Dr. Manner diagnoses Angela with dementia due to parkinsonism.

    _____

The following exercises provide practice in abstracting physicians' notes and learning to work with SOAP notes from our health care facility, *Taylor, Reader, & Associates*. These case studies (SOAP notes) are modeled on real patient encounters. Using the techniques described in this chapter, carefully read through the case studies and determine the most accurate ICD-10-CM code(s) and external cause code(s), if appropriate, for each case study.

TAYLOR, READER, & ASSOCIATES
A Complete Health Care Facility
975 CENTRAL AVENUE • SOMEWHERE, FL 32811 • 407-555-4321

PATIENT: WILSON, ANDREW
ACCOUNT/EHR #:   WILSAN001
DATE: 10/16/18

Attending Physician: John S. Warwick, MD

Despite being handsome, tall, personable, and an "A" student at a highly respected university, Andrew confided to me that he was struggling, in private, with a compulsive need to count to 100 every time he had a "bad thought." He stated that he did this to prevent the thoughts from taking over. He was finding it increasingly difficult to socialize with his friends without the need to, unobtrusively, wash his hands for fear of contamination. He began carrying antibacterial wipes for those occasions when he could not get to a sink. He had difficulty tolerating medication to help defuse these feelings, and he has found talk therapy to be of little benefit. He stated that he came to my office with his parents, desperately hoping to get some relief.

After a thorough 2½-hour evaluation, I diagnosed Andrew with OCD.

Diagnosis: Obsessive-compulsive disorder (OCD).

John S. Warwick, MD

JSW/pw   D: 10/16/18 09:50:16   T: 10/18/18 12:55:01

Determine the most accurate ICD-10-CM code(s).

_____

_____

_____

TAYLOR, READER, & ASSOCIATES
A Complete Health Care Facility
975 CENTRAL AVENUE • SOMEWHERE, FL 32811 • 407-555-4321

PATIENT: GARDNER, MAXINE
ACCOUNT/EHR #:   GARDMA001
DATE: 10/16/18

Attending Physician: Suzanne R. Taylor, MD

S: Maxine, a 47-year-old female, came to see me because her youngest son was going off to college, leaving her alone in a bad marriage. She stated that, over the last several weeks, she had begun having panic attacks whenever she thought about the upcoming separation from her son and the realization that she was headed for divorce. Cognitive behavioral therapy, followed by three different medications, still did not provide this patient with relief from these panic attacks.

O: I ordered blood work and found her CBC (complete blood count) showed that the size of her red blood cells (MCV) was slightly abnormal. The range was 80–100, and she was 101. I did some research and found that an elevated MCV could indicate a B_{12} deficiency, so I had Maxine do a Schilling test to see if that was the case. Sure enough, the result was abnormal.

A: Panic disorder without agoraphobia, vitamin B_{12} deficiency.

P: Rx B_{12} injections; patient to return in 10 days to 2 weeks.

Suzanne R. Taylor, MD

SRT/pw   D: 10/16/18 09:50:16   T: 10/18/18 12:55:01

Determine the most accurate ICD-10-CM code(s).

_____

_____

_____

TAYLOR, READER, & ASSOCIATES
A Complete Health Care Facility
975 CENTRAL AVENUE • SOMEWHERE, FL 32811 • 407-555-4321

PATIENT: WATSON, SAMUEL
ACCOUNT/EHR #: WATSSA001
DATE: 4/17/18

Attending Physician: Willard B. Reader, MD

Samuel, a 31-year-old male, has a successful career working in a forensic laboratory. He came to see me after his wife noticed his behavior. For the 3 years they have been married, she has noticed that every spring he exhibits 2 months of days of elevation followed by irritability. He sleeps for short periods of time, typically no more than 3 hours. He is more talkative and comes up with incredible, incessant ideas. His attention span is very limited, and he is easily distracted to another subject or item. I recognize these as the signs and symptoms of hypomania. Then it seems his mood levels off during the summer, but he becomes sad and hopeless as the season turns toward winter. This recall indicates winter depression.

After a complete psych workup, Sam is diagnosed with bipolar/seasonal affective disorder, moderate. I prescribe lithium carbonate, 600 mg tid, and light therapy during the winter months to help with the depressive episodes.

Diagnosis: Bipolar/seasonal affective disorder, moderate.

_____

Willard B. Reader, MD

WBR/pw   D: 4/17/18 09:50:16   T: 4/19/18 12:55:01

Determine the most accurate ICD-10-CM code(s).

_____

_____

_____

TAYLOR, READER, & ASSOCIATES
A Complete Health Care Facility
975 CENTRAL AVENUE • SOMEWHERE, FL 32811 • 407-555-4321

PATIENT: DUNKIN, CESAR
ACCOUNT/EHR #:   DUNKCE001
DATE: 10/16/18
Attending Physician: Suzanne R. Taylor, MD

Cesar, a 43-year-old male, is an accountant in his second marriage. He was referred by his therapist of 2 years, Ms. McKenna, for psychiatric evaluation and consideration of medication to treat worsening depression. At the initial interview, Cesar's wife, Francie, an attorney, was present to provide some history and perceptions. She was quite cooperative yet strangely detached. She answered all of the questions that I asked in a genuine manner, all the while working on paperwork. After ruling out any pathologic causes of Cesar's hopelessness and sadness, I performed a complete workup.

It gradually became clear that the source of Cesar's persistent depression was his wife's lack of accountability and responsibility in the marriage. While Francie said all the right things, she was frequently late for couples' sessions, with no notice (even though they both carry cell phones). She makes promises to Cesar with no follow through. Cesar had been raised by his parents to become a responsible provider for his family, with the emphasis on family. Francie's behavior resulted in Cesar's helplessness to achieve his dream, his lifelong expectation, of a satisfying marriage. This context (an uncooperative spouse, combined with a desire to make the marriage work) was powerful enough that Cesar's depressions were recurring repeatedly.

This came to a peak last week, when Cesar was in a hotel 1,500 miles from home, threatening suicide. After arranging for his safety, I made sure that he was escorted to a friend's home nearby the next morning. The next day, Cesar flew back and came directly from the airport to my office. He looked haggard and obviously sleep-deprived. He filled me in on the details of the episode, and I realized that the episode was again triggered by the ongoing helplessness he felt within the marriage. His wife, it turns out, had discontinued couples' therapy several weeks earlier and was clearly not engaged in Cesar's desire to improve the marriage. Cesar began feeling trapped between failure in a second marriage and powerlessness to improve the relationship. Suicide seemed to be a viable and reasonable exit strategy from the pain he was feeling.

Now Cesar wanted me to tell him whether he should stay out of the house or go back to his wife. Based on the sensitization and kindling models, as well as the learned helplessness and other models of depression, I advised Cesar that a change in his context was medically indicated and was my firm recommendation. His wife was creating a depressogenic (depression-inducing) context that neither a change in attitude nor medication could counterbalance. Cesar was experiencing continued depression caused by this context in which his level of control over the outcome was negligible, a context that was in conflict with his deep need to love and be loved. This led to more severe, frequent depression (sensitization, which could lead to kindling) and, of course, suicidal ideation. I advised him to stay out of the home. I stated that if he and Francie chose to, they could continue in couples' psychotherapy.

Diagnosis: Major depressive disorder, recurrent, moderate

Suzanne R. Taylor, MD

SRT/pw   D: 10/16/18 09:50:16   T: 10/18/18 12:55:01

Determine the most accurate ICD-10-CM code(s).

_____

_____

_____

TAYLOR, READER, & ASSOCIATES
A Complete Health Care Facility
975 CENTRAL AVENUE • SOMEWHERE, FL 32811 • 407-555-4321

PATIENT: JAMES, AVERY
ACCOUNT/EHR #: JAMEAV001
DATE: 10/20/18

Attending Physician: Willard B. Reader, MD

Avery, a 35-year-old female, came to see me upon recommendation from her obstetrician, Dr. Shoah. As a former vice president of a large retail chain, her transition to full-time mom had been very challenging. One of the first things she said to me was, "I was very high functioning until five years ago." This was important information because it gave me a baseline sense of who Avery was as a person in this regard.

She stated that during this most recent pregnancy (her third child), she was hospitalized with both preeclampsia and dehydration. Shortly after this birth, she realized that she had become depressed and constantly sad. About 18 months later, she had her first panic attack. After this, there was a whirlwind of treatments that never seemed to work. She was hospitalized four times for depression and panic attacks before her visit to me. During that time, she went through two courses of shock therapy (ECT) with minimal benefit. She was taking four medications: Clozaril, Depakote, Lorazepam, and Wellbutrin.

During the extended evaluation I conduct with patients (history and physical), Avery complained of migraines, deadening of emotion, extreme sedation, a 50-lb weight gain since being on medication, trouble falling asleep despite her medications, constipation/diarrhea, dry skin, peripheral edema, and impaired concentration. Her Beck Depression Inventory (BDI) was 29, indicating a depression of high-moderate severity.

A very careful history and charting revealed severe PMS (premenstrual syndrome): She was "agitated and hyper" in late luteal phase (end of the menstrual cycle) and repeatedly experienced mild-to-moderate depression in early follicular phase of her menstrual cycle (days 1–7). This was misinterpreted by her previous doctors as rapid cycling, and so they put her on valproic acid (often thought to help rapid-cycling bipolar disorder).

The history and physical strongly indicated adrenal output problems (salt craving, hyperpigmentation, orthostatic hypotension by history, low blood pressure in the office [110/70, 105/70] without orthostasis, hypoglycemia [weakness, headache, and irritability all relieved by food]). The physical exam also suggested hypothyroidism (decreased relaxation phase of her deep tendon reflexes). The adrenal gland and thyroid gland work closely together, so this was not surprising.

In reviewing Avery's family psychiatric history, it was clear that her maternal grandmother was an alcoholic and was diagnosed as bipolar. Her grandmother had one depression which was severe enough to require shock treatments (ECT), and she was later maintained on lithium. Avery's mother was described as impulsive and emotional. On the father's side, Avery's grandfather suffered from depression and alcoholism, as did her father and two uncles.

As a result of timed hormonal testing, we decided to use progesterone supplementation as a way to deal with the female hormone component of the mood and anxiety problems. Avery stated this really helped her. This positive response to the progesterone makes it immediately clear that stabilization of affective disorder would require hormonal intervention.

(*Continued*)

Further testing revealed that the mood cycling occurred in the context of numerous hormonal problems including:

a) Impaired glycemic control (secondary to medication and poor diet, lack of exercise)
b) Hypothyroidism (this was noted in her hospital chart but deemed "mild hypothyroidism not requiring treatment.")
c) Adrenal insufficiency
d) Low levels of melatonin
e) Ovarian dysfunction
f) Multiple nutrient deficiencies (l-tryptophan, B_6, phenylalanine, eicosapentaenoic acid), all known to create mood instability

From a psychological point of view, it was clear that Avery's self-esteem was severely affected by how bad she felt physically. Her repetitive uncontrollable monthly mood cycling, medication side effects, the transition to motherhood, and her identification with her grandmother, who had mental illness, negatively affected her sense of self. Avery was really terrified that she too would be mentally ill.

The treatment course consisted of correction of all of the above factors, and Avery remained on only one of her previous medications, her antidepressant, and I added a thyroid hormone. She engaged in ongoing therapy to help her with the motherhood role and her fear of being like her grandmother.

Diagnosis: Postpartum depression, panic disorder, hormonal imbalance

Willard B. Reader, MD

WBR/pw   D:10/20/18 09:50:16   T: 10/22/18 12:55:01

Determine the most accurate ICD-10-CM code(s).

_____

_____

_____

CODING NERVOUS SYSTEM CONDITIONS

9

Learning Outcomes
After completing this chapter, the student should be able to:

LO 9.1 Differentiate the types of nerves.

LO 9.2 Apply correctly the official guidelines for reporting dominant and nondominant sides.

LO 9.3 Identify the components of the central nervous system.

LO 9.4 Identify the components of the peripheral nervous system.

LO 9.5 Illuminate signs and symptoms of neurologic disorders.

LO 9.6 Apply correctly the official guidelines for reporting the medical necessity for pain management.

The most obvious function of the nervous system is to enable an individual to feel things—sensory touch and input. With this function, you are able to feel hot and cold, soft and hard, pleasure and pain. In addition to enabling the sense of feeling, the body's nervous system is also involved in the stimulation required for the musculoskeletal system to work. It is the brain that instructs muscles to contract so that you can sit up, cut a piece of paper, or walk down the street. Bundles of nerve fibers that instruct the activities of the cardiac muscles and smooth muscles, as well as gland function, are known as the **autonomic nervous system.** The nervous system is also responsible for the brain's ability to think, understand, remember, and perform other mental activities. This is why some mental disorders, such as dementia and epilepsy, are treated by neurologists.

The **central nervous system (CNS)** primarily involves two organs in the human body: the brain and the spinal cord. The **peripheral nervous system (PNS)** includes all the neurons, nerves, ganglia, and plexuses that reach outward from the CNS. Figure 9-1 illustrates these two systems.

LO 9.1 Types of Nerves

Every time you reach your hand out and touch something, **sensory (afferent) fibers** transmit sensory information to the CNS. Then sensory nerves forward that information to the brain or spinal cord. **Motor (efferent) fibers** contained within the motor nerves convey stimuli from the CNS to muscles and glands. Most nerve bundles are bound together by connective tissues and include both sensory and motor nerves. Those bundles of afferent and efferent nerves, specifically those that stimulate skeletal muscle and somatic tissue, are known as *somatic nerves.* The efferent nerves that regulate the dilation (opening) and constriction (closing) of blood vessels are known as *vasomotor nerves.* They support blood pressure activity.

Key Terms
Activities of daily living (ADLs)
Acute
Autonomic nervous system
Basal ganglia
Brain
Central nervous system (CNS)
Cerebellum
Cerebral hemispheres
Cerebral meninges
Chronic
Cranial nerves
Hypothalamus
Medulla oblongata
Motor (efferent fibers)
Neurologic function assessments
Peripheral nervous system (PNS)
Pons
Sensory (afferent) fibers
Spinal cord
Spinal nerves
Thalamus

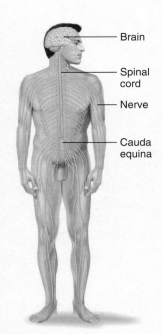

FIGURE 9-1 The Nervous System

Source: Booth et al., MA, 5e. Copyright © 2013 by McGraw-Hill. Figure 22-6b, p. 479

autonomic nervous system
The nerve fiber bundles that initiate automatic body functions, such as heart contraction.

central nervous system (CNS)
The brain and spinal cord.

peripheral nervous system (PNS)
Components of the nervous system other than the brain and spinal cord; includes ganglia and neurons.

sensory (afferent) fibers
Nerve fibers that carry information from a peripheral nerve to the central nervous system.

motor (efferent) fibers
Nerve fibers that carry information from a central organ to a peripheral site.

brain
An organ within the skull that controls body functions and external interactions; part of the central nervous system.

LO 9.2 Dominant and Nondominant Sides

Are you right-handed? If so, the right side of your body is considered your dominant side. Individuals who are left-handed have the left side of their bodies considered the dominant side. Then there are those who are ambidextrous (use both hands equally).

Patients suffering with *hemiplegia* (paralysis of one side of the body) or *hemiparesis* (weakness of one side of the body)—code category G81—will need documentation of whether the dominant side or nondominant side is affected. The same is required for a patient diagnosed with *monoplegia* (paralysis of one extremity, e.g.,one arm or one leg)—code category G83.

You may have no memory of a physician ever asking you whether you are right- or left-handed—I don't. While neurologists are trained to consider this, you may find this detail missing from the documentation. For such cases, querying the physician may not help because he or she may not know. ICD-10-CM Official Guidelines are here to help you determine the correct code when the affected (weakened or paralyzed) side is documented yet there is no indication of whether or not this is the patient's dominant side. The guidelines direct you:

- Documentation states right side is affected—report as dominant.
- Documentation states left side is affected—report as nondominant.

For those patients documented to be ambidextrous, whichever side is documented as affected should be reported as the patient's dominant side.

EXAMPLE

G81.12 Spastic hemiplegia affecting left dominant side
G83.14 Monoplegia of lower limb affecting left nondominant side

LO 9.3 Central Nervous System

The central nervous system (CNS) comprises the brain and the spinal cord.

The Brain

The **brain** functions as the control headquarters for the entire body. Some individuals incorrectly use the terms *brain* and *cerebrum* interchangeably; however, the cerebrum is actually only one part of the brain. Take a look at Figure 9-2.

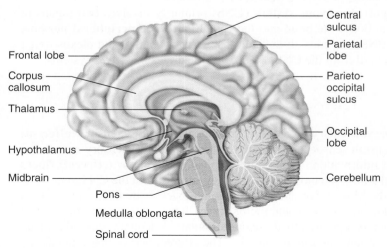

FIGURE 9-2 The Brain

Source: Booth et al., MA, 5e. Copyright © 2013 by McGraw-Hill. Figure 30-6, p. 599

The largest part of the brain, the *cerebrum* (consisting of the two cerebral hemispheres) controls sensory transmissions, motor activities, and intelligence. The parietal layer of the cerebrum is known as the *cerebral cortex* and is sometimes referred to as the *gray matter.* The deeper layers include the white matter (axons) and the **basal ganglia,** the control mechanism for coordination and stability. The lines that appear to separate the **cerebral hemispheres** into several lobes are called *fissures* and provide conductivity of nerve fibers (the *corpus callosum*) that enable communication between the sections. Each lobe has a specific responsibility for function in the body:

- *Frontal lobes* are responsible for voluntary muscle movements, motor areas for speech (Broca's area), personality, behavior, and intellect (critical thinking, memory, judgment), as well as autonomic (involuntary) functions, cardiac activities, and emotion.
- The *fissure of Rolando* (central sulcus) lies between the frontal lobes and the parietal lobes.
- *Parietal lobes* are responsible for interpretation and coordination of sensory information. The right parietal lobe processes sensory data from the left side of the body, and the left parietal lobe processes data from the right side. (Yes! From opposite sides.)
- The *fissure of Sylvius* (lateral sulcus) is the line between the temporal lobes and the frontal and parietal lobes.
- *Temporal lobes* are responsible for the senses (smell, taste, hearing) as well as interpretation of spoken language.
- The *parieto-occipital fissure* lies between the occipital lobe and the two parietal lobes.
- The *occipital lobe* processes visual impulses.

Below the corpus callosum sits the **thalamus,** the part of the brain responsible for transmitting impulses to the specific, appropriate part of the cerebellum, similar to a dispatcher. In addition, the thalamus is responsible for basic emotional responses such as fear, as well as for identifying likable and dislikable sensations. Beneath the thalamus is the **hypothalamus,** which is in charge of more autonomic responses such as body temperature control, appetite, blood pressure, respiration, stress reactions, and sleeping patterns.

Cerebral meninges are protective layers of membrane that insulate the brain. The three layers of the meninges are the *dura mater*—the parietal (outermost) layer; *arachnoid mater*—the center of the meninges that contains the cerebrospinal fluid (CSF); and *pia mater*—the deepest layer of the membrane, which contains a network of nerves and blood vessels. Atop the dura mater (between the dura mater and the skull) is the area known as the *epidural space.* Between the dura mater and the arachnoid mater is a space called the *subdural space,* and the area between the arachnoid mater and the pia mater is called the *subarachnoid space.* CSF is manufactured in the *choroid plexi* (plural of *plexus*) in the lateral (side) ventricles of the brain and held in all four cerebral ventricles and the spaces within the meninges until the fluid is absorbed back into the vascular system.

At the base of the brain, inferior to the cerebrum, is the area known as the **cerebellum.** The cerebellum coordinates motor activities with sensory impulses and maintains balance and muscle tone. For example, your sensory impulses inform you that something is hot, and the motor activity pulls your hand away from the heat source. The *brainstem* consists of the midbrain, the **pons,** and the **medulla oblongata.** The *reticular formation* (the thalamus, hypothalamus, midbrain, pons, and medulla oblongata) functions as an arousal process, supporting the awakened functions, and as a communications connector between the spinal cord and the brain.

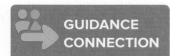

GUIDANCE CONNECTION

Review the ICD-10-CM Coding Guidelines, Section I.C.6, Chapter 6: **Diseases of the nervous system,** Subsection a, **Dominant/nondominant side**.

basal ganglia
Groups of nerve cell bodies involved with musculoskeletal movement.

cerebral hemispheres
The two halves of the cerebrum of the brain.

thalamus
A large oval mass responsible for relaying sensory impulses to and from the cerebral cortex.

hypothalamus
A part of the diencephalons of the brain; involved with controlling body temperature and the autonomic nervous system.

cerebral meninges
Three protective layers of membrane that insulate the brain.

cerebellum
The posterior portion of the brain responsible for controlling coordination and maintaining balance.

pons
The part of the posterior of the brain, superior to the medulla, that participates in brainstem functions.

medulla oblongata
The bottom portion of the brainstem, at the junction of the spinal cord; consists of nerves responsible for respiration, circulation, and other functions.

EXAMPLE

G46.3 Brain stem stroke syndrome

The Spinal Cord

The **spinal cord** is a part of the central nervous system located along the dorsal (posterior) surface of the torso. Starting at the brainstem (at the *foramen magnum*), the spinal cord is threaded through the center of the spinal vertebrae, within the *vertebral foramen,* and ends at the area around lumbar vertebra 1 or 2 (L1 or L2). It is protected by the vertebral body anteriorly (in the front) and the spinous process and pedicle posteriorly (at the back).

Spinal meninges, just like the cerebral meninges, are made up of a tri-layered membrane that lines the soft tissues of the CNS, protecting the spinal cord from the bones of the vertebrae. The three layers of the meninges are the *dura mater*—the parietal (outermost) layer; *arachnoid mater*—the center of the meninges that contains the CSF; and the *pia mater*—the deepest layer of the membrane, which contains a network of nerves and blood vessels.

There are two landmarks along the spinal cord that may be referred to in physician documentation. The *cervical enlargement* is a thickened area of the spinal cord containing peripheral nerves for the upper extremities. The *lumbar enlargement* is similar to the cervical enlargement, located lower on the column and housing the peripheral nerves for the lower extremities.

EXAMPLE

G12.0 Infantile spinal muscular atrophy, type 1 [Werdnig-Hoffman]

LO 9.4 Peripheral Nervous System

The peripheral nervous system (PNS) includes the cranial nerves and the spinal nerves. Somatic fibers are nerves that reach out into the skin as well as the skeletal muscles, while the autonomic fibers connect to the viscera (internal organs).

Cranial Nerves

Cranial nerves travel from the brain and brainstem throughout the body. ICD-10-CM refers to these nerves by their names. Understanding the functions of these nerves can support your determination of related, additional diagnoses involved with nerve damage and/or treatment.

The twelve pairs of cranial nerves (see Figure 9-3) each have specific responsibilities:

Olfactory nerves—cranial nerve I: This pair of nerves is located in the lining of the upper nasal cavity, and these nerves are related to the sense of smell.

Optic nerves—cranial nerve II: This pair of nerves transmits sensations from the eyes to the brain. These nerves are linked with vision.

Oculomotor nerves—cranial nerve III: Initiating in the center of the brain, this pair of nerves transmits to the orbit of the eyes and connects to the muscles that raise the eyelid and help to move the eye itself.

Trochlear nerves—cranial nerve IV: This pair, the smallest of the cranial nerves, transmits impulses to the fifth voluntary muscle, the muscle that enables the eye to move.

The midbrain is the reflex center for cranial nerves III and IV.

Trigeminal nerves—cranial nerve V: This pair of cranial nerves is the largest. These nerves extend from the pons area of the brain and include three sensory branches: the *ophthalmic branch* (transmitting impulses from the surface of the eye, tear glands, anterior scalp, forehead, and upper eyelids' skin), the *maxillary branch* (carrying impulses from the upper teeth, upper gum, upper lip, mucous

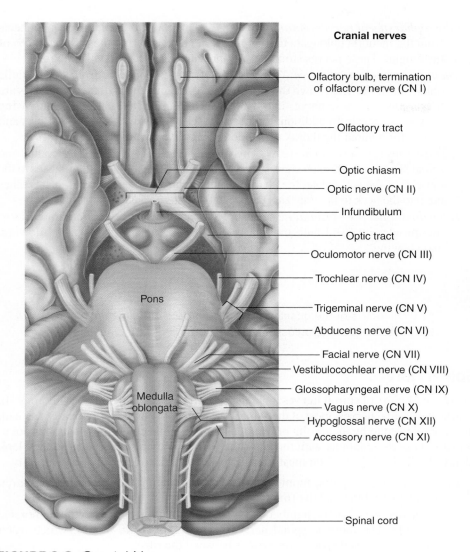

Cranial nerves

- Olfactory bulb, termination of olfactory nerve (CN I)
- Olfactory tract
- Optic chiasm
- Optic nerve (CN II)
- Infundibulum
- Optic tract
- Oculomotor nerve (CN III)
- Trochlear nerve (CN IV)
- Trigeminal nerve (CN V)
- Abducens nerve (CN VI)
- Facial nerve (CN VII)
- Vestibulocochlear nerve (CN VIII)
- Glossopharyngeal nerve (CN IX)
- Vagus nerve (CN X)
- Hypoglossal nerve (CN XII)
- Accessory nerve (CN XI)
- Spinal cord

Pons

Medulla oblongata

FIGURE 9-3 Cranial Nerves

Source: Michael McKinley and Valerie O'Loughlin, HUMAN ANATOMY, 1/e. © 2006 MHE. Figure 15.24, p. 475

lining of the palate, and facial skin), and the *mandibular branch* (carrying impulses from behind the ears, the lower jaw's skin, the lower teeth, lower gum, and lower lip, as well as making connections to the muscles of the floor of the mouth and the muscles that enable mastication [chewing]).

Abducens nerves—cranial nerve VI: This tiny pair of cranial nerves connects the pons, close to the medulla oblongata, with the orbit of the eye and transmits impulses to the muscle that assists with moving the eye.

Facial nerves—cranial nerve VII: This pair of cranial nerves, also originating at the pons, branches into the sides of the face and associates with the taste receptors on the anterior 60% of the tongue. Impulses are transmitted via this pair of nerves to the muscles used for facial expressions, and these nerves also stimulate excretions from both the salivary and tear glands.

Vestibulocochlear nerves—cranial nerve VIII: Each nerve of this pair has two specific branches: the vestibular and the cochlear. The vestibular branch connects with the inner ear and participates with the reflexes for maintaining equilibrium. The cochlear branch transmits impulses from the hearing receptors in the inner ear to the pons and medulla oblongata.

The pons is the reflex center for cranial nerves V through VIII.

Glossopharyngeal nerves—cranial nerve IX: This pair of cranial nerves connects from the medulla oblongata to the tonsils, the pharynx, and the posterior 35% of the tongue. These nerves stimulate the muscles involved with swallowing.

Vagus nerves—cranial nerve X: This pair of nerves connects from the medulla oblongata to the neck, down through the chest, and into the abdomen. Impulses are transmitted via these nerves into the laryngeal muscles to assist with swallowing as well as speech. In addition, the heart muscles, as well as smooth muscles and glands throughout the thorax and abdomen, receive impulses via these nerves.

Accessory nerves—cranial nerve XI: This pair of nerves has two branches: cranial and spinal. The cranial branch converges with a vagus nerve to transmit impulses to the muscles of the soft palate, the pharynx, and the larynx. The spinal branch reaches out into the neck to the trapezius muscle and the sternocleidomastoid muscle.

Hypoglossal nerves—cranial nerve XII: This pair of nerves transmits impulses to the muscles involved with moving the tongue to enable speaking, swallowing, and chewing.

EXAMPLE

G52.0 Disorders of the olfactory nerve (disorders of 1st cranial nerve)
G52.3 Disorders of hypoglossal nerve (disorders of 12th cranial nerve)

Spinal Nerves

spinal nerves
Nerves that extend from the spinal cord to the peripheral aspects of the body.

There are 31 pairs of **spinal nerves** that reach out from the spinal cord (see Figure 9-4). Unlike the cranial nerves, most of the spinal nerves are not named individually. Instead, they are referred to by their point of origin along the spinal column. Be cautious not to confuse these designations with those for the vertebrae themselves because they look identical: C1, T5, L3, etc. You must read the context of the documentation carefully.

Cervical nerves: 8 pairs, numbered C1–C8, originating from each of the seven cervical vertebrae and the first thoracic vertebra.

Thoracic nerves: 12 pairs, numbered T1–T12, originating from each of the thoracic vertebrae. The thoracic spinal nerves become *intercostal nerves,* which reach into the intercostal spaces (the spaces between the ribs).

Lumbar nerves: 5 pairs, numbered L1–L5, originating from the lumbar vertebrae.

Sacral nerves: 5 pairs, numbered S1–S5, originating from each of the original five sacral vertebrae.

Coccygeal nerves: 1 pair, originating at the coccyx.

You read earlier in this chapter that the spinal cord terminates at a point located between the L1 and L2 vertebrae. Here, you can see that these spinal nerves continue all the way down to the coccyx. These additional segments of nerves, located past the end of the spinal cord, are known collectively as the *cauda equina.*

The main segments of each of the other spinal nerves unite into multifaceted networks known as *plexuses.* There are three plexuses:

- Cervical plexus (C1–C4).
- Brachial plexus (C5–T1).
- Lumbosacral plexus (T12–S5), also referred to individually as the *lumbar plexus* and the *sacral plexus.*

EXAMPLE

G54.0 Brachial plexus disorders
G54.1 Lumbosacral plexus disorders

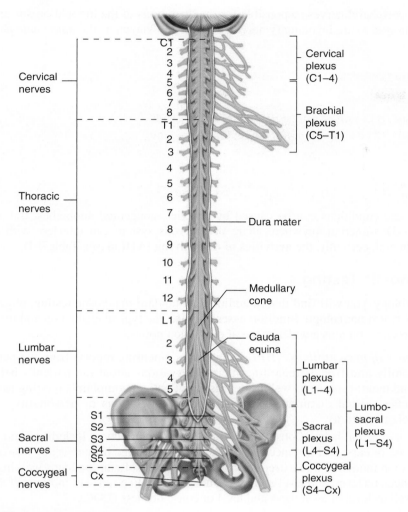

FIGURE 9-4 Spinal Nerves

Source: Booth et al., MA, 5e. Copyright © 2013 by McGraw-Hill. Figure 30-8, p. 602

Some spinal nerves are named. These nerves include:

Femoral nerve: the primary nerve transmitting to the muscles in the thigh.

Median nerve: a nerve that originates in the brachial plexus and reaches down the center of the upper extremity (arm).

Peroneal nerve: an offshoot of the sciatic nerve that reaches into the lateral part of the lower leg, on the side of the fibula bone.

Phrenic nerve: a cervical nerve that transmits impulses from C4 to the pericardium and motor signals to the diaphragm.

Pudendal nerve: the nerve connecting to the genital area.

Radial nerve: a nerve that originates from the cervical nerve and reaches down the medial (inner) side of the forearm and hand (thumb side).

Sciatic nerve: a nerve that originates from L2–S3 and passes through the thigh and down the lower extremity. At approximately the knee, the sciatic nerve divides into the peroneal nerve and the tibial nerve.

Tibial nerve: the nerve that branches from the sciatic nerve and reaches into the lower leg along the anterior side (along the tibia).

Ulnar nerve: a nerve that is a part of the brachial plexus and that branches to the skin and muscles along the lateral side of the forearm and hand (leading into the fifth digit [pinkie finger]).

The peripheral nerves responsible for the operations of the internal organs and the vascular system are involuntary nerves, collectively known as the *autonomic nervous system.*

EXAMPLE

> G57.01 Lesion of sciatic nerve, right lower limb
> G57.22 Lesion of femoral nerve, left lower limb

LO 9.5 Neurologic Disorders

Neurologic conditions can be caused by genetics, congenital anomalies, trauma, or disease. Dysfunction anywhere along the nervous system can interfere with organ function and, certainly, the **activities of daily living (ADLs)** (see Table 9-1).

Diagnostic Testing

In neurology, you will find that in addition to standard diagnostic testing, physicians often perform **neurologic function assessments.** The typical evaluation and management process contains a wider scope of evaluation points:

History of present illness (HPI) includes documenting reports from the patient's family and friends regarding their observations about the patient's behavior and mental status, as well as details about patient complaints relating to headaches, visual disturbances, mood swings, alterations of personality, and/or seizure activity.

Physical exam includes observation for physical dysfunction, including fluid in the nose or ears; performance of a prick test to determine if there is any loss of sensation (numbness) in extremities; and observation of gait (patient's walking, balance), reflexes, and level of motor function, including range of motion (ROM), as well as level of awareness and level of consciousness (LOC).

activities of daily living (ADLs)

Daily tasks involved in normal function: bathing, dressing, eating, mobility, and personal hygiene.

neurologic function assessments

Diagnostic examinations, observations, and questions/answers designed to evaluate the patient's neurologic function.

EXAMPLE

> Z02.2 Encounter for examination for admission to residential institution
> Z13.4 Encounter for screening for certain developmental disorders in childhood
> Z13.858 Encounter for screening for other nervous system disorders

TABLE 9-1 Activities of Daily Living

- Bathing and showering (washing the body)

- Dressing

- Eating/feeding (including chewing and swallowing)

- Functional mobility (moving from one place to another while performing activities)

- Personal hygiene and grooming (including brushing/combing/styling hair)

- Toilet hygiene (completing the act of urinating/defecating)

Source: US Department of Health and Human Services (1990) Measuring the Activities of Daily Living: Source: Comparisons Across National Surveys. Retrieved from http://aspe.hhs.gov/daltcp/reports/meacmpes.htm

The physician may also use tools such as the Glasgow Coma Scale (see Table 9-2) or the Stroke Assessment checklist, as well as tests such as PET scans, magnetic resonance imaging (MRI) (see Figure 9-5), computed tomography (CT) scans, skull x-rays, eletroencephalography (EEG), lumbar puncture, myelography, cerebral anteriography, brain scans, or electromyography.

TABLE 9-2 Glasgow Coma Scale

The eye opening part of the Glasgow Coma Scale has four scores:

- 4 indicates that the patient can open his eyes spontaneously.
- 3 is given if the patient can open his eyes on verbal command.
- 2 indicates that the patient opens his eyes only in response to painful stimuli.
- 1 is given if the patient does not open his eyes in response to any stimulus.

The best verbal response part of the test has five scores:

- 5 is given if the patient is oriented and can speak coherently.
- 4 indicates that the patient is disoriented but can speak coherently.
- 3 means the patient uses inappropriate words or incoherent language.
- 2 is given if the patient makes incomprehensible sounds.
- 1 indicates that the patient gives no verbal response at all.

The best motor response test has six scores:

- 6 means the patient can move his arms and legs in response to verbal commands.
- 5 is given if the patient responds to localized painful stimuli.
- 4 indicates the patient showed flexion-withdrawal.
- 3 means that flexion-abnormal (decorticate rigidity) is evidenced.
- 2 indicates the patient shows extension (decerebrate rigidity).
- 1 indicates that the patient shows no movement in response to stimuli.

The results of the three tests are added up to determine the patient's overall condition. A total score of 3 to 8 indicates a severe head injury, 9 to 12 indicates a moderate head injury, and 13 to 15 indicates a mild head injury.

Source: National Institute of Neurological Disorders and Stroke, National Institutes of Health. http://www.ninds.nih.gov/disorders/tbi/detail_tbi.htm

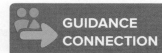

GUIDANCE CONNECTION

Review the ICD-10-CM Coding Guidelines, Section I.C.18, Chapter 18: **Symptoms, signs, and abnormal clinical and laboratory findings, not elsewhere classified,** Subsection e, **Coma scale,** for more input.

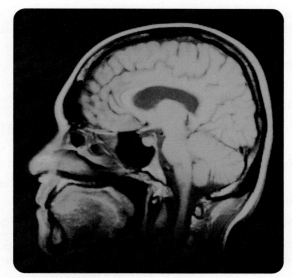

© Larry Mulvehill/Corbis

FIGURE 9-5 MRI Image of Brain

Inflammatory Conditions of the Central Nervous System

Bacteria and viruses can invade the nervous system and cause infection, malfunction, and, in some cases, death. Examples include encephalitis (inflammation of the brain tissue), myelitis (inflammation of the spinal cord), intracranial abscess, and, probably the most well-known condition, meningitis.

Meningitis is an inflammatory disease of the CNS. However, as a professional coder, you must know more than the fact that the patient is diagnosed with meningitis. Meningitis can be caused by a virus or a bacterial invader that you will need to identify from the documentation; this may be a virus such as enterovirus, herpes zoster, or leptospira or a bacteria such as *Haemophilus influenzae*, streptococcus, pneumococcus, staphylococcus, or *E. coli*, to name just a few. Each specific detail may lead you to a different code or require a second code.

EXAMPLE

G00.1 Pneumococcal meningitis

G00.8 Meningitis due to Escherichia coli (Other bacterial meningitis)

G03.0 Nonpyogenic meningitis

LET'S CODE IT! SCENARIO

Bruce Reed went to see Dr. Lockhart after returning from an exciting trip to South America. He confirmed that he had fallen and hit the back of his head during his trip and was now suffering with fever, headaches, and vomiting. He complained of becoming confused in familiar places, and at times he was unable to speak (aphasia). Tests confirmed Dr. Lockhart's diagnosis of intracranial epidural abscess caused by enterococcus.

Let's Code It!

Dr. Lockhart was able to confirm the diagnosis of *intracranial epidural abscess caused by enterococcus,* so let's begin with the first part and turn to the Alphabetic Index to look up "abscess." You can see a long, long list of additional descriptors indented below this entry. Take a minute to review the elements listed to see if any of them match what the physician wrote in the documented diagnosis.

Abscess

    Intracranial G06.0

Let's go to the Tabular List and begin reading at the three-character code category suggested here:

G06 Intracranial and intraspinal abscess and granuloma

Read the notation directly below this code. This is why it is always important to begin reading at the three-character code category.

Use additional code (B95–B97) to identify infectious agent

Remember that this tells you two very important things for accurately coding this diagnosis: (1) You will need another code, and (2) you will need to report this code (G06.-) first, followed by a second code to report the infectious agent (the "enterococcus" mentioned in Dr. Lockhart's notes), using a code from within the range B95–B97.

Go ahead and review all of the choices for the required fourth character for this code. Did you match this code to Dr. Lockhart's notes?

G06.0 Intracranial abscess and granuloma

Great! This code description does not match exactly; however, you can see one of the nonessential modifiers below it does match exactly.

Now let's turn to B95–B97 in the Tabular List, and see whether you can determine the second code needed to report the infectious agent (the pathogen). Remember to always begin reading at the three-character code category.

B95 Streptococcus, Staphylococcus, and Enterococcus as the cause of diseases classified elsewhere

Keep reading to determine the accurate fourth character:

B95.2 Enterococcus as the cause of diseases classified elsewhere

This matches the physician's documentation. For this encounter between Dr. Lockhart and Bruce Reed, you need to report:

G06.0 Intracranial abscess and granuloma

B95.2 Enterococcus as the cause of diseases classified elsewhere

Great job!

Hereditary and Degenerative Diseases of the Central Nervous System

Some nervous system conditions affect the function of the CNS and are linked to genetics or degeneration but not trauma. The patient may have a condition that is well known, such as Alzheimer's disease or dementia, or a lesser-known condition such as parkinsonism or Huntington's chorea.

As you have seen before, a diagnosis may seem to be complete but actually may not include enough information for a professional coder. For example, it is not enough to know the patient was diagnosed with dementia. To determine the most accurate code, you need more details, such as:

Frontotemporal dementia (Pick's disease) G31.01

Dementia with Lewy bodies (Lewy body dementia) G31.83

You may remember we discussed coding some forms of dementia in the Mental and Behavioral Disorders chapter of this textbook. The good news here is that the coding process you learned will help you get to the correct ICD-10-CM chapter, know which specific descriptors to look for in the documentation, and then lead you directly to the most accurate code.

LET'S CODE IT! SCENARIO

J.J. Fletcher, an 87-year-old female, came to see Dr. Keiser with complaints of increasing forgetfulness and difficulty remembering new information. She states virtually no ability to focus or concentrate. Her presentation confirms a deterioration in personal hygiene, and her appearance is somewhat disheveled. Her daughter insisted that she come to the doctor. After a neurologic exam, psychometric testing, a PET scan, and an EEG, Dr. Keiser diagnosed J.J. with late-onset Alzheimer's disease.

Dr. Keiser diagnosed J.J. with *Alzheimer's disease.* Let's turn to the Alphabetic Index in the ICD-10-CM book and find:

Disease
>> **Alzheimer's G30.9** *[F02.80]*

Read the list of additional descriptors indented below this. The specific code to report will change on the basis of documentation of behavioral disturbance, early onset, and/or late onset. What did Dr. Keiser document?

Disease
>> **Alzheimer's G30.9** *[F02.80]*
>>> **late onset G30.1** *[F02.80]*

Dr. Keiser stated nothing about behavioral disturbances, so this matches the notes. Let's turn to the Tabular List and begin reading at the three-character code:

G30 Alzheimer's disease

There is an *includes* note that identifies Alzheimer's dementia senile and presenile forms, a *use additional code* notation that explains the second code suggested in the Alphabetic Index listing, and an *Excludes1* note citing three diagnoses that are not reported from this code category. Do you see any of these diagnoses included in Dr. Keiser's documentation? No. Read all of the choices for the fourth character available in this code category, and determine which one best matches what Dr. Keiser wrote in J.J.'s notes:

G30.1 Alzheimer's disease with late onset

This matches the documentation exactly! Good job! Now you must go and investigate the second code suggested by the Alphabetic Index: F02.80. Remember, even though the Alphabetic Index gave us five characters, you must always begin reading at the three-character level:

F02 Dementia in other diseases classified elsewhere

Directly below this entry, you can see a notation to *code first* the underlying physiological condition, such as Alzheimer's disease. This is a great confirmation that you will need these two codes, and now you know the order in which to report them: G30.1 first, followed by the F02 code. Also, read carefully both the *Excludes1* and *Excludes2* notations. For J.J.'s encounter with Dr. Keiser, none of these apply. However, the next case you code may involve one of these diagnoses. Now is the best time to establish good coding habits.

Review the fourth-character choices. You will notice there is only one:

F02.8 Dementia in other diseases classified elsewhere

Now review the fifth-character choices. You have two. Which one matches Dr. Keiser's notes about J.J.? Dr. Keiser makes no mention at all about any behavioral disturbance.

F02.80 Dementia in other diseases classified elsewhere without behavioral disturbance

You have done a great job determining the two codes to report for Dr. Keiser's diagnosis of J.J.:

G30.1 Alzheimer's disease with late onset

F02.80 Dementia in other diseases classified elsewhere without behavioral disturbance

Diseases of the Peripheral Nervous System

The anatomy classes that you took will be very helpful when interpreting diagnoses involving the peripheral nervous system (PNS). These nerves run throughout the body from head to toe and are identified by names and numbered categories.

YOU CODE IT! CASE STUDY

Ronald Kling woke up and noticed that the left side of his face was weak and drooping. Saliva was dripping uncontrollably from his mouth, and he had a headache behind his left ear. After a thorough neurologic workup, Dr. Jonathan diagnosed him with Bell's palsy.

You Code It!

Go through the steps of coding and determine the code or codes that should be reported for this encounter between Dr. Jonathan and Ronald Kling.

Step 1: Read the case completely.

Step 2: Abstract the notes: Which key words can you identify relating to why Dr. Jonathan cared for Ronald?

_____

Step 3: Query the provider, if necessary.

Step 4: Code the diagnosis or diagnoses.

_____

Step 5: Code the procedure(s): Office visit.

Step 6: Link the procedure codes to at least one diagnosis code to confirm medical necessity.

Step 7: Back code to double-check your choices.

Answer:

Did you determine the correct code?

G51.0 Bell's palsy

Good job!

Treatments

As complex as the network of nerves that run through the body, the treatment plans for individuals with neurologic disorders vary greatly, from physical therapy to surgery. Discussed below are some of the most common disorders and what can be done to help the patient.

Hydrocephalus

When too much CSF accumulates in the ventricles and the body cannot absorb it back into the vascular system fast enough, the brain tissues can be damaged and lose the ability to function properly. This can occur in infants (a congenital anomaly: ICD-10-CM code category Q03, Congenital hydrocephalus), or it can develop in adults (code category G91, Hydrocephalus). The most common treatment for this condition is the surgical implantation of a ventriculoperitoneal shunt, which drains the excess fluid away from the brain and, via a connecting catheter, deposits the excess CSF in the peritoneal (abdominal) cavity, to be absorbed and eliminated from the body.

Cerebral Aneurysm

A cerebral aneurysm occurs when a weakness in the wall of a cerebral artery permits a bubble to form (code I67.1, Cerebral aneurysm, nonruptured). If (when) the bubble ruptures—code I60.7, Nontraumatic subarachnoid hemorrhage from unspecified intracranial artery (ruptured cerebral aneurysm)—the blood from the artery will flow out and create a subarachnoid hemorrhage (code I60.8, Other nontraumatic subarachnoid hemorrhage), disturbing the area's ability to function properly. Typically, the treatment is to prevent the possibility of rupture and hemorrhage by surgically repairing the weakness in that arterial wall. This can be done by wrapping the weak section with a muscle, clipping (resection), or ligating (tying) the artery.

Migraine Headaches

The two most frequent types of migraine headaches are the common migraine (ICD-10-CM code subcategory G43.0–) and the classical migraine (ICD-10-CM code subcategory G43.1–). Some patients will find treatment with pharmaceuticals, including ergotamine, metoclopramide, or naproxen. Antiemetics (to stop nausea and vomiting) may be helpful when these symptoms are present. As with most conditions, medications, such as propranolol, atenolol, amitriptyline, and clonidine, can work to prevent a migraine from developing.

Cerebrovascular Accident

Also known as a *stroke,* a cerebrovascular accident (CVA) is a suddenly occurring dysfunction of one or more cerebral blood vessels that prevents the supply of oxygen to cranial tissues (ICD-10-code category I63, Cerebral infarction). Often, this is caused by an embolus (blood clot) causing an obstruction in the artery or vein. The longer these tissues are denied oxygen, the greater the opportunity for necrosis (tissue death) or other serious damage. An estimated half-million people in the United States are struck with a CVA each year, and 50% result in fatalities. Time is critical for more positive outcomes, so patients need to receive treatment as quickly as possible. When administration can occur within 3 hours of the onset, tissue plasminogen activator (tPA), a clot-dissolving medication, has shown excellent results. Sequelae (late effects) of CVA (ICD-10-CM code category I69, Sequela of cerebrovascular disease) may require some types of physical and/or occupational therapy.

LET'S CODE IT! SCENARIO

Eric Springer was referred to Dr. Greenberg, a neurosurgeon, after his last brain MRI came back showing signs of an abundance of cerebrospinal fluid (CSF) in the ventricles of his brain. After taking a full history and examination, Dr. Greenberg determined that there was malabsorption of CSF in the brain—an official diagnosis of communicating hydrocephalus. Dr. Greenberg discussed the treatment options with Eric and his family.

Dr. Greenberg diagnosed Eric with *hydrocephalus*. Let's turn to the Alphabetic Index in the ICD-10-CM book and find:

Hydrocephalus (acquired) (external) (internal) (malignant) (noncommunicating) (obstructive) (recurrent) G91.9

This seems to match the notes, except included in the parenthetical nonessential modifiers is the term *noncommunicating*. When you look back at the notes, you can see that Dr. Greenberg diagnosed Eric with *communicating*—the opposite. So, you know that this code cannot be correct. There is still a long list of additional modifying terms indented below *hydrocephalus*. Read through all of the choices, and see if you can determine which one matches the documentation. Did you find:

Hydrocephalus
communicating G91.0

This matches the notes, so let's turn to the Tabular List (Volume 1) and begin reading at the three-character code:

G91 Hydrocephalus

There is an *includes* note that identifies acquired hydrocephalus, and an *Excludes1* note citing three diagnoses that are not reported from this code category. Do you see any of these diagnoses included in Dr. Greenberg's documentation? No. Read all of the choices for the fourth character available in this code category, and determine which one best matches what Dr. Greenberg wrote in Eric's notes:

G91.0 Communicating hydrocephalus

This matches the documentation exactly! Good job!

LO 9.6 Pain Management

Neurologists are among the health care professionals who most often treat pain because neurologic conditions involve the nerve endings and electrical impulses within the nervous system. There are physicians who specialize in pain management, although specialized training is not mandatory. **Acute** pain is determined by the severity of the pain and its impact on the patient's ability to function. The most common types of **chronic** pain include headache, low back pain, cancer pain, arthritis pain, neurogenic pain, and psychogenic pain. There is no specific time measurement to determine chronic pain. Therefore, the judgment of the physician, as stated in the documentation, is what differentiates acute pain from chronic pain. You must be careful not to assume a diagnosis of *chronic pain syndrome*. This condition is different from chronic pain, and its diagnosis may be reported (code G89.4) only when the attending physician specifically documents this condition.

Pain can be a very difficult thing to deal with clinically because it is not the same for every patient. Medically speaking, pain is an unpleasant sensation often initiated by tissue damage that results in impulses being transmitted to the brain via specific nerve fibers. It can be challenging for the patient to describe the level of intensity, and each individual patient's ability to cope with pain will vary greatly. Clinically speaking, pain can be diagnosed as acute, chronic, or both acute and chronic.

Most health care facilities use some type of pain scale from 0 to 10 (see Table 9-3) to help improve communication with patients. The zero indicates no pain at all, and the scale increases up to the number 10, representing excruciating, intolerable pain.

acute
Severe, intense.

chronic
Persisting for weeks, months, or years.

TABLE 9-3 Numeric Rating Scale for Pain

Numeric Rating	Meaning
0	No pain
1–3	Mild pain (nagging, annoying, interfering little with ADLs)
4–6	Moderate pain (interferes significantly with ADLs)
7–10	Severe pain (disabling; unable to perform ADLs)

Source: National Institutes of Health

Some facilities use a scale that includes illustrations to help patients accurately communicate what they are feeling.

Reporting Pain Separately

When the physician has documented a confirmed diagnosis and this condition is the underlying cause of the pain, pain should not be reported with a separate code. In these circumstances, the pain is considered to be an inclusive symptom. The exceptions to this guideline occur when:

- The principal purpose of the encounter is pain management and the encounter does not include treatment or management of the underlying condition.
- The pain is noted as acute and/or chronic, documenting that the pain suffered by the patient is above and beyond the level typical of the underlying condition.

ICD-10-CM provides code category G89, Pain, not elsewhere classified, from which to choose an appropriate code.

EXAMPLE

1. Sasha slipped during ice skating practice and broke her right ankle. After x-raying the ankle and applying the cast, Dr. Poppe gave her a prescription for pain medication. In this case, only the fractured ankle would be reported (S82.64xA, Nondisplaced fracture of lateral malleolus of right fibula, initial encounter for closed fracture). The pain is an inclusive symptom of the fracture.

2. Sasha came back to Dr. Poppe 10 days later complaining of unbearable pain and stating that the prescribed medication was not "doing the trick." Dr. Poppe discussed several management treatments for the acute pain with Sasha, and she agreed to try a different medication. This encounter was only for pain management. Dr. Poppe did not attend to the fracture at all. Therefore, this encounter would be reported with two codes:

   G89.11 Acute pain due to trauma
   S82.64xD Nondisplaced fracture of lateral malleolus of right fibula, subsequent encounter for fracture with routine healing

   A code from category G89 is reported to add details about the reason for this encounter with Dr. Poppe. The code for the fracture explains why Sasha had pain.

3. Ralph is diagnosed with chronic tension headaches due to the extreme pressures of his job. He told the doctor he could not stand the pain anymore and he needed help. This diagnosis would be reported with both of these codes:

   G89.29 Other chronic pain
   G44.229 Chronic tension-type headache, not intractable

The official guidelines state that if the pain is not specifically documented as acute or chronic, it should not be reported separately. The exceptions to this guideline include:

- *Post-thoracotomy pain:* G89.12 Acute post-thoracotomy pain (post-thoracotomy pain NOS); G89.22 Chronic post-thoracotomy pain.
- *Postprocedural pain:* G89.18 Other acute postprocedural pain (postprocedural pain NOS); G89.28 Other chronic postprocedural pain.
- *Neoplasm-related pain:* G89.3 Neoplasm related pain (acute)(chronic).
- *Central pain syndrome:* G89.0 Central pain syndrome.

In these four situations, the code from category G89 should be reported in addition to any other conditions related to the encounter.

Postprocedural Pain

As stated above, postprocedural pain would be reported with either G89.18 or G89.28, depending upon the physician's documentation of the pain as either acute or chronic. One of these codes may be reported only when the pain is documented as:

- More intense or lasting longer than the expected level of pain that is considered normal immediately after a surgical procedure.
- Not related to a detailed complication of the surgical procedure.

Site-Specific Pain Codes

There are many other code categories within ICD-10-CM used to report pain located in a specific anatomical site. Code category G89, Pain, not elsewhere classified, does not include any site-specific information. Anatomical site-specific code categories include:

> M54.5 Low back pain (lumbago)
>
> M79.602 Pain in left arm
>
> M79.672 Pain in left foot

Sequencing Pain Codes with Other Codes

To determine the proper sequencing of a code from category G89 with codes for site-specific pain or underlying conditions, the first question to be answered from the documentation is, "Why was this encounter necessary?" If the answer is for pain management, the code from category G89 should be first-listed or the principal diagnosis reported. If the encounter is for any other reason and the attention to pain management is secondary to the purpose for the encounter, then the first-listed or principal diagnosis code would report that other reason and the code from category G89 would be reported afterward.

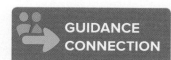

GUIDANCE CONNECTION

Review the ICD-10-CM Coding Guidelines, Section I.C.6, Chapter 6: **Diseases of the nervous system,** Subsection b, **Pain—category G89**.

LET'S CODE IT! SCENARIO

Kaitlyn Morrissey came in to see Dr. Catalano with complaints of extreme pain in her head. She stated that she was nauseous and irritable and that light made the pain even worse. Kaitlyn stated that these headaches seemed to happen every month, right before she got her menstrual period, and she couldn't take it anymore. She begged for something to help with the pain. After a full examination, Dr. Catalano diagnosed her with chronic premenstrual migraine.

Dr. Catalano diagnosed Kaitlyn with *premenstrual migraine headaches,* and pain management was the purpose of this visit to the physician. Let's turn to the ICD-10-CM Alphabetic Index and find:

Migraine (idiopathic) G43.909

There is a list of additional descriptors indented below this. Go back to the physician's notes. Did he describe the migraine with more detail? Yes, he stated her migraine was premenstrual. So look down the list and see if you can find a suggested code:

Migraine (idiopathic) G43.909

Premenstrual—*see* Migraine, menstrual

Menstrual G43.829

Perfect! Now, let's turn to code category G43 in the Tabular List:

G43 Migraine

Did you notice the notation below this code?

Use additional code for adverse effect, if applicable, to identify drug (T36–T50 with fifth or sixth character 5)

There is no mention of any drugs or adverse reactions in Dr. Catalano's documentation, so let's continue. Read the *Excludes1* note. Nothing there matches the physician's notes, so continue down the column and review *all* of the choices for the mandatory fourth character. Which one matches what Dr. Catalano wrote?

G43.8 Other migraine

There are fifth-character choices listed below this code, so you will have to look up the column and find the box containing the fifth-character choices. You will see the box directly below the three-character code category. Review the four choices. Which one matches?

G43.82 Menstrual migraine, not intractable

Good. There was no mention that Kaitlyn was having an intractable migraine. Read the notation beneath this code classification:

Code also associated premenstrual tension syndrome (N94.3)

There was no mention of this in Dr. Catalano's notes on Kaitlyn. Review the choices for the sixth character:

G43.829 Menstrual migraine, not intractable, without mention of status migrainosus

Do you also need to include a code from the G89 code category? Check the Official Guidelines, specifically Section 1.c.6.b(1)(b), **Use of category G89 codes in conjunction with site specific pain codes.** You will see that it states, *"If the code describes the site of the pain, but does not fully describe whether the pain is acute or chronic, then both codes should be assigned."* Terrific! Dr. Catalano documented that Kaitlyn's pain was chronic, and code G43.829 does not include that specific detail. That's the answer to that question, so go and review all of the possible codes from code category G89 to determine the most accurate code to report:

G89.29 Other chronic pain

You have one last task to complete. Now that you have two codes to report Dr. Catalano's reasons for caring for Kaitlyn during this encounter, you need to determine the correct sequence in which to report these codes. Refer again to that guideline, and the next part tells you, *"If the encounter is for pain control or pain management, assign the code from category G89 followed by the code identifying the specific site of pain."* You know from the notes that the reason for this encounter was pain management, so again you know that the correct codes and the correct order to report the reason why Dr. Catalano cared for Kaitlyn during this encounter are:

G89.29 Other chronic pain

G43.829 Menstrual migraine, not intractable, without mention of status migrainosus

Good job!

Chapter Summary

Many different circumstances and situations can be the cause of malfunction anywhere in the nervous system. As with any other organ system or diagnosis, professional coding specialists should never assume. Everything you need to report these conditions accurately is in the physician's documentation. If it is not, you must query the physician.

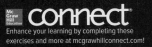
Enhance your learning by completing these
exercises and more at mcgrawhillconnect.com!

Using Terminology

Match each key term to the appropriate definition.

_____ **1.** LO 9.6 Severe, intense.

_____ **2.** LO 9.3 An organ within the skull that controls body functions and external interactions; part of the central nervous system.

_____ **3.** LO 9.3 Three protective layers of membrane that insulate the brain.

_____ **4.** LO 9.3 Groups of nerve cell bodies involved with musculoskeletal movement.

_____ **5.** LO 9.3 A part of the diencephalons of the brain; involved with controlling body temperature and the autonomic nervous system.

_____ **6.** LO 9.3 A large oval mass responsible for relaying sensory impulses to and from the cerebral cortex.

_____ **7.** LO 9.3 Nerve fibers that carry information from a peripheral nerve to the central nervous system.

_____ **8.** LO 9.6 Persisting for weeks, months, or years.

_____ **9.** LO 9.3 The posterior portion of the brain responsible for controlling coordination and maintaining balance.

_____ **10.** LO 9.3 The nerve fiber bundles that initiate automatic body functions, such as heart contraction.

_____ **11.** LO 9.3 The brain and spinal cord.

_____ **12.** LO 9.3 Nerve tissue that runs through the vertebral bodies along the dorsal aspect of the torso and from which peripheral nerves extend.

_____ **13.** LO 9.4 Twelve pairs of nerves, each having specific responsibilities that extend directly from the brain and brainstem.

_____ **14.** LO 9.3 Nerve fibers that carry information from a central organ to a peripheral site.

_____ **15.** LO 9.3 Components of the nervous system other than the brain and spinal cord; includes ganglia and neurons.

A. Acute
B. Autonomic nervous system
C. Basal ganglia
D. Brain
E. Central nervous system (CNS)
F. Cerebellum
G. Cerebral meninges
H. Chronic
I. Cranial nerves
J. Hypothalamus
K. Motor (efferent) fibers
L. Peripheral nervous system (PNS)
M. Sensory (afferent) fibers
N. Spinal cord
O. Thalamus

Checking Your Understanding

Choose the most appropriate answer for each of the following questions.

1. LO 9.1/9.3 The brain and spinal cord compose the

   a. peripheral nervous system.
   b. central nervous system.
   c. cerebral hemispheres.
   d. medulla oblongata.

2. LO 9.3 The nerve fiber bundles that initiate automatic body functions are known as the

   a. central nervous system.
   b. peripheral nervous system.
   c. autonomic nervous system.
   d. cranial nerves.

3. LO 9.1 _____ transmit sensory information to the CNS.

    a. afferent fibers.
    b. efferent fibers.
    c. motor fibers.
    d. cerebral fibers.

4. LO 9.3 The control center of the entire body is the

    a. cerebral hemispheres.
    b. cerebrum.
    c. thalamus.
    d. brain.

5. LO 9.3 The landmark(s) along the spinal cord that may be referred to in physician documentation is (are)

    a. the cervical enlargement.
    b. the lumbar enlargement.
    c. the enter of the meninges.
    d. the cervical enlargement and the lumbar enlargement.

6. LO 9.4 There are _____ pairs of cranial nerves that travel from the brain throughout the body.

    a. 31.
    b. 25.
    c. 12.
    d. 8.

7. LO 9.5 All of the following are examples of inflammatory conditions of the central nervous system *except*

    a. encephalitis.
    b. meningitis.
    c. dementia.
    d. intracranial abscess.

8. LO 9.5 Huntington's chorea is an example of a(n)

    a. inflammatory disease of the CNS.
    b. trauma of the CNS.
    c. hereditary disease of the CNS.
    d. disease of the PNS.

9. LO 9.6 A severe, intense pain is known as

    a. chronic.
    b. acute.
    c. nagging.
    d. interferon.

10. LO 9.6 The Official Guidelines state that if the pain is not specifically documented as acute or chronic, it should not be reported separately. The exceptions to this guideline include all of the following *except*

    a. post-thoracotomy pain.
    b. neoplasm-related pain.
    c. tension headaches.
    d. central pain syndrome.

Applying Your Knowledge

1. LO 9.3 What is the central nervous system (CNS) composed of? _____

   _____

2. LO 9.4 What is the peripheral nervous system (PNS) composed of? _____

   _____

3. LO 9.3 Explain the difference between the sensory (afferent) fibers and the motor (efferent) fibers. _____

   _____

4. LO 9.3 What is the largest part of the brain, and what is its function? _____

   _____

5. LO 9.3 List five of the responsibilities of the frontal lobes. _____

   _____

6. LO 9.3 Explain the responsibility of the parietal lobes, and identify which side each lobe controls. _____

   _____

7. LO 9.3 Explain the function of the cerebral meninges. Then name the layers of the cerebral meninges. and explain
   in what order they are positioned. _____

   _____

8. LO 9.5 List three ADLs. _____

   _____

9. LO 9.5 Differentiate between an inflammatory and a hereditary/degenerative type of diseases of the nervous system. Give an example of each type. _____

   _____

10. LO 9.6 Explain the difference between acute and chronic pain. _____

    _____

Using the techniques described in this chapter, carefully read through the case studies and determine the most accurate ICD-10-CM code(s) and external cause code(s), if appropriate, for each case study.

1. Marja Aarnio, a 62-year-old female, presents today for a spinal puncture. The procedure was performed; however, there were complications, which leads to a diagnosis of cerebrospinal fluid leak from spinal puncture.

   _____

2. George Baumgartner, a 9-year-old male, is brought in by his parents for his sports participation physical examination. Dr. Grimm notes lack of muscle strength and tone on George's right dominant side. George is diagnosed with flaccid hemiplegia.

   _____

3. Robert Tucker, a 58-year-old male, presents today with pain and weakness in his left leg. After an examination and testing, Robert is diagnosed with sciatic neuropathy.

   _____

4. Heather Southard, a 16-year-old female, comes in today to see Dr. Xylas. Heather says she is having difficulty opening her mouth, is experiencing jaw pain, and is grinding her teeth. Dr. Xylas diagnoses Heather with orofacial dyskinesia.

   _____

5. Keith Gallop, an 18-year-old male, presents today with his parents. Keith comes in with the left side of his face drooping. Keith states that it began yesterday afternoon. After an examination and tests, Keith is diagnosed with Bell's palsy.

   _____

6. Pam Yandle, a 65-year-old female, is brought in by her daughter. Pam's daughter is concerned because she has noticed that her mother has become absentminded and forgetful and becomes confused easily outside her home. After a thorough examination, Dr. Causey diagnoses Pam with early onset Alzheimer's disease.

   _____

7. Lola Wozniak, a 31-year-old female, presents today with sudden intense pain in the eyes, lips, nose, scalp, forehead, and jaw. A thorough examination is completed, and Dr. Dingle diagnoses Lola with trigeminal neuralgia.

   _____

8. Alfonso Edmonds, a 56-year-old male, comes in today with the complaint of restless sleep and sleepiness during the daytime. He also states that his wife has told him his snoring has gotten much worse in the past few weeks. Alfonso is diagnosed with obstructive sleep apnea.

_____

9. Kayla Eller, a 68-year-old female, comes in today with the complaint of a severe, pounding headache on the left half of her head. It has lasted for approximately 36 hours. She admits to some nausea and light sensitivity. Dr. Sutton diagnoses Kayla with a persistent migraine aura headache.

_____

10. Frank Norris, a 45-year-old male, presents today with the complaints of quivering, feeling stiff, moving slowly, and having difficulty standing straight. Frank is diagnosed with vascular parkinsonism.

_____

11. Zena Medlock, a 45-year-old female, comes to see Dr. Algernon due to pain in her right arm. Patient states the pain is stabbing and burning and the limb is extremely sensitive to touch. Zena is diagnosed with complex regional II pain syndrome.

_____

12. Steve Solomon, a 4-year-old male, is brought in by his parents today for a well-baby check. Dr. Torrance notes overall muscle weakness, poor muscle tone, and limpness. Steve is diagnosed with childhood type II spinal muscular atrophy.

_____

13. Janet Woods, a 38-year-old female, comes in to see Dr. Albertson with the complaint of weakness while chewing and trying to swallow. After an examination and testing, Janet is diagnosed with myasthenia gravis.

_____

14. Betty Mays, a 31-year-old female, comes in today to see Dr. Jacobs. Betty complains of muscle weakness in her legs and arms. Betty also states that for the past day she has had difficulty maintaining her posture and walking. Dr. Jacobs completes a thorough examination and diagnoses Betty with acute ascending myelitis.

_____

15. Bennie Noble, a 21-year-old male, presents today with a headache, fever, and neck stiffness. After an examination, Dr. Taylor diagnoses Bennie with meningitis due to Gram-negative bacteria.

_____

The following exercises provide practice in abstracting physicians' notes and learning to work with SOAP notes from our health care facility, *Taylor, Reader, & Associates.* These case studies (SOAP notes) are modeled on real patient encounters. Using the techniques described in this chapter, carefully read through the case studies and determine the most accurate ICD-10-CM code(s) and external cause code(s), if appropriate, for each case study.

TAYLOR, READER, & ASSOCIATES
A Complete Health Care Facility
975 CENTRAL AVENUE • SOMEWHERE, FL 32811 • 407-555-4321

PATIENT: LEWIS, COLLETTE
ACCOUNT/EHR #:   LEWICO001
DATE: 10/17/18

Attending Physician: Willard B. Reader, MD

S: This is a 10-year-old female who is brought into the office by her parents with a chief complaint of clumsiness and blurred vision. She had been well until approximately two weeks ago, when she noticed a loss of sensation and strength in her left leg, a rapid deterioration in vision, and a decrease in coordination. There is no history of fever, vomiting, or seizures. One year prior to this event, she presented to the hospital with poor coordination, dizziness, and headaches. A left hemiplegia was noted as well as an asymmetric gait. A full recovery was made 5 days later, and she was discharged from the hospital without further treatment or a definite diagnosis.

O: VS are normal. Her weight, height, and head circumference are all at the 50th percentile. She is alert but subdued. Her HEENT exam is notable for severe visual loss and pale optic discs on funduscopy. Her heart, lungs, and abdomen are normal. She is noted to have a hyporeflexive paraparesis on the left.

    I admitted her into the hospital. A CT scan shows slightly enlarged ventricles, and an MRI scan shows multiple lesions in the periventricular white matter and cerebellum. Pattern visual evoked responses showed markedly delayed latencies. She is treated with corticosteroids, and a full recovery within a few weeks is expected.

A: Multiple sclerosis (MS)

P: Continue to follow and treat with traditional medication.
    Research any alternative or complementary medications and/or methods.

Willard B. Reader, MD

WBR/pw   D: 10/17/18 09:50:16   T: 10/19/18 12:55:01

Determine the most accurate ICD-10-CM code(s).

_____

_____

_____

TAYLOR, READER, & ASSOCIATES
A Complete Health Care Facility
975 CENTRAL AVENUE • SOMEWHERE, FL 32811 • 407-555-4321

PATIENT: FLETCHER, LACY
ACCOUNT/EHR #:   FLETLA001
DATE: 10/17/18

Attending Physician: Suzanne R. Taylor, MD

S: This is a 2-year-old female who appeared to be recovering from an upper respiratory infection when she developed vomiting. Her grandmother may have given her aspirin, but she was supposed to have taken acetaminophen. She initially presents to the emergency department with irritability and restlessness. She subsequently develops convulsions, which are treated with anticonvulsants, and she is admitted to the PICU.

O: VS T 37.8, P 100, R 50, BP 110/70, oxygen saturation 99% in room air. Height, weight, head circumference are at the 50th percentile. She is agitated and not cooperative. Head shows no signs of external trauma. Pupils are equal and reactive to light. Conjunctiva are clear, sclera nonicteric. EOMs cannot be fully tested, but they are conjugate. TMs are normal. Mouth is not easily examined. Neck reveals no adenopathy. She is agitated, so it is not possible to be certain that her neck is supple. Heart regular without murmurs. Lungs are clear. Abdomen is flat with normal bowel sounds. It is difficult to tell if she has any hepatosplenomegaly. No definite tenderness. No inguinal hernias are present. She moves all extremities. Reflexes are not testable because of her agitation.

Labs: Serum bilirubin: normal. Serum AST and ALT: increased. Serum ammonia: increased. Prothrombin time: prolonged. A CT scan of the brain is obtained which shows cerebral edema.
Her neurologic symptoms rapidly worsen and she becomes unresponsive. She is intubated and put on mechanical ventilation. Reye's syndrome is suspected. A confirmatory liver biopsy reveals diffuse, small lipid deposits in the hepatocytes (microvesicular steatosis) without significant necrosis or inflammation. The findings are consistent with the diagnosis of Reye's syndrome.

A: Reye's syndrome

P: Continue to follow and treat

_____

Suzanne R. Taylor, MD

SRT/pw   D: 10/17/18 09:50:16   T: 10/18/18 12:55:01

Determine the most accurate ICD-10-CM code(s).

_____

_____

_____

TAYLOR, READER, & ASSOCIATES
A Complete Health Care Facility
975 CENTRAL AVENUE • SOMEWHERE, FL 32811 • 407-555-4321

PATIENT: MILLER, NATASHA
ACCOUNT/EHR #:   MILLNA001
DATE: 10/16/18

Attending Physician: John S. Warwick, MD

S: This is a 12-year-old female brought to the ER by her mother with a chief complaint of leg weakness. One week prior, she had a fever of 101.4F with vomiting and diarrhea. After 3 days, the vomiting and diarrhea resolved. She was doing well until this morning when she fell while trying to get out of bed and could not stand or walk without support. She denies headache, blurred vision, tinnitus, vertigo, dysphagia, and incontinence. No history of toxic ingestion. Her immunizations are up to date. While in the ER, she complains that her arms feel week.

O: VS T 37.0, P 84, R 24, BP 102/64. Height and weight are at the 25th percentile. She is alert, slightly fearful, but cooperative. HEENT: She has no nystagmus and no papilledema. Her extraocular movements are intact. Pupils are equal and reactive to light. No facial weakness or asymmetry is present. Heart, lung, and abdomen exams are normal.

Neuro: Strength 4/5 in the upper extremities, 3/5 in the lower extremities. DTRs 1–2+ in the upper extremities and absent in the lower extremities. Sensation is intact in all extremities. Cerebellar function is normal except for the weakness. No cranial nerve abnormalities are noted. She refuses to walk.
   CBC, electrolytes, BUN, creatinine, glucose, calcium, and liver function tests are normal. Urine toxicology screen is negative. A lumbar puncture is performed. Opening pressure is normal. CSF analysis shows protein 146 mg/dL (high), glucose 70 mg/dL, 5 WBC/mm^3, 1 RBC/mm^3, and Gram stain shows no WBCs and no organisms.
   An MRI of the brain and spinal cord is normal. She is started on IVIG, and over the next few days, she slowly regains strength in her arms and legs. However, she still requires assistance with walking at the time of discharge.

A: Guillain-Barre syndrome (GBS)

P: She is referred to a rehabilitation hospital to continue outpatient physical therapy.

John S. Warwick, MD

JSW/pw   D: 10/16/18 09:50:16   T: 10/18/18 12:55:01

Determine the most accurate ICD-10-CM code(s).

_____

_____

_____

TAYLOR, READER, & ASSOCIATES
A Complete Health Care Facility
975 CENTRAL AVENUE • SOMEWHERE, FL 32811 • 407-555-4321

PATIENT: WANG, JUI LI
ACCOUNT/EHR #:   WANGJU01
DATE: 10/16/18

Attending Physician: John S. Warwick, MD

S: The patient was last seen on September 10 and presents today to discuss the results of the MRI.

O: The MRI scan of the brain demonstrates the patient has hydrocephalus with transependymal edema.

A: The patient has normal pressure hydrocephalus.

P: Patient requires a ventricular shunt placement. I have explained to the patient and his family the shunt procedure, its indications, risks, benefits, and alternatives in detail, including the risk of bleeding, infection, injury to the brain tissue with hemorrhages, stroke, paralysis, blindness, coma, or even death. All of their questions have been answered. No guarantees have been given. I have advised that the patient will need to have medical clearance from his primary care physician, Dr. Torman. Once we have the medical clearance, we can schedule him for surgery.

_____

John S. Warwick, MD

JSW/pw   D: 10/16/18 09:50:16   T: 10/18/18 12:55:01

Determine the most accurate ICD-10-CM code(s).

_____

_____

_____

TAYLOR, READER, & ASSOCIATES
A Complete Health Care Facility
975 CENTRAL AVENUE • SOMEWHERE, FL 32811 • 407-555-4321

PATIENT: BINYON, ROSE
ACCOUNT/EHR #:   BINYRO001
DATE: 10/16/18

Attending Physician: Suzanne R. Taylor, MD

S: This patient is a 6-month-old female brought into the office as a new patient for a well-baby visit. Her family moved here recently from Asia, where she was born. There were no prenatal or postnatal complications, and she has had no significant medical problems since birth.

Family History: Positive for her father, who has a condition in which his body is covered with fleshy small growths, similar to skin tags, and on the father's side, there are several family members with same warty growths, seizures, and high blood pressure.

O: VS are normal. Her growth parameters are in the 25th to 50th percentiles. Her examination is otherwise unremarkable except for multiple coffee-colored spots on her trunk and abdomen.

A: Neurofibromatosis, type I

P: Schedule parents for a follow-up visit tomorrow to discuss this further.

_____

Suzanne R. Taylor, MD

SRT/pw   D: 10/16/18 09:50:16   T: 10/18/18 12:55:01

Determine the most accurate ICD-10-CM code(s).

_____

_____

_____

10

CODING DISEASES OF THE EYE AND ADNEXA

Learning Outcomes

After completing this chapter, the student should be able to:

LO 10.1 Identify the components of the optical system.

LO 10.2 Distinguish between idiopathic and traumatic effects on the eyes.

LO 10.3 Report the various types of corneal dystrophy.

LO 10.4 Recognize inclusive signs and symptoms in glaucoma.

LO 10.5 Explain the impact of co-morbidities and underlying conditions on vision.

LO 10.6 Apply coding guidelines for reporting hypertensive retinopathy.

Key Terms

Accommodation

Blepharitis

Bulbar conjunctiva

Cataract

Choroid

Ciliary body

Cone

Conjunctivitis

Cornea

Corneal dystrophy

Dacryocystitis

Extraocular muscles

Glands of Zeis

Glaucoma

Iris

Keratitis

Lacrimal apparatus

Lens

Meibomian glands

Moll's glands

The five senses, as you know, are touch, taste, smell, sight, and hearing. The sense of touch is realized in the skin—a part of the integumentary system. Taste is done in the mouth—a part of the digestive system. And smell is the olfactory process in the nose—a part of the respiratory system. The other two senses are the function of their own individual systems within the body: The auditory system, which enables the sense of hearing, will be discussed in the next chapter. The optical system, which enables the sense of sight or vision, is considered one of the most complex organ systems in the body. This chapter will help you discover why.

Loss of sight, or even the reduction of vision, has both social and economic impact on the patient and his or her family. In the United States, it is estimated that 14 million people aged 12 and over have some type of visual impairment, and about 61 million adults are believed to be at high risk for acute vision loss.

LO 10.1 Optical System Anatomy

There are two recesses in the human skull, each known as an **orbit,** or eye socket (see Figure 10.1). Within this bony conical orbit sits the contents of the eye, the structure of which is very complex and consists of many inter-active components.

EXAMPLE

H05.022 Osteomyelitis of left orbit
H05.321 Deformity of right orbit due to bone disease

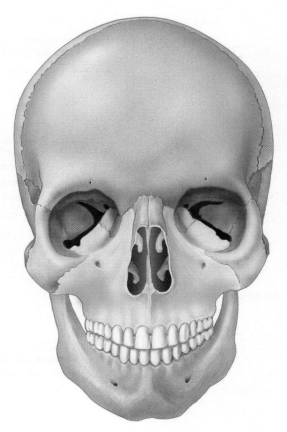

FIGURE 10-1 Bony Conical Orbit within the Human Skull

Source: David Shier et al., HOLE'S HUMAN ANATOMY & PHYSIOLOGY, 12/e. © 2010 MHE. Figure 7.17, pg. 209

Interior of the Eye

The organ that is commonly referred to as the *eye* (see Figure 10-2) consists of the eyeball, the optic nerves, the extraocular muscles, the cranial nerves, the blood vessels, orbital adipose (fat), and the lacrimal system.

The Sclera The outer protective layer of the eyeball is known as the **sclera.** It consists of a dense, white fibrous layer of tissue. At the anterior (front) of the eyeball, approximately at the superior aspect (above, or the top) and the inferior aspect (below, or the bottom) of the anterior chamber, the sclera meets the cornea. This meeting point is known as the *limbus* or *corneoscleral junction* (*corneo* = cornea + *-scleral* = sclera). As the sclera comes around the back (posterior) of the eyeball, the sclera connects to the *dural sheath* (also referred to as the *lamina cribrosa*) of the optic nerve.

The Cornea The portion of the sclera at the medial anterior aspect (the middle of the front) of the eyeball is called the **cornea.** It is a curved, multilayer, transparent, and avascular (no blood vessels) segment of this structure (see Figure 10-3). The cornea's only function within the eye is to refract light rays. There are five layers that make up the cornea:

- *Epithelium:* the location of sensory nerves.
- *Bowman's membrane:* the location of epithelial cells.
- *Stroma:* the supporting tissue that makes up 90% of the corneal structure.
- *Descement's membrane:* elastic fibers.
- *Endothelium:* cells that help to maintain proper hydration of the cornea to keep it moist.

orbit
The bony cavity in the skull that houses the eye and its ancillary parts (muscles, nerves, blood vessels).

sclera
The membranous tissue that covers all of the eyeball (except the cornea); also known as *the white of the eye.*

cornea
Transparent tissue covering the eyeball; responsible for focusing light into the eye and transmitting light.

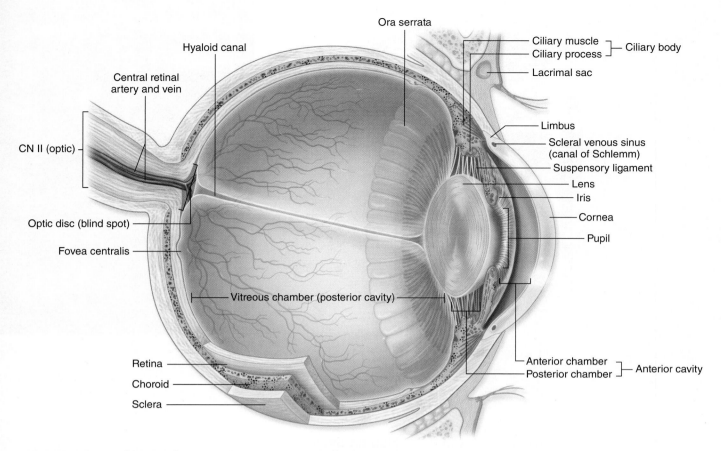

FIGURE 10-2 Orbital Septum (View from the Right Side)

Source: Michael McKinley and Valerie O'Loughlin, HUMAN ANATOMY, 1/e. © 2006 MHE. Figure 19.12b, p. 582

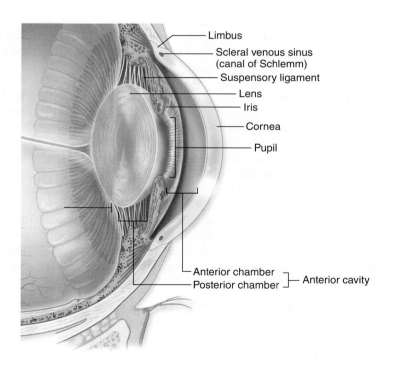

FIGURE 10-3 The Cornea

Source: Michael McKinley and Valerie O'Loughlin, HUMAN ANATOMY, 1/e. © 2006 MHE. Figure 19.12b, p. 582

The posterior (back) surface of the cornea is coated in an aqueous humor that keeps intraocular pressure at a consistent volume and rate of outflow.

The Uveal Tract The **uveal tract** is the middle layer of the eye; it has three sections: the **iris** (in the anterior), followed by the **ciliary body,** and the **choroid** in the posterior. Together, the parts of the uvea improve the contrast of the image created by the retina. The uvea accomplishes this by reducing the light reflected within the eye while absorbing outside light as it is transmitted through the sclera. The uvea is also responsible for providing nutrition to the eye structure and exchanging gases (see Figure 10.4).

When you look into someone's eyes, the **pupil** is the black center and the iris is the colored part: the blue, green, brown, or hazel. The iris is the mechanism that controls the amount of light that enters the eye through the pupil. So, when in bright light, the iris contracts the pupil to reduce the amount of light traveling into the eye, thereby preventing damage internally. In a dark room, the iris will widen the pupil to allow in as much light as possible, to permit the eye to better distinguish objects.

The ciliary body lies from the root of the iris to the ora serrate and creates the aqueous humor. The choroid, the most substantial portion of the uveal tract, contains blood vessels that are connected by the suprachoroid externally on the outside and by Bruch's membrane internally.

uveal tract
The middle layer of the eye, consisting of the iris, ciliary body, and choroid.

iris
The round, pigmented muscular curtain in the eye.

ciliary body
The vascular layer of the eye that lies between the sclera and the crystalline lens.

choroid
The vascular layer of the eye that lies between the retina and the sclera.

pupil
The opening in the center of the iris that permits light to enter and continue on to the lens and retina.

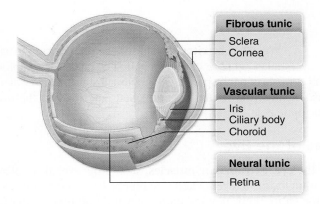

Fibrous tunic
- Sclera
- Cornea

Vascular tunic
- Iris
- Ciliary body
- Choroid

Neural tunic
- Retina

FIGURE 10-4 The Interior of the Eye

Source: Michael McKinley and Valerie O'Loughlin, HUMAN ANATOMY, 1/e. © 2006 MHE. Figure 19.12a, p. 582

retina
A membrane in the back of the eye that is sensitive to light and functions as the sensory end of the optic nerve.

rod
An elongated, cylindrical cell within the retina that is photo-sensitive in low light.

cone
A receptor in the retina that is responsible for light and color.

The Retina The **retina,** the area of the eye that contains nerve endings, is responsible for receiving visual images and forwarding these images to the brain for analysis (see Figure 10.4). The choroid is lightly attached to the retinal pigment epithelium (RPE) and is adjacent to the rods and cones that function as light receptors. The **rods** are located throughout the retina and are responsible for detecting movement so that you can see when something in front of you is moving. There are three types of **cones** that, together, provide designation for up to 150 shades of color: one type of cone reacts to red light, one to blue-violet light, and the third to green light. Isn't it amazing that you can go into a paint store and see 500 different colors, yet the eye can really only interpret up to 150? The eye combines the light wavelengths to enable perception of a multitude of colors.

EXAMPLE

H33.23 Serous retinal detachment, bilateral
H34.812 Central retinal vein occlusion, left eye
H35.061 Retinal vasculitis, right eye

lens
A transparent, crystalline segment of the eye, situated directly behind the pupil, that is responsible for focusing light rays as they enter the eye and travel back to the retina.

accommodation
Adaptation of the eye's lens to adjust for varying focal distances.

The Lens The **lens** of the eye is located at the anterior of the vitreous chamber (see Figure 10.4). The lens is a semipermeable membrane that is transparent, avascular (contains no blood vessels), and biconvex. The lens goes through what's called **accommodation,** which is the process of changing shape to accomplish seeing objects both near and far. To view objects that are close (near vision), the lens reshapes to a spherical body, the pupil contracts, and the eyes converge (come toward the middle). When looking at something at a distance (far vision), the lens flattens out, the eyes straighten, and the pupils dilate (open wider). As individuals get older, the lens gets tired of accommodating and is not as flexible as it used to be. This makes it more likely the lens may get stuck in the near-vision shape, meaning the individual is near-sighted and may need corrective lenses (eyeglasses or contact lenses) to enable him or her to see far away. When somebody is farsighted, the lens gets stuck in the flattened position and the individual will need corrective lenses to see close-up.

EXAMPLE

H27.111 Subluxation of lens, right eye
H27.122 Anterior dislocation of lens, left eye

vitreous chamber
The interior segment of the eye that contains the vitreous body.

The Vitreous Chamber The **vitreous chamber,** also referred to as the *posterior chamber* of the eye, makes up 65% of the eyeball. The chamber establishes the shape of the eyeball and consists of a transparent gelatinous substance (99% water, 1% insoluble protein) that rests against the retina. It is attached anteriorly to the *ora serrate* and posteriorly to the optic disc.

The Muscles of the Eye

extraocular muscles
The muscles that control the eye.

The muscles of the eye, **extraocular muscles,** secure the eyeball in place and control its movement within the orbit (eye socket) (see Figure 10.5). These muscles are the busiest muscles in the entire body, moving more than 100,000 times every day. They are:

- *Inferior rectus muscle:* presses the eyeball downward and adducts and rotates the eyeball laterally (outward).

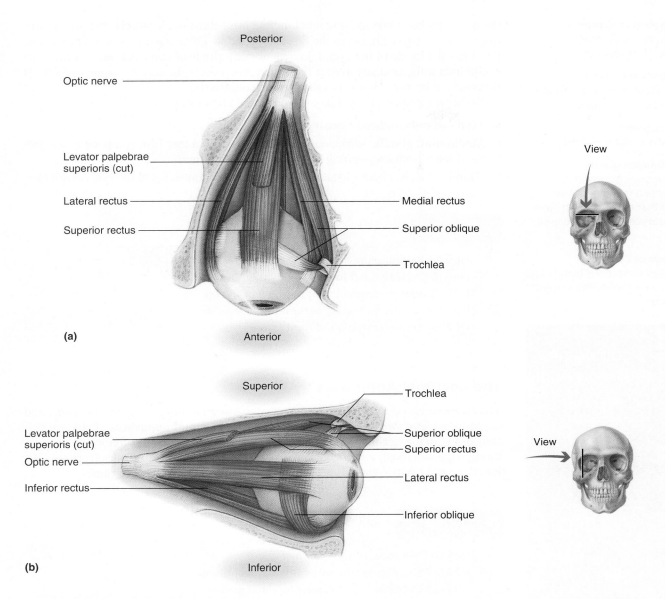

FIGURE 10-5 Extraocular Muscles

Source: Booth et al., MA, 5e. Copyright © 2013 by McGraw-Hill. Figure 35-5, p. 675

- *Superior rectus muscle:* raises the eyeball upward as well as adducts and rotates the eyeball medially (inward).
- *Medial rectus muscle:* also pulls the eye medially (inward).
- *Lateral rectus muscle:* also pulls the eye laterally (outward).
- *Inferior oblique muscle:* turns the eye laterally (outward) and depresses the eye.
- *Superior oblique muscle:* turns the eye medially (inward) and elevates the eye.

The Exterior of the Eye

The **palpebrae** (eyelids) cover the eyeballs to protect them from injury and environmental invaders as well as to maintain the proper level of moisture. Some people think eyelids are made of epidermis, like regular skin; however, they are really composed of connective tissue. The *levator palpebrae muscle superioris* (*levator* = lift; *palpebrae* = eyelids; muscle; *superioris* = above) is responsible for opening and closing

palpebrae
The eyelids.

palpebral conjunctiva
A mucous membrane that lines the palpebrae.

bulbar conjunctiva
A mucous membrane on the surface of the eyeball.

moll's glands
Ordinary sweat glands.

meibomian glands
Sebaceous glands that secrete a tear film component that prevents tears from evaporating so that the area stays moist.

glands of Zeis
Altered sebaceous glands that are connected to the eyelash follicles.

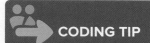

CODING TIP

You may be thinking, "Hey, wait a minute. You just taught us that *palpebrae* is the medical term for eyelid. And yet here in the code description, it says 'eyelid,' the English word." That's very true. However, the reason you need to learn that the term *palpebrae* means eyelid is because when your physician is writing operative notes or procedure notes, he or she may use the term *palpebrae,* and if you're not familiar with that and you don't know what it means, you won't know how to code this.

lacrimal apparatus
A system in the eye that consists of the lacrimal glands, the upper canaliculi, the lower canaliculi, the lacrimal sac, and the nasolacrimal duct

the upper eyelid, while the fascia behind the orbicularis oculi muscle (the orbital septum) creates a barrier between the lids and the orbit. There is a thin mucous membrane that lines the inside of the eyelid, known as the **palpebral conjunctiva;** this lines the eyelid internally, creasing over at the fornix, and covers the surface of the eyeball. At that point, it becomes known as the **bulbar conjunctiva.**

Within the palpebrae (eyelids), there are three types of glands:

- **Moll's glands:** ordinary sweat glands.
- **Meibomian glands:** sebaceous glands that secrete a tear film component that prevents tears from evaporating so that the area stays moist.
- **Glands of Zeis:** altered sebaceous glands that are connected to the eyelash follicles.

EXAMPLE

H00.024 Hordeolum internum left upper eyelid
H00.15 Chalazion left lower eyelid
H01.112 Allergic dermatitis of right lower eyelid
H02.031 Senile entropion of right upper eyelid
H02.131 Senile ectropion of right upper eyelid

The Lacrimal Apparatus

The *lacrimal glands,* the *upper canaliculi,* the *lower canaliculi,* the *lacrimal sac,* and the *nasolacrimal duct* are together known as the **lacrimal apparatus.** Tears are created in the main lacrimal gland and then flow through several excretory ducts, pass through the canaliculi and the lacrimal sac, and continue down the nasolacrimal duct into the nasal cavity—the nose. This is why when you cry, your nose runs.

EXAMPLE

H04.111 Dacryops of right lacrimal gland
H04.122 Dry eye syndrome of left lacrimal gland
H04.133 Lacrimal cyst, bilateral lacrimal glands

Optical System—Related Abbreviations

There are many abbreviations related directly to the optical system that may be used by your health care providers in their documentation. Some of the most common abbreviations are:

OD = right eye
OS = left eye
OU = each eye
ACC = accommodation
PERRLA = pupils equal, round, reactive to light and accommodation
VA = visual acuity
VF = visual field
REM = rapid eye movements
ARMD = age-related macular degeneration

Arnie Rogers, a 9-year-old male, was brought to see Dr. Amatage by his mother because his eyelid was swollen and he was running a fever. Upon examination, edema and erythema (redness) of the right eyelid were observed. Hyperemia of the orbital tissues was also noted, as were matted eyelashes. Arnie admitted pain and stated it was difficult to move his eye. Ophthalmic exam followed by CT scan of the orbital tissues denied a tumor and confirmed preseptal cellulitis. WBC lab test confirmed Streptococcus pneumoniae as the involved pathogen. Dx. Orbital cellulitis, right eye.

Let's Code It!

Dr. Amatage confirmed Arnie's diagnosis of *orbital cellulitis* of the *right eye* caused by *Streptococcus pneumoniae.* Let's begin in the Alphabetic Index, looking up the primary condition, cellulitis:

Cellulitis (diffuse)(phlegmonous)(septic)(suppurative) L03.90

Notice the long list of anatomical sites beneath this listing. See if you can find anything that matches Dr. Amatage's documentation:

Cellulitis (diffuse)(phlegmonous)(septic)(suppurative) L03.90

Orbit, orbital H05.01-

That's great! Let's turn in the Tabular List to begin reading at the three-character code category:

H05 Disorders of orbit

There is an *Excludes1* notation. Read it and determine if this has anything to do with Dr. Amatage's care for Arnie. No, it doesn't—great! So continue reading and review all of the fourth-character options. Which one matches Dr. Amatage's diagnosis of Arnie?

H05.0 Acute inflammation of orbit

Good work! Now review the choices for a fifth and then sixth character. Which do you determine most accurately matches the physician's diagnosis?

H05.011 Cellulitis of right orbit

This is terrific and reports the primary diagnosis. However, it does not tell the entire story about Arnie's condition, does it? You have lab results that identify the pathogen that caused this inflammation as *Streptococcus pneumoniae.* You need to report this detail as well. Turn to the Alphabetic Index to find this suggestion:

Streptococcus, streptococcal—*see also* condition pneumoniae, as cause of disease classified elsewhere B95.3

Remember, you are reporting that the *Streptococcus pneumoniae* caused the orbital cellulitis. Turn to the Tabular List and read the code description thoroughly and completely:

B95.3 Streptococcus pneumoniae as the cause of diseases classified elsewhere

H05.011 Cellulitis of right orbit

B95.3 Streptococcus pneumoniae as the cause of diseases
    classified elsewhere

Good job!

LO 10.2 Diseases of the Optical System

Diseases of the Eyelid, Lacrimal System, and Orbit

blepharitis
Inflammation of the eyelid.

Staphylococcal blepharitis, also known as ulcerative **blepharitis,** is a condition in which the rims of the eyelids become inflamed and appear red. Most often, this condition is chronic and affects bilaterally, as well as simultaneously to the upper and lower lids. In addition to the redness, dry scales and ulcerations may form. Early treatment employing warm compresses along with the use of an antibiotic ophthalmic ointment can be successful.

EXAMPLE

H01.011 Ulcerative blepharitis right upper eyelid

*B95.61 Methicillin susceptible Staphylococcus aureus infection as the cause
    of diseases classified elsewhere

(*When on the job, be certain to check the pathology report to determine if the *Staphylococcus aureus* is methicillin-susceptible, methicillin-resistant, or other.)

dacryocystitis
Lacrimal gland inflammation.

Dacryocystitis is lacrimal gland inflammation (*dacry/o* = lacrimal sac or duct + *cyst* = sac + *itis* = inflammation). This may be caused by a blockage of the tear ducts and can be acute and/or chronic. Research shows that *Staphylococcus aureus*—or, on occasion, beta-hemolytic streptococci—is the pathogen responsible for acute dacryocystitis inflammation, whereas the chronic condition is more often caused by *Streptococcus pneumoniae* or, on occasion, a fungal infection such as *actinomyces* or *Candida albicans.* Constant tearing is the most obvious sign of both the acute and chronic condition. Tenderness and other signs of inflammation may also be evident.

EXAMPLE

H04.321 Acute dacryocystitis of right lacrimal passage
H04.413 Chronic dacryocystitis of bilateral lacrimal passage

proptosis
Bulging out of the eye; also known as *exophthalmos.*

Exophthalmos, also known as **proptosis,** is an abnormal displacement of the eyeball. Most often, ophthalmic Graves' disease is the underlying condition that results in the eyeball bulging outward while the eyelids retract backward, bilaterally. Trauma, such as ethmoid bone fracture, may cause a unilateral diagnosis. Edema, hemorrhage, thrombosis, or varicosities may also cause exophthalmos, either unilaterally or bilaterally.

YOU CODE IT! CASE STUDY

Geneva Randan, a 27-year-old female, came in to Dr. Mosby complaining of swelling, pain, and redness on her left eyelid. She was pretty certain it was a stye, but it was so painful, she had to ask for help. Dr. Mosby examined her and confirmed a diagnosis of hordeolum externum of the left lower eyelid (commonly known as a stye).

You Code It!

Go through the steps of coding, and determine the code or codes that should be reported for this encounter between Dr. Mosby and Geneva.

Step 1: Read the case completely.

Step 2: Abstract the notes: Which key words can you identify relating to why Dr. Mosby cared for Geneva?

_____

Step 3: Query the provider, if necessary.

Step 4: Code the diagnosis or diagnoses.

_____

Step 5: Code the procedure(s): Office visit.

Step 6: Link the procedure codes to at least one diagnosis code to confirm medical necessity.

Step 7: Back code to double-check your choices.

Answer:

Did you determine the correct code to be:

H00.015 Hordeolum externum left lower eyelid

Disorders of the Conjunctiva

Conjunctivitis, commonly known as *pink eye,* actually refers to an inflammation of the conjunctiva of the eye. The most common signs and symptoms include swelling, itching, burning, and redness of the conjunctiva as well as the palpebral conjunctiva (lining of the eyelids).

A pathogen (bacterium or virus), allergic reactions, environmental irritants, a contact lens product, eyedrops, or eye ointments may all be an underlying cause of conjunctivitis. This condition is highly contagious (easily spread from one person to another).

Mucopurulent conjunctivitis is evident by mucus and pus produced by the inflammation, whereas *atopic conjunctivitis* is most often caused by allergies. Yet, be careful:

conjunctivitis
Inflammation of the conjunctiva.

Vernal conjunctivitis is the result of an allergic reaction to seasonal allergens, such as pollen or mold.

EXAMPLE

H10.022 Other mucopurulent conjunctivitis, left eye
H10.211 Acute toxic conjunctivitis, right eye
H10.44 Vernal conjunctivitis

pterygium
A flap of thick-tissue, often triangularly shaped, abnormal growth on the conjunctiva.

A **pterygium** is a pinkish, triangular-shaped growth of tissue on the cornea, yet it is considered to be a disorder of the conjunctiva. This condition is generally unnoticeable unless it becomes inflamed from an invasion of dust and other air pollutants. In cases where the growth interferes with vision, it may be removed surgically. However, this surgery is not often performed because the condition frequently recurs.

Pterygia are more common in sunny climates and among adults aged 20 to 40 years. While unconfirmed scientifically, the condition is believed to be caused by excessive exposure to ultraviolet (UV) light from the sun.

EXAMPLE

H11.023 Central pterygium of eye, bilateral
H11.061 Recurrent pterygium of right eye

LO 10.3 Disorders of the Sclera, Cornea, Iris, and Ciliary Body

keratitis
An inflammation of the cornea, typically accompanied by an ulceration.

Keratitis, an inflammation and ulceration of the cornea, may be instigated by any type of pathogen: bacterium, virus, or fungus. When caused by herpes simplex virus, type 1, the diagnosis is dendritic corneal ulcer (herpesviral keratitis). Typically it is a unilateral condition, and initial signs and symptoms include reduced visual clarity, tearing, photophobia, and varying levels of pain (anywhere from mild discomfort to acute pain). Treatment most often consists of prescription eyedrops or ointment. Lack of treatment might result in irreversible blindness.

EXAMPLE

B00.52 Herpesviral keratitis
H16.111 Macular keratitis, right eye

corneal dystrophy
Growth of abnormal tissue on the cornea, often related to a nutritional deficiency.

Corneal dystrophy occurs when one or more parts of the cornea develop an accumulation of cloudy material, resulting in the loss of normal clarity. There are over 20 varieties of corneal dystrophies, all of which share several characteristics:

• Genetic (inherited).
• Bilateral.
• Not the result of external causes, such as injury or diet.
• Develop gradually.
• Onset limited to a single layer of the cornea, with the disorder spreading later to the others.
• No known manifestations or underlying conditions.

Some of the most common corneal dystrophies include Fuchs' dystrophy (endothelial corneal dystrophy), keratoconus, lattice dystrophy, and map-dot-fingerprint (epithelial corneal) dystrophy.

EXAMPLE

H18.51 Endothelial corneal dystrophy
H18.52 Epithelial (juvenile) corneal dystrophy
H18.54 Lattice corneal dystrophy
H18.612 Keratoconus, stable, left eye

LET'S CODE IT! SCENARIO

Saul Ruben, a 33-year-old male, came in to see Dr. Jadan with complaints of pain in his left eye upon blinking, photophobia, and increased tearing. He has also noticed some blurring. He states he hasn't been able to put his contact lenses in for several days. Dr. Jadan examined Saul, and fluorescein dye dropped into the conjunctival sac stained the outline of the ulcer, the entire outer rim of the cornea. Dr. Jadan diagnosed Saul with a ring corneal ulcer of the left eye.

Let's Code It!

Dr. Jadan diagnosed Saul with a *ring corneal ulcer* of the *left eye*. In the Alphabetic Index, let's look at the main term—*ulcer:*

Ulcer, ulcerated, ulcerating, ulceration, ulcerative

Find the term *cornea* in the long list below. Then, in the list indented beneath *cornea,* determine the most accurate match to Dr. Jadan's notes:

Ulcer, ulcerated, ulcerating, ulceration, ulcerative

Cornea H16.00-

Ring H16.02-

Now to the Tabular List—let's check out the top of the code category:

H16 Keratitis

Are you in the wrong place? Remember that earlier, when you learned about keratitis, you learned it is an inflammation and ulceration of the cornea. Double-check, though, to be certain. Do you see a confirmation that you are in the correct location?

H16.0 Corneal ulcer

Whew! Now review the options for fifth and sixth characters to see if you can determine an accurate code:

H16.022 Ring corneal ulcer, left eye

That matches perfectly!

Disorders of the Lens

cataract
Clouding of the lens or lens capsule of the eye.

A **cataract** is the gradual opacity (clouding) of the lens or lens capsule of the eye, which causes a reduction of vision. Many individuals perceive this to be a condition of the elderly; however, cataracts can occur at any age, including being present at birth. Patients with diabetes mellitus are especially prone to developing cataracts. Complicated cataracts are most often an idiopathic condition, caused by a preexisting condition such as diabetes mellitus or hypoparathyroidism. However, this condition can also be caused by trauma, especially after a foreign body has injured the lens.

Ophthalmoscopy examination, or a slit-lamp exam, can be used to confirm the presence of a cataract by enabling the observation of a dark area in the normally consistent red reflex of the lens. Treatment of a cataract is an outpatient procedure with little to no recovery time. Without treatment, this condition results in blindness—in fact, it is the leading cause of blindness in the United States.

EXAMPLE

H25.11 Age-related nuclear cataract, right eye
H26.012 Infantile and juvenile cortical, lamellar, or zonular cataract, left eye
Q12.0 Congenital cataract

YOU CODE IT! CASE STUDY

Denny Chowe, a 45-year-old male, was tightening the rope holding a load on the bed of his pickup truck when the rope broke suddenly. His fist, clenching the rope, snapped backward, hitting him in the right eye. The pain was difficult for him to deal with, so his friends brought him to the emergency department. After examination, Dr. Emmatt diagnosed Denny with an anterior dislocation of his right eye lens. He was taken up to the procedure room.

You Code It!

Go through the steps of coding, and determine the code or codes that should be reported for this encounter between Dr. Emmatt and Denny Chowe.

Step 1:   Read the case completely.

Step 2:   Abstract the notes: Which key words can you identify relating to why Dr. Emmatt cared for Denny Chowe?

_____

Step 3:   Query the provider, if necessary.

Step 4:   Code the diagnosis or diagnoses.

_____

Step 5:   Code the procedure(s): Emergency department visit.

Step 6:   Link the procedure codes to at least one diagnosis code to confirm medical necessity.

Step 7:   Back code to double-check your choices.

Answer:

Did you determine the correct code to be:

H27.121 Anterior dislocation of lens, right eye

Disorders of the Choroid and Retina

Retinal detachment is the separation of the outer retinal pigment epithelium (RPE) from the neural retina, creating a space immediately beneath the retina. This subretinal space then fills with fluid (liquid vitreous) and obstructs the flow of choroidal blood (which supplies oxygen and nutrients to the retina). Signs and symptoms include floaters (floating black spots) as well as photopsia (recurring flashes of light). Without treatment, a gradual loss of vision, often described as a curtain, will reduce the visual field. Examination with an ophthalmoscope, after full dilation, will show the retina as gray and opaque instead of its normal transparent appearance.

retinal detachment
A break in the connection between the retinal pigment epithelium layer and the neural retina.

EXAMPLE

H33.012 Retinal detachment with single break, left eye
H33.021 Retinal detachment with multiple breaks, right eye
H33.21 Serous retinal detachment, right eye

LO 10.4 Glaucoma

Glaucoma is a malfunction of the fluid pressure within the eye; the pressure rises to a level that can cause damage to the optic disc and nerve. Treatment can successfully prevent blindness or any vision loss from resulting. Glaucoma is essentially categorized as either open angle or closed angle:

glaucoma
The condition that results when poor draining of fluid causes an abnormal increase in pressure within the eye, damaging the optic nerve.

- *Open angle:* a slowly developing, chronic condition that typically has no signs or symptoms until very advanced.
- *Closed angle:* a painful condition with a sudden onset and rapidly progressing vision loss.

The treating physician should include in the documented diagnosis of glaucoma the current stage of development of this condition: mild stage (evidence of changes in the aqueous outflow system of the eye), moderate stage (elevated intraocular pressure), or severe stage (atrophy of the optic nerve and loss of the visual field). For unusual circumstances, there is also an option to report indeterminate stage. This is reported with the seventh character for glaucoma codes.

EXAMPLE

H40.11x3 Primary open-angle glaucoma, severe stage
H40.2221 Chronic angle-closure glaucoma, left eye, mild stage

LO 10.5 Co-morbidities and Underlying Conditions

An ophthalmologist can evaluate patients' health beyond just their vision. An eye exam can reveal signs of diabetes, hypertension, cardiovascular concerns, lupus, multiple sclerosis, and even some malignancies. The reason lies with the fact that, via the

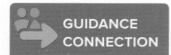

GUIDANCE CONNECTION

Review the ICD-10-CM Coding Guidelines, Section I.A.5, **7th characters,** for more information.

TABLE 10-1 Chronic Conditions among Older Adults with and without Vision Loss

| Condition | Vision Impairment + Co-morbid Condition | | Chronic Conditions for All Aged 65+ | |
	Estimated Population*	%	Estimated Population*	%
Depression				
Mild/Moderate	3,260,000	57.2	14,359,000	43.7
Severe	351,000	6.2	8,323,000	2.5
No Risk	2,087,000	36.6	17,824,000	54.0
Diabetes	1,243,000	22.3	4,928,000	15.2
Hearing Impairment	3,033,000	52.3	12,850,000	38.9
Heart Problems	2,146,000	42.9	10,247,000	31.0
Hypertension	3,468,000	61.0	17,555,000	53.3
Joint Symptoms	3,563,000	69.1	15,936,000	55.7
Stroke	879,000	15.5	2,808,000	8.5

*Rounded to nearest 1,000.

Source: Centers for Disease Control and Prevention, "Vision Loss and Comorbid Conditions," www.cdc.gov/visionhealth/basic_information/vision_loss_comorbidity.htm. Adapted from J. E. Crews, G. C. Jones, and J. H. Kim, "Double Jeopardy: Source: The Effects of Comorbid Conditions among Older People with Vision Loss," *Journal of Visual Impairment and Blindness* 100 (2006), pp. 824–848.

eye, a physician can directly observe arteries and veins without having to perform an invasive procedure. In addition, it can work the other way: There are some chronic conditions that manifest themselves with optical concerns and sometimes vision loss (see Table 10-1).

Diabetic Retinopathy

retinopathy
Degenerative condition of the retina.

Patients diagnosed with diabetes mellitus are at risk for ophthalmic manifestations of their improper glucose levels. Diabetic **retinopathy** is the most common; it is a condition that causes damage to the tiny blood vessels inside the retina (*retina* + *-pathy* = disease). Signs and symptoms include:

- Blurry or double vision.
- Rings around lights.
- Flashing lights.
- Blank spots.
- Dark or floating spots (commonly known as *floaters*).
- Pain in one or both eyes.
- Sensation of pressure in one or both eyes.
- Difficulty in seeing things peripherally (out of the corners of the eyes).
- Macular edema occurs when fluid and protein deposits collect on or beneath the macula (a central area of the retina), resulting in swelling (edema). The swelling then causes the macula to thicken, distorting the person's central vision.

Diabetic retinopathy progresses through four stages of development:

1. Mild nonproliferative retinopathy (microaneurysms).
2. Moderate nonproliferative retinopathy (blockage in some retinal vessels).
3. Severe nonproliferative retinopathy (more vessels are blocked, depriving the retina from blood supply).
4. Proliferative retinopathy (most advanced stage).

When diagnosis and treatment are implemented in the early stages, vision loss can be reduced. Therefore, individuals with diabetes mellitus are encouraged to get regular eye exams. Diabetic retinopathy is one of the leading causes of blindness in U.S. adults, affecting more than 4 million Americans.

EXAMPLE

E10.321 Type 1 diabetes mellitus with mild nonproliferative diabetic retinopathy with macular edema

E11.36 Type 2 diabetes mellitus with diabetic cataract

LO 10.6 Hypertensive Retinopathy

Patients with hypertension (high blood pressure) can develop damage to the retina because of the unusually high pressure of the blood traveling through the vessels. This condition is known as *hypertensive retinopathy*. The higher the pressure and the longer this condition has been ongoing, the more severely the retina may be harmed. Signs and symptoms most evident for those with hypertensive retinopathy include:

- Double vision
- Dimmed vision
- Blindness (vision loss)
- Headaches

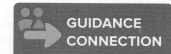

GUIDANCE CONNECTION

Review the ICD-10-CM Coding Guidelines, Section I.C.9, Chapter 9: **Diseases of the circulatory system,** Subsection a(5), **Hypertensive retinopathy,** for more input.

EXAMPLE

H35.031 Hypertensive retinopathy, right eye

H35.032 Hypertensive retinopathy, left eye

Chapter Summary

One of the five senses, vision is involved in virtually every aspect of one's life. This incredible complex organ system captures light and transmits it via interactive anatomical sites to the optic nerve and into the brain for evaluation and interpretation. Even though it is protected by the skull, the optical system is still susceptible to the invasions of pathogens (bacteria, viruses, fungi); can be damaged by trauma; and can be impacted by other environmental issues, such as UV light rays from the sun.

CHAPTER 10 REVIEW
Coding Diseases of the Eye and Adnexa

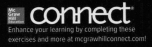

Enhance your learning by completing these
exercises and more at mcgrawhillconnect.com!

Using Terminology

Match each key term to the appropriate definition.

Part One

_____ 1. LO 10.1 A membrane in the back of the eye that is sensitive to light and functions as the sensory end of the optic nerve.

_____ 2. LO 10.1 An elongated, cylindrical cell within the retina that is photosensitive in low light.

_____ 3. LO 10.1 A receptor in the retina that is responsible for light and color.

_____ 4. LO 10.1 The membranous tissue that covers the entire eyeball (except the cornea); also known as *the white of the eye.*

_____ 5. LO 10.1 Transparent tissue covering the eyeball; responsible for focusing light into the eye and transmitting light.

_____ 6. LO 10.1 The vascular layer of the eye that lies between the retina and the sclera.

_____ 7. LO 10.1 A transparent, crystalline segment of the eye, situated directly behind the pupil, that is responsible for focusing light rays as they enter the eye and travel back to the retina.

_____ 8. LO 10.1 The opening in the center of the iris that permits light to enter and continue on to the lens and retina.

_____ 9. LO 10.1 The bony cavity in the skull that houses the eye and its ancillary parts (muscles, nerves, and blood vessels).

_____ 10. LO 10.1 The round, pigmented muscular curtain in the eye.

A. Choroid
B. Cones
C. Cornea
D. Iris
E. Lens
F. Orbit
G. Pupil
H. Retina
I. Rod
J. Sclera

Part Two

_____ 1. LO 10.1 The eyelids.

_____ 2. LO 10.1 Sebaceous glands that secrete a tear film component that prevents tears from evaporating so that the area stays moist.

_____ 3. LO 10.1 The vascular layer of the eye that lies between the sclera and the crystalline lens.

_____ 4. LO 10.1 The interior segment of the eye that contains the vitreous body.

_____ 5. LO 10.1 Altered sebaceous glands that are connected to the eyelash follicles.

_____ 6. LO 10.1 A system in the eye that consists of the lacrimal glands, the upper canaliculi, the lower canaliculi, the lacrimal sac, and the nasolacrimal duct.

_____ 7. LO 10.1 A mucous membrane that lines the palpebrae.

_____ 8. LO 10.1 Adaptation of the eye's lens to adjust for varying focal distances.

_____ 9. LO 10.1 Ordinary sweat glands.

_____ 10. LO 10.1 The muscles that control the eye.

_____ 11. LO 10.1 A mucous membrane on the surface of the eyeball.

_____ 12. LO 10.1 The middle layer of the eye, consisting of the iris, ciliary body, and choroid.

A. Accommodation
B. Bulbar conjunctiva
C. Ciliary body
D. Extraocular muscles
E. Glands of Zeis
F. Lacrimal apparatus
G. Meibomian glands
H. Moll's glands
I. Palpebral conjunctiva
J. Palpebrae
K. Uveal tract
L. Vitreous chamber

Checking Your Understanding

Choose the most appropriate answer for each of the following questions.

1. LO 10.1 All of the following are part of the senses *except*
   a. smell.
   b. taste.
   c. sight.
   d. digestion.

2. LO 10.1 The bony cavity in the skull that houses the eye and its ancillary parts is known as the
   a. orbit.
   b. rods.
   c. retina.
   d. sclera.

3. LO 10.1 The membranous tissue that covers all of the eyeball except the cornea is known as the
   a. rods.
   b. retina.
   c. sclera.
   d. cones.

4. LO 10.1 The transparent tissue covering the eyeball, responsible for focusing light into the eye and transmitting light, is known as the
   a. retina.
   b. cornea.
   c. sclera.
   d. iris.

5. LO 10.1 The round, pigmented muscular curtain in the eye is known as the
   a. retina.
   b. sclera.
   c. cornea.
   d. iris.

6. LO 10.1 The opening in the center of the iris that permits light to enter and continue on to the lens and retina is known as the
   a. iris.
   b. pupil.
   c. rods.
   d. cornea.

7. LO 10.1 A membrane in the back of the eye that is sensitive to the light and functions as the sensory end of the optic nerve is known as the

a. iris.
b. rods.
c. retina.
d. cones.

8. LO 10.1 An elongated, cylindrical cell within the retina that is photosensitive in low light is known as a

a. rod.
b. cone.
c. retina.
d. lens.

9. LO 10.1 A transparent, crystalline segment of the eye, situated directly behind the pupil, that is responsible for focusing light rays as they enter the eye and travel back to the retina is known as the

a. rods.
b. cones.
c. lens.
d. retina.

10. LO 10.1 The muscles that control the eye are known as

a. intraocular.
b. extraocular.
c. palpebrae.
d. vitreous.

Applying Your Knowledge

1. LO 10.1 List the components of the organ that is commonly referred to as the *eye*. _____

   _____

2. LO 10.1/10.2 Explain the impact of visual dysfunction. _____

   _____

3. LO 10.1 What is the function of the sclera? What is another common term for the sclera? _____

   _____

4. LO 10.1 List the five layers that make up the cornea. _____

   _____

5. LO 10.1 What is the function of the pupil? _____

   _____

6. LO 10.1 Explain the difference between rods and cones. _____

   _____

7. LO 10.1 Explain accommodation. _____

   _____

8. LO 10.1 Describe the lacrimal apparatus and its function. _____

   _____

YOU CODE IT! Practice

Chapter 10: Coding Diseases of the Eye and Adnexa

Using the techniques described in this chapter, carefully read through the case studies and determine the most accurate ICD-10-CM code(s) and external cause code(s), if appropriate, for each case study.

1. Bennie Whacker, a 38-year-old female, presents today with a pus-filled lump on her left lower eyelid that is very tender and painful. Dr. Henson diagnoses Bennie with a furuncle of the eyelid.

   _____

2. Randy Bonner, a 33-year-old male, comes in today for his annual physical. Dr. Greene notes Randy's pupils are dilated without cause. Randy is diagnosed with mydriasis.

   _____

3. Jeff Stokes, a 17-year-old male, comes in today complaining of difficulty seeing three-dimensional images. Dr. Rabon diagnoses Jeff with refractive amblyopia, bilaterally.

   _____

4. Jamie Faber, a 9-year-old female, is brought in today by her father. Jamie has cracking and peeling skin around her left eye. Dr. Robert diagnoses Jamie with xeroderma of the left upper eyelid.

   _____

5. Noel Walker, an 8-year-old male, is brought in today by his mother. Noel is complaining that it hurts when he moves his eyes. After testing, Noel is diagnosed with optic papillitis, bilaterally.

   _____

6. Allen Watts, a 29-year-old male, presents today with eye pain and headaches. Dr. Avalon diagnoses Allen with hypopyon, bilaterally.

   _____

7. Sydney Yarborough, a 43-year-old female, comes in today with the complaint of loss of vision in her right eye. After testing, Sydney is diagnosed with intermittent angle-closure glaucoma, right eye.

   _____

8. Stacia Hogue, a 73-year-old female, presents today because she feels like she has a loss of vision in both eyes. Dr. West diagnoses Stacia with age-related (senile) nuclear cataracts, bilaterally.

   _____

9. John Veillette, a 27-year-old male, presents today with the complaint that his left eye feels heavy and he can see sudden flashes of light. John is diagnosed with retinal detachment with a giant retinal tear, left eye.

   _____

10. Felicia Collen, a 27-year-old female, presents today with blurry vision. Dr. Faber diagnoses Felicia with a vitreous hemorrhage.

    _____

11. Harry Pugh, a 7-year-old male, is brought in today because his eyes are very red and watering. Harry is diagnosed with acute mucopurulent folliculae conjunctivitis.

    _____

12. Michelle Adams, a 6-month-old female, presents today with her right eye turning inward. Michelle is diagnosed with convergent monocular esotropia with a V pattern.

    _____

13. Tyheira Knight, a 48-year-old female, comes in today to see Dr. Stevens. Tyheira complains her right lower eyelid is swollen and her eye is sensitive to light. Dr. Stevens diagnoses Tyheira with chalazion of the right lower eyelid.

    _____

14. Donald Arrants, a 3-year-old male, is brought in today by his parents for a well-child checkup. Dr. Bryan notes involuntary eye movement and diagnoses Don with dissociated nystagmus.

    _____

15. Jane Brenan, a 16-year-old female, is brought in by her mother to see Dr. Trainer. Jane has a lump on her right eyelid, and it is tender and red. Dr. Trainer diagnoses Jane with hordeolum externum, right upper eyelid.

    _____

YOU CODE IT! Application
Chapter 10: Coding Diseases of the Eye and Adnexa

The following exercises provide practice in abstracting physicians' notes and learning to work with SOAP notes from our health care facility, *Taylor, Reader, & Associates*. These case studies (SOAP notes) are modeled on real patient encounters. Using the techniques described in this chapter, carefully read through the case studies and determine the most accurate ICD-10-CM code(s) and external cause code(s), if appropriate, for each case study.

TAYLOR, READER, & ASSOCIATES
A Complete Health Care Facility
975 CENTRAL AVENUE • SOMEWHERE, FL 32811 • 407-555-4321

PATIENT: HAGIN, CHARLES
ACCOUNT/EHR #:   HAGICH001
DATE: 10/17/18

Attending Physician: Willard B. Reader, MD

S: Charles is a 6-month-old male brought in by his parents for a well-child examination. No past history for eye problems; he tracks well and reaches for objects. His parents deny any crossing of the eyes when he looks at objects from a distance; however, his mother has a history of a lazy eye, which was surgically corrected.

O: Vital signs are normal for age. His red reflex and corneal light reflex tests are normal. Cover test is negative for strabismus. His extraocular movements appear intact; he is able to follow objects 180 degrees.

A: Normal eye examination

P: Next appointment at 9 months old or earlier prn

Willard B. Reader, MD

WBR/pw   D: 10/17/18 09:50:16   T: 10/19/18 12:55:01

Determine the most accurate ICD-10-CM code(s).

_____

_____

_____

TAYLOR, READER, & ASSOCIATES
A Complete Health Care Facility
975 CENTRAL AVENUE • SOMEWHERE, FL 32811 • 407-555-4321

PATIENT: DeWALT, RONNIE
ACCOUNT/EHR #:   DEWARO001
DATE: 10/17/18

Attending Physician: Suzanne R. Taylor, MD

S: Ronnie presents today with a red, irritated right eye and decreased vision.

O: History of Present Illness: A 74-year-old male presented to our office with a 1-day history of conjunctival injection and mild discomfort in his right eye (OD). He had a known history of pigmentary glaucoma that was treated with a combined procedure of cataract extraction/posterior-chamber intraocular lens (PCIOL) and trabeculectomy with mitomycin C in the right eye five years earlier. His visual acuity had decreased from 20/125 (5 months previously) to 20/250 OD on presentation.

    Past Ocular History: Pigmentary glaucoma (OD), age-related macular degeneration in both eyes (OU), and lattice degeneration (OU). The patient had suffered a severe retinal detachment in the left eye (OS) with very poor residual vision despite treatment with a scleral buckle procedure.
    Medical History: Hypertension, thyroidectomy.
    Medications: Latanoprost OD qhs, Synthroid, and Buspar.
    Family History: Noncontributory.
    Social History: The patient denies alcohol and tobacco use.
    Exam, Ocular:

- Visual acuity, with correction: OD—20/250; OS—Light perception.
- Intraocular pressure: OD—5mmHg.
- External and anterior segment examination, OD: Conjunctival hyperemia with papillary reaction. There were 3+ cells (per high-power field) visible in the anterior chamber with a small (0.75-mm) hypopyon. The right eye had an elevated, thin avascular bleb with a small infiltrate visible within the bleb. The bleb had a positive Seidel test.
- Dilated fundus exam (DFE), OD: 2+ vitreous cell with a hazy view. Visible retina appeared to be normal.

    Course: I performed aqueous and vitreous taps, administered intravitreal vancomycin and ceftazidime, and prescribed hourly topical, fortified gentamycin and vancomycin drops.
    The patient responded well to the combination of intravitreal and topical antibiotics. His visual acuity has returned to baseline, and the bleb leak resolved in 2 months.

A: Bleb-related endophthalmitis

P: Next appointment 2 months or earlier prn

Suzanne R. Taylor, MD

SRT/pw   D: 10/17/18 09:50:16   T: 10/18/18 12:55:01

Determine the most accurate ICD-10-CM code(s).

_____

_____

_____

TAYLOR, READER, & ASSOCIATES
A Complete Health Care Facility
975 CENTRAL AVENUE • SOMEWHERE, FL 32811 • 407-555-4321

PATIENT: WALTERS, JANICE
ACCOUNT/EHR #:   WALTJA001
DATE: 10/17/18

Attending Physician: John S. Warwick, MD

S: Janice is an 8-year-old female brought in to the ER by her parents with moderately severe right-eye pain 6 hours after riding her bicycle through some low hanging leaves from a tree at the nearby public park. She didn't notice the tree branches until a few leaves hit her in the face. She has no bleeding lacerations. I was called in for the ophthalmologic consultation by the attending physician, Dr. Morgan.

O: VS are normal. She does not want to open her right eye because of discomfort. Some anesthetic eyedrops are instilled into her right eye. She complains that it burns a lot, and she begins to cry. After 10 minutes, she is able to open her eye. Her visual acuity was 20/20 in the left eye and 20/30 in the right eye. Her pupils are equal and reactive. Her conjunctiva is slightly infected. No hyphema is visible. A drop of saline is placed on a fluorescein paper strip. This drop is then touched to her lower eyelid so fluorescein dye flows over the surface of her eye. With an ultraviolet light, a 0.5-cm linear abrasion is seen in the lateral aspect of her right cornea.

A: Corneal abrasion

P: Her eye is rinsed with saline to remove excess fluorescein. A single drop of homatropine is instilled into her right eye, and a pressure eye patch is applied. She is instructed to take over-the-counter analgesics for pain.

_____

John S. Warwick, MD

JSW/pw   D: 10/16/18 09:50:16   T: 10/18/18 12:55:01

Determine the most accurate ICD-10-CM code(s).

_____

_____

_____

TAYLOR, READER, & ASSOCIATES
A Complete Health Care Facility
975 CENTRAL AVENUE • SOMEWHERE, FL 32811 • 407-555-4321

PATIENT: BURTON, LONNIE
ACCOUNT/EHR #:   BURTLO001
DATE: 10/17/18

Attending Physician: Willard B. Reader, MD

S: Lonnie is an 80-year-old male who was referred by Dr. Tellmon due to recurrent episodes of blurry vision and hyphema in his left eye. Each episode was associated with high intraocular pressure.

O: Past Medical History: Significant for bilateral cataract extraction and lens implantation 19 years ago.

Exam: His BCVA was 20/20 OU, and pressures were 20 OU. In the left eye, he had 2+ cells, a patent PI, a sulcus PCIOL in the vertical position, an intact posterior capsule, and an area of blood staining between optic and capsule. In the right eye, there was no cell or flare, two patent PIs, and ACIOL in the vertical position, and an open posterior capsule. There was no rubeosis, transillumination defects OU, pseudophakodonesis or pseudoexfoliation OU. Gonioscopy revealed open structures 360 degrees OU with no PAS. A UBM revealed the inferior haptic of the left eye sulcus IOL pressing on the ciliary body/iris junction. The superior haptic was OK.

A: Uveitis-glaucoma-hyphema (UGH) syndrome OS

P: Treatment of UGH syndrome is discussed with patient. He requests time to discuss this with his daughter, who lives in another state. He will return in 1 week.

_____

Willard B. Reader, MD

WBR/pw   D: 10/17/18 09:50:16   T: 10/19/18 12:55:01

Determine the most accurate ICD-10-CM code(s).

_____

_____

_____

TAYLOR, READER, & ASSOCIATES
A Complete Health Care Facility
975 CENTRAL AVENUE • SOMEWHERE, FL 32811 • 407-555-4321

PATIENT: KLINE, JODIE
ACCOUNT/EHR #:   KLINJO001
DATE: 10/17/18

Attending Physician: Suzanne R. Taylor, MD

S: Jodie is a 30-year-old female who has been referred for bilateral macular lesions.

O: History of Present Illness: Patient was found to have bilateral macular lesions on routine examination. She has no visual complaints and denies any history of "night blindness." Her family history is negative for eye diseases.
    Patient Medical History: Healthy.
    Family History: Noncontributory.
    Exam:

- Best corrected visual acuities: 20/25 OD & OS
- Color Vision: normal
- Pupils: normal
- VF: full to CF OU
- EOM: normal
- IOP: normal OU
- SLE: normal

A: Best vitelliform macular dystrophy
P: CNVM.
    Genetic testing.
    Visual potential is usually very good.

_____

Suzanne R. Taylor, MD

SRT/pw   D: 10/17/18 09:50:16   T: 10/18/18 12:55:01

Determine the most accurate ICD-10-CM code(s).

_____

_____

_____

CODING DISEASES OF THE AUDITORY SYSTEM (EARS)

11

Learning Outcomes
After completing this chapter, the student should be able to:

LO 11.1 Identify the components of the auditory system.

LO 11.2 Enumerate the multiple causes of hearing loss.

LO 11.3 Outline the signs and symptoms of hearing loss.

LO 11.4 Recognize the testing implemented to evaluate hearing.

LO 11.5 Correctly report the most common auditory dysfunctions.

LO 11.6 Interpret treatment options of those with hearing loss.

The mechanics of the auditory system—enabling the ability to hear sounds—is not as complex as that of the optical system, but it is important, nonetheless (see Figure 11-1). When an individual suffers from hearing loss or deafness, it can impede the ability to communicate with others.

LO 11.1 The Anatomy of the Ear

External Ear

The part of the ear that is visible on the sides of your head is a segment of the **external ear** (outer ear). The *pinna* (helix) at the top and the *earlobe* (lobule) at the bottom simulate a cupped or conical effect as a way to capture sounds (see Figure 11-2) and funnel them into the ear via the *external auditory canal*. The size and shape of this portion of the auditory system is designed to create an acoustic effect that will enhance the vibrations entering the passageway to the middle ear on their way to the brain.

> ### EXAMPLE
>
> H60.01 Abscess of right external ear
> H60.552 Acute reactive otitis externa, left ear

Middle Ear

The innermost part of the external auditory canal—the beginning of the **middle ear**—is the *tympanic membrane* (the eardrum). As the vibrations (sounds) approach the tympanic membrane, it vibrates. The vibrations pass through the *tympanic cavity* that contains the three bones known collectively as the **ossicles: malleus, incus,** and **stapes.** The stapes vibrates against the oval window portion of the ear to continue the transmission of the vibrations into the inner ear, specifically, the perilymphatic fluid (see Figure 11-2).

Key Terms
Cerumen
Conductive hearing loss
Decibel (dB)
External ear
Incus
Inner ear
Labyrinth
Malleus
Middle ear
Ossicles
Sensorineural hearing loss
Stapes

external ear
The portion of the auditory system that includes the pinna (helix), earlobe, and external auditory canal.

middle ear
A membrane-lined cavity that transmits sound waves from the eardrum to the inner ear.

ossicles
The three small bones within the middle ear: the incus, the malleus, and the stapes.

malleus
The small bone within the middle ear that resembles a hammer and transfers sound waves from the eardrum to the incus.

incus
The small bone within the middle ear that is shaped like an anvil and transfers sound waves from the malleus to the stapes.

stapes
The small bone within the middle ear that is shaped like a stirrup and transmits sound waves from the incus to the inner ear.

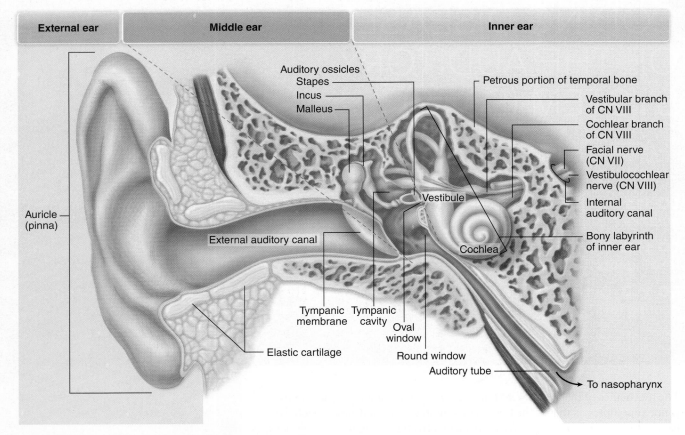

FIGURE 11-1 The Anatomy of the Human Ear

Source: Michael McKinley and Valerie O'Loughlin, HUMAN ANATOMY, 1/e. © 2006 MHE. Figure 19.21, p. 595

inner ear
The innermost and most complex segment of the auditory system; contains the semicircular canals, vestibule, and cochlea and is responsible for transmitting sound to the auditory nerve and maintaining equilibrium.

sensorineural hearing loss
Damage to the nerves that detect sound in the ear; damage may occur by trauma, pathogen, or congenital anomaly.

cerumen
A yellow waxy substance secreted into the ear canal.

conductive hearing loss
A problem in the outer or middle ear that interferes with the passage of sound waves.

labyrinth
A sequence of canals located within the inner ear that is responsible for maintaining equilibrium.

The *auditory tube,* also known as the *eustachian tube,* connects the nasopharynx to the middle ear.

> ## EXAMPLE
>
> H65.04 Acute serous otitis media, recurrent, right ear
> H68.112 Osseous obstruction of Eustachian tube, left ear

Inner Ear

The inner ear has two functions: assistance in the hearing process and maintenance of equilibrium.

To continue the hearing process, the vibrations pass from the stapes of the middle ear into the **inner ear** through the fluid receptor in the *cochlea* that inspires the hair cells of the *organ of Corti* to move. This motion of the hair cells converts into nerve impulses that are sent through the vestibular branch of the acoustic nerve (eighth cranial nerve) to the cerebellum of the brain. Continuous loud noises or music can damage the hair cells and cause permanent **sensorineural hearing loss.** Impacted **cerumen** (earwax), external or middle ear infection (otitis externa or otitis media), or a perforated eardrum may result in **conductive hearing loss**—reduction of hearing due to a malfunction in the external and/or middle ear.

The components of the inner ear, particularly the *vestibule* and the **labyrinth,** are also responsible for sustaining balance and equilibrium via the fluid located in the *semicircular canals (labyrinth).* When the body moves, the fluid moves and activates the nerve cells within these canals (see Figure 11-3).

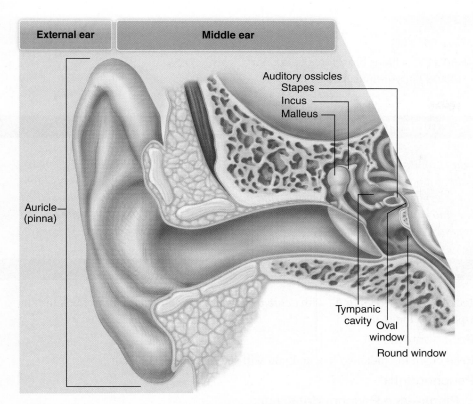

FIGURE 11-2 The External Ear and Middle Ear

Source: Michael McKinley and Valerie O'Loughlin, HUMAN ANATOMY, 1/e. © 2006 MHE. Figure 19.21, p. 595

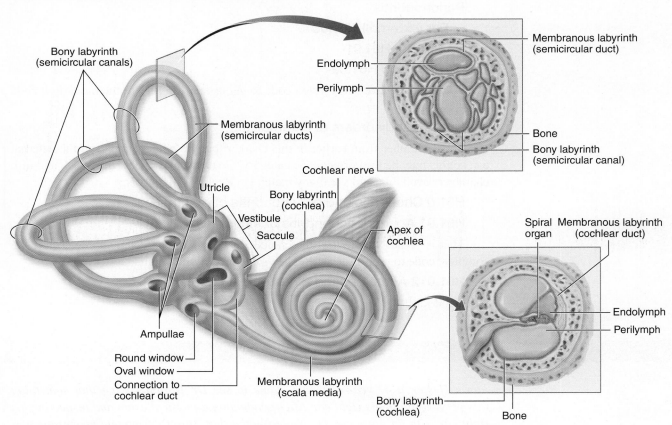

FIGURE 11-3 The Internal Ear

Source: Michael McKinley and Valerie O'Loughlin, HUMAN ANATOMY, 1/e. © 2006 MHE. Figure 19.23, p. 597

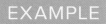
LET'S CODE IT! SCENARIO

Galinda Hamille, a 27-year-old female, was at a club and met a guy doing ear piercings. She got a piercing through the cartilage of her upper left ear. Now, 3 days later, her ear is erythematous (red), swollen, and painful to the touch. Dr. Reckey examined her ear and diagnosed her with acute perichondritis of the left pinna. He prescribed fluoroquinoline with a semisynthetic penicillin and told her to come back in 2 weeks.

Let's Code It!

Dr. Reckey diagnosed Galinda with *acute perichondritis of the left pinna.* Let's turn in the Alphabetic Index to find:

Perichondritis

Read down the indented list, and you will see that *pinna* is listed:

Perichondritis
Pinna—*see* Perichondritis, ear

However, this is giving us a directive not a code to look back up the list to:

Perichondritis
Ear (external) H61.00
Acute H61.01-
Chronic H61.02-

OK, now we have a suggested code to get us started. Turn to the three-digit code category suggested here:

H61 Other disorders of external ear

You remember from earlier in this chapter that the pinna is a part of the external ear, so this may be the correct code category. Go ahead and review the fourth and fifth characters available, and see if any match Dr. Reckey's diagnosis.

H61.0 Chondritis and perichondritis of external ear
H61.01 Acute perichondritis of external ear

That is great. Now review the choices for the sixth character, and determine the complete code to report for Dr. Reckey's encounter with Galinda.

H61.012 Acute perichondritis of left external ear

Good job!

YOU CODE IT! CASE STUDY

Aaron Hester, a 41-year-old male, came to see Dr. Nation feeling that something was very wrong in his right ear. After conducting a physical exam and inspecting his right ear with an otoscope, Dr. Nation noted that Aaron's tympanic membrane was inflamed. Blisters within the middle ear were filled with blood. He drained the blisters, and the culture of the fluid showed that Haemophilus influenzae *was the infectious agent. Dx. Bullous myringitis, right ear.*

You Code It!

Go through the steps of coding, and determine the code or codes that should be reported for this encounter between Dr. Nation and Aaron.

Step 1: Read the case completely.

Step 2: Abstract the notes: Which key words can you identify relating to why Dr. Nation cared for Aaron?

_____

Step 3: Query the provider, if necessary.

Step 4: Code the diagnosis or diagnoses.

_____

Step 5: Code the procedure(s): Office visit.

Step 6: Link the procedure codes to at least one diagnosis code to confirm medical necessity.

Step 7: Back code to double-check your choices.

Answer:

Did you determine the correct code to be:

H73.011 Bullous myringitis, right ear

B96.3 Hemophilus influenza [H. influenza] as the cause of diseases classified elsewhere

Did you remember the second code to report the infectious agent? Good job!

LET'S CODE IT! SCENARIO

Margaret Ionie, a 33-year-old female, was having a terrible time with dizziness. She states that she has also had a problem keeping her balance. A complete examination by Dr. Wallace confirmed a diagnosis of bilateral aural vertigo.

Let's Code It!

Dr. Wallace confirmed a diagnosis of *bilateral aural vertigo*. Turn to the Alphabetic Index and find:

Vertigo R42

Wait. Before you turn to the Tabular List, review the additional terms shown in the indented list.

Vertigo R42

    Aural H81.31-

This matches the diagnosis documented by Dr. Wallace much closer, doesn't it? Let's check this out in the Tabular List, of course, beginning at the code category:

H81 Disorders of vestibular function

Directly below this is an *Excludes1* notation. Do either of these diagnoses relate to Dr. Wallace's notes about Margaret? No. Good. Continue reading to review the available choices for fourth and fifth characters. Did you find:

H81.31 Aural vertigo

Perfect! Just one more thing: Take a look at Dr. Wallace's documentation and determine which ear or ears are affected. Now you can report with confidence that Margaret's diagnosis is:

H81.313 Aural vertigo, bilateral

Good work!

LO 11.2 Diagnosing Hearing Loss

Causes of Hearing Loss

There are several things that might contribute to loss of hearing: genetics and congenital anomalies, pathogens, and external causes that may be traumatic or environmental.

Genetics and Congenital Anomalies Causing Hearing Loss During gestation, some infections, such as rubella, herpes, or toxoplasmosis, are known to possibly cause deafness in the fetus. In addition, congenital anomalies may cause a malformation of any of the ear structures, and there are over 400 genetic conditions that have been identified as causing genetic hearing loss. Most often, these circumstances result in sensorineural hearing loss.

> ### EXAMPLE
>
> P00.2 Newborn (suspected to be) affected by maternal infectious and parasitic diseases
> Q16.5 Congenital malformation of inner ear
> H91.1 Presbycusis
> H93.25 Central auditory processing disorder (Congenital auditory imperception)

Psychogenic (Hysterical) Hearing Loss Sometimes a traumatic event can be so upsetting to an individual that it results in neurologic symptoms that have no organic cause. This is a psychiatric disorder that was formerly called "hysteria."

> ### EXAMPLE
>
> F44.6 Conversion disorder with sensory symptom or deficit (psychogenic deafness)

Idiopathic Causes of Hearing Loss Cerumen (earwax) serves an important function within the ear canal. It protects the skin of the ear canal; protects the middle ear from bacteria, fungi, insects, and water; and enables cleaning and lubrication. However, too much cerumen can build up in the canal and form an obstruction, blocking the entrance of sound waves and causing sudden conductive hearing loss. Recurrent ear infections can result in scarring of the tympanic membrane, reducing its ability to transmit sounds into the middle ear.

EXAMPLE

H61.22 Impacted cerumen, left ear
H91.21 Sudden idiopathic hearing loss, right ear

YOU CODE IT! CASE STUDY

Annette Yertelle, a 39-year-old female, felt something in her ear. She was having problems hearing in her left ear and felt very uncomfortable. When Dr. Eammes asked her, she stated that it felt like something was inside her ear. Upon inspection with the otoscope, Dr. Eammes diagnosed a polyp in her middle ear.

You Code It!

Go through the steps of coding, and determine the code or codes that should be reported for this encounter between Dr. Eammes and Annette.

Step 1: Read the case completely.

Step 2: Abstract the notes: Which key words can you identify relating to why Dr. Eammes cared for Annette?

_____

Step 3: Query the provider, if necessary.

Step 4: Code the diagnosis or diagnoses.

_____

Step 5: Code the procedure(s): Office visit.

Step 6: Link the procedure codes to at least one diagnosis code to confirm medical necessity.

Step 7: Back code to double-check your choices.

Answer:

Did you determine the correct code to be:

H74.42 Polyp of left middle ear

Terrific!

Trauma and External Causes of Hearing Loss The ear is well protected, for the most part, by the skull; however, trauma can still damage it and interfere with the proper transmission of sound. Fireworks set off too close to a person's ear, explosions, and even standing too close to the amplifiers at a rock concert can result in a loss of hearing. A skull fracture might also cause injury to the ear structures or nerves. While you might not have thought about this, some medications and drugs can result in ototoxic hearing loss. Ototoxic medications—including gentamicin (an aminoglycoside antibiotic) and cisplatin and carboplatin (both cancer chemotherapy drugs)—may cause permanent hearing loss. Others—such as aspirin and other salicylate pain relievers, quinine (which is used to treat malaria), and some loop diuretics—are known to result in temporary hearing loss.

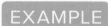

> ### EXAMPLE
>
> H83.3x1 Noise effects on right inner ear
> H91.03 Ototoxic hearing loss, bilateral
> S09.21xA Traumatic rupture of right ear drum

Remember, whenever an external cause is documented, you must include the additional codes to explain how the injury or poisoning occurred.

> ### EXAMPLE
>
> T36.8x5A Adverse effect of other systemic antibiotics, initial encounter
> W36.1xxA Explosion and rupture of aerosol can

GUIDANCE CONNECTION

Review the ICD-10-CM Coding Guidelines, Section I.C.20, Chapter 20: **External causes of morbidity,** for more input.

Sound Levels

Walk down the street and you can hear construction equipment or the siren from a passing ambulance that may cause you to cover your ears to lessen the discomfort. Your neighbor revs his motorcycle as he drives past your house, or you go to the airport to see your parents off on a flight for vacation and you wait as the jet takes off into the sky. What is "loud"? And what is so loud that it could damage your hearing? Take a look at Table 11-1 to see the decibel (dB) levels of some of the sounds of everyday life.

LO 11.3 Signs and Symptoms of Hearing Loss

While each individual will notice loss of hearing in a different way, these are the most common complaints:

- Hearing speech and other sounds as muffled.
- Having difficulty understanding conversations, particularly when in a crowd or in a noisy place (e.g., a restaurant).
- Frequently asking others to speak more slowly, clearly, and loudly.
- Turning up the volume of the television or radio.
- No longer engaging in conversation.
- Avoiding some social settings.

LO 11.4 Diagnostic Testing

Once a patient has become aware of problems with hearing, the physician will often review the complete patient, family, and social history (PFSH) and perform diagnostic testing to determine the issue. Some of the tests are discussed below.

Basic or General Screening Test The physician has the patient cover one ear at a time and evaluates how well spoken words and other sounds at varying volumes are heard.

Tuning Fork Test A tuning fork is a two-pronged, metal instrument that vibrates and produces a sound when struck. A physician can use it to determine some hearing

TABLE 11-1 Common Sounds

Sound	Noise Level (dB)	Effect
Boom cars	145	
Jet engines (near)	140	
Shotgun firing Jet takeoff (100–200 ft)	130	
Rock concerts (varies)	110–140	Threshold of pain begins around 125 dB.
Oxygen torch	121	
Discotheque/boom box Thunderclap (near)	120	Threshold of sensation begins around 120 dB.
Stereos (over 100 watts)	110–125	
Symphony orchestra Power saw (chainsaw) Pneumatic drill/jackhammer	110	Regular exposure to sound over 100 dB for more than 1 minute risks permanent hearing loss.
Snowmobile	105	
Jet flyover (1,000 ft.)	103	
Electric furnace area Garbage truck/cement mixer	100	No more than 15 minutes of unprotected exposure recommended for sounds between 90 and 100 dB.
Farm tractor	98	
Newspaper press	97	
Subway, motorcycle (25 ft)	88	Very annoying.
Lawn mower, food blender Recreational vehicles, TV	85–90 70–90	85 dB is the level at which hearing damage (8 hr) begins.
Diesel truck (40 mph, 50 ft)	84	
Average city traffic Garbage disposal	80	Annoying; interferes with conversation; constant exposure may cause damage.
Washing machine	78	
Dishwasher	75	
Vacuum cleaner, hair dryer	70	Intrusive; interferes with telephone conversation.
Normal conversation	50–65	
Quiet office	50–60	Comfortable hearing levels are under 60 dB.
Refrigerator humming	40	
Whisper	30	Very quiet.
Broadcasting studio	30	
Rustling leaves	20	Just audible.
Normal breathing	10	

Source: Decibel table developed by the National Institute on Deafness and Other Communication Disorders, National Institutes of Health, Bethesda, Maryland 20892. January 1990. Retrieved from https://www.nidcd.nih.gov/health/education/teachers/pages/common_sounds.aspx

loss when caused by damage to the eardrum and/or the ossicles, which are supposed to vibrate with the transmission of sound through the middle ear, or damage to the sensors and/or nerves of the inner ear.

Pure Tone Hearing Tests Most often performed by an audiologist, this test involves sending varying ranges of sounds and tones at multiple volumes to earphones worn by the patient. A chart, known as an *audiogram* (see Figure 11-4a), is used to

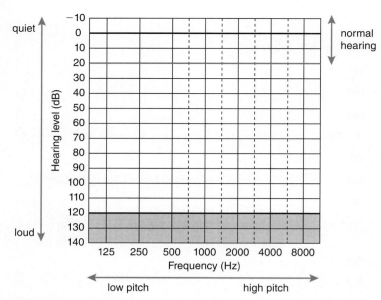

FIGURE 11-4a Audiogram

Source: Harp casenotes. Retrieved from http://en.wikipedia.org/wiki/File:Audio23.jpg

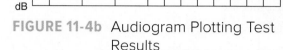

FIGURE 11-4b Audiogram Plotting Test Results

Source: Welleschik. Retrieved from http://en.wikipedia.org/wiki/File:Tonaud_w_norm.jpg

decibel (dB)
Unit of measurement used to determine the intensity, or loudness, of sound.

document the patient's ability to hear sounds at various **decibels (dB).** After the test, the patient's results are charted (see Figure 11-4b).

The results of the audiogram can then be evaluated to determine the level of hearing loss, if any. The audiologist and/or otologist (a physician specializing in treating the ears) will review the audiogram and look at details related to the patient's hearing, including:

Frequency or pitch: measured in hertz (Hz). The frequencies most often used during these tests range from low pitch (left side of the audiogram) to high pitch (right side of the audiogram). The vertical columns on the chart represent the hertz, typically 125, 250, 500, 1,000, 2,000, 4,000, and 8,000 Hz.

Intensity: measured in decibels (dB). This part of the assessment identifies the volume heard—from soft sounds to loud. The horizontal lines of the audiogram track the patient's acknowledged sounds. Audiologists tend to measure volumes from zero dB (soft sounds) up to 120 dB (extremely loud sounds). Hearing loss is classified in degrees of hearing from normal to profound. This determination is evaluated using the standard hearing thresholds—the softest a sound was heard at a specific frequency (see Table 11-2).

Laterality: Naturally, each ear is assessed separately. When bilateral headphones are used during the test, the industry norm is to identify the results of the right ear with a circle or triangle and the left ear's results with the letter "x" or a square.

TABLE 11-2 Degrees of Hearing Loss

Indication of Hearing Loss	Hearing Threshold (dB)
Normal hearing	0–20
Mild hearing loss	21–40
Moderate hearing loss	41–55
Moderately severe hearing loss	56–70
Severe hearing loss	71–90
Profound hearing loss	91 and above

Source: http://www.hopkinsmedicine.org/hearing/hearing_testing/understanding_audiogram.html

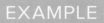

EXAMPLE

Z01.10 Encounter for examination of ears and hearing without abnormal findings
Z13.5 Encounter for screening for eye and ear disorders

LO 11.5 Most Common Auditory Dysfunctions

Otitis media is the inflammation of the middle ear. There are various types of this condition: suppurative and nonsuppurative, acute and chronic. While otitis media is common in children, it is not exclusively a childhood condition. Interestingly, the cases of this diagnosis increase during the winter, while there is an increase of otitis externa (inflammation of the external ear) in the summer. A lack of treatment for otitis media can result in a perforation of the tympanic membrane. Antibiotic therapy is the first-line standard of care. ICD-10-CM code category H66, Suppurative and unspecified otitis media, requires additional characters to report details including acute or chronic, suppurative or nonsuppurative, and with or without rupture of the eardrum, as well as laterality.

Endolymphatic hydrops (Ménière's disease) is a dysfunction of the labyrinth (semi-circular canals). Signs and symptoms include vertigo, sensorineural hearing loss, and tinnitus. A feeling of fullness within the ear is not uncommon. Pharmaceutical treatment with atropine, diphenhydramine, meclizine, or diazepam is the standard of care and will depend upon the frequency and severity of attacks. Report this diagnosis with ICD-10-CM code H81.0, Ménière's disease, with an additional character to identify laterality.

Otosclerosis is a condition of increasing growth of spongy bone in the otic capsule. This growth interferes with the travel of sound vibrations from the tympanic membrane to the cochlea, causing a progressive deterioration of hearing. This condition is seen most frequently in adults between the ages of 18 and 35, and it is more prevalent in females. Report this condition with ICD-10-CM code category H80, Otosclerosis, with additional characters to identify the specific location within the ear as well as laterality. Treatment may include a stapedectomy—excision of the stapes.

Tumors of the ear canal include osteomas and sebaceous cysts and can grow large enough to interfere with hearing. Should the growth become infected, the patient may develop a fever and other signs of inflammation, including pain. While these tumors rarely become malignant, pain might indicate a malignancy. Examination with an otoscope can typically confirm this diagnosis, although a biopsy would be required to confirm benign or malignant status.

EXAMPLE

C30.1 Malignant neoplasm of middle ear (malignant neoplasm of inner ear)
C44.212 Basal cell carcinoma of skin of right ear and external auricular canal
D14.0 Benign neoplasm of middle ear, nasal cavity and accessory sinuses
D23.22 Other benign neoplasm of skin of left ear and external auricular canal

LO 11.6 Treatment Options

A cochlear implant is a small, complex electronic device that can help to provide a sense of sound. The implant consists of two parts:

- A microphone, sound processor, and transmitter are placed behind the ear, externally.
- A receiver is surgically implanted, with an electrode system containing electronic circuits, near the auditory nerve that passes along the received signals to the brain. (see Figure 11-5).

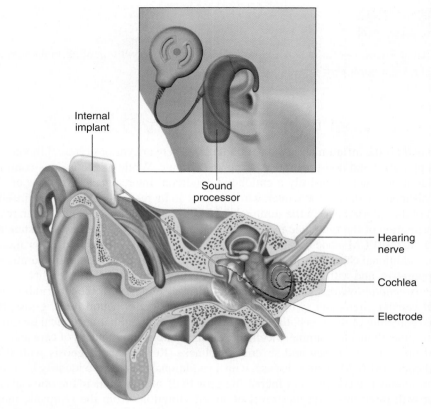

Internal
implant

Sound
processor

Hearing
nerve

Cochlea

Electrode

FIGURE 11-5 Cochlear Implant

While this process simulates natural hearing, in a fashion, it is not exactly the same. Not all patients can be helped with a cochlear implant. A physician will make this determination based on some of these qualifications:

- Severe to profound bilateral sensorineural hearing loss.
- A functional auditory nerve.
- Hearing loss of approximately 70 decibels or more for at least a short time.
- Strong speech, language, and communication skills (infants and young children with a family willing to work toward speech and language skills with therapy).
- Insufficient benefit from other kinds of hearing aids.
- No medical contraindications for surgery.
- Realistic expectations about results.
- Support of family and friends.
- Post-cochlear-implant aural rehabilitation resources in place.

Chapter Summary

The auditory (hearing) system enables the human body to hear—one of only two senses that have their own organ systems. The auditory system passes along sound vibrations captured by the external ear, through the middle ear and the inner ear, to the cerebellum for interpretation.

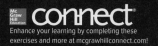
Enhance your learning by completing these
exercises and more at mcgrawhillconnect.com!

Using Terminology

Match each key term to the appropriate definition.

_____ **1.** LO 11.1 The small bone within the middle ear that is shaped like a stirrup and transmits sound waves from the incus to the inner ear.

_____ **2.** LO 11.1 The most complex segment of the auditory system; contains the semicircular canals, vestibule, and cochlea.

_____ **3.** LO 11.1 The small bone within the middle ear that is shaped like an anvil and transfers sound waves from the malleus to the stapes.

_____ **4.** LO 11.1 A problem in the outer or middle ear that interferes with the passage of sound waves.

_____ **5.** LO 11.1 The small bone within the middle ear that resembles a hammer and transfers sound waves from the eardrum to the incus.

_____ **6.** LO 11.1 The three small bones within the middle ear: the incus, the malleus, and the stapes.

_____ **7.** LO 11.1 The portion of the auditory system that includes the pinna (helix), earlobe, and external auditory canal.

_____ **8.** LO 11.1 A membrane-lined cavity that transmits sound waves from the eardrum to the inner ear.

_____ **9.** LO 11.1 Damage to the nerves that detect sound in the ear; damage may occur by trauma, pathogen, or congenital anomaly.

_____ **10.** LO 11.1 A yellow waxy substance secreted into the ear canal.

A. Cerumen
B. Conductive hearing loss
C. External ear
D. Incus
E. Inner ear
F. Malleus
G. Middle ear
H. Ossicles
I. Sensorineural hearing loss
J. Stapes

Checking Your Understanding

Choose the most appropriate answer for each of the following questions.

1. LO 11.1 All of the following are part of the external ear *except*

  a. pinna.
  b. earlobe.
  c. incus.
  d. external auditory canal.

2. LO 11.1 What is the collective term for the incus, malleus, and stapes?

  a. hammer.
  b. ossicles.
  c. helix.
  d. anvil.

3. LO 11.1 The malleus in the middle ear resembles a(n)

  a. anvil.
  b. stirrup.
  c. pinna.
  d. hammer.

4. LO 11.1 The auditory tube is also known as the

   a. eustachian tube.
   b. tympanic tube.
   c. external ear tube.
   d. sensorineural tube.

5. LO 11.1 A problem in the outer or middle ear that interferes with the passage of sound waves is known as

   a. inner ear hearing loss.
   b. conductive hearing loss.
   c. sensorineural hearing loss.
   d. organ of Corti hearing loss.

6. LO 11.2 Which of the following could cause permanent hearing loss?

   a. listening regularly to a music CD at 65 dB.
   b. regularly vacuuming the house at 70 dB.
   c. regularly hearing jet engines for more than 1 minute at 140 dB.
   d. regular office noise at 55 dB.

7. LO 11.1 A yellow waxy substance secreted into the ear canal is known as

   a. organ of Corti.
   b. stapes.
   c. aural.
   d. cerumen.

8. LO 11.3 Which of the following would be a sign of hearing loss?

   a. enjoying social settings.
   b. having difficulty understanding conversation.
   c. speaking clearly.
   d. watching TV at 60 dB.

9. LO 11.4 The hearing threshold for moderately severe hearing loss is

   a. 20 dB and below.
   b. 41 to 55 dB.
   c. 56 to 70 db.
   d. 91 dB and above.

10. LO 11.5 Auditory dysfunction of the labyrinth is known as

   a. otitis media.
   b. endolymphatic hydrops.
   c. otosclerosis.
   d. tumors of the ear canal.

Applying Your Knowledge

1. LO 11.1 List the components of the external ear. _____

_____

2. LO 11.1 Explain the function of the middle ear. _____

_____

3. LO 11.1 List the three small bones within the middle ear. _____

_____

4. LO 11.1 Explain the function of the inner ear. _____

_____

5. LO 11.4 List three diagnostic tests for hearing problems. _____

_____

6. LO 11.3 List four signs of hearing loss. _____

_____

7. LO 11.4 Explain an audiogram, who administers it, and what it is testing. _____

_____

Using the techniques described in this chapter, carefully read through the case studies and determine the most accurate ICD-10-CM code(s) and external cause code(s), if appropriate, for each case study.

1. Paul Younkins, a 29-year-old male, comes in today to see Dr. Evans. Paul complains of dizziness and hearing difficulty. After a thorough examination, Dr. Evans diagnoses Paul with a right labyrinthine fistula.

   _____

2. Janice Walker, a 31-year-old female, presents today with a discharge from her right ear and admits to some hearing loss. After an examination, Dr. Anderson diagnoses Janice with external ear cholesteatoma.

   _____

3. Michael Pomeroy, a 34-year-old male, presents today with the complaint of clicks or cracking sounds in his head. Dr. Burgess can hear an audible bruit from Michael's right ear. Michael is diagnosed with objective tinnitus.

   _____

4. Gee Gee Eller, a 43-year-old female, presents today complaining of hearing loss in her right ear. She fell and hit her head yesterday afternoon. After a thorough examination, Dr. Hogue diagnoses Gee Gee with acquired stenosis of the external ear canal secondary to trauma.

   _____

5. Ernest Polk, a 63-year-old male, presents today complaining of ringing in his ears. Ernest admits to sensitivity to noises and pressure in both ears. Ernest is diagnosed with Ménière's disease, bilaterally.

   _____

6. Steve Jordan, a 15-year-old male, is brought in today by his father. Steve has been complaining that he is having a hard time hearing at school. He has also had several ear infections lately. Dr. Chatterley diagnoses Steve with bilateral surfer's ear (exostosis of the external ear canal).

   _____

7. Kitty Bowman, a 6-year-old female, is brought in today by her parents. Kitty has an earache. After a thorough examination, Kitty is diagnosed with acute nonsuppurative serous otitis media.

   _____

8. Kenny Hope, a 31-year-old male, presents today with left ear pain. Kenny is diagnosed with chronic seromucinous otitis media.

_____

9. Peggy Lewis, a 4-year-old female, is brought in today by her mother. Peggy has an earache in both ears. This is Peggy's third ear infection in 8 months. Dr. Lee diagnoses Peggy with acute serous otitis media, bilateral, recurrent.

_____

10. Elijah Maple, a 28-year-old male, presents today with a bad right earache. After a thorough examination Dr. Levan diagnoses Elijah with chronic tubotympanic suppurative otitis media with central perforation of the tympanic membrane.

_____

11. Dorothy McDonald, a 48-year-old female, comes in today to see Dr. Park with the complaint of swelling behind her left ear. She admits to the area being tender, and she has some headaches. Dr. Park diagnoses Dorothy with acute mastoiditis.

_____

12. Kimberly Pierson, a 7-year-old female, is brought in today by her parents to see Dr. Phillips. Kimberly had the mumps last year and has been having difficulty with her hearing in her left ear. Dr. Phillips performs a Weber test and diagnoses Kimberly with sensorineural deafness, unilateral.

_____

13. Keith Rabon, a 28-year-old male, comes in today with the complaint of hearing loss in his left ear. Dr. Jeffords examines his left ear canal, which was found to be completely occluded with cerumen. Dr. Jeffords diagnoses Keith with a cerumen impaction.

_____

14. Lisa Williams, a 72-year-old female, comes in today with the complaint of hearing difficulty. Lisa admits that it is becoming harder to follow conversations, and she needs to turn the volume up when she is watching television. Dr. Zeigler diagnoses Lisa with presbycusis, bilaterally.

_____

15. Tommy Hanson, a 12-year-old male, is brought in by his mother because Tommy is complaining that his left ear hurts and he won't let her touch his ear due to the discomfort. Tommy is diagnosed with external ear cellulitis.

_____

The following exercises provide practice in abstracting physicians' notes and learning to work with SOAP notes from our health care facility, *Taylor, Reader, & Associates*. These case studies (SOAP notes) are modeled on real patient encounters. Using the techniques described in this chapter, carefully read through the case studies and determine the most accurate ICD-10-CM code(s) and external cause code(s), if appropriate, for each case study.

TAYLOR, READER, & ASSOCIATES
A Complete Health Care Facility
975 CENTRAL AVENUE • SOMEWHERE, FL 32811 • 407-555-4321

PATIENT: UNGER, REBECCA
ACCOUNT/EHR #:   UNGERE001
DATE: 10/16/18

Attending Physician: Suzanne R. Taylor, MD

S: Rebecca Unger, a 65-year-old woman, presented with a 3-year history of progressive hearing loss in the right ear. She had no prior history of ear infections or ear surgery. She denied any vertigo or dizziness. She had no family history of hearing loss. She denied any pain, numbness, or weakness. She had no significant medical history and no history of significant sun exposure or head and neck malignancies.

O: Upon examination, her right ear canal was completely occluded with skin debris not consistent with simple cerumen. Attempts at removing the debris in the office were limited by the patient's severe discomfort.

   The audiogram showed a maximum conductive hearing loss on the right and normal hearing on the left.

   Imaging included a CT scan that showed only opacification of the external ear canal with no evidence for bone erosion.

   The patient was taken to the operating room, at which time the debris was again visualized to be flaky and keratinaceous. A portion of this was traced back to the anterior portion of the cartilaginous ear canal, where it appeared to be adherent to the skin. There were no areas of ulceration or granulation tissue. This lesion was removed en block and sent to frozen pathology, at which time no carcinoma was identified. There was some irregular-appearing tissue along the tympanic membrane, and for this reason this was also removed and sent with the specimen. The patient underwent a tympanoplasty without any complications.

   Final pathology, however, revealed squamous cell carcinoma. The patient was then taken for a lateral temporal bone resection and external ear canal closure.

A: Squamous cell carcinoma of the external ear canal, right

P: Will continue to follow patient closely

Suzanne R. Taylor, MD

SRT/pw   D: 10/16/18 09:50:16   T: 10/18/18 12:55:01

Determine the most accurate ICD-10-CM code(s).

_____

_____

_____

TAYLOR, READER, & ASSOCIATES
A Complete Health Care Facility
975 CENTRAL AVENUE • SOMEWHERE, FL 32811 • 407-555-4321

PATIENT: COMPANO, DARREN
ACCOUNT/EHR #:   COMPDA001
DATE: 10/16/18

Attending Physician: Suzanne R. Taylor, MD

S: Darren Compano, a 9-year-old male, is brought in today by his parents. Darren is complaining that his right ear hurts and is throbbing. Darren seems to be in moderate discomfort.

O: VS normal.
    Past medical history: noncontributory.
    Review of systems: negative.
    Ear exam: Left ear is within normal range. Right ear pinna, antihelix: a lump is noted, swollen and inflamed. It appears to be a localized collection of blood. Dr. Taylor evacuates the blood from the area and applies a pressure bandage.

A: Auricle hematoma

P: Rx: antibiotics
    Return appointment in 10 to 14 days to check skin and cartilage reconnection.

_____

Suzanne R. Taylor, MD

SRT/pw   D: 10/16/18 09:50:16   T: 10/18/18 12:55:01

Determine the most accurate ICD-10-CM code(s).

_____

_____

_____

TAYLOR, READER, & ASSOCIATES
A Complete Health Care Facility
975 CENTRAL AVENUE • SOMEWHERE, FL 32811 • 407-555-4321

PATIENT: MILLER, TYRELL
ACCOUNT/EHR #:   MILLTY001
DATE: 10/16/18

Attending Physician: John S. Warwick, MD

S: Tyrell Miller, a 51-year-old male, first presented to the office 12 years ago with a recurrent left-sided cholesteatoma for which he had previously undergone five separate surgeries, including a mastoidectomy. By the time he was first seen in our office, he had a left-sided complete facial paralysis (6/6 House Brackmann scale) and a severe-to-profound sensorineural hearing loss.

O: Over the subsequent 10 years, he underwent three different skull base surgeries (most recently in 2013) for recurrent left-sided cholesteatoma using a combination of transcochlear, translabyrinthine, and infralabyrinthine approaches. He had extensive cholesteatoma adherent to the dura, internal carotid artery, jugular bulb, facial nerve, and eroding through the otic capsule, necessitating closure of his external auditory canal. He was routinely followed with imaging, and subsequent procedures were done based on his symptoms and growth of the cholesteatoma on imaging. His facial movement never returned, and reconstructive options were discussed over the course of his care.

   The patient continued to be bothered by his complete left-sided facial paralysis. EMG testing confirmed nonfunctional motor end plates. After a detailed discussion of the different reconstructive options, the patient underwent a left hypoglossal facial nerve anastomosis, sural nerve graft, and tensor fascia lata sling to reconstruct the left side of his face in January 2014. This procedure involved connecting part of the 12th cranial nerve to the facial nerve stump via a cable graft nerve, which was the sural nerve in this patient's case. I also harvested the fascia overlying the thigh muscle to pull up the sagging side of his left lower face. The goal of the surgery was to restore facial tone and ultimately symmetry to his face. He was discharged home several days after the operation. He had some left lower leg paresthesias from the sural nerve donor site, which resolved over the following 2 months.

A: Cholesteatoma, recurrent

P: Will keep patient under close observation and monitoring with periodic CT scans given the adherence of the cholesteatoma to critical structures.

_____

John S. Warwick, MD

JSW/pw   D: 10/16/18 09:50:16   T: 10/18/18 12:55:01

Determine the most accurate ICD-10-CM code(s).

_____

_____

_____

TAYLOR, READER, & ASSOCIATES
A Complete Health Care Facility
975 CENTRAL AVENUE • SOMEWHERE, FL 32811 • 407-555-4321

PATIENT: CARDOSA, LAWRENCE
ACCOUNT/EHR #:   CARDLA001
DATE: 8/16/18

Attending Physician: Willard B. Reader, MD

S: Lawrence Cardosa, a 6-year-old boy, is accompanied to the office by his dad. He is in distress, holding his ear and crying intermittently. Dad states that Larry has been complaining of pain in his ear for 3 days and yesterday complained that the pain was worse with movement of his ear or when he is eating. He has noted no discharge from the ear, and he has not been running a fever.

    Patient has been spending the summer at a local day camp, swimming in the pool every day and playing T-ball. Dad recalls no exposure to ticks or poison ivy/oak. There is a cat at home, which has been present since Larry was an infant. His appetite is good and he is normally "very energetic." Both parents are smokers.

O: Past medical history: Normal childhood development. History of frequent middle ear infections as well as exertional asthma. History of mild seasonal allergies.

    Medications: Occasional oral antibiotic for otitis media in the past year and intermittent use of an asthma inhaler. Dad stated that Mom has been giving Larry baby aspirin for the past few days for pain relief.
    Physical examination: Afebrile fit young boy in obvious distress.
    Ears: Canal is red and swollen. No fluid or discharge noted. On visual exam, no pus or debris is present in the canal. Eardrum appears intact.

A: Swimmer's ear, bilateral

P: Recommended Burow's solution.
    Instructed patient to refrain from swimming or washing hair for a few days.

_____

Willard B. Reader, MD

WBR/pw   D: 8/16/18 09:50:16   T: 8/18/18 12:55:01

Determine the most accurate ICD-10-CM code(s).

_____

_____

_____

TAYLOR, READER, & ASSOCIATES
A Complete Health Care Facility
975 CENTRAL AVENUE • SOMEWHERE, FL 32811 • 407-555-4321

PATIENT: MYERS, JENNIFER
ACCOUNT/EHR #:   MYERJE001
DATE: 10/16/18

Attending Physician: John S. Warwick, MD

S: Jennifer Myers, a 46-year-old female, presents today with fever and ear pain.

O: T 100.5, BP 142/85, R 20, P 80. Pupils are equal, round, and reactive. Oxygen saturation is 98%.
Dr. Warwick documents Jennifer is in obvious discomfort. She admits to a pain level of 4 on a scale
of 0–10. Dr. Warwick notes discharge from Jennifer's left ear.

    Past medical history: noncontributory.
    Review of systems: negative.
    Medications: none.

A: Acute suppurative otitis media, attic perforation of the tympanic membrane

P: Rx: AMOX, ibuprofen
    Follow up with patient in 10 days.

John S. Warwick, MD

JSW/pw   D: 10/16/18 09:50:16   T: 10/18/18 12:55:01

Determine the most accurate ICD-10-CM code(s).

_____

_____

_____

CODING CIRCULATORY CONDITIONS

12

Learning Outcomes   *After completing this chapter, the student should be able to:*

LO 12.1 Name the components of the circulatory system.

LO 12.2 Discern the included signs and symptoms of cardiovascular disease.

LO 12.3 Interpret the difference between elevated blood pressure and hypertension.

LO 12.4 Accurately code the known manifestations of hypertension.

LO 12.5 Apply the guidelines correctly to code the sequelae of CVA.

LO 12.6 Code the sequela of cerebrovascular disease accurately.

The circulatory (cardiovascular) system (Figure 12-1) includes the heart, arteries, and veins and has the job of circulating blood to carry oxygen to cells throughout the body and waste products away from those cells. This network touches and affects every area of the body, from hair and tissues to organ function.

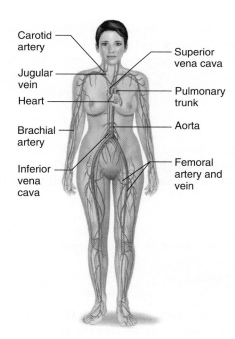

FIGURE 12-1 The Cardiovascular System

Source: Booth et al., MA, 5e. Copyright © 2013 by McGraw-Hill. Figure 22-6b, p. 479

Key Terms

Angina pectoris

Atherosclerosis

Atrium

Cerebral infarction

Cerebrovascular accident (CVA)

Edema

Elevated blood pressure

Embolus

Gestational hypertension

Hypertension

Hypotension

Infarction

Myocardial infarction

NSTEMI

Secondary hypertension

STEMI

Thrombus

Vascular

Ventricle

LO 12.1 Circulatory System Anatomy

The center of your body, and some say the center of the soul, is the heart. Like the engine in a car, this small organ promotes nourishment to all components, from your head to your toes, as it pumps oxygen-rich blood through your arteries to every cell in the body. After utilizing the oxygen brought by the arteries, your cells discard carbon dioxide that is carried by your veins back up to the heart so your respiratory system can eventually expel this gas. Of course, your cardiovascular system is not this simple, as you will learn in this chapter. This simplistic overview is used to illustrate the extensive span of this system.

As mentioned in the introduction, the cardiovascular system is composed of the heart and blood vessels (arteries and veins) that lead to and from the heart. The average adult has about 11 pints (approximately 5.5 liters) of blood in his or her system. Together, the components of the cardiovascular system will pump these 11 pints through the body every minute.

The Heart

The heart beats approximately once every second (60 beats per minute). Each beat is a compression—the heart contracting to force blood through it and out through the aorta to travel through the body delivering oxygen (see Figure 12-2). Let's investigate this in detail, from the beginning.

The heart is divided into four chambers:

atrium
A chamber that is located in the top half of the heart and receives blood.

- Right **atrium**
- Left atrium

The two atria (plural of *atrium*) are located in the top half of the heart. These thinly walled empty chambers fill with blood that is returning to the heart. The cardiac septum, specifically the atrial septum, lies between the right and left atria.

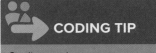

CODING TIP

Cardiovascular:
cardio = heart +
-vascular = vessels (veins and arteries).

EXAMPLE

I23.6 Thrombosis of atrium, auricular appendage, and ventricle as current complications following acute myocardial infarction

I23.1 Atrial septal defect as current complication following acute myocardial infarction

ventricle
A chamber that is located in the bottom half of the heart and receives blood from the atrium.

- Right **ventricle**
- Left ventricle

The two ventricles are located in the bottom half of the heart. The blood passes from the atrium through a valve into the ventricle. The cardiac septum, specifically the ventricular septum, lies between the right and left ventricles.

EXAMPLE

I23.2 Ventricular septal defect as current complication following acute myocardial infarction

I49.01 Ventricular fibrillation

Between each of these chambers, and between the chambers and the vessels that carry blood away from the heart, are valves (see Figure 12-3). Like doors, these valves open to permit blood to flow out, and then they close to prevent any backflow of blood. The *chordae tendineae* connect the *mitral valve* and the *tricuspid valve* to the floor of the ventricles to secure their positions. The *pulmonary valve* and the *aortic valve* function in the same manner as double doors—opening in the center and closing again to prevent backflow into the ventricles.

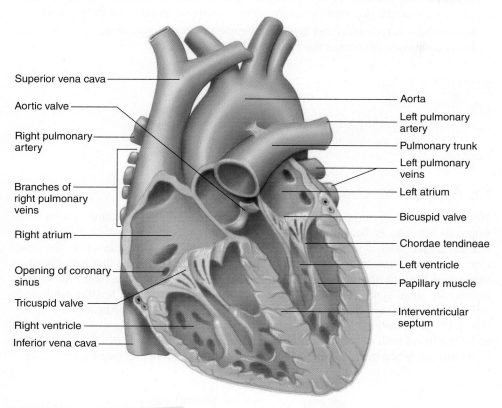

FIGURE 12-2 The Heart

Source: David Shier et al., HOLE'S HUMAN ANATOMY & PHYSIOLOGY, 12/e. © 2010 MHE. Figure 15.6b, p. 558

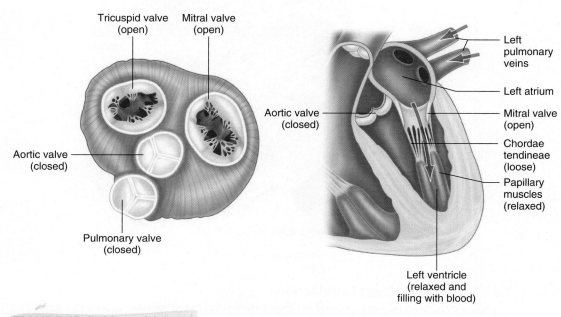

FIGURE 12-3 Heart Valves

The heart is wrapped and protected by the *pericardium,* a fluid-filled sac, consisting of three layers:

- *Endocardium* is the innermost layer, constructed of epithelium and connective tissues. Specialized cardiac muscle fibers known as *Purkinje fibers* are contained in the interior ventricular walls, just below the endocardium.
- *Myocardium,* the middle layer, is thick and is made of cardiac muscle tissue. It provides strength to power the contractions that move blood through the heart.
- *Epicardium* is the outermost layer, constructed of serous membrane to protect the heart and lessen friction as the heart moves with each beat.

EXAMPLE

I40.0 Infective myocarditis [infection of the myocardium]
I33.0 Acute and subacute infective endocarditis

Conduction Mechanisms

How does the heart make itself beat (contract)? The cardiac conduction system feeds impulses into the myocardium by way of special cardiac muscle tissue fibers. The sinoatrial (SA) node is situated right below the epicardium, at the site where the superior vena cava connects to the right atrium. The cells of this node instigate impulses that travel through the myocardium and incite the cardiac muscle fibers to contract around the atrial syncytium surrounding the right and left atria. A healthy adult node will send 70 to 80 impulses a minute and sets the pace for the heartbeat (the contractions). For this reason, it is known as the *pacemaker.* This is the natural pacemaker, not to be confused with a mechanical device, also called a "pacemaker," that is designed to do this job when the SA node is unable to perform consistently (see Figure 12-4).

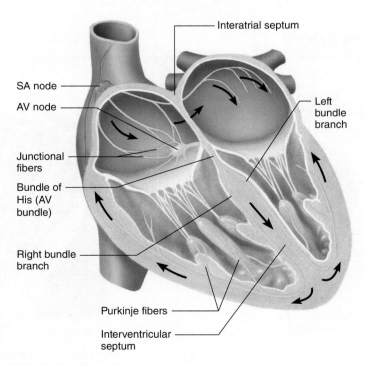

FIGURE 12-4 Heart Conduction

Source: David Shier et al., HOLE'S HUMAN ANATOMY & PHYSIOLOGY, 12/e. © 2010 MHE. Figure 15.18, p. 567

The atrioventricular (AV) node receives the impulse next. Located beneath the endocardium at the inferior aspect of the interatrial septum, the impulse is delayed from continuing to the ventricles so the atria have the time to contract completely, emptying their contents. Once the impulse arrives at the distal aspect of the AV node, it continues into the AV bundle, also known as the *bundle of His,* a cluster of large fibers. The bundle splits off into two separate branches (left and right) traveling through the ventricular septum and branching off into the Purkinje fibers that reach around the ventricles into the papillary muscles.

> ## EXAMPLE
>
> I51.1   Rupture of chordae tendineae, not elsewhere classified
> I23.5   Rupture of papillary muscle as current complication following acute myocardial infarction

The Circulatory System

Here's how the whole system works: Once the blood has delivered oxygen to the cells via the arteries, the veins bring back the carbon dioxide in the blood (deoxygenated blood) toward the heart. The blood flows via the inferior vena cava and the superior vena cava (large veins carrying the deoxygenated blood) into the right atrium. Once full, the right atrium contracts to push the blood through the tricuspid valve into the right ventricle. When full, the right ventricle contracts and pushes the blood through the pulmonary valve into the pulmonary trunk, which then divides into the right and left pulmonary arteries, taking the blood to the lungs, where it releases the carbon dioxide and picks up oxygen.

The oxygenated blood from the lungs travels through the pulmonary veins into the left atrium of the heart. When it contracts, the left atrium pushes the blood through the mitral (bicuspid) valve into the left ventricle. From here, the left ventricle contractions push this oxygen-rich blood out through the aortic valve into the aorta (a large artery) to deliver oxygen throughout the body and begin the process all over again. *Note:* The first two arteries that branch off the aorta are known as the *coronary arteries.* These vessels bring oxygen to the heart itself. Coronary veins carry deoxygenated blood from the heart tissues back into the right atrium.

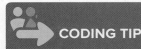

CODING TIP

Arteries = blood vessels that carry oxygenated blood from the heart to the tissues and cells throughout the body. Veins = blood vessels that carry deoxygenated blood, along with carbon dioxide and cell waste, away from the tissues and cells throughout the body and back to the heart.

Cardiovascular Dysfunction

Circulatory conditions are very serious because they affect the flow of blood and, therefore, the delivery of oxygen. While problems with circulation can affect a patient of any age, older individuals are more susceptible to such conditions. This is because as the body ages, the strength and elasticity of blood vessels decrease and become less efficient. In addition, long-term improper nutrition and lack of cardiovascular exercise take their toll and contribute to the circulatory system's inability to do its job.

LO 12.2 Signs and Symptoms of Cardiovascular Disease

There are many distinct disorders that affect the components of the cardiovascular system. Some signs and symptoms that are frequently seen are the following:

- *Angina,* also referred to as *angina pectoris,* is pain in the upper chest, often caused by a lack of oxygen being provided to a part of the heart. For example: I20.0 Unstable angina.

- *Cardiac arrest* means the heart actually stops beating. Typically, this happens suddenly and may be brought on by many different things, including a myocardial infarction (heart attack), electric shock (such as from wiring or lightning), drug interaction, drug overdose, or trauma. For example: I46.2 Cardiac arrest due to underlying cardiac condition.
- *Dyspnea* indicates that the patient is having trouble breathing (short of breath). When due to cardiac problems, this is reported as I50.1, Left ventricular failure.
- *Dysrhythmia,* or *arrhythmia,* refers to an irregular heartbeat. The set of signs includes *tachycardia* (rapid heartbeat, more than 100 beats per minute) as well as *bradycardia* (abnormally slow heartbeat, less than 60 beats per minute). A short-term version of tachycardia may be *palpitations,* a condition in which the patient feels a very rapid heartbeat that lasts only a few minutes. Palpitations are a temporary condition that may be caused by another condition, such as anxiety, whereas tachycardia is an ongoing malfunction of the heart. For example: R00.1, Sinoatrial bradycardia, or R00.2, Palpitations.
- **Edema** is swelling due to an accumulation of fluid in the tissues. It may be observed in the patient's legs, abdominal cavity, or other portions of the body. For example: R60.0 Localized edema.

edema
An overaccumulation of fluid in the cells of the tissues.

LO 12.3 Hypotension and Hypertension

Blood Pressure

The force with which blood travels through your veins and arteries must have enough pressure to ensure the cycle of oxygenation and carbon dioxide is maintained properly. Blood pressure that is too low—a condition known as **hypotension** (*hypo* = low or under + *tension* = pressure)—can result in organs and tissue cells being unable to function. In hypotension, the patient has lower-than-normal blood pressure. Low blood pressure indicates an inadequate flow of blood and, therefore, inadequate oxygen to the brain, heart, and other vital organs. Lightheadedness and dizziness can occur in a person with hypotension.

Some medications, such as antianxiety drugs and diuretics, can cause hypotension, as can alcohol and narcotics. Conditions such as advanced diabetes, dehydration, or arrhythmia can also result in a patient suffering from hypotension. When blood pressure is too high—a condition known as **hypertension** (*hyper* = high or over + *tension* = pressure)—the force of the pressure can actually damage organs and tissues as the blood rushes through.

A health care professional will use a sphygmomanometer (blood pressure machine) to measure a patient's blood pressure and will document the results in two numbers. For example: A patient's blood pressure is documented in the chart as 125/85. The number 125 represents the systolic pressure, and the number 85 is the diastolic pressure (see Table 12-1).

Systolic pressure (SP) is the measure of the maximum push of blood being forced into an artery from the ventricle during a cardiac contraction. This is the top number of a reported blood pressure.

Diastolic pressure (DP) is the measure of the pressure of blood left in the arteries in between ventricular contractions. This is the bottom number of a reported blood pressure.

Hypertension is a condition that millions of people must deal with every day and is a major cause of death. According to the Centers for Disease Control and Prevention (CDC), 31% of all American adults—67 million people—have high blood pressure. These numbers include more women than men and a greater prevalence of individuals over 65 years of age. There are estimates that only about one-third have been officially diagnosed and are getting treatment. It is believed that as many as 50% of all people over age 60 are included in these numbers.

Statistics show that hypertension has caused 35,000 deaths and has been a contributing factor in another 180,000 deaths. The risk of heart disease is increased 300%

hypotension
Low blood pressure; systolic blood pressure below 90 mmHg and/or diastolic measurements of lower than 60 mmHg.

hypertension
High blood pressure, usually a chronic condition; often identified by a systolic blood pressure above 140 mmHg and/or a diastolic blood pressure above 90 mmHg.

TABLE 12-1 Blood Pressure Levels

Systolic/Diastolic Measurement (mmHg)	Diagnosis
< 90/60	Hypotension
90–120/60–80	Normal
120–139/80–89	Prehypertension
140–159/90–99	Hypertension stage 1
160–179/100–109	Hypertension stage 2
180–209/110–119	Hypertension stage 3
210/120 +	Hypertension stage 4

by the presence of hypertension, and the risk of stroke is increased 700%. Research proves that African-Americans are at a much higher risk of hypertension and its effects than any other racial or ethnic group.

Hypertension versus Elevated Blood Pressure

For coders, the first rule when coding hypertension is that the attending physician must specifically state the diagnosis of *hypertension*. The patient may simply have **elevated blood pressure** with no diagnosis of hypertension (code R03.0) rather than the actual chronic disorder of hypertension.

Among the many causes of hypertension are the following:

- An underlying disorder such as renal disease or Cushing's syndrome.
- Chronic emotional stress.
- A sedentary lifestyle.
- Excessive diet of sodium.
- Family history of hypertension.
- Postmenopausal state.
- Advancing age.
- Excessive use of alcohol.
- Obesity.
- African-American ancestry.

elevated blood pressure
An occurrence of high blood pressure; an isolated or infrequent reading of a systolic blood pressure above 140 mmHg and/or a diastolic blood pressure above 90 mmHg.

Primary Hypertension Hypertension frequently shows no signs and symptoms, other than continuous high blood pressure measurements, until the condition alters **vascular** function in the heart, brain, and/or kidneys. This effect is similar to what would happen if the pressure level at which water flows through the pipes in your home increased: High pressure can break a dish in your kitchen sink and make a mess. Patients with high blood pressure, specifically diagnosed as *hypertension,* are known to suffer manifestations of this condition, including damage to the heart and kidneys. Hypertension causes the heart to work harder than normal and can result in left ventricular hypertrophy and subsequently can cause left-sided heart failure or right-sided heart failure, as well as pulmonary edema (excess fluid in the tissues).

A diagnosis will typically come from trending—charting the blood pressure readings over time (an excellent tool in most electronic health record software programs). In addition, a physician can support a diagnosis of hypertension with other data derived from a variety of sources:

- *Auscultation* (listening to sounds with a stethoscope) over the abdominal aorta as well as the carotid, renal, and femoral arteries may reveal bruits (an abnormal sound created by blood flowing past an obstruction; also known as *turbulent flow*).

vascular
Referring to the vessels (arteries and veins)

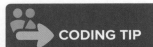
- *Ophthalmoscopy* (examination of the interior of the eye) may reveal arteriovenous nicking.
- *Patient history* may include a family history of hypertension.
- *Chest x-ray* may reveal cardiomegaly (enlargement of the heart).
- *Echocardiography* may show left ventricular hypertrophy (*hyper* = high or over + −*trophy* = growth).
- *Electrocardiogram* (ECG or EKG) may show ischemia (shortage of oxygen due to reduced or restricted blood flow).

When the documentation includes a specific diagnosis of hypertension, you, the coder, will need more information to accurately report this diagnosis.

Essential Hypertension Essential (primary) hypertension is the usual type of hypertension. Code category I10 is used for any diagnosis written by the physician that is stated as high blood pressure, arterial hypertension, benign hypertension, malignant hypertension, primary hypertension, or systemic hypertension.

Most often, essential hypertension can be kept under control with diet (including avoiding high-sodium foods) and medication (e.g., angiotensin-converting enzyme, or ACE, inhibitors, diuretics, and beta-blockers).

LET'S CODE IT! SCENARIO

Sarah Curtis, a 63-year-old female, came to see Dr. Leffert. She was complaining of occasional dizziness and a headache. After a complete examination, Dr. Leffert diagnosed Sarah with idiopathic systemic hypertension.

Let's Code It!

Dr. Leffert diagnosed Sarah with *idiopathic systemic hypertension.* Let's turn to the Alphabetic Index and find the key term *hypertension* and begin reading. If you look down the alphabetic listing under *hypertension,* you will see no listing for *idiopathic* or *systemic.* So go back to the very first entry for this key term, "Hypertension, hypertensive," and read the words shown in parentheses following that entry.

Do you see the words *(idiopathic)* and *(systemic)* included? Both of the adjectives used by Dr. Leffert in his diagnostic statement are in the listing. Therefore, the diagnosis code for Sarah Curtis's current diagnosis is I10. Turn to the Tabular List to double-check.

I10 Essential (primary) hypertension

Perfect!

LO 12.4 Common Hypertensive Manifestations

Hypertension with Heart Disease

When a patient has heart disease or heart failure and also has hypertension, you must carefully examine the words used by the physician in the description.

1. Heart condition *due to* hypertension.
2. *Hypertensive* heart condition.
3. Heart condition *with* hypertension.

If the physician states that the heart condition is "due to" hypertension or describes the heart condition as "hypertensive," then you will use one code from the I11 category to report the diagnosis. This documented statement of cause and effect is required to report the condition with an I11 code.

However, when a patient is documented as having hypertension and having a heart condition but there is no specific cause-and-effect terminology identifying that the heart condition was caused by the hypertension (such as "*with* hypertension"), you are not to use a code from code category I11. In such cases, you are to code these two conditions separately, reporting I10 in addition to the code for the heart condition.

GUIDANCE CONNECTION

Review the ICD-10-CM Coding Guidelines, Section I.C.9, Chapter 9: **Diseases of the circulatory system,** Subsection a(1), **Hypertensive with heart disease.**

EXAMPLE

Hypertensive heart disease without heart failure I11.9
Benign hypertension with acute carditis I10, I51.89
Myocarditis due to malignant hypertension without heart failure I11.9

Hypertensive Heart Disease with Heart Failure

In cases where the physician states that the patient has heart failure due to hypertension, you will need to:

1. Use the appropriate fourth character, as shown in the Tabular List under category I11.
2. Use an additional code to specify the type of heart failure from category I50.-.

ICD-10-CM includes a notation directing you to "use additional code to identify type of heart failure (I50.−)" to remind you.

CODING TIP

The question you need to answer when coding a patient with both hypertension and heart disease is this: Did the hypertension cause the heart condition?
If the answer is yes, code from category I11, Hypertensive heart disease.
If the answer is no, you will need two codes, reporting the hypertension and the heart condition separately.

EXAMPLE

Congestive heart failure due to benign hypertension I11.0, I50.3

LET'S CODE IT! SCENARIO

Jared Rainey, a 41-year-old male, was diagnosed with congestive heart failure due to benign hypertension. Dr. Sanders wrote a prescription for medication and scheduled follow-up tests.

Let's Code It!

Jared was diagnosed with *congestive heart failure due to benign hypertension.* You should remember, from earlier in this chapter, that when the diagnostic statement is written "heart condition *due to* hypertension," the guidelines state that only one code, from category I11, is used.

Turn to the Tabular List for I11:

I11 Hypertensive heart disease
Includes any condition in I51.4–I51.9 due to hypertension

This description fits perfectly. Now we must look at the fourth character. Dr. Sanders wrote "congestive heart failure," bringing us to:

I11.0 Hypertensive heart diseases with heart failure
Use additional code to identify type of heart failure (I50.−)

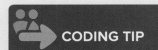

CODING TIP

Determine what type of heart failure the patient has so you can report it with an additional code.

Does the documentation identify the specific type of heart failure? Yes, Dr. Sanders indicated that Jared has congestive heart failure. Let's turn to:

I50 Heart failure

Read the notation under the code:

Code first:

heart failure due to hypertension (I11.0)

This is the book's way of reinforcing the guideline as well as the notation that you found beneath I11. Continue reading, and you see that the second code you need to include for Jared's diagnosis is:

I50.9 Heart failure, unspecified (Congestive heart failure NOS)

You need to show both codes for the visit between Jared and Dr. Sanders:

I11.0 Hypertensive heart diseases with heart failure

I50.9 Heart failure, unspecified

Good work!

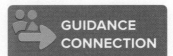

GUIDANCE CONNECTION

Review the ICD-10-CM Coding Guidelines, Section I.C.9, Chapter 9: **Diseases of the circulatory system,** Subsection a(2), **Hypertensive chronic kidney disease**.

Hypertensive Chronic Kidney Disease

When a diagnosis of hypertensive chronic kidney disease is documented, you will report a combination code, as appropriate. In such cases, a cause-and-effect relationship between the hypertension and the kidney disease does not need to be specifically stated by the physician. The mere existence of both conditions in the same body at the same time is enough to report them together. You will need the documentation to specify the stage of the chronic kidney disease to determine the correct code in ICD-10-CM. Code category I12 is to be used for reporting a patient with a diagnosis of hypertensive chronic kidney disease.

The fourth-character choices are:

I12.0 Hypertensive chronic kidney disease with stage 5 chronic kidney disease or end stage renal disease

I12.9 Hypertensive chronic kidney disease with stage 1 through stage 4 chronic kidney disease or unspecified chronic kidney disease

You can see that beneath each of these codes is a notation:

Beneath I112.0:

Use additional code to identify the stage of chronic kidney disease (N18.5, N18.6)

Beneath I112.9:

Use additional code to identify the stage of chronic kidney disease (N18.1–N18.4, N18.9)

As always, in cases where the physician does not document the specific stage, you have to query him or her before choosing an unspecified code.

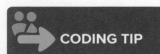

CODING TIP

If you can't find the information in the documentation as to what stage of kidney disease the patient has, query the doctor.

Samuel Mannion, a 41-year-old male, is admitted to Barton Hospital for observation with a diagnosis of stage 3 chronic renal disease due to benign hypertension.

You Code It!

Go through the steps of coding, and determine the code or codes that should be reported for Samuel Mannion's admission into the hospital.

Step 1:   Read the case completely.

Step 2:   Abstract the notes: Which key words can you identify relating to why Barton Hospital provided services to Samuel?

_____

Step 3:   Query the provider, if necessary.

Step 4:   Code the diagnosis or diagnoses.

_____

Step 5:   Code the procedure(s): Hospital observation evaluation and management.

Step 6:   Link the procedure codes to at least one diagnosis code to confirm medical necessity.

Step 7:   Back code to double-check your choices.

Answer:

Did you determine the diagnosis codes to be:

I12.9 **Hypertensive chronic kidney disease with stage 1 through stage 4 chronic kidney disease or unspecified chronic kidney disease**

N18.3 Chronic kidney disease, stage 3 (moderate)

Hypertensive Heart and Chronic Kidney Disease

If the patient is diagnosed with both hypertensive heart disease and hypertensive chronic kidney disease, you will choose one combination code from category I13. Now, there has been great emphasis on telling you never to assume. You are permitted to code only what you know for a fact from the documentation. But, as you know, every rule has an exception, and this is it. The Official Guidelines state that you *"may assume the relationship between the hypertensive heart disease and hypertensive renal disease even if the physician does not state this relationship in the diagnosis."*

You will still need to confirm that a cause-and-effect relationship is specified for the hypertension and the heart condition, even though the cause-and-effect relationship between the hypertension and the kidney disease does not have to be specified. The additional-character choices for code I13 will identify whether the patient is documented to have:

- Heart failure or not.
- Stage 1, 2, 3, or 4 chronic kidney disease or unspecified stage.
- Stage 5 chronic kidney disease, or ESRD.

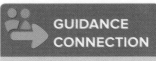

GUIDANCE CONNECTION

Review the ICD-10-CM Coding Guidelines, Section I.C.9, Chapter 9: **Diseases of the circulatory system,** Subsection a(3), **Hypertensive heart and chronic kidney disease**.

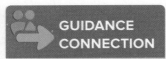

GUIDANCE CONNECTION

Review the ICD-10-CM Coding Guidelines, Section I.C.9, Chapter 9: **Diseases of the circulatory system**, Subsection a(6), **Hypertension, secondary**.

In addition to using this code, you will also need a code for the specific type of heart failure and another to report the stage of the kidney disease. ICD-10-CM includes notations under code I13 to remind you of the additional coding:

Use additional code to identify type of heart failure (I50.−)

Use additional code to identify stage of chronic kidney disease (N18.−)

YOU CODE IT! CASE STUDY

Daisy Farewald, a 55-year-old female, is seen at Barton Hospital with a diagnosis of congestive heart failure due to hypertensive heart disease. Ms. Farewald responds positively to Lasix therapy. She is also diagnosed with stage 1 chronic renal disease.

You Code It!

Go through the steps of coding, and determine the code or codes that should be reported for Daisy Farewald's admission into the hospital.

Step 1: Read the case completely.

Step 2: Abstract the notes: Which key words can you identify relating to why Barton Hospital provided services to Daisy Farewald?

_____

Step 3: Query the provider, if necessary.

Step 4: Code the diagnosis or diagnoses.

_____

Step 5: Code the procedure(s): IV therapies.

Step 6: Link the procedure codes to at least one diagnosis code to confirm medical necessity.

Step 7: Back code to double-check your choices.

Answer:

Did you determine the diagnosis codes to be:

I13.0 Hypertensive heart and chronic kidney disease with heart failure and stage 1 through stage 4 chronic kidney disease or unspecified chronic kidney disease

I50.3 Diastolic (congestive) heart failure

N18.1 Chronic kidney disease, stage 1

Secondary Hypertension

There are occasions when instead of hypertension causing other conditions (manifestations) in the patient, another condition or a medication may cause hypertension. Medications, such as corticosteroids (e.g., prednisone), antidepressants (e.g., Sinequan), and hormones (e.g., Estrace), or diseases, such as Cushing's syndrome or scleroderma, may trigger a hypertensive condition. When the hypertensive condition is generated by, or secondary to, another disease or medication, the condition is called **secondary hypertension.**

secondary hypertension
The condition of hypertension caused by another condition or illness.

The involvement of renal disease as an underlying cause of hypertension, also known as *renovascular hypertension*, may be diagnosed as a result of testing, including:

- *Urinalysis* showing protein levels and red and white blood cells indicating glomerulonephritis (inflammation of small blood vessels in the kidneys).
- *Excretory urography* that reveals renal atrophy (wasting away of a kidney), pointing to chronic renal disease, or a shortening of one kidney, which may indicate unilateral renal disease.
- *Blood tests for serum potassium levels* (measuring the levels of potassium in the blood) that show levels below the normal measure of 3.5 mEq/L, which can indicate primary hyperaldosteronism (*hyper* = high or over + *aldosterone* = a hormone produced by the adrenal cortex that prompts the kidney to preserve sodium and water).

Hypertension is coded as secondary when the physician uses terms such as "due to" an underlying disease, "resulting from" another condition, or other descriptors that point to another disease or condition. In such cases, you will need two codes:

1. The underlying condition
2. The type of secondary hypertension (I15.*x*)

EXAMPLE

I15.0 Renovascular hypertension

I15.1 Hypertension secondary to other renal disorders

I15.2 Hypertension secondary to endocrine disorders

I15.8 Other secondary hypertension

I15.9 Secondary hypertension, unspecified

There is a notation to "code also underlying condition." Note that sequencing is not identified in this notation. Therefore, you will need to report the two codes based on the sequencing guidelines in the Official Guidelines, Section II, which will guide you in determining the principal diagnosis code. So the order in which you will list the two codes is determined by the answer to the question, "Why did the patient come to see the physician today?"

LET'S CODE IT! SCENARIO

Samantha Dennis, a 63-year-old female, came to see Dr. Wiley in his office. She was having headaches and bouts of dizziness. After a physical examination, a urinalysis, and blood work, he diagnosed her with benign hypertension. Dr. Wiley's notes stated that her hypertension was the result of her existing diagnosis of pituitary-dependent Cushing's disease.

Let's Code It!

Dr. Wiley diagnosed Samantha with *benign hypertension due to pituitary-dependent Cushing's disease.* This means that Cushing's disease caused Samantha's hypertension. First, go to the Alphabetic Index, and look under *hypertension.* Look down the indented column until you see "due to" (which is the same as "result of" stated in the physician's notes). Now, look at the indented listing under "due to"; you will see no listing for "Cushing's disease." So "specified disease" is a strong consideration.

You can also keep looking down the column until you see "secondary" specified NEC I15.8. Both paths take you to the same suggested code:

Hypertension
Due to
> **Endocrine disorders I15.2**

Now let's check this code in the Tabular List:

I15.2 Hypertension secondary to endocrine disorders

Did you remember that the pituitary gland is a component of the endocrine system? Now, one more thing: Even though there is no notation, don't you think something is missing? That's right—a code for the Cushing's disease. In the Alphabetic Index, you see the following under *Cushing's:*

Cushing's
> **Syndrome or disease E24.9**
>> **Pituitary-dependent E24.0**

In the Tabular List, you will see:

E24 Cushing's syndrome

Next, there is an *Excludes1* note:

Excludes1 congenital adrenal hyperplasia (E25.0)

Just because Samantha is 63 years old does not mean this isn't a congenital condition. However, Dr. Wiley provides no documentation stating that her Cushing's disease is congenital, so this *excludes* note does not apply to this patient for this encounter.

E24.0 Pituitary-dependent Cushing's disease

The claim form you complete for Samantha's encounter with Dr. Wiley today will show:

I15.2 Hypertension secondary to endocrine disorders
E24.0 Pituitary-dependent Cushing's disease

In what order should these codes be listed? Samantha's claim will list the hypertension first (I15.2) because it was the symptoms of the hypertension (headaches, dizziness) that brought Samantha to Dr. Wiley's office for this encounter.

Hypertension and Pregnancy

When a pregnant woman has a diagnosis of hypertension, you will first need to determine from the documentation whether she developed hypertension before or after conception.

A woman with a preexisting diagnosis of hypertension who then becomes pregnant will be reported with the appropriate code from the O10, Pre-existing hypertension complicating pregnancy, childbirth, and the puerperium, code category. This code reports this situation clearly. Reflecting the structure of I10, this code category also is subdivided, as identified by the fourth character reporting the specific hypertensive manifestation, if any:

O10.0 Pre-existing essential hypertension complicating pregnancy, childbirth, and the puerperium

O10.1 Pre-existing hypertensive heart disease complicating pregnancy, childbirth, and the puerperium

O10.2 Pre-existing hypertensive chronic kidney disease complicating pregnancy, childbirth, and the puerperium

O10.3 Pre-existing hypertensive heart and chronic kidney disease complicating pregnancy, childbirth, and the puerperium

O10.4 Pre-existing secondary hypertension complicating pregnancy, childbirth, and the puerperium

However, if the hypertension is diagnosed as **gestational hypertension,** or transient hypertension, you will report a code from O13, Gestational [pregnancy-induced] hypertension without significant proteinuria. This is not unusual and generally means that the hypertension will go away after the baby is born.

O13.1 Gestational [pregnancy-induced] hypertension without significant proteinuria, first trimester

O13.2 Gestational [pregnancy-induced] hypertension without significant proteinuria, second trimester

O13.3 Gestational [pregnancy-induced] hypertension without significant proteinuria, third trimester

Should the woman's diagnosed hypertension cause problems directly related to the pregnancy or complicating the pregnancy, you will choose the best, most appropriate code from Chapter 15, Pregnancy, Childbirth, and the Puerperium (O00–O9A).

gestational hypertension
Hypertension that develops during pregnancy and typically goes away once the pregnancy has ended.

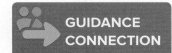

GUIDANCE CONNECTION

Review the ICD-10-CM Coding Guidelines, Section I.C.9, Chapter 9: **Diseases of the circulatory system,** Subsection a(7), **Hypertension, transient**.

EXAMPLE

O11.3 Pre-existing hypertension with pre-eclampsia, third trimester
O16.1 Unspecified maternal hypertension, first trimester

LET'S CODE IT! SCENARIO

Carla Jennings, a 23-year-old female, is 20 weeks pregnant. Dr. Jacoby diagnoses her with gestational hypertension. Even though there is no evidence of proteinuria, he is concerned about the effect of the condition on her pregnancy and writes a prescription.

Let's Code It!

Carla Jennings has *gestational hypertension*. Her hypertensive condition is complicating her pregnancy. Turn to the term *hypertension* in the Alphabetic Index, and look down the column of adjectives below the primary term *hypertension*. You see:

Hypertension

Complicating

    Pregnancy

        Gestational (pregnancy-induced) (transient)(without proteinuria) O13.–

That matches Dr. Jacoby's notes. Now you must turn to the Tabular List to confirm the code *and* determine the correct fourth character:

O13 Gestational [pregnancy-induced] hypertension without significant proteinuria

Now turn to the first page of Chapter 15 in ICD-10-CM to see the definitions of the trimesters. You can see the information:

1st trimester—less than 14 weeks, 0 days

2nd trimester—14 weeks, 0 days to less than 28 weeks, 0 days

3rd trimester—28 weeks, 0 days until delivery

Carla is in her 20th week, so she is in her 2nd trimester. This points us to the correct fourth character of 2. The code to be used for this visit between Dr. Jacoby and Carla Jennings is:

O13.2 Gestational [pregnancy-induced] hypertension without significant proteinuria, second trimester

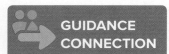

Review the ICD-10-CM Coding Guidelines, Section I.C.9, Chapter 9: **Diseases of the circulatory system,** Subsection a(5), **Hypertensive retinopathy.**

Hypertensive Retinopathy

Retinopathy is a degenerative disease of the eye, most specifically the retina. The condition can be caused by diabetes, hypertension, or other circumstances. In cases where the patient is diagnosed with hypertensive retinopathy due to hypertension, you will need two codes to thoroughly report the patient's condition.

Your first code is from the subcategory H35.03-, Hypertensive retinopathy. This code requires a sixth character to identify which eye is affected:

H35.031 Hypertensive retinopathy, right eye

H35.032 Hypertensive retinopathy, left eye

H35.033 Hypertensive retinopathy, bilateral

Then you will need an additional code to identify the type of hypertension that caused the retinopathy. Choose that code from the I10–I15 range. There is a reminder notation for you, shown beneath code H35.0:

Code also any associated hypertension (I10.−)

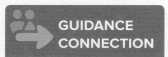

Review the ICD-10-CM Coding Guidelines, Section I.C.9, Chapter 9: **Diseases of the circulatory system,** Subsection a(4), **Hypertensive cerebrovascular disease.**

Hypertensive Cerebrovascular Disease

Patients with cerebrovascular disease due to hypertension will have two codes assigned. The first code will report the cerebrovascular disease, a code from the I60–I69 range. The second code will identify the hypertension, using the appropriate code from the I10–I15 range. Both the guidelines and a notation under the category heading shown directly above code I60 remind you of the necessity for a second code. You can see that the notation also instructs you as to which order to place the codes:

Use additional code to identify presence of hypertension (I10–I15)

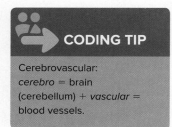

Cerebrovascular:
cerebro = brain (cerebellum) + *vascular* = blood vessels.

Heather Harper, a 47-year-old female, came to see Dr. Azevedo because she was experiencing headaches and problems with her vision. Heather was diagnosed with essential benign hypertension 3 years ago. After a thorough physical examination and further questioning about her visual disturbances, Dr. Azevedo ordered a CT scan of her head and a few other tests. The test results indicate that Heather has hypertensive encephalopathy.

You Code It!

Carefully review Dr. Azevedo's notes on his visit with Heather, along with the test results. Determine the best, most appropriate diagnosis code or codes.

Step 1: Read the case completely.

Step 2: Abstract the notes: Which key words can you identify relating to why Dr. Azevedo spent time caring for Heather?

_____

Step 3: Query the provider, if necessary.

Step 4: Code the diagnosis or diagnoses.

_____

Step 5: Code the procedure(s): Office visit evaluation and management, CT scan.

Step 6: Link the procedure codes to at least one diagnosis code to confirm medical necessity.

Step 7: Back code to double-check your choices.

Answer:

Did you determine the diagnosis codes to be:

I67.4 Hypertensive encephalopathy

I10 Essential hypertension

Good job!

Other Circulatory Conditions

LO 12.5 CVA and Cerebral Infarction

A **cerebrovascular accident (CVA)** is technically considered a condition of the neurologic system, yet this diagnosis is reported with codes included in this subsection (codes I60–I67) because a CVA is the result of an obstruction in a cerebral blood vessel. A cerebrovascular accident, also known as a *stroke,* is the result of a thrombus or embolism getting lodged in a cerebral vessel and preventing blood from flowing through the area. There are times when the blockage (occlusion) resolves quickly, either on its own or from the administration of blood-thinning medication (tPA), making the event short-lived. This is known as an *ischemic* attack (code category I63). In some cases, the obstruction causes a backup of blood that subsequently bursts through

cerebrovascular accident (CVA)
Rupture of a blood vessel causing hemorrhaging in the brain or an embolus in a blood vessel in the brain causing a loss of blood flow; also known as *stroke.*

the vessel wall and a hemorrhage floods the area of the brain. This is known as a *hemorrhagic* attack (code category I61).

While a cerebrovascular accident is not technically the same as a **cerebral infarction,** the term *CVA* is frequently used to indicate a cerebral infarction. An **infarction** occurs when the occlusion created by the thrombus deprives surrounding tissue of oxygen and the cells die (necrosis).

You will need to abstract details from the documentation to determine the correct code category:

I61 Nontraumatic intracerebral hemorrhage

I63 Cerebral infarction (Occlusion and stenosis of cerebral arteries, resulting in cerebral infarction)

I65 Occlusion and stenosis of precerebral arteries, not resulting in cerebral infarction

I66 Occlusion and stenosis of cerebral arteries, not resulting in cerebral infarction

It can happen that a cerebrovascular hemorrhage or infarction is brought about by a medical procedure, most typically surgery. When the procedure is plainly identified as the cause of the infarction, you have to use two codes. The first code will be:

I97.810 Intraoperative cerebrovascular infarction during cardiac surgery

I97.811 Intraoperative cerebrovascular infarction during other surgery

I97.820 Postprocedural cerebrovascular infarction during cardiac surgery

I97.821 Postprocedural cerebrovascular infarction during other surgery

As noted below code I97.8, you will need an additional code to identify the exact complication. The second code will identify the exact nature of the infarction, and you will choose it from the I60–I67 range, as appropriate, according to the notes.

Heart Failure

A diagnosis of heart failure is serious; however, it does not mean the heart has totally "failed" to function. Also known as *congestive heart failure (CHF),* this condition is characterized by the inability of the individual's heart to pump a sufficient quantity of blood throughout the body. This can cause fluid to back up into the lungs, resulting in respiratory problems, such as shortness of breath and fatigue. In addition, fluid might build up in the lower extremities, causing edema (swelling) in the feet, ankles, and legs. In some patients, the edema can become so acute (severe) that they may have pain and trouble walking.

According to the National Heart, Lung, and Blood Institute, approximately 5 million people in the United States have been diagnosed with heart failure. The institute estimates that this condition contributes to as many as 30,000 deaths each year.

There are several types of heart failure:

Left heart failure indicates an insufficiency of the heart's left ventricle. This malfunction results in the accumulation of fluid in the lungs. When this happens, patients may also develop respiratory problems.

Right heart failure, secondary to left heart failure, is diagnosed when the heart cannot pump and circulate the blood needed throughout the body. Patients with this diagnosis may develop hypertension, congestion, edema, and fluid collection in the lungs.

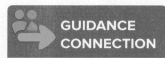

GUIDANCE CONNECTION

Review the ICD-10-CM Coding Guidelines, Section I.C.9, Chapter 9: **Diseases of the circulatory system,** Subsection c, **Intraoperative and postprocedural cerebrovascular accident.**

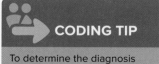

CODING TIP

To determine the diagnosis code for heart failure, you need to know:

- What type of heart failure?
- Is it acute or chronic?

Systolic heart failure occurs when the contractions of the ventricles are too weak to push the blood through the heart.

Diastolic heart failure is the result of a ventricle of the heart being unable to fill as it should.

Combined systolic and diastolic heart failure means that the function of the heart is weak and unable to process blood properly.

CODING TIP

When a condition, such as right heart failure, causes the patient to develop another condition, such as hypertension, that other condition may be referred to as a *secondary condition*. For example, if Mary developed hypertension due to her right heart failure, you would report the hypertension as *secondary hypertension*.

YOU CODE IT! CASE STUDY

Ellyn Carrera, an 81-year-old female, came to see her cardiologist, Dr. Odem, to follow up on her CHF. The edema (swelling) of her legs has improved, but she continues to have dyspnea (shortness of breath) with mild exertion. No syncope (fainting) at this time. Dx: Chronic diastolic congestive heart failure.

You Code It!

Look at Dr. Odem's notes for Ellyn Carrera, and determine the best, most appropriate code or codes.

Step 1: Read the case completely.

Step 2: Abstract the notes: Which key words can you identify relating to why Dr. Odem spent time caring for Ellyn?

_____

Step 3: Query the provider, if necessary.

Step 4: Code the diagnosis or diagnoses.

_____

Step 5: Code the procedure(s): Office visit for evaluation of CHF.

Step 6: Link the procedure codes to at least one diagnosis code to confirm medical necessity.

Step 7: Back code to double-check your choices.

Answer:

Did you determine the diagnosis code to be:

I50.32 Chronic diastolic (congestive) heart failure

Good job!

Myocardial Infarction

When a part of the heart muscle deteriorates, or actually dies, that muscle can no longer function properly. This malfunction within a person's heart, known as a **myocardial infarction (MI),** will cause persistent pain in the chest, left arm, jaw, and neck; fatigue; nausea; vomiting; and shortness of breath. These signs and symptoms can be confirmed by an electrocardiogram (EKG), blood tests measuring the serial serum enzyme levels, and/or an echocardiogram. An ST elevation myocardial infarction (**STEMI**) is a heart event during which the coronary artery is completely blocked by a **thrombus** or **embolus.** The ST segment is a specific range seen in an EKG (ECG). A nontransmural myocardial infarction (**NSTEMI**) indicates that only a portion of the artery is occluded (blocked).

myocardial infarction (MI)
Malfunction of the heart due to necrosis or deterioration of a portion of the heart muscle; also known as a *heart attack.*

STEMI
An ST elevation myocardial infarction—a heart event during which the coronary artery is completely blocked by a thrombus or embolus.

thrombus

A blood clot in a blood vessel; plural = *thrombi*.

embolus

A thrombus that has broken free from the vessel wall and is traveling freely within the vascular system.

NSTEMI

A nontransmural myocardial infarction—a heart event during which the coronary artery is partially occluded (blocked).

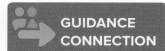

GUIDANCE CONNECTION

Review the ICD-10-CM Coding Guidelines, Section I.C.9, Chapter 9: **Diseases of the circulatory system**, Subsection e(1), **Acute myocardial infarction (AMI)**.

A thrombus is a blood clot that has attached itself to the wall of a blood vessel. If left untreated, it may cause a blockage, preventing blood from flowing through the vessel. In addition, there is always concern that the clot will detach and float through the vessel and pass through an organ. A detached clot is known as an *embolus;* it can get stuck as it passes through an organ and can completely prevent blood from moving through. The greatest danger occurs when an embolus travels into the lung or the heart, potentially causing death.

EXAMPLE

I26.02 Saddle embolism of pulmonary artery with acute cor pulmonale

Another important aspect of a diagnosis of MI is whether or not this is the first time this patient has experienced this event. When the patient is documented as having had an acute myocardial infarction (AMI) within the last 4 weeks (28 days) and it is the second event, it is reported with a code describing a "subsequent" MI. When the previous MI is documented either as a "healed MI" or as a past MI without any current signs or symptoms, this is reported with I25.2 Old myocardial infarction.

EXAMPLE

I21.11 ST elevation (STEMI) myocardial infarction involving right coronary artery

I22.2 Subsequent non-ST elevation (NSTEMI) myocardial infarction

YOU CODE IT! CASE STUDY

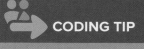

CODING TIP

To determine the code for a diagnosis of MI, you will need to know:

- What specific part of the heart was affected by the infarction?
- Has this patient been treated for an MI before? If so, how long ago?
- Is this infarction a STEMI or an NSTEMI?

Jason is sitting in the stands watching his son play softball when all of a sudden he feels a severe pain in his chest. He is having difficulty taking a breath, and the pain is radiating down his left arm. He arrives at the ED via ambulance, and Dr. Alexis and nurses work on him, taking blood and doing an EKG. Dr. Alexis determines that Jason had an ST elevation myocardial infarction (STEMI) of the inferolateral wall. Once he is stabilized, Jason is admitted into the hospital and transferred to the ICU.

You Code It!

Go through the steps of coding, and determine the code or codes that should be reported for this encounter between Dr. Alexis and Jason.

Step 1: Read the case completely.

Step 2: Abstract the notes: Which key words can you identify relating to why Dr. Alexis cared for Jason?

_____

Step 3: Query the provider, if necessary.

Step 4: Code the diagnosis or diagnoses.

_____

Step 5: Code the procedure(s): ED encounter and admission to ICU.

Step 6: Link the procedure codes to at least one diagnosis code to confirm medical necessity.

Step 7: Back code to double-check your choices.

Answer:

Did you determine the correct code to be:

I21.19 ST elevation (STEMI) myocardial infarction involving other coronary artery of inferior wall (Inferolateral transmural (Q wave) infarction (acute))

Deep Vein Thrombosis

Earlier in this chapter, you learned about thrombi and emboli—blood clots that develop within the blood vessels. Deep vein thrombi can block the blood flow, causing venous insufficiency and affecting the ability of oxygen to get to the tissues, not only in the heart, as we discussed their involvement with myocardial infarctions, but throughout the entire body. A lack, or reduction, of blood flow can cause edema, congestion, necrosis, and pain. In addition, there is the danger that the blood clot can break loose and travel within the veins and arteries (embolism), causing damage to internal organs, blocking oxygen from the lungs (pulmonary embolism), or blocking off blood flow through the heart.

Reporting a diagnosis of deep vein thrombosis (DVT) will require you to know a few specifics to determine the most accurate code:

- Is the condition identified as acute or chronic?
- Where (the specific anatomical site) has the thrombus been located?

EXAMPLE

I82.412 Acute embolism and thrombosis of left femoral vein
I82.543 Chronic embolism and thrombosis of tibial vein, bilateral

Atherosclerotic Coronary Artery Disease (ACAD)

Atherosclerosis, also known as *arteriosclerosis,* is a stricture or stenosis of an artery (e.g., code I70.0 Atherosclerosis of aorta) that may require the placement of a stent (a wire mesh tube inserted to support the walls of the artery and keep them open). You have probably heard about this in some commercials on television that talk about the buildup of plaque in the arteries and the damage that may result. Atherosclerosis (*athero* = artery + *sclerosis* = narrowing) is the condition of plaque-lined arteries. The plaque builds up on the inner walls of the arteries, thereby narrowing the passageway and reducing the flow of blood. Remember that arteries carry oxygenated blood from the heart to the tissues and cells throughout the body.

In coronary artery disease (CAD), plaque collects specifically within the coronary arteries (arteries within the heart); the heart itself becomes oxygen-deprived. This means there will be a greater potential for a stroke (CVA), a heart attack, or death. According to the National Heart, Lung, and Blood Institute, CAD is the number-one cause of death in the United States.

A patient may first be alerted to reduced flow of blood to the heart muscle by angina. **Angina pectoris** is an event of acute chest pain caused by an insufficient supply of oxygen to an area of the heart. This condition may be treated with medication, such as Isordil or Nitrostat (sublingual nitroglycerin), drugs categorized as vasodilators that

atherosclerosis
A condition resulting from plaque buildup on the interior walls of the arteries, causing reduced blood flow; also known as *arteriosclerosis.*

angina pectoris
Chest pain.

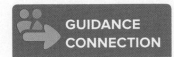

GUIDANCE CONNECTION

Review the ICD-10-CM Coding Guidelines, Section I.C.9, Chapter 9: **Diseases of the circulatory system,** Subsection b, **Atherosclerotic coronary artery disease with angina.**

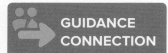
GUIDANCE CONNECTION

Review the ICD-10-CM Coding Guidelines, Section I.C.9, Chapter 9: **Diseases of the circulatory system,** Subsection d, **Sequelae of cerebrovascular disease.**

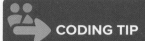
CODING TIP

There is a note in the Tabular List, directly under code I69, that reads:

Note: Category I69 is to be used to indicate conditions in I60–I67 as the cause of sequela. The "sequelae" include conditions specified as such or as residuals which may occur at any time after the onset of the causal condition.

You will see similar notes in other locations as well. They can be confusing to understand. What the note above means is this: When you read in the patient's chart that he or she was previously diagnosed with a condition that was originally reported with any of the codes in the range I60–I67 and, during this visit, the doctor documents that the patient currently has a neurologic deficit, such as paralysis or dysphasia, that is a result of that earlier condition, you will use a code from category I69 to report the new condition—the neurologic deficit.

dilate arterial walls, making it easier for blood to flow smoothly. When hypertension is also present, a calcium channel blocker, such as Norvasc or Vascor, may be prescribed instead. Report this with a code from category I20, Angina pectoris, with a required additional character for the specific type of angina, and use an additional code to report the underlying cause.

LO 12.6 Sequelae of Cerebrovascular Disease

The sequelae, or late effects, of cerebrovascular disease are coded differently from other sequelae.

ICD-10-CM provides a series of combination codes in category I69, Sequela of cerebrovascular disease. It is not unusual for patients who are poststatus CVA to suffer with neurologic deficits that last past the initial onset of the condition. In such cases, the physician must connect the dots and specifically identify the current condition as a sequela, or late effect, of the cerebrovascular issue.

Should the patient be diagnosed with neurologic deficits from both a previous cerebrovascular condition *and* a current cerebrovascular accident (CVA), you are permitted to use both a code from the I60–I67 range *and* a code from the I69 category.

When there are no neurologic deficits present and the patient has a personal history of cerebrovascular disease, you should use a code from subcategory Z86.7-, Personal history of diseases of the circulatory system, and not code I69. Remember, you will only code that history when it has been documented that the physician addressed the condition during the current encounter.

LET'S CODE IT! SCENARIO

Priscilla Lewis goes to see Dr. Belman. She was diagnosed with a cerebral embolism 3 months ago that has now been resolved. She explains that she has been having difficulty putting words together to make a sentence and it seems to be getting worse. After examination, Dr. Belman diagnoses her with post-cerebral embolic dysphasia.

Let's Code It!

Priscilla has been diagnosed with *post-cerebral embolic dysphasia.* This is one way the physician may state that the dysphasia is a late effect of the cerebral embolism she had before.

Turn to the ICD-10-CM Alphabetic Index and look up the term *dysphasia.*

There is one code suggested: R47.02. In the Tabular List, find the beginning of this code category:

R47 Speech disturbances, not elsewhere classified

Dysphasia is a speech disturbance—a problem speaking—so that is OK, so far. There is nothing in the *Excludes1* note that relates to this patient. As you read down, you see that fourth and fifth characters are required, so continue reading the column until you get to:

R47.0 Dysphasia and aphasia

R47.02 Dysphasia

This is where the Alphabetic Index pointed you, so look closely at this code. Below it is another *Excludes1* note, which tells you that this code does not include a diagnosis of *dysphasia due to a late effect of cerebrovascular accident* and directs you to the codes in the I69 code category.

Excludes1 dysphasia following cerebrovascular disease (I69.- with final characters -21)

Go back to the physician's notes (the scenario). The documentation doesn't state that Priscilla had cerebrovascular disease; it states that she had a cerebral embolism. Is this the same thing, or is it unrelated to this notation?

This is the same thing: A cerebral embolism is a type of CVA. When you look it up, you will see that a cerebral embolism is reported with code I66.9, clearly in the range of I60–I67. This means you will report the dysphasia from a code in the I69 category.

Therefore, this *Excludes1* note applies to this encounter, and you must turn to code I69 to determine the correct code to report Priscilla's diagnosis. The notation directly under I69, Sequela of cerebrovascular disease, confirms that you are in the right place now. Read down and determine the code:

I69.821 Dysphasia following other cerebrovascular disease

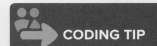

CODING TIP

Read carefully! *Dysphasia* (ending in "sia") means impaired speech, and *dysphagia* (ending in "gia") means difficulty swallowing. Another word that is close is *dysplasia*, which means abnormal cell growth. Big difference!

YOU CODE IT! CASE STUDY

Andrew Hogan, a 77-year-old male, was brought into the recovery room after having a craniectomy for the drainage of an intracranial abscess. Dr. Greenwald's notes indicate that Andrew had a postoperative intracranial hemorrhage showing an acute subdural hematoma.

You Code It!

Look at Dr. Greenwald's notes for Andrew Hogan, and determine the best, most appropriate code or codes.

Step 1: Read the case completely.

Step 2: Abstract the notes: Which key words can you identify relating to why Dr. Greenwald spent time caring for Andrew Hogan?

_____

Step 3: Query the provider, if necessary.

Step 4: Code the diagnosis or diagnoses.

_____

Step 5: Code the procedure(s): Craniectomy.

Step 6: Link the procedure codes to at least one diagnosis code to confirm medical necessity.

Step 7: Back code to double-check your choices.

Answer:

Did you determine the diagnosis codes to be:

I97.821 Postprocedural cerebrovascular infarction during other surgery

I62.01 Nontraumatic acute subdural hemorrhage

Good job!

Other Cardiovascular Conditions

Hypercholesterolemia (*hyper* = high + *cholesterol* + *emia* = in the blood) indicates that plaque is accumulating in the arteries, causing them to narrow. This narrowing (stenosis) reduces the amount of blood that flows through the vessel, causing strain on the heart and other organs in addition to causing an interruption of the delivery of oxygen and the removal of carbon dioxide. This diagnosis is reported with code E78.0, Pure hypercholesterolemia.

In addition to diet and exercise modification, antilipemic drugs, such as Lipitor or Zocor, may be prescribed to decrease the lipid (fat) blood level. If these actions are not sufficient, a PTCA percutaneous transluminal coronary angioplasty (PTCA) may be performed. During a PTCA, a catheter is threaded through the artery to the site of the plaque buildup. A balloon on the tip of the catheter is expanded, compacting the plaque against the walls of the artery, thereby reducing the blockage.

Atrial fibrillation is a condition in which the atria, instead of contracting to push blood through to the ventricles, shudder or tremble. This results in incomplete emptying of the atria, leaving blood to collect and sometimes clot. Episodes of paroxysmal atrial tachycardia (PAT), a rapid heart rate that can go as high as 150 or 200 beats per minute, can occur. Anticoagulants (drugs that prevent clotting) and/or thrombolytics (clot-dissolving drugs) are often prescribed. For example: code I48.2 Chronic atrial fibrillation.

Mitral valve prolapse is a rather common abnormality that prevents the mitral valve from closing properly (the mitral valve is the gateway between the left atrium and the left ventricle). It may develop or be influenced by other conditions, including hyperthyroidism, congenital heart lesions, or Marfan syndrome. For example: code I34.1 Nonrheumatic mitral (valve) prolapse. In acute cases, a valve replacement may be required.

Chapter Summary

Cardiovascular conditions initially may be treated within the specialty of a cardiologist. However, the manifestations of heart failure and heart disease can affect the patient anywhere in the body—from the brain to the feet. Blood vessels extend throughout the body, from the large aorta to the tiny capillaries, delivering oxygen and transporting carbon dioxide back to the lungs so it can be released. When something goes awry, the health of the entire body, as well as the patient's quality of life, can be negatively affected.

Hypertension is a condition that you may encounter, as a professional coder, while working for a family physician, an internist, a gerontologist, or a cardiologist. It can be a very dangerous condition and can cause many co-morbidities and manifestations. As complex as the condition is, so is the coding of the diagnosis. As with all other situations, it must be diagnosed and documented by the attending physician. Read the notes carefully, and query the physician when necessary to get all the specifics that you need to code accurately.

CHAPTER **12** REVIEW
Coding Circulatory Conditions

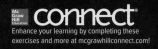

Enhance your learning by completing these exercises and more at mcgrawhillconnect.com!

Using Terminology

Match each key term to the appropriate definition.

_____ **1.** LO 12.5 A heart attack.

_____ **2.** LO 12.1 Upper chambers of the heart that receive blood returning to the heart.

_____ **3.** LO 12.1 Lower chambers of the heart that push blood away from the heart.

_____ **4.** LO 12.4 The condition of hypertension caused by another condition or illness.

_____ **5.** LO 12.3 An occurrence of high blood pressure; an isolated or infrequent reading.

_____ **6.** LO 12.5 A stroke.

_____ **7.** LO 12.5 A heart event during which the coronary artery is completely blocked by a thrombus or embolus.

_____ **8.** LO 12.1 Heart.

_____ **9.** LO 12.5 A blood clot in a blood vessel.

_____ **10.** LO 12.4 Hypertension that develops during pregnancy and typically goes away once the pregnancy has ended.

_____ **11.** LO 12.5 A thrombus that has broken free from the vessel wall and is traveling freely within the vascular system.

_____ **12.** LO 12.5 An area of dead tissue (necrosis) in the brain, caused by a blocked or ruptured blood vessel.

_____ **13.** LO 12.5 A heart event during which the coronary artery is partially occluded (blocked).

_____ **14.** LO 12.3 Veins and arteries.

_____ **15.** LO 12.3 Low blood pressure.

_____ **16.** LO 12.3 High blood pressure.

A. Atrium

B. Cerebral infarction

C. Cerebrovascular accident (CVA)

D. Elevated blood pressure

E. Embolus

F. Gestational hypertension

G. Hypertension

H. Hypotension

I. Myocardial infarction (MI)

J. NSTEMI

K. Secondary hypertension

L. STEMI

M. Thrombosis

N. Ventricle

O. Cardio

P. Vascular

Checking Your Understanding

Choose the most appropriate answer for each of the following questions.

1. LO 12.3 Hypertension is a

  a. genetic condition.

  b. contagious condition.

  c. chronic condition.

  d. terminal condition.

2. LO 12.3 When the patient's records indicate a current blood pressure reading of 150/100 and no diagnosis is related to that factor, you should

  a. code elevated blood pressure.

  b. query the physician.

  c. code hypertension.

  d. code history of hypertension.

3. LO 12.3 Essential hypertension can usually be controlled with
   a. proper diet.
   b. certain medications.
   c. surgery.
   d. both proper diet and certain medications.

4. LO 12.4 If the patient has a diagnosis of heart failure due to hypertension, you will need to
   a. use the appropriate fourth character, as shown in the Tabular List under category I11.
   b. use an additional code to specify the type of heart failure from category I50.
   c. use code I10.
   d. use both the appropriate fourth character, as shown in the Tabular List under category I11, and an additional code to specify the type of heart failure from category I50.

5. LO 12.5 A heart event during which the coronary artery is completely blocked by a thrombus or embolus is called a(n)
   a. myocardial infarction.
   b. thrombus.
   c. nontransmural myocardial infarction.
   d. ST elevation myocardial infarction.

6. LO 12.4 A diagnosis of secondary hypertension means you will code
   a. the underlying condition only.
   b. the hypertension only.
   c. the underlying condition code and the hypertension code.
   d. the hypertension code first and then the underlying condition code.

7. LO 12.4 When a pregnant woman is diagnosed with hypertension, you must determine
   a. if it is gestational hypertension.
   b. if it is an infarction.
   c. if it is transient hypertension.
   d. if it is familial.

8. LO 12.6 A patient with no neurologic deficits and who had a previous diagnosis of cerebrovascular disease (which has since resolved) should be reported with a code from
   a. the I60–I69 range.
   b. the I69 code category.
   c. Z86.7-.
   d. none of these.

9. LO 12.4 A diagnosis of hypertension
   a. occurs with other conditions only.
   b. will often affect the treatment of almost any other condition.
   c. is always coded with other conditions.
   d. is temporary.

10. LO 12.3 A physician can support a diagnosis of hypertension with all of the following data *except*
   a. auscultation over the abdominal aorta.
   b. EKG.
   c. chest x-ray.
   d. ACE.

Applying Your Knowledge

1. LO 12.1 What are the components of the circulatory system? _____

   _____

2. LO 12.1 List the four chambers of the heart. _____

   _____

3. LO 12.3 Differentiate between systolic pressure and diastolic pressure. _____

   _____

4. LO 12.3 What is the difference between hypertension and elevated blood pressure? _____

   _____

5. LO 12.4 What is gestational hypertension? _____

   _____

6. LO 12.5 Explain the difference between STEMI and NSTEMI. _____

   _____

Using the techniques described in this chapter, carefully read through the case studies and determine the most accurate ICD-10-CM code(s) and external cause code(s), if appropriate, for each case study.

1. Sarah Linscott, a 37-year-old female, was diagnosed with benign hypertension due to a brain tumor.

   _____

2. David Nguyen, a 53-year-old male, is diagnosed with unspecified hypertension due to renal artery stenosis.

   _____

3. Dr. Sirianni diagnosed Gordon Baxa with secondary malignant hypertension due to Cushing's disease.

   _____

4. Robert Hall, a 61-year-old male, was diagnosed with accelerated hypertension.

   _____

5. Pauline Robinson, a 27-year-old obese female, was diagnosed with intermittent vascular hypertensive disease.

   _____

6. Glenn Livingston, a 79-year-old male, was diagnosed with heart failure due to benign hypertension.

   _____

7. Vanessa Dostoimov, a 67-year-old female, was diagnosed with hypertrophy of the heart due to malignant hypertension.

   _____

8. Angelo Vila, a 75-year-old male, was diagnosed with angina decubitus with hypertension.

   _____

9. Kathy Griffo, a 41-year-old obese female, was diagnosed with hyperpiesia.

   _____

10. Dennis Timmons, a 63-year-old male, came to see Dr. Maricella because he was not feeling well. Dennis was diagnosed with hypertension 2 years ago, and over the last week his medication didn't appear to be working. Dr. Maricella diagnosed Dennis with uncontrolled hypertension and wrote a new prescription.

_____

11. Rhoda Grindstaff, an 81-year-old female, has been seeing Dr. Sesna for several years. She is now diagnosed with congestive heart failure due to hypertension.

_____

12. Gary Allen, a 59-year-old male, has been diagnosed with retinopathy due to benign hypertension, controlled.

_____

13. Melinda Monahan, a 49-year-old female, has been diagnosed with benign hypertensive renal failure with stage 3 chronic kidney disease.

_____

14. Gray Morrisetti, a 77-year-old male, was brought into the emergency department (ED) by ambulance. Dr. Archer diagnosed him with vertebrobasilar artery syndrome.

_____

15. Lorelei Manning, a 33-year-old female, was rushed to the hospital after her CT scan showed a nonruptured cerebral aneurysm.

_____

YOU CODE IT! Application
Chapter 12: Coding Circulatory Conditions

The following exercises provide practice in abstracting physicians' notes and learning to work with SOAP notes from our health care facility, *Taylor, Reader, & Associates*. These case studies (SOAP notes) are modeled on real patient encounters. Using the techniques described in this chapter, carefully read through the case studies and determine the most accurate ICD-10-CM code(s) and external cause code(s), if appropriate, for each case study.

TAYLOR, READER, & ASSOCIATES
A Complete Health Care Facility
975 CENTRAL AVENUE • SOMEWHERE, FL 32811 • 407-555-4321

PATIENT: CHEN, MELONIE
ACCOUNT/EHR #:   CHENME001
DATE: 08/11/18

Attending Physician: Willard B. Reader, MD

S: Pt is an 81-year-old female who suffered a stroke last week. Her daughter is concerned about the patient's dysphasia. Evidently her speech has been impaired as a result of the stroke. The daughter notes that the patient has been unable to speak properly, having trouble forming sentences and finding the right word.

O: Ht 5′1″ Wt. 135 lb. R 19. T 98.6. BP 145/93 Physical examination: unremarkable.

A: Dysphasia, late effect of a CVA.

P: 1. Pt to return PRN
   2. Referral to physical therapist

Willard B. Reader, MD

WBR/pw   D: 08/11/18 09:50:16   T: 08/13/18 12:55:01

Determine the most accurate ICD-10-CM code(s).

_____

_____

_____

TAYLOR, READER, & ASSOCIATES
A Complete Health Care Facility
975 CENTRAL AVENUE • SOMEWHERE, FL 32811 • 407-555-4321

PATIENT:	JACKELLSOHN, BRANDON
ACCOUNT/EHR #:	JACKBR002
DATE:	11/04/18

ADMITTING DIAGNOSES: Deep venous thrombosis (DVT) right leg
Urinary tract infection (UTI)
Parkinson's disease

FINAL DIAGNOSES: Acute DVT, right
UTI
Parkinson's disease

HOSPITAL COURSE: The patient had presented to the office with pain in right leg, discomfort, and also some foul-smelling urine. He was evaluated, and Doppler studies of the leg confirmed DVT suggestive of infection. The patient was started on Levaquin and Lovenox subcu 1 mg per kg twice a day, and in 2 days the patient was symptomatic both with his urinary symptoms and with pain in the calf. His physical examination revealed his vital signs stable. He is afebrile. Lungs clear. Heart rhythm regular.

Neurologic examination: Tremors and rigidity secondary to Parkinson's disease. Rest is unremarkable. His Doppler studies were positive for right popliteal vein thrombosis and some flow abnormalities in superficial femoral vein. He did have a pelvic sonogram suggesting an enlarged prostate and questionable intraluminal. Kidney showed normal right kidneys. Simple cyst lower pole of left kidney. His symptoms improved.

PT, INR on the day of discharge was 14.4 and 1.1 His UA was positive for blood, negative for leukocyte esterase, nitrites, and WBC. His CHEM-7 showed sodium of 140, potassium 4.1, chloride 102, CO_2 31, sugar 112, BUN 15 and creatinine 0.9. WBC 5,300, H&H 15.5 and 45.8. Platelets 116,000. He was discharged home.

DISPOSITION: Arrange for home health.

Arrange for follow-up with his primary physician in 1 week. He will need patient evaluation for repeat urine and possible urology consultation for prostate and questionable bladder mass.

Suzanne R. Taylor, MD

SRT/pw   D: 11/04/18 09:50:16   T: 11/07/18 12:55:01

Determine the most accurate ICD-10-CM code(s).

_____

_____

_____

TAYLOR, READER, & ASSOCIATES
A Complete Health Care Facility
975 CENTRAL AVENUE • SOMEWHERE, FL 32811 • 407-555-4321

PATIENT: FRONNETH, VALERIE
ACCOUNT/EHR #: FRONVA001
DATE: 08/21/18

Attending Physician: Willard B. Reader, MD

S: Pt is a 61-year-old female who comes in today complaining of syncope, angina, and dyspnea. She states that the symptoms began approximately 5 days ago. Pt has essential hypertension, diagnosed 2 years ago. She has been successful in keeping the hypertension under control with diet and exercise.

O: Ht 5'7" Wt. 173 lb. R 18. T 98.6. BP 155/95 Blood tests, UA, CBC, and EKG are ordered. Results indicate the development of renal sclerosis (stage 5) with benign hypertension. Evidence also shows left ventricular failure and acute systolic heart failure.

A: Renal sclerosis with benign hypertension; left ventricular failure and acute systolic heart failure

P: 1. Pt to return PRN
   2. Referral for renal dialysis evaluation

Willard B. Reader, MD

WBR/pw   D: 08/21/18 09:50:16   T: 08/23/18 12:55:01

Determine the most accurate ICD-10-CM code(s).

_____

_____

_____

TAYLOR, READER, & ASSOCIATES
A Complete Health Care Facility
975 CENTRAL AVENUE • SOMEWHERE, FL 32811 • 407-555-4321

PATIENT: HARRIS, FELIX
ACCOUNT/EHR #:   HARRFE001
DATE: 08/23/18

Attending Physician: Willard B. Reader, MD

S: Pt is a 57-year-old male coming in to discuss the results of testing done 2 days ago at our imaging center.

O: Ht 5′7″ Wt. 173 lb. R 18. T 98.6. BP 155/95 I explain to the patient and his wife that the test results show a narrowing of the basilar, carotid, and vertebral arteries on his left side. Stricture of these arteries branching into the brain is shown to be the cause of the symptoms he discussed with me at our last encounter, including headaches, dizziness, and reduced mental acuity. Currently, there is no cerebral infarction. We discussed a variety of treatment options, and they both agreed to a referral for a surgical consult to investigate the insertion of a shunt.

A: Stenosis of precerebral arteries, including the basilar, carotid, and vertebral arteries

P: 1. Pt to return PRN
   2. Referral for surgical consult for shunt placement

_____

Willard B. Reader, MD

WBR/pw   D: 08/23/18 09:50:16   T: 08/28/18 12:55:01

Determine the most accurate ICD-10-CM code(s).

_____

_____

_____

TAYLOR, READER, & ASSOCIATES
A Complete Health Care Facility
975 CENTRAL AVENUE • SOMEWHERE, FL 32811 • 407-555-4321

PATIENT: SCHOLAL, AMIR
ACCOUNT/EHR #:   SCHOAM001
DATE: 08/03/18

Attending Physician: Willard B. Reader, MD

Pt is a 59-year-old male who entered the hospital because of weakness, dry mouth, no energy. The patient claimed that he has been very weak, drinking water, but has not been passing enough water. His blood pressure was elevated, and he has been having pain in the left side of the face.

PMH: In 2008, he had a segment of coccyx removed. He had bladder suspension operation in 1995 and has a history of arrhythmias.

    The patient has been placed in the past on Norpace and Pronestyl. He was changed to Tenormin. The patient has had trouble with some swelling of the ankles.

    The electrocardiogram shows a sinus rhythm with premature ventricular contractions.

FH: The family history is contributory by longevity. Father died of stroke. There is a lot of cancer in the family.

CURRENT MEDICATIONS: Inderal; Ativan; Zestril

ALLERGIES: NKA

FINAL DIAGNOSES:
    1. Acute myocardial infarction—anterior wall
    2. Systemic arterial hypertension
    3. Cardiomegaly with chronic systolic CHF
    4. Cardiac arrhythmia

Willard B. Reader, MD

WBR/pw   D: 08/03/18 09:50:16   T: 08/05/18 12:55:01

Determine the most accurate ICD-10-CM code(s).

_____

_____

_____

CODING RESPIRATORY CONDITIONS

13

Learning Outcomes *After completing this chapter, the student should be able to:*

LO 13.1 Identify the components of the respiratory system.

LO 13.2 Discern the various underlying causes of respiratory disorders.

LO 13.3 Accurately code any involvement of tobacco in the patient's respiratory disorder.

LO 13.4 Determine the details needed to code pneumonia and influenza correctly.

LO 13.5 Accurately code chronic obstructive pulmonary disease (COPD) diagnoses and manifestations.

LO 13.6 Determine the appropriate use of external codes when applicable to respiratory conditions.

As you know, breathing is a crucial part of life; the average person breathes approximately 25,000 times each day. The human body accomplishes this function via the respiratory system that is designed to process oxygen (O_2) and carbon dioxide (CO_2). The respiratory system includes many anatomical sites, beginning with the nose and continuing down the windpipe to the lungs and the bronchi. The central nervous system controls respiration from the lateral medulla oblongata of the brainstem.

Respiration is the term used for what is commonly known as breathing and consists of two parts: **inspiration** (bringing oxygen into the body and delivering it into the circulatory system, which then distributes the oxygen to the cells throughout the body), and **expiration** (getting rid of carbon dioxide).

LO 13.1 Anatomy of the Respiratory System

The respiratory system is referred to in two segments: the upper respiratory system and the lower respiratory system (see Figure 13-1).

The Upper Respiratory System

The upper respiratory system includes the nose, nasal cavity, nasal conchae, paranasal sinuses, internal nares, nasopharynx, and the pharynx.

The respiratory system begins with your nose. Even though many people breathe through their mouths, the oral cavity is officially part of the digestive system and not the respiratory system. When you breathe in (inspire) through your nose, the air will pass in through your external nares (commonly known as *nostrils*) and travel into the nasal cavity, a hollow area behind the nose, which is laterally separated by the **nasal septum,** creating the right and left nasal cavities. Have you ever heard of someone diagnosed with a *deviated septum* (code J34.2, Deviated nasal septum)?

Key Terms

Alveolar sac
Bronchi
Bronchioles
Chronic obstructive
    pulmonary disease (COPD)
Diaphragm
Epiglottis
Exacerbation
Expiration
Influenza
Inspiration
Larynx
Lungs
Nasal septum
Paranasal sinuses
Pleura
Pneumonia
Pneumothorax
Respiration
Respiratory disorder
Status asthmaticus
Trachea

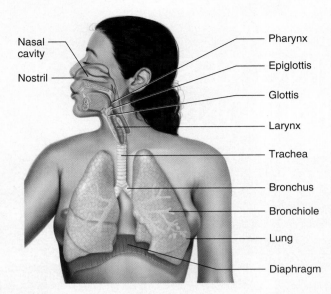

FIGURE 13-1 The Respiratory System

Source: Booth et al., MA, 5e. Copyright © 2013 by McGraw-Hill. Figure 29-1 (a), p. 582

In that condition, this nasal divider is bent and therefore does not separate the cavity equally right and left. When one side is narrower, it is more difficult to bring in the necessary quantity of air and oxygen. The smallest amount of swelling or mucous buildup can cause a total blockage. To repair this condition, a procedure called a *rhinoplasty* (*rhino* = nose + *plasty* = repair) is performed.

The **paranasal sinuses** (see Figure 13-2), air-filled cavities within the skull above and behind the nose, are lined with a mucous membrane. The maxillary, frontal, ethmoidal, and sphenoidal sinuses are included in this group. The air continues to flow down, entering the pharyngeal area, commonly known as the *throat*. The pharynx begins behind the nose (the nasopharynx) and continues down behind the oral cavity (the oropharynx) to the laryngopharynx (near the larynx).

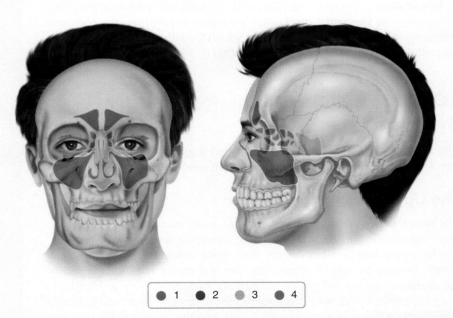

● 1   ● 2   ● 3   ● 4

FIGURE 13-2 Paranasal Sinuses: (1) frontal sinuses, (2) ethmoid sinuses (ethmoidal air cells), (3) sphenoid sinuses, (4) maxillary sinuses

This is the journey air and oxygen travel from the nose through the upper respiratory tract to the larynx—the beginning of the lower respiratory tract.

EXAMPLE

J32.0 Chronic maxillary sinusitis
J33.0 Polyp of nasal cavity

LET'S CODE IT! SCENARIO

Gayle Permanente, a 19-year-old female, was feeling very congested in her chest and was having trouble breathing. She went to see Dr. Matlock at the school clinic. After a complete PE and blood tests, he diagnosed her with an acute upper respiratory infection.

Let's Code It!

Dr. Matlock diagnosed Gayle with *acute upper respiratory infection.* In the Alphabetic Index, turn to *infection, respiratory, upper,* and find:

Infection
Respiratory (tract) NEC J98.8
Upper (acute) NOS J06.9

Turn to code J06 in the Tabular List, and check the description:

J06 Acute upper respiratory infections of multiple or unspecified sites

Read the *Excludes1* note. Does it relate to Gayle's diagnosis? No, so keep reading down the column. Which fourth character best reports Gayle's condition?

J06.9 Acute upper respiratory infection, unspecified

Good job!

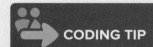

CODING TIP

Why is this unspecified code description acceptable? In this code description, "unspecified" means that there is no confirmation of exactly where in the upper respiratory system the infection is located. Take a look again at the list of anatomical sites included in the upper respiratory system and you can see that this is reasonable.

The Lower Respiratory System

The lower respiratory system includes the larynx, trachea, bronchi, lungs, bronchioles, and alveoli.

The **epiglottis** sits on top of the **larynx** (which includes the thyroid and cricoid cartilage, also referred to as the *rima glottidis*). The epiglottis is a flap of cartilage that opens to permit air to travel into the larynx and closes to prevent food particles and liquids from entering the larynx and ultimately the lungs. Food particles in the lungs can create severe breathing problems and can provide a breeding ground for bacteria that cause infection.

The air continues through the larynx into the **trachea.** At a point, approximately at the center of the chest (thoracic cavity), the trachea forks into two parts, identified as the left and right primary **bronchi.** The bronchi enter the left and right lungs, respectively, and continue to branch out into smaller **bronchioles.** Each bronchiole branches out into a smaller tubelike structure called the *alveolar duct* that ends with the **alveolar sac.** The sacs are surrounded by a fishnetlike network of capillaries from the pulmonary vein and pulmonary artery to enable the exchange of gases (oxygen and carbon dioxide)—the primary purpose of the respiratory system.

epiglottis
A flap made of cartilage that covers the superior end of the larynx.

larynx
A tubular organ that connects from the pharynx to the trachea; commonly known as the voice box.

trachea
Tubular membrane that connects the larynx to the bronchi; commonly known as the windpipe.

bronchi
Bilateral air passageways that connect the trachea to the lungs.

bronchioles
Bilateral tubes, small branches of the bronchi, leading to the air sacs.

alveolar sac
A tiny bubble, grouped in clusters at the end of each bronchiole, that holds air.

lungs
Bilateral lobed organs that function like balloons, expanding on inspiration and deflating on expiration.

This structure is similar to the branches of a tree. The trachea is like the trunk of a tree, branching out its limbs (the bronchi). Each limb then has its branches (the bronchioles), whose twigs (the alveolar ducts) blossom with buds (the alveolar sacs).

The **lungs,** located in the lower respiratory tract, are within the thoracic cavity and represent the largest portion of the respiratory system. The ribs form a protective cage around the lungs, meeting at the sternum in the anterior medial (front center) of the thorax. The diaphragm sits inferior to the lungs.

EXAMPLE

J04.10 Acute tracheitis without obstruction
J21.1 Acute bronchiolitis due to human metapneumovirus

The Lungs As you can see in Figure 13-3, the lungs are composed of two hemispheres: the right lung and the left lung. The right lung is subdivided into three segments: the superior lobe, the middle lobe, and the inferior lobe. The superior lobe is posterior to the first rib and the top of the sternum. It is separated from the middle lobe by the horizontal fissure. The middle lobe is behind the fifth rib, and the seventh rib protects the distal end of the inferior lobe. These two lobes (middle and inferior) are separated by the right oblique fissure. The left lung has only two lobes: the superior and the inferior. The left oblique fissure (an angular crack) separates these lobes.

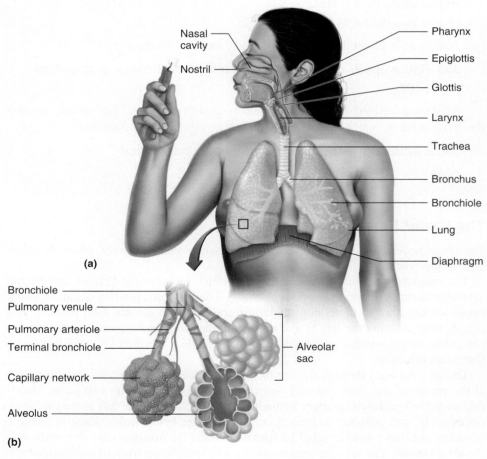

FIGURE 13-3 The Lungs

Source: Booth et al., MA, 5e. Copyright © 2013 by McGraw-Hill. Figure 29-1 (a), p. 582

The exterior surface of the lungs is covered by the *visceral* **pleura,** the inner layer of a lubricated membrane, and the *parietal* pleura along the inside of the chest wall. This lubrication (slippery fluid), which is contained in the intrapleural space, hinders friction between the internal surface of the ribs and the lungs when they expand after inhalation.

pleura
A double-layered membrane that envelops the lungs and lines the chest wall.

EXAMPLE

J90 Pleural effusion not elsewhere classified

Diaphragm Along the inferior aspect of the lungs lies the **diaphragm** (see Figure 13-4). This is a membrane, fortified with muscle, that separates the thoracic and abdominal cavities. In addition to being a divider, the diaphragm assists with respiration. During inspiration, the diaphragm contracts and shifts downward, providing more room for the lungs to expand and take in more air. Once inspiration is complete, the diaphragm slackens and the lungs return to their natural shape and size.

diaphragm
A transverse muscle that divides the torso between the chest and the abdomen; its motion aids respiration.

Respiratory Disorders

Respiratory disorders can be caused by many things, including trauma, genetics, environmental concerns, congenital anomalies, and infection. Regardless of the underlying cause, having difficulty bringing oxygen into the lungs and getting carbon dioxide out of the body can interfere with the patient's quality of life—and, actually, the ability to live life at all.

respiratory disorder
A malfunction of the organ system relating to respiration.

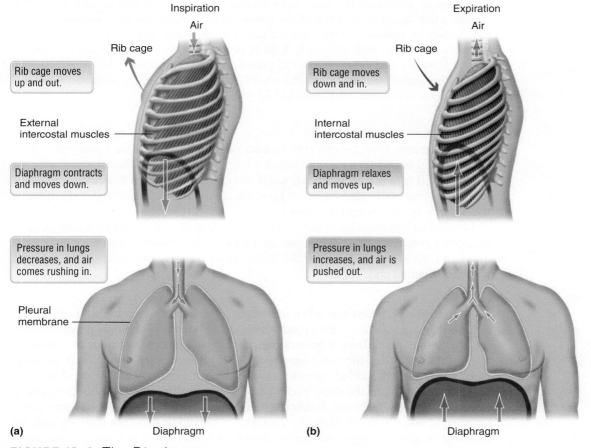

FIGURE 13-4 The Diaphragm

Source: Booth et al., MA, 5e. Copyright © 2013 by McGraw-Hill. Figure 29-3, p. 584

LO 13.2 Underlying Causes of Respiratory Disorders

As stated earlier in this section, respiratory conditions can have many different causes. Some of these causes are discussed below.

Congenital Anomalies Respiratory distress and cyanosis are the two most frequent manifestations of congenital anomalies of the lungs, usually identified within the child's first 24 months. The most common congenital respiratory disorder is *pulmonary hypoplasia,* a situation in which the lung does not form completely or forms improperly. When you are reporting this condition, ICD-10-CM requires you to determine from the documentation whether the pulmonary hypoplasia is a result of short gestation (i.e., prematurity), reported with code P28.0, Primary atelectasis of newborn (pulmonary hypoplasia associated with short gestation), or not—reported with code Q33.6, Congenital hypoplasia and dysplasia of lung.

The most common cause of neonate mortality is respiratory distress syndrome (RDS) and is seen most often in premature births. RDS can be fatal within 72 hours if not treated. Mechanical ventilation improves patient outcomes. Idiopathic RDS is reported with code P22.0 for a *newborn* or code J80 for *acute RDS in a child or adult patient.* Remember, the definition of a neonate (newborn) is one who is age 28 days or younger.

Genetic Disorders Alpha-1 antitrypsin deficiency is a genetic condition that may cause respiratory dysfunction as well as liver disease. Individuals with an alpha-1 antitrypsin deficiency often will develop emphysema, with the first signs and symptoms appearing in adulthood (between ages 20 and 50). Cystic fibrosis is another genetic condition that causes malfunction of the mucous glands and results in progressive damage to the lungs. A mutation of the BMPR2 gene causes pulmonary arterial hypertension, a genetic condition with extremely high hypertension specifically in the pulmonary artery. Dyspnea and fainting are symptoms of this condition. *Primary pulmonary arterial hypertension* is reported with code I27.0, while *secondary pulmonary arterial hypertension* is reported with code I27.2.

Manifestations of Another Disease Measles, as well as the adenovirus, may cause obliterative bronchiolitis (J44.9). Left-sided heart failure can cause pulmonary edema (J81.0 or J81.1), an accumulation of fluid in the lung. The administration of diuretics will help reduce the fluid, while vasodilators are given to decrease vascular resistance. High concentrations of oxygen, via cannula or facemask, will help improve the delivery of oxygen into the tissues.

Pleurisy, an inflammation of the parietal and visceral pleurae, is usually a complication of another condition, such as pneumonia, lupus erythematosus, pulmonary infarction, trauma to the chest, or tuberculosis. *Tuberculous pleurisy,* for example, is reported with combination code A15.6.

Trauma Car accidents and other activities can result in trauma to the chest, throat, or nose that can interfere with a patient's ability to breathe. Traumatic pneumothorax (S27.0xx-) may result from a penetrating chest wound or can occur due to a medical misadventure during the insertion of a central venous line or thoracic surgery. During a pneumothorax, air accumulates between the parietal and visceral pleurae, reducing the space in the chest cavity and thereby limiting the room the lungs have to expand during inhalation. When the lungs cannot expand properly, oxygen cannot be brought down into the lungs far enough, so breathing becomes difficult and the exchange of gases (oxygen and carbon dioxide) is hindered. Blunt trauma to the chest, or a penetrating wound, can also cause hemothorax, in which blood (instead of air, as in pneumothorax) fills the pleural cavity. Report this condition with code J94.2, Hemothorax.

Environment Whether the element is natural, such as volcanic dust from an erupting volcano or dander from cats, or human-made, such as asbestos in the ceiling (J61), respiratory dysfunction can be caused by the world around us. Legionnaires' disease, an aerobic Gram-negative bacillus, is transmitted through the air—for example, through air-conditioning systems (J67.7). Men are more susceptible than women. Administration of antibiotics, specifically erythromycin, is the primary treatment, along with fluid replacement and oxygen administration, if necessary. When a patient is diagnosed with coal worker's pneumoconiosis, another environmentally caused lung disease, this is reported with code J60, Coal worker's pneumoconiosis, along with code Y92.64, Mine or pit as the place of occurrence of the external cause, and Y99.0, Civilian activity done for income or pay.

Lung Infections Both bacteria and viruses can cause respiratory disorders. Bacterial pneumonia (J15.-), community-acquired pneumonia, nosocomial (originating in a hospital) pneumonia, viral pneumonia (J12.-), and opportunistic pneumonia (affecting individuals with compromised immunities) are common examples of respiratory infection. In addition, bronchitis (inflammation of the bronchi) (J20.-) and influenza (J09.- or J10.-) are also frequently seen, particularly in children and the elderly. Viruses affecting the pulmonary parenchyma result in interstitial pneumonia (J84.9). Mycobacterium tuberculosis, acquired by inhaling aerosols, has been seen more often in the last several years, especially in patients who are HIV-positive and have developed AIDS. When an HIV-positive patient is diagnosed with tuberculosis affecting the lungs, this condition would be reported with code B20, HIV, followed by code A15.0, Tuberculosis of the lung.

Lifestyle Behaviors Smoking cigars and cigarettes is known to cause respiratory disorders, including lung cancer. In addition, sedentary lifestyles can encourage the creation of thrombi in the legs. What does that have to do with the lungs? A dislodged thrombus becomes an embolus that can travel through the pulmonary artery into the lungs, becoming a pulmonary embolus. An acute pulmonary embolism NOS is reported with code I26.99; however, several other details are required for a complete code.

LO 13.3 Tobacco Involvement

One set of elements that has become required is the reporting of tobacco use, abuse, and/or dependence. For example, at the start of ICD-10-CM Chapter 10, Diseases of the respiratory system (J00–J99), there is a notation that applies to all codes within:

> **Use additional code, where applicable, to identify:**
> **Exposure to environmental tobacco smoke (Z77.22)**
> **Exposure to tobacco smoke in the perinatal period (P96.81)**
> **History of tobacco use (Z87.891)**
> **Occupational exposure to environmental tobacco smoke (Z57.31)**
> **Tobacco dependence (F17.-)**
> **Tobacco use (Z72.0)**

Surely you know that tobacco use can be a risk factor to the development of respiratory illness. ICD-10-CM makes it easier to collect data on tobacco use. To do so, you need to understand what the terms *exposure, use, abuse, dependence,* and *history* really mean.

- *Exposure* means that the patient has been in contact with, or in close proximity to, a source of tobacco smoke in such a way that the harmful effects of this agent may impact the patient. When it comes to health care issues, this would apply to an individual who does not use tobacco products but lives or works with someone who smokes, resulting in the patient's breathing in secondhand tobacco smoke on an ongoing basis. If this individual develops a respiratory disease as a result of this environment, you would include a code to report this exposure.

EXAMPLE

Z77.22 Contact with and (suspected) exposure to environmental tobacco smoke (acute)(chronic)[Exposure to second hand tobacco smoke]

- *Use* is the term that identifies that the patient smokes tobacco on a regular basis, taken by his or her own initiative, even though the substance is known to be a detriment to one's health. There are no obvious clinical manifestations.

EXAMPLE

V72.0 Tobacco use

- *Abuse* describes the patient's habitual smoking of tobacco, taken by his or her own initiative, even though the substance is known to be a detriment to one's health. Clinical manifestations are evident as signs and symptoms develop. The patient deals with a daily fixation on obtaining and smoking tobacco with virtually everything else in life becoming secondary.

EXAMPLE

F17.218 Nicotine dependence, cigarettes, with other nicotine-induced disorders

- *Dependence* indicates the patient's compulsive, continuous smoking of tobacco that has resulted in significant clinical manifestations as well as the physiological need for the substance to function normally. Any interruption results in signs and symptoms of withdrawal, occurring within a continuous 12-month time frame.

EXAMPLE

F17.220 Nicotine dependence, chewing tobacco, uncomplicated

- *History* describes a patient who has successfully quit using tobacco products.

EXAMPLE

Z87.891 Personal history of tobacco dependence

Diagnostic Testing

Imaging of the chest is often the first diagnostic test when a respiratory concern arises. In addition to an x-ray, under certain conditions the physician may also order a computed tomography (CT) scan, angiography, magnetic resonance angiography (MRA), positron emission tomography (PET), or an ultrasound to provide imaging of the lower respiratory tract. Lung scans (scintiphotography) check ventilation and perfusion in order to assess the presence of a pulmonary embolus, but a pulmonary artery angiography, which locates a pulmonary embolus by injecting dye into the pulmonary artery, is considered the gold-standard test for this purpose.

Endoscopic diagnostic procedures, such as a bronchoscopy or a mediastinoscopy, can be helpful because the physician can view the area directly, excise tissue for a biopsy, or wash to remove secretions. A sputum culture can be taken using tracheal aspiration or a natural contraction (cough). A thoracentesis uses a long needle to remove fluid from the pleura for pathologic assessment.

Pulmonary function tests measure lung volume and flow rates. A spirometer may be used to document the volume of air brought in during inspiration and expelled during expiration. A peak flow meter permits a tangible determination of the greatest flow of air during forced expiration.

Arterial blood gas analysis evaluates the patient's ability to exchange gases (oxygen and carbon dioxide) within the lungs. Capnography can provide insights to identify $PaCO_2$ (partial pressure of arterial carbon dioxide), while oximetry measures O_2 saturation.

Pleural Disorders

The pleura is made up of two membranes: the visceral pleura—a thin membrane that coats the outside of the lung; and the parietal pleura—a membrane that lines the inside of the thoracic (chest) cavity. *Pleurisy,* also known as *pleuritis,* identifies the presence of inflammation on one or both of the pleural membranes. This condition can cause pain to the patient with each breath. A virus is most often the cause. To report pleurisy, the Alphabetic Index provides a long list of possibilities that lead to a surprisingly short number of codes:

A15.6 Tuberculous pleurisy

J10.1 Influenza due to other identified influenza virus with other respiratory manifestations

R09.1 Pleurisy

J90 Pleurisy with effusion, not elsewhere classified

S27.63XA Injury to the pleura, laceration of pleura, initial encounter

(*Note:* Of course, you remember that with code S27.63XA an external cause code should be reported to identify how the injury happened, as well as the place of occurrence.)

The very narrow space between the two pleural membranes is referred to as the *pleural space* or *pleural cavity.* Normally, this space contains a tiny amount of fluid, just enough to enable the visceral pleura and the parietal pleura to move and function without irritation. If excess air or fluid gets into this space, it can cause pressure on the lung and prevent the patient from inhaling because the lung does not have the room required to expand as the oxygen is brought in. Pleural space disorders include:

Pleural effusion: The presence of excess fluid in the pleural cavity, frequently a manifestation of congestive heart failure.

J94.0 Other pleural effusion

J91.0 Malignant pleural effusion

P28.89 Newborn pleural effusion

Pneumothorax: The presence of excess air or gases in the pleural space, typically caused by respiratory disease such as chronic obstructive pulmonary disorder (COPD) or tuberculosis (TB).

pneumothorax
A condition in which air or gas is present within the chest cavity but outside the lungs.

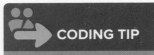
J93.81 Chronic pneumothorax

J86.9 Pyothorax without fistula (empyema) [an infection within the pleural space]

Hemothorax: An accumulation of blood in the pleural cavity, most often caused by an injury to the thoracic cavity (the chest).

J94.2 Hemothorax

Pulmonary Embolism

As you probably remember, an embolus is the medical term for a blood clot (thrombus) or other tiny piece of bone marrow fat (most often created by high cholesterol) that travels within the bloodstream. During its passage through the body, this embolus can get stuck in an artery and block the flow of blood through that area. When this occurs in the lungs, it is called a *pulmonary embolism.*

The presence of a pulmonary embolism can create serious problems for the patient, including dyspnea (shortness of breath), pain, and/or hemoptysis (coughing up blood). Over the course of time, a pulmonary embolism can result in permanent damage to the lung as well as damage to the organs being denied oxygen because of the blockage. A pulmonary embolism can also cause an infarction (necrotic tissue) due to the lack of oxygen to the cells. A large clot, or cluster of several clots, can result in the patient's death.

I26.02 Saddle embolus of pulmonary artery with acute cor pulmonale

I27.82 Chronic pulmonary embolism

LET'S CODE IT! SCENARIO

Gray Silverheels, a 3-year-old male, was brought to his pediatrician, Dr. Hancock, with an odd-sounding cough and chest congestion. He had the measles just a short time prior. After a complete PE and the appropriate tests, Dr. Hancock diagnosed Gray with the croup.

Let's Code It!

Gray was diagnosed with *the croup.* Let's turn to the Alphabetic Index:

Croup, croupous (catarrhal) (infective) (inflammatory) (nondiphtheritic) J05.0

The Tabular List confirms:

J05 Acute obstructive laryngitis [croup] and epiglottitis

You can see a *use additional code* notation beneath this code category directing you to "identify the infectious agent." Notice that *croup* is included, in brackets. This is the common term for the medical diagnosis of acute obstructive laryngitis. However, this is not what Gray was diagnosed with, so keep reading down the column to review the choices for the required fourth character:

J05.0 Acute obstructive laryngitis

Good job!

Infectious Respiratory Diseases

Respiratory Syncytial Virus Infections

While most adults and teenagers suffer only mild symptoms (similar to a cold), respiratory syncytial virus infection (RSV) can cause serious problems for infants. Similar to other infectious diseases, RSV can be spread from person to person by touching an infected person or by coming in contact with an infected object like a toy or a tabletop. Upon infection, infants can have difficulty breathing, a stuffy nose, and fever. RSV is actually the pathogen that causes respiratory illness in young children such as pneumonia or acute bronchitis.

B97 Viral agents as the cause of diseases classified elsewhere

Read down the column to review your choices for the required fourth character.

B97.4 Respiratory syncytial virus (RSV) as the cause of diseases classified elsewhere

This code looks perfect except for one thing. Did you read the note directly above code B95 that states:

> NOTE: These categories are provided for use as supplementary or additional codes to identify the infection agent(s) in diseases classified elsewhere.

So, if the notes state that the child has pneumonia due to RSV, you would first list the pneumonia followed by B97.4.

Pulmonary Fibrosis

Fibrosis is the creation of extra fibrous tissue (also known as *scar tissue*) in response to inflammation or irritation. When this abnormal process occurs in the lungs, it is called *pulmonary fibrosis*. This development of thickened tissue reduces the flexibility of the lung sac, making it harder for the lungs to expand with inspiration and contract for expiration. Idiopathic pulmonary fibrosis may also be referred to as cryptogenic fibrosing alveolitis, diffuse interstitial fibrosis, idiopathic interstitial pneumonitis, and Hamman-Rich syndrome.

Pulmonary fibrosis may be caused by another disease, such as tuberculosis, or develop as a result of debris inhaled from an environment, such as the dust that may be breathed in by sand blasters or coal miners during their work. Pulmonary fibrosis is also associated as a side effect of certain medications.

J84.10 Pulmonary fibrosis, unspecified

YOU CODE IT! CASE STUDY

Tyrell Watermann, a 59-year-old male, has been suffering with chronic inflammation of his left bronchus. He admits to previous crack cocaine use, but denies current use. He complains of a dry, hacking, paroxysmal cough and occasional dyspnea lasting at least 5 months. Chest x-ray and pulmonary function tests lead Dr. Zachman to diagnose Tyrell with idiopathic pulmonary fibrosis due to mucopurulent chronic bronchitis. Tyrell is placed on oxygen therapy immediately.

You Code It!

Go through the steps of coding, and determine the diagnosis code or codes that should be reported for this encounter between Dr. Zachman and Tyrell Watermann.

Step 1: Read the case completely.

Step 2: Abstract the notes: Which key words can you identify relating to why Dr. Zachman cared for Tyrell?

_____

Step 3: Query the provider, if necessary.

Step 4: Code the diagnosis or diagnoses.

_____

Step 5: Code the procedure(s): Office visit.

Step 6: Link the procedure codes to at least one diagnosis code to confirm medical necessity.

Step 7: Back code to double-check your choices.

Answer:

Did you determine the correct codes?

J84.112 Idiopathic pulmonary fibrosis

J41.1 Mucopurulent chronic bronchitis

Terrific!

LO 13.4 Pneumonia and Influenza

Pneumonia

pneumonia
An inflammation of the lungs.

Pneumonia is a serious infection of the lung parenchyma (tissue) and typically hinders the exchange of gases. When an individual with normal, healthy lungs contracts pneumonia, the expectation of a complete recovery is good. However, early treatment is important. Even with this good news, pneumonia is one of the top 10 leading causes of death in the United States. A virus, bacterium, fungus, or other type of protozoan can cause pneumonia. You have to know which type of pneumonia the patient has contracted in order to code it accurately.

VIRAL PNEUMONIA

- Influenza
- Adenovirus
- Respiratory syncytial virus
- Measles (rubeola)
- Chickenpox (varicella)
- Cytomegalovirus

BACTERIAL PNEUMONIA

- Streptococcus (*Streptococcus pneumoniae*)
- Klebsiella
- Staphylococcus

PROTOZOAN PNEUMONIA

- *Pneumocystis carinii*

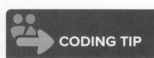

CODING TIP

Note that these examples of pneumonia codes are both combination codes reporting both the condition (pneumonia) and the pathogen (adenovirus or Klebsiella). Not all pneumonia codes are combination codes, so you may need to remember to use an additional code to identify the pathogen.

Aspiration pneumonia is a specific type of condition that results from the patient vomiting and then inhaling gastric or oropharyngeal contents into the trachea and/or lungs.

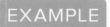

> J12.0 Adenoviral pneumonia
> J15.0 Pneumonia due to Klebsiella pneumoniae

Influenza

Influenza, the formal term for what is commonly known as the *flu* or the *grippe,* is a highly contagious and serious illness. It is a respiratory tract infection that can affect individuals of all ages, but is most dangerous to young children, the elderly, and those who have chronic diseases, because these individuals have immune systems that are more sensitive and more susceptible. To code a diagnosis of influenza correctly, you have to know what virus is involved:

influenza
An acute infection of the respiratory tract caused by the influenza virus.

> J09- Influenza due to certain identified influenza viruses
> J10- Influenza due to other identified influenza virus
> J11- Influenza due to unidentified influenza virus

Pneumonia as a Manifestation of HIV

In some cases, pneumonia *may be* a manifestation of HIV infection. Therefore, if the notes report that the patient has also been diagnosed with HIV-positive status, you have to include:

> B20 Human immunodeficiency virus (HIV) disease

Code B20 should be listed first, followed by the appropriate pneumonia code. There are other types of pneumonia that may have other underlying diseases. Read the notations carefully.

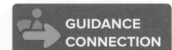

GUIDANCE CONNECTION

Review the ICD-10-CM Coding Guidelines, Section I.C.10, Chapter 10: **Diseases of the respiratory system,** Subsection c, **Influenza due to avian influenza virus (avian influenza)**.

LET'S CODE IT! SCENARIO

Mason Dominey, a 15-year-old male, came to see Dr. Siplin with a complaint of a sore throat, fever, cough, chills, and malaise. Dr. Siplin examined Mason, took a chest x-ray, and did a WBC count. After reviewing the results of the exam and tests, Dr. Siplin diagnosed Mason with adenovirus pneumonia.

Let's Code It!

Dr. Siplin identified Mason's health concern as *adenovirus pneumonia*. The Alphabetic Index will direct you to:

> Pneumonia
>> Adenoviral J12.0

Will the Tabular List confirm that it is the correct code? Turn to:

> J12 Viral pneumonia, not elsewhere classified

There are no notations or directions, so keep reading to review all of the choices for the required fourth character:

> J12.0 Adenoviral pneumonia

You will remember that when there is an infectious organism involved, you must code it. Dr. Siplin's notes identify it as the adenovirus. Should you use an additional code or not?

Professional coding specialists are responsible for relating the entire story with all specific details applicable to the diagnosis. This one combination code tells both the condition *and* the infectious organism. There is no reason to provide a second code to repeat the same information. Therefore, the code on Mason's claim form will be J12.0 alone.

LO 13.5 Chronic Obstructive Pulmonary Disease

chronic obstructive pulmonary disease (COPD)
An ongoing obstruction of the airway.

One of the most common respiratory disorders that you may code is **chronic obstructive pulmonary disease (COPD).** It is estimated that as much as 10% of the world population over age 40 has a lung disorder that is parallel with COPD. COPD is distinguished by restricted airflow. It is not fully reversible and, therefore, is a leading cause of disability and death. Clinically, there are three types of COPD:

- Chronic bronchitis
- Emphysema
- Asthma

EXAMPLE

J40 Bronchitis, not specified as acute or chronic
J41 Simple and mucopurulent chronic bronchitis
J42 Unspecified chronic bronchitis
J43 Emphysema
J44 Other chronic obstructive pulmonary disease
J45 Asthma

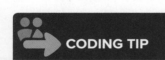

CODING TIP

Never, never, never, never code out of the Alphabetic Index. *Always* confirm the code by reading the complete description in the Tabular List.

The diagnoses in the COPD section can be particularly complex. You will need to be very diligent as you read the terms in the physician's notes and those included in the code descriptions. It is, as always, crucial that you refer to the index and then verify the code in the Tabular List.

LET'S CODE IT! SCENARIO

Peggy Newman, a 63-year-old female, quit smoking 2 years ago after a two-pack-a-day habit that lasted 40 years. She came to see Dr. Michaels with an insidious onset of dyspnea, tachypnea, and malaise. PE showed use of her accessory muscles for respiration. Dr. Michaels took a chest x-ray, EKG, RBC count, and pulmonary function test. The results directed a diagnosis of panlobular emphysema.

Let's Code It!

Dr. Michaels diagnosed Peggy with *panlobular emphysema*. The Alphabetic Index shows:

Emphysema

    Panlobular J43.1

Go to the Tabular List to confirm this code:

J43 Emphysema

Read the *use additional code* notation carefully, as well as the *Excludes1* note. Does either of them relate to Peggy's condition? Yes, the note to *use additional code* for "history of tobacco use" applies. First, keep reading and review all of the choices for the required fourth character:

J43.1 Panlobular emphysema

Now let's follow the lead to the code for "history of tobacco use." Turn to code Z87:

Z87 Personal history of other diseases and conditions
Z87.891 Personal history of nicotine dependence

Now you have two codes to report the story of why Dr. Michaels cared for Peggy:

J43.1 Panlobular emphysema
Z87.891 Personal history of nicotine dependence

Exacerbation and Status Asthmaticus

You may notice that some of the codes in this section have the designation for acute **exacerbation** of asthma, COPD, or other related condition. It is a clinical term and can be assigned only by the attending physician.

Acute exacerbation of asthma indicates an increase in the severe nature of a patient's asthmatic condition. The patient may be suffering from wheezing or shortness of breath, commonly called an *asthma attack*. **Status asthmaticus,** however, is a life-threatening condition and is a diagnosis indicating that the patient is not responding to therapeutic procedures. If a patient is diagnosed with status asthmaticus *and* COPD or acute bronchitis, the status asthmaticus should be the first-listed code. As a life-threatening condition, it is considered to be the diagnosis with the greatest severity and follows the sequencing rules that you learned earlier. In addition, status asthmaticus, being the more severe condition, will override an additional diagnosis of acute exacerbation of asthma.

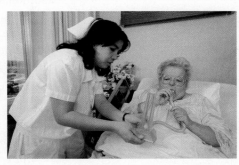
© Larry Mulvehill/Corbis

exacerbation
An increase in the severity of a disease or its symptoms.

status asthmaticus
The condition of asthma that is life-threatening and does not respond to therapeutic treatments.

LET'S CODE IT! SCENARIO

Nita Kinnerson, a 57-year-old female, has a history of intermittent dyspnea and wheezing. She comes today to see Dr. Hall with complaints of tachypnea, chest tightness, and a cough with thick mucus. The results of Dr. Hall's PE, the chest x-ray, sputum culture, EKG, pulmonary function tests, and an arterial blood gas analysis indicate moderate, persistent asthma with COPD, with exacerbation.

Let's Code It!

Dr. Hall's diagnosis of Nita's condition is *moderate, persistent asthma with COPD, with exacerbation.* This is also referred to as *chronic obstructive asthma.* Let's turn to the Alphabetic Index and look up:

Asthma
With

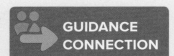

GUIDANCE CONNECTION

Review the ICD-10-CM Coding Guidelines, Section I.C.10, Chapter 10: **Diseases of the respiratory system,** Subsection a, **Chronic obstructive pulmonary disease (COPD) and asthma**.

Chronic obstructive pulmonary disease J44.9

> With
>
> > Exacerbation (acute) J44.1

That's great, it matches perfectly. Turn in the Tabular List to:

J44 Other chronic obstructive pulmonary disease

You can see "chronic obstructive asthma" in the INCLUDES list. Also notice the instruction to *code also* type of asthma, if applicable (J45.-).

First, let's look at the options for the fourth character for this first code:

J44.0 Chronic obstructive pulmonary disease with acute lower respiratory infection

J44.1 Chronic obstructive pulmonary disease with (acute) exacerbation

J44.9 Chronic obstructive pulmonary disease, unspecified

You can see that J44.1 matches. Terrific! Now let's turn to J45 to determine the additional code for the asthma.

Go back to Dr. Hall's notes and determine if Nita's asthma is documented as mild, moderate, or severe and if her condition is intermittent or persistent. Then match all of the options within code category J45 to determine which code is accurate:

J45.41 Moderate persistent asthma with (acute) exacerbation

One more detail to address: Certainly you saw the *use additional code* notation regarding tobacco exposure, use, dependence, or history. Is there documentation that Nita was a smoker? No! Good for her (and good for you). Now you have the codes to report this encounter:

J44.1 Chronic obstructive pulmonary disease with (acute) exacerbation

J45.41 Moderate persistent asthma with (acute) exacerbation

Good job!

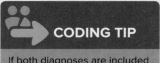

CODING TIP

If both diagnoses are included in the notes—status asthmaticus *and* acute exacerbation of asthma—use only one asthma code, for status asthmaticus. Do not use two asthma codes.

YOU CODE IT! CASE STUDY

Roger Samuels, a 57-year-old male, was brought into the emergency department (ED) by ambulance because he was having a severe asthma attack. His wife, Roxan, stated that he was diagnosed with asthma about 2 years prior. This attack began 5 days ago and has not responded to his inhaler, his regular asthma pills, or any other treatment. Dr. Hunter diagnosed Roger with acute exacerbation of late-onset severe, persistent asthma with status asthmaticus.

You Code It!

Go through the steps of coding, and determine the diagnosis code or codes that should be reported for this encounter between Dr. Hunter and Roger Samuels.

Step 1:   Read the case completely.

Step 2:   Abstract the notes: Which key words can you identify relating to why Dr. Hunter cared for Roger?

Step 3: Query the provider, if necessary.

Step 4: Code the diagnosis or diagnoses.

Step 5: Code the procedure(s): ED visit.

Step 6: Link the procedure codes to at least one diagnosis code to confirm medical necessity.

Step 7: Back code to double-check your choices.

Answer:

Did you determine the correct code?

J45.52 Severe persistent asthma with status asthmaticus

You are really getting good at this!

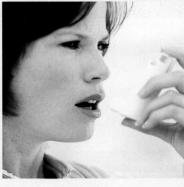

© Stockdisk/Punchstock

LO 13.6 Respiratory Conditions Requiring External Cause Codes

Earlier in this text, you learned about external cause codes and how to determine whether they are necessary. There are respiratory conditions that may require external cause codes to explain how, and sometimes where, an external condition was involved in causing this health problem. Some of these conditions are:

J39.8 Cicatrix of trachea might need an external cause code to identify it as a late effect of an injury or poisoning.

J67 Farmers' lung might need an external cause code for a workers' compensation claim.

J68 Respiratory conditions due to inhalation of chemicals, gases, fumes and vapors would need an external cause code to identify the chemical.

J70 Respiratory conditions due to other external agents would need an external cause code to identify the external cause of the condition.

J95.811 Postprocedural pneumothorax would need an external cause code to identify that it was a postoperative condition.

External Cause Codes

When a patient has been injured traumatically, been poisoned or had an adverse reaction, been abused or neglected, or experienced other harm as a result of an external cause, you will need to report the details of the event so that you tell the whole story. In addition to reporting the other codes, you will also need to report codes that explain:

- *Cause of the injury,* such as a car accident or a fall off a ladder.
- *Place of the occurrence,* such as the park or the kitchen.
- *Activity during the occurrence,* such as playing basketball or gardening.
- *Patient's status,* such as paid employment, on-duty military, or leisure activity.

Refer back to Chapter 2 to remind yourself about reporting external cause codes whenever you are reporting an injury or poisoning.

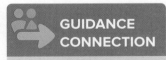

GUIDANCE CONNECTION

Review the ICD-10-CM Coding Guidelines, Section I.C.20, Chapter 20: **External causes of morbidity,** for more input.

Corrine Alexander, a 28-year-old female, worked in a veterinary clinic. After a very sick stray animal was brought in, she was instructed by her boss to disinfect the floor of the clinic by mopping it with straight bleach. It was cold outside, so all the doors and windows were closed tightly, and Corrine began to have trouble breathing. She went immediately to Dr. Borman's office, where, after examination and tests, he diagnosed her with acute chemical bronchitis.

Let's Code It!

Dr. Borman diagnosed *acute chemical bronchitis.* In the Alphabetic Index:

Bronchitis

Acute chemical (due to gases, fumes, or vapors) J68.0

Will the Tabular List confirm this suggested code?

J68 Respiratory conditions due to inhalation of chemicals, gases, fumes and vapors

Did you notice that there are two notations: *Code first* (T51–T65) to identify cause and *use additional code* to report the associated respiratory condition. Keep reading down the column to:

J68.0 Bronchitis and pneumonitis due to chemicals, gases, fumes and vapors (chemical bronchitis (acute))

Next, you must report how and where Corrine was exposed to the chemical. Let's go the Alphabetic Index for external cause codes and look up how Corrine was injured by the bleach—she inhaled the chemical:

Inhalation

Liquid air, hydrogen, nitrogen W93.12

The above is not an exact match, but it appears to be the closest description. Let's turn to the Tabular List:

W93.12x- Inhalation of liquid air

This does not match Corrine's situation at all. Let's go back to the external cause code Alphabetic Listing:

Inhalation

Poisonous gas—*see* Table of Drugs and Chemicals

Turn to the Table of Drugs and Chemicals, and look down the first column to find *bleach:*

Bleach NEC

Reading across this line, in the column titled "Poisoning accidental," you will see the suggested poisoning code. Remember: If the condition was not an adverse reaction to properly prescribed and taken medication, it is reported as a poisoning. The code suggested on the line for bleach is T54.91.

Now turn to the Tabular List to confirm the most accurate code. Let's begin with the poisoning code:

T54 Toxic effect of corrosive substances

There are no notations or directives, so keep reading to find the most accurate fourth, fifth, and sixth characters:

T54.91xA Toxic effect of unspecified corrosive substance, accidental (unintentional), initial encounter

This does look like the best choice.

In addition, Corrine was at work when the exposure happened, so you will need an external cause code to report where she was at the time of her injury. The External Cause Code Alphabetic Index will direct you:

Place of occurrence if accident—see Accident (to), occurring (at) (in)

Turn to *Accident,* and find:

Place of occurrence

Hospital Y92.239

There is no specific listing for *veterinary clinic.* However, *hospital* does come the closest. Let's turn to the code in the Tabular List and check the description:

Y92.232 Corridor of hospital as the place of occurrence of the external cause

Well, that really does hit the target. Remember, the code is being included to explain that Corrine was hurt at work; such information is most often required to support a workers' compensation claim.

The three codes on Corrine's report are:

J68.0 Bronchitis and pneumonitis due to chemicals, gases, fumes and vapors (chemical bronchitis (acute))

T54.91xA Toxic effect of unspecified corrosive substance, accidental (unintentional), initial encounter

Y92.232 Corridor of hospital as the place of occurrence of the external cause

Respiratory Failure

Respiratory failure identifies that a patient's lungs are not working efficiently. The result may be a reduced intake of oxygen or an excess of carbon dioxide that is not thoroughly being expelled from the lungs, or both. You have learned throughout this chapter about the problems that can occur in the body when it does not get enough oxygen, a condition called *hypoxemic respiratory failure,* or when there is too much carbon dioxide, a condition called *hypercapnic respiratory failure.*

Respiratory failure can be a manifestation of a respiratory disease such as COPD. In addition, certain injuries can affect a patient's ability to breathe. For example, a spinal cord injury may involve damage to the nerves that control breathing. A drug or alcohol overdose can also have an impact on the nervous system in a manner that affects the nervous system's ability to properly control respiration. Code choices include:

J96.0- Acute respiratory failure

J96.1- Chronic respiratory failure

J96.2- Acute and chronic respiratory failure

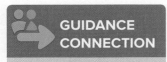

GUIDANCE CONNECTION

Review the ICD-10-CM Coding Guidelines, Section I.C.10, Chapter 10: **Diseases of the respiratory system,** Subsection b, **Acute respiratory failure**.

The physician may diagnose the patient with acute respiratory failure as a primary diagnosis when it meets the requirements to be first-listed as directed in the Official Guidelines. More typically, you will find that respiratory failure will be a secondary diagnosis, as mentioned previously.

Ventilator-Associated Pneumonia

When a patient needs help breathing because of a malfunction in the respiratory system, he or she may be placed on a ventilator, a machine that will, essentially, complete respiration. While the patient is hooked up to the machine, which uses a tube placed into the patient's throat, pathogens can travel directly into the patient's lungs, potentially resulting in the development of ventilator-associated pneumonia (VAP). The attending physician must specifically document the diagnosis of VAP before you can report code J95.851. Only the physician can link the ventilator with the infection. If the documentation is not clear, you must query the physician for clarification.

Beneath this code is a *use additional code* notation reminding you that you will need to report a second code to identify the specific organism responsible for this infection. Also, an *Excludes1* notation directs you to report code P27.8 instead if the patient is a newborn.

Chapter Summary

Sadly, most people take breathing for granted . . . until they cannot do it without difficulty or pain. You have to know how to code respiratory conditions accurately whether you are working for a family physician, a pediatrician, or a pulmonologist. In addition, respiratory conditions might be present in a patient of an immunologist; allergist; or ear, nose, and throat (ENT) specialist.

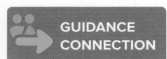

GUIDANCE CONNECTION

Review the ICD-10-CM Coding Guidelines, Section I.C.10, Chapter 10: **Diseases of the respiratory system,** Subsection d, **Ventilator associated pneumonia**.

CHAPTER 13 REVIEW
Coding Respiratory Conditions

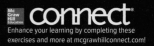

Enhance your learning by completing these
exercises and more at mcgrawhillconnect.com!

Using Terminology

Match each key term to the appropriate definition.

Part One

_____ 1. LO 13.1 Bilateral tubes, small branches of the bronchi, leading to the air sacs.

_____ 2. LO 13.1 A double-layered membrane that envelops the lungs and lines the chest wall.

_____ 3. LO 13.1 A ridge of bone and cartilage that forms a barrier between the left and right nares.

_____ 4. LO 13.1 Tubular membrane that connects the larynx to the bronchi; commonly known as the *windpipe*.

_____ 5. LO 13.1 A tubular organ that connects from the pharynx to the trachea.

_____ 6. LO 13.1 A flap made of cartilage that covers the superior end of the larynx.

_____ 7. LO 13.1 Bilateral air passageways that connect the trachea to the lungs.

_____ 8. LO 13.1 Bilateral facial sinuses.

_____ 9. LO 13.1 A transverse muscle that divides the torso between the chest and the abdomen; its motion aids respiration.

_____ 10. LO 13.1 Bilateral lobed organs that function like balloons, expanding on inspiration and deflating on expiration.

_____ 11. LO 13.1 A tiny bubble, grouped in clusters at the end of each bronchiole, that holds air.

A. Alveolar sac
B. Bronchi
C. Bronchioles
D. Diaphragm
E. Epiglottis
F. Larynx
G. Lungs
H. Nasal septum
I. Paranasal sinuses
J. Pleura
K. Trachea

Part Two

_____ 1. LO 13.1 The physical process of acquiring oxygen.

_____ 2. LO 13.5 An increase in the severity of a disease or its symptoms.

_____ 3. LO 13.4 An acute infection of the respiratory tract caused by the influenza virus.

_____ 4. LO 13.1 The physical process of acquiring oxygen and releasing carbon dioxide.

_____ 5. LO 13.1 The physical process of expulsing carbon dioxide.

_____ 6. LO 13.5 An ongoing obstruction of the airway.

_____ 7. LO 13.3 A condition in which air or gas is present within the chest cavity but outside the lungs.

_____ 8. LO 13.1 A malfunction of the organ system relating to respiration.

_____ 9. LO 13.4 An inflammation of the lungs.

_____ 10. LO 13.5 The condition of asthma that is life-threatening and does not respond to therapeutic treatments.

A. Chronic obstructive pulmonary disease (COPD)
B. Exacerbation
C. Expiration
D. Influenza
E. Inspiration
F. Pneumonia
G. Pneumothorax
H. Respiration
I. Respiratory disorder
J. Status asthmaticus

Checking Your Understanding

Choose the most appropriate answer for each of the following questions.

1. LO 13.2 Respiratory disorders can be
   a. genetic.
   b. environmental.
   c. congenital.
   d. all of these.

2. LO 13.3 When a known infectious organism is involved in a respiratory condition, code
   a. only the infectious organism.
   b. both the known organism and the respiratory condition.
   c. only the respiratory condition.
   d. a personal history code.

3. LO 13.4 When the cause of pneumonia is an underlying disease such as HIV or whooping cough, the codes should be sequenced:
   a. pneumonia first, underlying disease second.
   b. pneumonia only.
   c. underlying disease only.
   d. underlying disease first, pneumonia second.

4. LO 13.5 COPD stands for
   a. chronic obstructive pneumonia dyspnea.
   b. chronic olfactory pharyngitis disease.
   c. chronic other pneumonic disease.
   d. chronic obstructive pulmonary disease.

5. LO 13.5 One of the three types of COPD is
   a. sinusitis.
   b. pneumonia.
   c. emphysema.
   d. pharyngitis.

6. LO 13.5 If the diagnostic statement includes both status asthmaticus and acute exacerbation of asthma,
   a. code only the status asthmaticus.
   b. code only the acute exacerbation of asthma.
   c. code both status asthmaticus and acute exacerbation with two codes.
   d. these two diagnoses cannot be in the same patient at the same time.

7. LO 13.5 A patient diagnosed with chronic obstructive pulmonary disease with acute exacerbation would be coded with
   a. J44.
   b. J44.0.
   c. J44.1.
   d. J44.9.

8. LO 13.6 Respiratory conditions need external cause codes

    a. never.
    b. sometimes.
    c. always.
    d. only if there is an external cause for the condition.

9. LO 13.6 An external cause code might be needed to support

    a. a workers' compensation claim.
    b. a liability claim.
    c. none of these.
    d. both a workers' compensation claim and a liability claim.

10. LO 13.2/13.4/13.6 Code the diagnosis of pneumonitis due to inhalation of lubricating oil, unintentional, initial encounter.

    a. T52.0X1A.
    b. J69.1.
    c. T52.0X1A, J69.1.
    d. J69.1, T52.0X1A.

Applying Your Knowledge

1. LO 13.1 What are the two segments of the respiratory system? _____

_____

2. LO 13.1 List the components of the upper respiratory system. _____

_____

3. LO 13.1 List the components of the lower respiratory system. _____

_____

4. LO 13.1 Differentiate between respiration, inspiration, and expiration. _____

_____

5. LO 13.3 In relation to tobacco involvement, explain the difference between *exposure, use, abuse, dependence,* and *history.* _____

_____

6. LO 13.5 What does COPD stand for? Explain the condition, and include the clinical types of COPD. _____

_____

7. LO 13.5 Differentiate between exacerbation and status asthmaticus. _____

_____

8. LO 13.6 Explain why a respiratory condition might require an external cause code. Include an example. _____

_____

Using the techniques described in this chapter, carefully read through the case studies and determine the most accurate ICD-10-CM code(s) and external cause codes, if appropriate, for each case study.

1. Scott Merlman, a 36-year-old male, is admitted into the hospital with chest pain and shortness of breath. After a thorough examination and the appropriate tests, he is diagnosed with chronic obstructive pulmonary disease.

   _____

2. Beth Ramos, a 26-year-old female, was brought into the ED suffering a severe asthma attack. Dr. Porter gave her an injection for rapid desensitization after determining that she was having an allergic reaction that affected her bronchial asthma.

   _____

3. Edward Agmata, a 13-year-old male, is brought in today by his mother with the complaint that Edward has been sneezing and has a stuffed nose. Dr. Kristine diagnosed him with allergic rhinitis and ordered testing to discover the allergen.

   _____

4. Ronine Fabrere, a 29-year-old male, is HIV-positive, asymptomatic. Ronine was just admitted with organic pneumonia.

   _____

5. Gigi Warner, a 47-year-old female, was diagnosed with chronic bronchitis 6 months ago and is on medication. This morning, she came to see Dr. Lorrel because she was coughing and having difficulty breathing. Dr. Lorrel admitted her into the hospital with a diagnosis of chronic obstructive pulmonary disease with acute exacerbation.

   _____

6. Trudy Benington, a 3-year-old female, was brought to the ED by her mother. Trudy had a cough and fever, and her eyes were tearing. She was complaining that her eyes were itchy and burning. After a thorough examination and chest x-ray, Dr. Minister diagnosed her with an upper respiratory infection with bilateral acute conjunctivitis.

   _____

7. Gerald Fontaine, an 18-year-old male, came to see Dr. Brown with complaints of a fever and postnasal drip. After the exam, Dr. Brown diagnosed Gerald with chronic sinusitis.

   _____

8. Erin Bishoff, a 59-year-old female, was admitted to the hospital with a diagnosis of complete bilateral paralysis of the vocal cords.

_____

9. Feona Fennell, a 41-year-old female, has had centrilobular emphysema for over a year. Dr. Orton admits her today to the hospital with a diagnosis of aspiration pneumonia with pneumonia due to *Staphylococcus aureus* (MSSA).

_____

10. Garrett Church, a 33-year-old male, presents today with chest congestion and discomfort. Dr. Peterson also notes the patient is wheezing and is short of breath. Garret is admitted to the hospital and is diagnosed with pneumonia. He also has COPD with acute bronchitis.

_____

11. Faith Dutton, a 21-year-old female, comes to see Dr. Fraiser with complaints of a headache and sinus congestion. Dr. Fraiser diagnoses her with acute and chronic maxillary sinusitis.

_____

12. Sean Dublin a 29-year-old male, has a history of cystic fibrosis. Sean presents today with the complaint of chest pain and breathlessness. After a thorough examination and chest x-ray, Dr. Alvin diagnoses Sean with a secondary spontaneous pneumothorax.

_____

13. Joy Carter, a 21-year-old female, comes in today with a nosebleed. She was playing basketball at the local sports area and was struck in the face by the basketball. After an examination, Dr. Jordan diagnoses Joy with a deviated nasal septum.

_____

14. Clay Logan, a 12-year-old male, is brought in by his parents. Clay is complaining of a sore throat, fever, cough, and headaches. Dr. Anderson diagnoses Clay with hypertrophic tonsillitis, bilaterally.

_____

15. Meredith Chester, a 35-year-old female, presents today with chest congestion and chest pain. Dr. Hayden diagnoses her with interlobar pleurisy.

_____

The following exercises provide practice in abstracting physicians' notes and learning to work with SOAP notes from our health care facility, *Taylor, Reader, & Associates.* These case studies (SOAP notes) are modeled on real patient encounters. Using the techniques described in this chapter, carefully read through the case studies and determine the most accurate ICD-10-CM code(s) and external cause code(s), if appropriate, for each case study.

TAYLOR, READER, & ASSOCIATES
A Complete Health Care Facility
975 CENTRAL AVENUE • SOMEWHERE, FL 32811 • 407-555-4321

PATIENT: COOPER, MARION
ACCOUNT/EHR #:   COOPMA001
DATE: 07/16/18

Attending Physician: Suzanne R. Taylor, MD

Pt presented to the ED normotensive with respirations of 10 and without any cyanosis. The Pt is currently awake and alert. She is on the ACUD mode on the ventilator, breathing approximately 10 times per minute. She does seem disoriented and does not appear to be as lucid as she had been when she first arrived, although there is no obvious focal neurologic deficit. The Pt appears to be staring to the ceiling and was able to answer some questions, but was confused. She did speak over the ventilator but was following commands appropriately. She denied any pain and she was disoriented.

The patient's blood gases showed a compensated respiratory acidosis, and she was supporting stable vital signs and was afebrile. BP 153/71. Sinus tachycardia on the monitor at about 127 beats per minute. Lung fields are clear to auscultation and percussion.

DIAGNOSES: 1. Respiratory failure, chronic
                        2. Sinus tachycardia

PLAN/RECOMMENDATIONS:
                        1. 100% ventilator support for the time being
                        2. Continue nutrition with PulmoCare at 60 cc an hour
                        3. Follow up laboratory

Suzanne R. Taylor, MD

SRT/pw   D: 07/16/18 09:50:16   T: 07/18/18 12:55:01

Determine the most accurate ICD-10-CM code(s).

_____

_____

_____

TAYLOR, READER, & ASSOCIATES
A Complete Health Care Facility
975 CENTRAL AVENUE • SOMEWHERE, FL 32811 • 407-555-4321

PATIENT: MCLEOD, WINSTON
ACCOUNT/EHR #:   MCLEWI001
DATE: 08/11/18

Attending Physician: Willard B. Reader, MD

S: Pt is a 23-month-old male who almost drowned in the swimming pool at his home 2 days ago. He is experiencing rapid, shallow breathing and dyspnea.

O: Hypoxemia is apparent. Chest sounds, crackles, and rhonchi indicate fluid accumulation. Tachycardia and restlessness are also evident. ABG (arterial blood gas) analysis shows respiratory acidosis; serial chest x-rays show bilateral infiltrates.

A: Acute respiratory distress

P: Oxygen hood to supply warm, humidified, oxygen-enriched gases

_____

Willard B. Reader, MD

WBR/pw   D: 08/11/18 09:50:16   T: 08/13/18 12:55:01

Determine the most accurate ICD-10-CM code(s).

_____

_____

_____

TAYLOR, READER, & ASSOCIATES
A Complete Health Care Facility
975 CENTRAL AVENUE • SOMEWHERE, FL 32811 • 407-555-4321

PATIENT: CUMMINGS, LINDA
ACCOUNT/EHR #:   CUMMLI001
DATE: 07/16/18

Attending Physician: Suzanne R. Taylor, MD

S: This Pt is a 66-year-old female who presents today with complaints of dyspnea on exertion, and coughing.
    I last saw this patient 1 year ago.

O: Ht 5'3" Wt. 157 lb. R 15. BP 145/95. P90 thready. Chest: tachycardia, tachypnea, dependent crackles. HEENT: neck vein distention. Coughing produces frothy, bloody sputum. Skin is cold, clammy, diaphoretic, and cyanotic. ABG analysis shows hypoxia. Chest x-ray shows diffuse haziness of the lung fields.

A: Acute pulmonary edema

P: 1. Administer high concentrations of oxygen by a cannula
    2. Rx Lasix

_____

Suzanne R. Taylor, MD

SRT/pw   D: 07/16/18 09:50:16   T: 07/18/18 12:55:01

Determine the most accurate ICD-10-CM code(s).

_____

_____

_____

TAYLOR, READER, & ASSOCIATES
A Complete Health Care Facility
975 CENTRAL AVENUE • SOMEWHERE, FL 32811 • 407-555-4321

PATIENT: CLYDE, NELSON
ACCOUNT/EHR #:   CLYDNE001
DATE: 09/15/18

Attending Physician: Willard B. Reader, MD

S: This new Pt is a 23-year-old male who presents with complaints of fever and recurrent chills. He states that he has a cough producing rusty, bloody, viscous sputum (Pt states "like currant jelly"). He states his breathing is difficult and shallow, and he noticed that his lips and fingernails appear bluish. Pt recently moved here from Detroit. He was found to be HIV-positive 2 years ago and is on pharmaceutical therapy.

O: HEENT: Cyanosis of lips confirms hypoxemia. Chest: respirations are shallow and grunting. Chest x-ray shows consolidation in the upper lobe causing bulging of fissures; WBC count is elevated; sputum culture and Gram stain show Gram-negative cocci Klebsiella.

A: Pneumonia due to Klebsiella, HIV positive

P: Admit to hospital. Recommend surgical clearing. Begin antimicrobial agent therapy.

Willard B. Reader, MD

WBR/pw   D: 09/15/18 09:50:16   T: 09/17/18 12:55:01

Determine the most accurate ICD-10-CM code(s).

_____

_____

_____

TAYLOR, READER, & ASSOCIATES
A Complete Health Care Facility
975 CENTRAL AVENUE • SOMEWHERE, FL 32811 • 407-555-4321

PATIENT: CONDRON, CLARENCE
ACCOUNT/EHR #:   CONDCL001
DATE: 11/25/18

Attending Physician: Willard B. Reader, MD

S: This new Pt is a 35-year-old male complaining of a cough with a foul-smelling sputum, dyspnea, excessive sweating, and chills.

PMH: Pt has poor oral hygiene. Missing teeth and inflamed gums have gone untreated for years due to his fear of the dentist. He states that a few months ago, he had a bout of pneumonia. He self-medicated but hasn't felt right since then.

O: Chest: Auscultation reveals crackles and decreased breath sounds. Chest x-ray shows localized infiltrate with one clear space containing air-fluid. Blood cultures, Gram stain, and sputum culture identify leukocytosis.

A: Abscess of the lung, putrid

P: Begin antibiotic therapy immediately

_____

Willard B. Reader, MD

WBR/pw   D: 11/25/18 09:50:16   T: 11/27/18 12:55:01

Determine the most accurate ICD-10-CM code(s).

_____

_____

_____

14

CODING DISEASES OF THE DIGESTIVE SYSTEM

Learning Outcomes *After completing this chapter, the student should be able to:*

LO 14.1 Identify the components of the digestive system.

LO 14.2 Enumerate the medical necessity for endoscopic procedures.

LO 14.3 Define the various anatomical sites that may develop a digestive ulcer.

LO 14.4 Distinguish various types of hernias.

LO 14.5 Use additional codes to report alcohol abuse and dependence, as required.

LO 14.6 Code accurately the presence of cholecystitis with other disorders of the gallbladder.

Key Terms

Accessory organs

Alimentary canal

Anus

Ascending colon

Cecum

Cheeks

Cholelithiasis

Common bile duct

Descending colon

Duodenum

Edentulism

Esophagus

Fundus

Gallbladder

Gangrene

Hemorrhage

Hernia

Ileum

Jejunum

Lingual tonsils

You experience the workings of your digestive system every day. Liquids and solids enter your body and provide nourishment to the cells, tissues, and organs so that they have the energy to function. The digestive system, as illustrated in Figure 14-1, starts at the mouth and ends at the anus.

LO 14.1 The Digestive System

The complex mechanisms that permit our bodies to function require energy. This energy is extracted from nourishment and is a requirement for life. The old saying "You are what you eat" may not be specifically accurate, but without food and drink we cannot exist. The digestive system is referred to in two parts: the alimentary canal and the accessory organs.

The Alimentary Canal

The **alimentary canal** is the direct path through the body from the mouth to the anus. This pathway includes the mouth, pharynx, esophagus, stomach, small intestine, large intestine, rectum, and anus.

Mouth Virtually all nourishment enters the body at the mouth, also referred to as the **oral cavity.** The components within this area include the lips, cheeks, tongue, lingual tonsils, hard and soft palates, uvula, palatine tonsils, pharyngeal tonsils, and teeth (see Figure 14-2).

The **lips** form the entranceway into the oral cavity and the alimentary canal. Their mobility and flexibility aids in the formation of sounds to enable speech. In addition, they can close the mouth to prevent food from falling out while it is being chewed (masticated).

The **cheeks** form an area, as they meet the gingiva, that is known as the *buccal cavities.* This may sound familiar if you watch any of the legal or science shows on television in which analysts ask a suspect for a buccal swab and run a cotton swab along the inside of the person's cheek (buccal

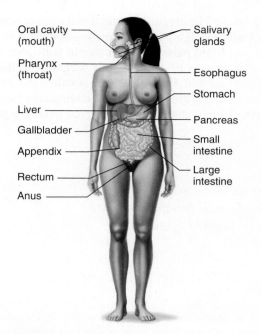

FIGURE 14-1 The Digestive System

Source: Booth et al., MA, 5e. Copyright © 2013 by McGraw-Hill. Figure 22-6a, p. 478

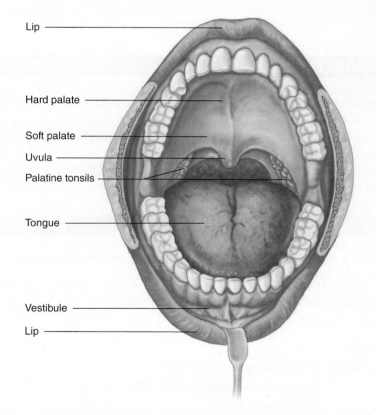

FIGURE 14-2 The Oral Cavity (Human Mouth)

Source: David Shier et al., HOLE'S HUMAN ANATOMY & PHYSIOLOGY, 12/e. © 2010 MHE. Figure 17.5, p. 657

area of the mouth). The inner lining of the cheek is made up of moist, stratified squamous epithelium cells.

The **tongue** does more than help you form the sounds of speech. It helps rotate food particles around into position so the teeth, particularly the molars, can grind the food

alimentary canal
The digestive pathway from the oral cavity to the anus.

oral cavity
The opening in the face that begins the alimentary canal and is used for the input of nutrition; also known as the *mouth*.

lips
A muscular structure around the external area of the oral cavity.

cheeks
The walls of the oral cavity that form both sides of the face; the buccal area.

tongue
Sensory organ attached to the bottom of the mouth; enables speech, eating, and tasting.

to enable swallowing safely. The tongue is secured at the hyoid bone in the posterior of the mouth and has a surface of lymphatic tissue masses known as the **lingual tonsils.** When you touch the roof (hard palate) of your mouth with your tongue, you can see a membrane below that appears to connect your tongue with the *sublingual glands* along the bottom of your mouth. This membrane is called the *lingual frenulum.* You may find that some medications are administered sublingually (under the tongue). For example, nitroglycerin, 0.3 mg tablet: 1 tab *sublingual* to relieve pain.

EXAMPLE

D00.02 Carcinoma in situ of buccal mucosa
K05.11 Chronic gingivitis, non-plaque induced
K14.0 Glossitis (abscess of the tongue)

EXAMPLE

Ursula brought her 6-month-old son, Judah, to Dr. Rodriquez, his pediatrician, because he had been crying all night long. It seemed nothing she or her husband could do calmed him. After examination, Dr. Rodriquez diagnosed Judah with teething syndrome and provided Ursula with several ways to help the family through this experience. This diagnosis is reported with code K00.7, Teething syndrome.

LET'S CODE IT! SCENARIO

*Gene Oteri, a 53-year-old male, comes in to see his dentist, Dr. Petris. He knew that he had periodontitis for a while, but now his teeth on the lower right side of his mouth are really bothering him. Dr. Petris did a full evaluation and found that five teeth on the lower right were so loose that they came out with little encouragement. Dr. Petris determined that Gene has partial loss (**edentulism**) of teeth due to periodontal disease, class 1.*

edentulism
Absence of teeth.

Let's Code It!

Gene lost five teeth due to periodontal disease. Let's turn to the Alphabetic Index and find the key term of the diagnosis:

Edentulism—*see* Absence, teeth, acquired

Turn to:

Absence

    Teeth, tooth (congenital) K00.0

        Acquired (complete) K08.109

        Partial K08.409

            Class I K08.401

            Class II K08.402

            Class III K08.403

            Class IV K08.404

Also take note of the listings within this long list for the loss of teeth due to caries (dental cavities), periodontal disease, trauma, or another specified cause. These will take you to other specific codes.

Refer to the physician's documentation and read that Gene was diagnosed with *partial class I edentulism,* so let's turn to the Tabular List and find:

K08 Other disorders of teeth and supporting structures

Read the *Excludes2* notation carefully. Does it have anything to do with this encounter? No! Great, so now review all the choices for the required fourth character, and determine which one most accurately reports the diagnosis:

K08.4 Partial loss of teeth

There are *Excludes1* and *Excludes2* notes here. Read them carefully, and reread Dr. Petris's documentation. Nothing there matches. Next, you must review the options for fourth and fifth characters.

K08.42 Partial loss of teeth due to periodontal diseases

Check the documentation. Dr. Petris wrote that Gene's loss of teeth was caused by the periodontitis, and it was class 1. Review all of the choices, and determine the most accurate code:

K08.421 Partial loss of teeth due to periodontal diseases, class I

Good work!

On each side at the back of the tongue are collections of lymphatic tissue known as the **palatine tonsils.** These tonsils are named so because of their location at the back of the mouth where the hard and soft palates begin to curve into the throat. If you work in a pediatrician's office, you will get to know this part of the oral cavity well, as *tonsillitis* (inflammation/infection of the palatine tonsils) is common with children. The drop-shaped appendage hanging in the posterior of your throat, called the **uvula,** helps to modulate tones during speech.

Pharyngeal tonsils (adenoids) sit on the posterior wall of the pharynx and are also made of lymphatic tissue. When these tonsils are enlarged and cause problems with respiration through the nasal cavity, they may be surgically removed.

The health of an individual's oral cavity can provide insights to the patient's complete health. Even further, poor oral health can have a negative impact on the heart and other organ systems. Good oral health care, including brushing and flossing every day, enables the balance of good and bad bacteria in the mouth. When bad bacteria cultivate out of control, tooth decay and diseases of the gum can develop. The bacteria, when left unchecked by improper care, can enter the bloodstream, carried by saliva flow, and contribute to the progress of conditions such as cardiovascular disease, diabetes, and endocarditis. Such bacteria have also been linked to premature delivery and low-birth-weight neonates (see Table 14-1).

Salivary Glands As the teeth and tongue are breaking down food in preparation for the journey down the alimentary canal, three sets of major **salivary glands** (the parotid, submandibular, and sublingual glands) secrete saliva to moisten and bind the food particles. This begins the chemical digestion of carbohydrates, dissolves foods so their flavor can be appreciated, and helps enable swallowing of the food particles. In addition, saliva helps to clean the teeth and mouth after the particles leave the oral cavity.

palatine tonsils
Lymphoid tissue situated at the entrance to the throat, bilaterally.

uvula
Hanging, fleshy tissue suspended from the soft palate at the opening of the throat.

pharyngeal tonsils
Lymphoid nodules located on the wall of the pharynx, bilaterally.

salivary glands
Three sets of bilateral exocrine glands that secrete saliva: parotid glands, submaxillary glands, and sublingual glands.

TABLE 14-1 Health Conditions Connected to Poor Oral Hygiene

Disease of the gums of the mouth, known as *periodontal disease,* has been shown to affect the health of other organs throughout the body. Some examples include:	
Cardiovascular system	• Increased risk of stroke • Increased risk of fatal heart attack • Increased risk of cardiovascular disease • Increased risk of clotting disorder
Respiratory system	Bacteria from mouth, dental plaque buildup, and throat can contribute to pneumonia and other lung diseases.
Musculoskeletal system	Increased risk of osteopenia.
Endocrine system	Interference with control of diabetes mellitus.
Reproductive system	• During gestation, mothers with advanced periodontitis are at increased risk for premature and/or underweight neonates. • Microbes from periodontitis can cross through the placenta and expose the fetus to infection.

EXAMPLE

K11.0 Atrophy of salivary gland

K11.4 Fistula of salivary gland

pharynx
The section of the tubular organ that leads from the oral cavity to the esophagus.

Pharynx Posterior to the nose and mouth lies the **pharynx,** an open cavity that leads down to the esophagus. This section of the human anatomy serves two important systems: the respiratory system (when inhalation is in process) and the digestive system (when food and drink are ingested). The pharynx (see Figure 14-3) is referred to in three sections:

- *Nasopharynx* refers to the segment of the pharynx that lies behind the nasal cavity. It permits air, taken in through the nose, to travel down toward the lungs for respiration.
- *Oropharynx* refers to the segment of the pharynx that lies behind the oral cavity—inferior to the nasopharynx and posterior to the soft palate. When food and liquids are ingested through the mouth, they will travel down the oropharynx on the way to the esophagus. Note that the oropharynx is open to the nasopharynx, a fact that explains why laughing too hard while drinking causes milk to come out of your nose.
- *Hypopharynx,* also called the *laryngopharynx,* is the segment of the pharynx inferior to the oropharynx and posterior to the larynx. This is the lowest third of the pharynx and the portion that connects to the esophagus. This is the fork in the road, so to speak, for food and liquid and for air. Air will continue to the lungs via the larynx and trachea. At the superior end of the larynx is the *epiglottis,* a flap that closes the path to the larynx and trachea, thereby directing food and liquid down the esophagus to the stomach. On occasion, the epiglottis does not close properly, causing an individual to "swallow the wrong way" and have food or liquid enter the larynx and trachea. This results in a cough reflex, the body's way of trying to stop the food particles or liquid from getting into the lungs.

EXAMPLE

A69.1 Fusospirochetal pharyngitis

J31.2 Chronic pharyngitis

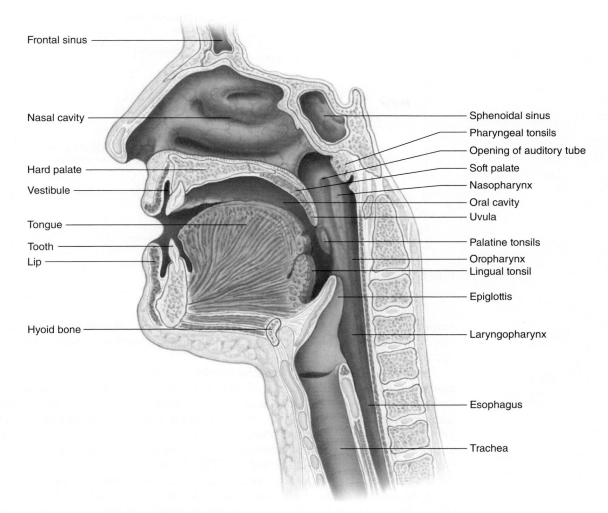

FIGURE 14-3 The Upper Digestive System

Source: David Shier et al., HOLE'S HUMAN ANATOMY & PHYSIOLOGY, 12/e. © 2010 MHE. Figure 17.7, p. 658

Labels in figure:
Frontal sinus
Nasal cavity
Hard palate
Vestibule
Tongue
Tooth
Lip
Hyoid bone
Sphenoidal sinus
Pharyngeal tonsils
Opening of auditory tube
Soft palate
Nasopharynx
Oral cavity
Uvula
Palatine tonsils
Oropharynx
Lingual tonsil
Epiglottis
Laryngopharynx
Esophagus
Trachea

Esophagus The tubelike structure that connects the hypopharynx to the stomach is known as the **esophagus.** As you can see in Figure 14-3, the esophagus lies parallel and posterior to the trachea. Just as the epiglottis blocks food and liquid from entering the trachea, the esophagus has its own gateway, called the *upper esophageal sphincter,* to restrict the entrance of air into the stomach. A **sphincter** is a circular muscle that can open or close an opening. There are several sphincters along the alimentary canal.

A second esophageal sphincter is located at the juncture between the esophagus and the stomach (the lower esophageal sphincter). This sphincter is designed to prevent the contents of the stomach from splashing back up into the esophagus. When this sphincter does not function properly, the patient might experience chronic heartburn, nausea, and possibly a sore throat. This may lead to a diagnosis of gastroesophageal reflux disease (GERD), reported with code K21.9, Gastro-esophageal reflux disease without esophagitis. One test used to diagnose a patient suspected of having GERD is an esophagogastroduodenoscopy (EGD). Left untreated, GERD may develop into Barrett's esophagus (code K22.70, Barrett's esophagus without dysplasia), which might be treated with gastroesophageal fundoplication.

Stomach The next organ along the alimentary canal is the **stomach.** As stated earlier, the stomach connects to the esophagus at the lower esophageal sphincter in the cardiac region of the stomach, also known as the *cardia.* To the left, the stomach curves upward creating the fundic region, or **fundus.** A fundus is defined as a domed

esophagus
The tubular organ that connects the pharynx to the stomach for the passage of nourishment.

sphincter
A circular muscle that contracts to prevent passage of liquids or solids.

stomach
A saclike organ within the alimentary canal designed to contain nourishment during the initial phase of the digestive process.

fundus
The section of an organ farthest from its opening.

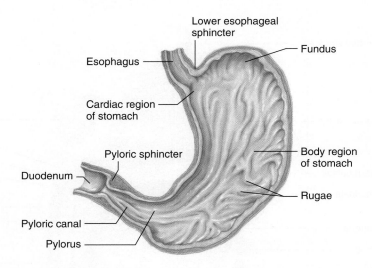

FIGURE 14-4 The Stomach

Source: David Shier et al., HOLE'S HUMAN ANATOMY & PHYSIOLOGY, 12/e. © 2010 MHE. Figure 17.17, p. 666

portion of a hollow organ that sits the farthest from, above, or opposite an opening. As you can see in Figure 14-4, the fundus of the stomach is located superior to (above) the opening to the esophagus.

The lining of the stomach, a mucous membrane, contains gastric glands that secrete gastric juices. As with the function of saliva in the processing of food in the mouth, the gastric juices support the extraction of nutritional elements in the contents that entered from the esophagus. Mucous cells coat the internal wall of the stomach to prevent the gastric juices from digesting it. When this coating is flawed, the patient might develop a gastric (peptic) ulcer, a condition in which the acids in the stomach actually eat a hole in the lining and wall of the stomach. This diagnosis is reported with code K25.9, Gastric ulcer, unspecified as acute or chronic, without hemorrhage or perforation.

As the shape of the stomach's body curves downward, the inside of the curve on the side of the cardia is referred to as the *lesser curvature,* and the outside curve, coming down from the fundus, is referred to as the *greater curvature.* The lower portion of the stomach narrows as it nears the duodenum and connects to the small intestine. The pyloric sphincter is located here to control the emptying of the contents of the stomach into the lower half of the digestive system.

EXAMPLE

K31.1 Adult hypertrophic pyloric stenosis
K31.3 Pylorospasm, not elsewhere classified

Small Intestine The inferior aspect of the pyloric sphincter is the **duodenum,** the first segment of the small intestine. The duodenum curves around like the letter "C," with the pancreas tucked in the center. The hepatopancreatic sphincter, also called the *sphincter of Oddi,* is the connection point between the duodenum, the pancreatic duct, and the common bile duct that comes from the gallbladder and the liver.

As the duodenum trails into that last portion, at the bottom of the "C," it curves around and becomes the **jejunum,** the segment of the small intestine that twists and turns throughout the abdomen (see Figure 14-5). The **mesentery** is a membrane that connects to the jejunum like a spider web filled with blood vessels, nerves, and lymphatic vessels to provide nourishment to the intestine. On the anterior side of the abdominal cavity, coming from the greater curvature of the stomach down to the anterior of the jejunum like a protective curtain, is a double fold of the peritoneum called the *greater omentum.*

duodenum
The first segment of the small intestine, connecting the stomach to the jejunum.

jejunum
The segment of the small intestine that connects the duodenum to the ileum.

mesentery
A fold of a membrane that carries blood to the small intestine and connects it to the posterior wall of the abdominal cavity.

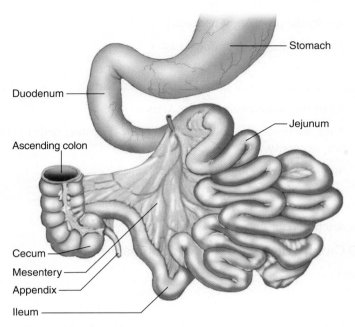

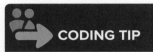

FIGURE 14-5 The Lower Alimentary Canal

Source: David Shier et al., HOLE'S HUMAN ANATOMY & PHYSIOLOGY, 12/e. © 2010 MHE. Figure 17.31 p. 680

The last segment of the small intestine is the **ileum.** The ileum connects to the **cecum,** the bridge to the large intestine via the ileocecal sphincter. This sphincter controls the passage of material from the small intestine into the large intestine.

ileum
The last segment of the small intestine.

cecum
A pouchlike organ that connects the ileum with the large intestine; the point of connection for the vermiform appendix.

EXAMPLE

K29.80 Duodenitis without bleeding
K31.5 Obstruction of duodenum

YOU CODE IT! CASE STUDY

Esther Levine, a 31-year-old female, came to see Dr. Premann with symptoms of persistent diarrhea and ongoing right lower-quadrant (RLQ) abdominal pain. Lab work showed an increased white blood cell count and erythrocyte sedimentation rate. A barium enema showed string sign. A biopsy confirmed a diagnosis of Crohn's disease of the jejunum.

You Code It!

Go through the steps of coding, and determine the code or codes that should be reported for this encounter between Dr. Premann and Esther Levine.

Step 1:   Read the case completely.

Step 2:   Abstract the notes: Which key words can you identify relating to why Dr. Premann cared for Esther?

Step 3: Query the provider, if necessary.

Step 4: Code the diagnosis or diagnoses.

_____

Step 5: Code the procedure(s): Office visit.

Step 6: Link the procedure codes to at least one diagnosis code to confirm medical necessity.

Step 7: Back code to double-check your choices.

Answer:

Did you determine the correct code to be:

K50.00 Crohn's disease of the small intestine

Good job!

Large Intestine The colon is also known as the large intestine. As you look at the illustration (see Figure 14-6), you might wonder why it is considered large when the small intestine seems to be so much longer. This distinction has nothing to do with length; the large intestine has a larger diameter.

You may notice that the two terms, _colon_ and _large intestine,_ are used almost interchangeably. In reality, they are technically not the same thing. The large intestine consists of the cecum, the vermiform appendix, the colon, the rectum, and the anus. The colon represents the majority of the large intestine. Let's take a look at the parts of the large intestine.

Starting at the cecum, the colon frames the abdomen almost like the beltway around Washington, D.C., and is referred to in four segments.

The ileum of the small intestine connects to the **ascending colon** on the right side of the large intestine at the cecum. The **vermiform appendix,** a rounded tubular appendage, protrudes from the end of the cecum. The ascending colon stretches upward from the cecum to just below the liver in the superior aspect of the abdomen. At this point, this tubular structure makes a sharp left turn, known as the _hepatic flexure_ (named because of the proximity to the liver) and runs across to the left side. This section is known as the **transverse colon** because it traverses across the abdomen (_transverse_ = across). On the left side, the colon turns downward at a curve known as the _splenic flexure_ (named because of the proximity to the spleen), becoming the **descending colon.** It continues down until it slightly curves, just above the pelvis, and becomes the **sigmoid colon.**

The large intestine turns again, downward. This area is called the **rectum** (rectal vault), and it leads directly into the anal canal. At the distal end of the anal canal, the _internal and external anal sphincters_ form the **anus**—the opening to the outside.

ascending colon
The portion of the large intestine that connects the cecum to the hepatic flexure.

vermiform appendix
A long, narrow mass of tissue attached to the cecum; also called _appendix._

transverse colon
The portion of the large intestine that connects the hepatic flexure to the splenic flexure.

descending colon
The segment of the large intestine that connects the splenic flexure to the sigmoid colon.

sigmoid colon
The dual-curved segment of the colon that connects the descending colon to the rectum; also referred to as the _sigmoid flexure._

rectum
The last segment of the large intestine, connecting the sigmoid colon to the anus.

anus
The portion of the large intestine that leads outside the body.

EXAMPLE

K51.20 Ulcerative (chronic) proctitis without complications
K56.41 Fecal impaction of the intestine
K35.3 Acute appendicitis with localized peritonitis

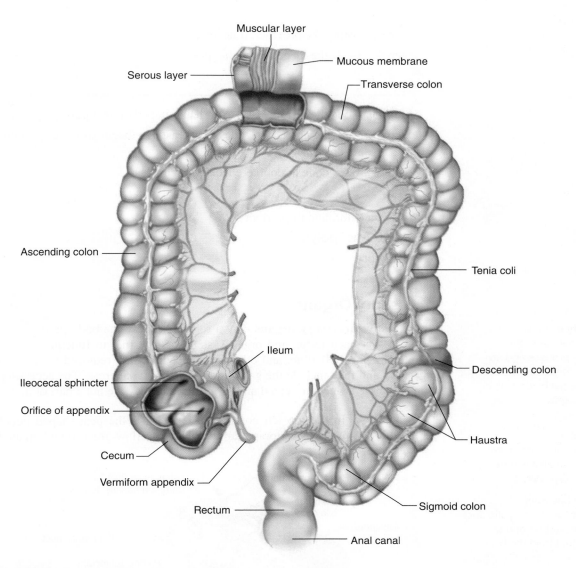

FIGURE 14-6 The Large Intestine (Colon)

Source: David Shier et al., HOLE'S HUMAN ANATOMY & PHYSIOLOGY, 12/e. © 2010 MHE. Figure 17.43 p. 687

YOU CODE IT! CASE STUDY

Theda Richter, a 37-year-old female, was brought into the procedure room so Dr. Charne could remove her anal polyps.

You Code It!

Go through the steps of coding, and determine the code or codes that should be reported for this encounter between Dr. Charne and Theda Richter.

Step 1: Read the case completely.

Step 2: Abstract the notes: Which key words can you identify relating to why Dr. Charne cared for Theda Richter?

Step 3: Query the provider, if necessary.

Step 4: Code the diagnosis or diagnoses.

Step 5: Code the procedure(s): Surgical removal of anal polyps

Step 6: Link the procedure codes to at least one diagnosis code to confirm medical necessity.

Step 7: Back code to double-check your choices.

Answer:

Did you determine the correct code?

K62.0 Anal polyp

Good job!

Accessory Organs

accessory organs
Organs that assist the digestive process and are adjacent to the alimentary canal: the gallbladder, liver, and pancreas.

gallbladder
A pear-shaped organ that stores bile until it is required to aid the digestive process.

common bile duct
The juncture of the cystic duct of the gallbladder and the hepatic duct from the liver.

The digestive **accessory organs** play a role in the way the body processes food and water so that each tissue and organ system has the fuel to function. These organs secrete enzymes, alkaline, and other substances that are required for the process of digestion, and they include the gallbladder, liver, and pancreas. The accessory organs connect to the alimentary canal and support it, but they are not a part of it.

Gallbladder In the top left corner of Figure 14-7, the pear-shaped pouch is the **gallbladder.** This sac is a storage tank for bile, a yellow-green liquid created by the

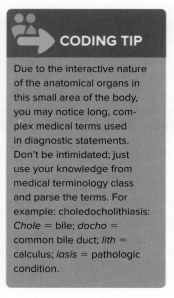

CODING TIP

Due to the interactive nature of the anatomical organs in this small area of the body, you may notice long, complex medical terms used in diagnostic statements. Don't be intimidated; just use your knowledge from medical terminology class and parse the terms. For example: choledocholithiasis: *Chole* = bile; *docho* = common bile duct; *lith* = calculus; *iasis* = pathologic condition.

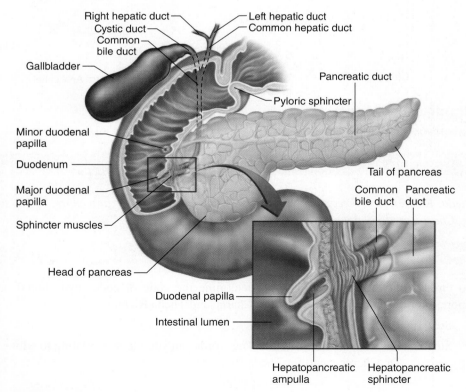

FIGURE 14-7 Accessory Organs

Source: David Shier et al., HOLE'S HUMAN ANATOMY & PHYSIOLOGY, 12/e. © 2010 MHE. Figure 17.23 p. 672

liver and used by the body to assist in the digestive process. When required, the gall-bladder contracts to release bile into the duodenum via the **common bile duct** and the hepatopancreatic ampulla. The common bile duct is the juncture where the *hepatic duct* (which comes from the liver) meets the *cystic duct* (which comes from the gall-bladder). At the *hepatopancreatic sphincter,* both the common bile duct and the pancreatic duct meet to continue into the duodenum.

Liver The **liver** is an almost triangular-shaped organ (see Figure 14-8) located in the right upper quadrant (RUQ) of the abdominal cavity, beneath the diaphragm, anterior to the stomach and pancreas. As the largest gland in the body, it performs many functions, including regulating blood sugar levels and aiding the digestive process by secreting bile to the gallbladder. The liver cleans the blood of toxins; metabolizes proteins, fats, and carbohydrates; and manufactures some blood proteins.

Pancreas Situated posterior to the stomach, tucked inside a curve of the duodenum, is the **pancreas.** The section of the pancreas adjacent to the duodenum, called the *head of the pancreas,* extends to the center section (the body of the pancreas), which extends to the tail of the pancreas, which forms almost a fingerlike shape. The **pancreatic islets** (the islets of Langerhans) create glucagon and insulin, as well as other hormones, and secrete them into the bloodstream. Similar to the gallbladder, the pancreas manufactures certain digestive enzymes that pass into the duodenum via the pancreatic duct (see Figure 14-7).

Malfunction of the pancreas may lead to various health problems, including pancreatic cancer, pancreatitis, cystic fibrosis, and diabetes mellitus. One of the most dangerous concerns about the impact on the body of conditions of the pancreas is that signs and symptoms are few and nonspecific, making diagnosis difficult. For example, there is actually a treatment for pancreatic cancer. However, due to lack of signs and symptoms that typically promote early identification and treatment, diagnosis is not often realized until the malignancy has metastasized to other organs and cannot be halted.

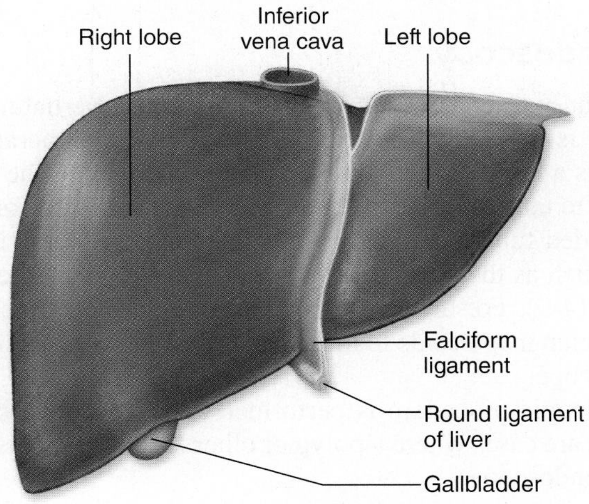

liver
The organ, located in the upper right area of the abdominal cavity, that is responsible for regulating blood sugar levels; secreting bile for the gallbladder; metabolizing fats, proteins, and carbohydrates; manufacturing some blood proteins; and removing toxins from the blood.

pancreas
A large gland responsible for creating digestive enzymes.

pancreatic islets
Cells within the pancreas that secrete insulin and other hormones into the bloodstream.

FIGURE 14-8 The Liver (Anterior View)

Source: Michael McKinley and Valerie O'Loughlin, HUMAN ANATOMY, 1/e. © 2006 MHE. Figure 26.18, p. 815

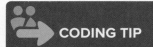
Diagnostic Testing

Pathology and Laboratory

Diagnostic lab tests to identify problems in the liver or pancreas may be ordered by the physician, including:

Glucose (fasting)	Lower than 70mg/dL may indicate liver disease.
	Higher than 99 mg/dL may indicate pancreatitis.
Blood urea nitrogen (BUN)	Higher than 20 mg/dL may indicate liver disease.
Calcium	Lower than 8.5 mg/dL may indicate pancreatitis.
Protein	Lower than 6.3 g/dL may indicate liver disease.
	Higher than 7.9 g/dL may indicate liver disease.
Albumin	Lower than 3.9 g/dL may indicate liver disease.
Bilirubin	Higher than 1.9 mg/dL may indicate liver disease or bile duct disorder.
Amylase	Abnormal levels may indicate a pancreatic disorder.
Alkaline phosphatase (ALP)	Higher than 147 IU/L may indicate liver cancer or bile duct obstruction.
Alanine aminotransferase (ALT)	Higher than 37 IU/L may indicate hepatitis.
Aspartate aminotransferase (AST)	Higher than 34 IU/L may indicate hepatitis.

LO 14.2 Endoscopy

Due to the fact that both ends of the alimentary canal have natural openings to the outside, endoscopy is frequently used for both diagnostic and therapeutic purposes.

An endoscope is a flexible tube with a camera mounted on the end. Small attachments can be used to take biopsies of suspicious tissues or to perform excisions, ablations, or other needed functions. This instrument can be inserted into naturally open anatomical sites, such as the nose, mouth, or anus, to visualize internal aspects of the body (see Figure 14-9). For areas less conducive to visualization through a natural opening, the physician may decide to make a small incision in the skin just big enough to insert the endoscope.

When an endoscopic procedure is performed as a preventive measure, such as a colonoscopy, there are cases where a polyp or other type of lesion is removed using an attachment to the endoscope.

Of course, there are times when the lesion within the colon or other anatomical area may be too flat or small to extirpate. The physician may, then, ablate or fulgurate the lesion.

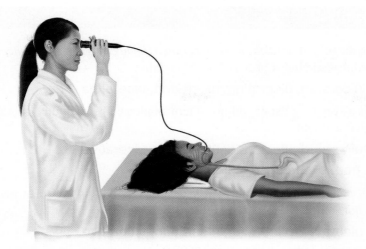

FIGURE 14-9 A Peroral Endoscopy (Endoscope Inserted through the Patient's Mouth)

Digestive Conditions

LO 14.3 Ulcers

An ulcer is a sore or hole in the tissue. Ulcers can occur externally, such as a decubitus ulcer, or they can form internally. The terms used to document an internal ulcer in the digestive system may include:

- Ulcer of esophagus
- Gastric ulcer (in the lining of the stomach)
- Duodenal ulcer
- Gastrojejunal ulcer

You will notice that these descriptors identify the location of the ulcer, such as the esophagus, the stomach, or the jejunum.

Further description of these ulcers may include known complications resulting from an ulcer in this segment of the upper digestive system: **perforation** and **hemorrhage.**

perforation
An atypical hole in the wall of an organ or anatomical site.

hemorrhage
Excessive or severe bleeding.

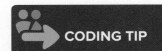
CODING TIP

If a medication caused the ulcer, an external cause code will be required to identify the specific drug and whether or not it was taken for therapeutic purposes.

LET'S CODE IT! SCENARIO

Pauline Ochoa had been taking aspirin several times a day every day for pain in her knees. Her husband, John, came home and found her lying on the kitchen floor. Emergency medical services (EMS) brought her to the ED. Tests revealed an acute perforated, hemorrhaging peptic ulcer due to chronic use of aspirin.

Pauline was diagnosed with an *acute perforated, hemorrhaging peptic ulcer,* so let's turn to the Alphabetic Index of ICD-10-CM and find:

Ulcer, ulcerated, ulcerating, ulceration, ulcerative

There is a very long list of additional terms indented beneath this main listing, so read through it and find:

Ulcer, ulcerated, ulcerating, ulceration, ulcerative
peptic (site unspecified) K27.9

Beneath *peptic* is another indented list. Is there anything here that matches the physician's notes?

Ulcer, ulcerated, ulcerating, ulceration, ulcerative
peptic (site unspecified) K27.9
with
hemorrhage K27.4
and perforation K27.6
acute K27.3
with
hemorrhage K27.0
and perforation K27.2

Hmmm. The good news is that all of these choices are within one code category, K27, so let's turn to the Tabular List and begin reading at:

K27 Peptic ulcer, site unspecified

Use additional code to identify alcohol abuse and dependence (F10.-)

Read the *Includes* and *Excludes1* notes, as well as the *use additional code* notation. Then read down and review all of the choices for the required fourth character. Which one matches the physician's notes the best?

K27.2 Acute peptic ulcer, site unspecified, with both hemorrhage and perforation

Excellent!
Are you done? No. Remember that notation beneath the code category?

Use additional code to identify alcohol abuse and dependence (F10.-)

Was there any mention of alcohol abuse or alcohol dependence in the documentation? No. However, you do know that aspirin caused this ulcer. There is no notation, but remember that your job is to tell the *whole* story. So you will need to find an external cause code to report which drug caused Pauline's peptic ulcer. Aspirin is a drug, so let's turn to the Table of Drugs and Chemicals and find the name of the drug that caused Pauline's peptic ulcer in the first column ("Substance"): aspirin. Look across the line to the code listed in the column under "Adverse Effect." Remember that Pauline was taking the aspirin for therapeutic use—a medical reason. This shows code T39.015.

Let's turn to the T codes in the Tabular List and begin reading at:

T39 Poisoning by, adverse effect of and underdosing of nonopioid analgesics, antipyretics and antirheumatics

Notice that beneath this code category is a notation:

The appropriate 7th character is to be added to each code from category T39

> **A** initial encounter
>
> **D** subsequent encounter
>
> **S** sequela

Remember this is here for reference later. But first you need the fourth, fifth, and sixth characters. Read down and review all of the choices. Which one matches most accurately?

T39.015- Adverse effect of aspirin

Great! Now you need that seventh character. Go back to the documentation. Is this the first time that Pauline is being treated by this physician for this diagnosis? She is in the emergency department, so, yes, this is the initial encounter. Now you have two codes to report Pauline's condition:

K27.2 Acute peptic ulcer, site unspecified, with both hemorrhage and perforation

T39.015A Adverse effect of aspirin, initial encounter

LO 14.4 Hernias

A **hernia** is a condition that is created when a tear or opening in a muscle permits a part of an internal organ to push through. Due to the nature of one anatomical part squeezing through a hole in another site, the blood supply can be cut off to the section stuck in that opening. When that happens, the tissue might become necrotic (deteriorate and die) and/or develop **gangrene.** In addition, this condition can create an **obstruction** in the structure or organ, preventing the normal flow of material.

There are several types of hernias, or anatomical sites that can be susceptible to herniation:

- *Hiatal* (esophageal) hernia may occur when a portion of the stomach pokes through an opening in the diaphragm; congenital diaphragmatic hernias are considered birth defects and reported from the Congenital malformations section of ICD-10-CM.
- *Umbilical* hernia may occur when the muscle around the navel (belly button) does not close completely, permitting an internal organ to protrude.
- *Incisional* hernia is a defect that may occur at the site of a previous abdominal surgical opening (scar tissue).
- *Inguinal* hernias, more common in men, appear in the groin area.
- *Femoral* hernias, more common in women, appear in the upper thigh.

hernia
A condition in which one anatomical structure pushes through a perforation in the wall of the anatomical site that normally contains that structure.

gangrene
Necrotic tissue resulting from a loss of blood supply.

obstruction
A blockage or closing.

YOU CODE IT! CASE STUDY

Jeffrey Gilberts, a 31-year-old male, is brought in for Dr. Gensin to surgically repair his left inguinal hernia created during gestation by a peritoneal sac improperly closing.

You Code It!

Go through the steps of coding, and determine the code or codes that should be reported for this encounter between Dr. Gensin and Jeffrey Gilberts.

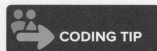
Step 1: Read the case completely.

Step 2: Abstract the notes: Which key words can you identify relating to why Dr. Gensin cared for Jeffrey?

_____

Step 3: Query the provider, if necessary.

Step 4: Code the diagnosis or diagnoses.

_____

Step 5: Code the procedure(s): Surgical repair of inguinal hernia.

Step 6: Link the procedure codes to at least one diagnosis code to confirm medical necessity.

Step 7: Back code to double-check your choices.

Answer:

Did you determine the correct code?

K40.90 Unilateral inguinal hernia, without obstruction or gangrene, not specified as recurrent

Good job!

LO 14.5 Hepatitis

Hepatitis (*hepa-* = liver; *-itis* = inflammation or disease) is a swelling of the liver that causes a reduction in function. Most often, hepatitis is caused by a virus, resulting in a diagnosis that includes the specific type of inflammation, such as hepatitis A, hepatitis B, and so on. (For more details on this condition, see chapter 4 Coding Infectious Diseases).

There are cases when drugs and alcohol can lead to this same diagnosis. Identified as acute or chronic nonviral hepatitis, most patients will exhibit signs and symptoms very similar to viral hepatitis, including nausea, vomiting, and jaundice (yellowing of the skin). Take a look at the *use additional code* notation beneath code category K70:

> **Alcoholic liver disease:**
>> **Use additional code to identify: alcohol abuse and dependence (F10.-)**

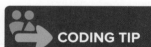
EXAMPLE

B18.2 Chronic viral hepatitis C
K70.10 Alcoholic hepatic failure without coma
K76.4 Peliosis hepatis

Cirrhosis

After a person suffers with chronic hepatic disease, fibrotic tissue may form on hepatic cells causing scarring, known as *cirrhosis of the liver*. This condition may be caused by injury as well. The scar tissue impairs the normal function of the liver and can result in easy bruising or bleeding, abdominal swelling, lower extremity edema, and possibly kidney failure. There is evidence that approximately 5% of patients suffering with cirrhosis will develop liver cancer.

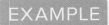

EXAMPLE

K743 Primary biliary cirrhosis

LO 14.6 Cholecystitis

Cholecystitis is the medical term for inflammation of the gallbladder (*chole* = bile; *cyst* = fluid filled sac; *-itis* = inflammation). In cases where the disease affects the bile duct rather than the gallbladder, the diagnosis is cholangitis.

Calculi can accumulate in this area and harden into small rocks (stones) that may block the flow of bile from the gallbladder. This condition is known as **cholelithiasis.** This may occur with or without cholecystitis, changing the code used to report the condition.

cholelithiasis
Gallstones.

EXAMPLE

K80.70 Calculus of gallbladder and bile duct without cholecystitis without obstruction
K81.1 Chronic cholecystitis

Chapter Summary

The organs included in the digestive system run from the head to the bottom of the torso. Therefore, several different health care specialists may be involved in caring for patients with digestive disorders, depending upon where the abnormality is located. Health care issues within the digestive system can occur as the result of a congenital anomaly, a traumatic event, or dietary influence. This means that there may be times when an external cause code is required to be included so that you can tell the whole story about the reasons why (the medical necessity) this patient was cared for.

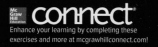

Using Terminology

Match each key term to the appropriate definition.

Part One

_____ **1.** LO 14.1 The section of the tubular organ that leads from the oral cavity to the esophagus.

_____ **2.** LO 14.1 Cells within the pancreas that secrete insulin and other hormones into the bloodstream.

_____ **3.** LO 14.1 A large gland responsible for creating digestive enzymes.

_____ **4.** LO 14.1 The last segment of the small intestine.

_____ **5.** LO 14.1 A saclike organ within the alimentary canal designed to contain nourishment during the initial phase of the digestive process.

_____ **6.** LO 14.1 A long, narrow mass of tissue attached to the cecum; also called *appendix*.

_____ **7.** LO 14.1 The last segment of the large intestine, connecting the sigmoid colon to the anus.

_____ **8.** LO 14.1 Sensory organ attached to the bottom of the mouth; enables speech, eating, and tasting.

_____ **9.** LO 14.1 The tubular organ that connects the pharynx to the stomach for the passage of nourishment.

_____ **10.** LO 14.1 The walls of the oral cavity that form both sides of the face; the buccal area.

_____ **11.** LO 14.1 The organ, located in the upper right area of the abdominal cavity, that is responsible for regulating blood sugar levels; secreting bile for the gallbladder; metabolizing fats, proteins, and carbohydrates; manufacturing some blood proteins; and removing toxins from the blood.

_____ **12.** LO 14.1 The portion of the large intestine that leads outside the body.

_____ **13.** LO 14.1 A muscular structure around the external area of the oral cavity.

_____ **14.** LO 14.1 The first segment of the small intestine, connecting the stomach to the jejunum.

_____ **15.** LO 14.1 The segment of the small intestine that connects the duodenum to the ileum.

A. Anus
B. Cheeks
C. Duodenum
D. Esophagus
E. Ileum
F. Jejunum
G. Lips
H. Liver
I. Pancreas
J. Pancreatic islets
K. Pharynx
L. Rectum
M. Stomach
N. Tongue
O. Vermiform appendix

Part Two

_____ **1.** LO 14.1 A pouchlike organ that connects the ileum with the large intestine; the point of connection for the vermiform appendix.

_____ **2.** LO 14.1 Lymphoid tissue located at the root of the tongue, bilaterally.

_____ **3.** LO 14.1 The digestive pathway from the oral cavity to the anus.

_____ **4.** LO 14.1 The segment of the large intestine that connects the splenic flexure to the sigmoid colon.

_____ **5.** LO 14.1 The portion of the large intestine that connects the hepatic flexure to the splenic flexure.

A. Alimentary canal
B. Ascending colon
C. Cecum
D. Common bile duct
E. Descending colon
F. Lingual tonsils
G. Oral cavity
H. Palatine tonsils

_____ 6. LO 14.1 The juncture of the cystic duct of the gallbladder and the hepatic duct from the liver.

_____ 7. LO 14.1 Lymphoid tissue situated at the entrance to the throat, bilaterally.

_____ 8. LO 14.1 The portion of the large intestine that connects the cecum to the hepatic flexure.

_____ 9. LO 14.1 Lymphoid nodules located on the wall of the pharynx, bilaterally.

_____ 10. LO 14.1 The dual-curved segment of the colon that connects the descending colon to the rectum; also referred to as the *sigmoid flexure*.

_____ 11. LO 14.1 The opening in the face that begins the alimentary canal and is used for the input of nutrition; also known as the *mouth*.

_____ 12. LO 14.1 Three sets of bilateral exocrine glands that secrete saliva: parotid glands, submaxillary glands, and the sublingual glands.

I. Pharyngeal tonsils
J. Salivary glands
K. Sigmoid colon
L. Transverse colon

Part Three

_____ 1. LO 14.4 A blockage or closing.

_____ 2. LO 14.3 An atypical hole in the wall of an organ or anatomical site.

_____ 3. LO 14.1 Organs that assist the digestive process and are adjacent to the alimentary canal: the gallbladder, liver, and pancreas.

_____ 4. LO 14.6 Gallstones.

_____ 5. LO 14.1 A fold of a membrane that carries blood to the small intestine and connects it to the posterior wall of the abdominal cavity.

_____ 6. LO 14.1 A circular muscle that contracts to prevent passage of liquids or solids.

_____ 7. LO 14.1 A pear-shaped organ that stores bile until it is required to aid the digestive process.

_____ 8. LO 14.1 The section of an organ farthest from its opening.

_____ 9. LO 14.1 Absence of teeth.

_____ 10. LO 14.4 A condition in which one anatomical structure pushes through a perforation in the wall of the anatomical site that normally contains that structure.

_____ 11. LO 14.4 Necrotic tissue resulting from a loss of blood supply.

_____ 12. LO 14.3 Excessive or severe bleeding.

A. Accessory organs
B. Cholelithiasis
C. Edentulism
D. Fundus
E. Gallbladder
F. Gangrene
G. Hernia
H. Hemorrhage
I. Mesentery
J. Obstruction
K. Perforation
L. Sphincter

Checking Your Understanding

Choose the most appropriate answer for each of the following questions.

1. LO 14.1 The digestive system includes the
   a. Liver.
   b. Larynx.
   c. Heart.
   d. Coccyx.

2. LO 14.1 The duodenum, jejunum, and ileum are all parts of the

   a. Esophagus.
   b. Liver.
   c. Small intestine.
   d. Large intestine.

3. LO 14.3 The term *hemorrhage* means

   a. Atypical hole.
   b. Obstruction.
   c. Liver.
   d. Excessive bleeding.

4. LO 14.5 Cirrhosis of the liver can be caused by

   a. Abuse of alcohol.
   b. Trauma.
   c. Disease.
   d. All of these.

5. LO 14.4 A hiatal hernia occurs at the

   a. Esophagus.
   b. Small intestine.
   c. Surgical site.
   d. Groin.

6. LO 14.1 The digestive system begins at the

   a. Mouth.
   b. Esophagus.
   c. Stomach.
   d. Small intestine.

7. LO 14.1 The transverse colon lies between the

   a. Ascending colon and the hepatic flexure.
   b. Hepatic flexure and the splenic flexure.
   c. Splenic flexure and the sigmoid colon.
   d. Sigmoid colon and the anus.

8. LO 14.6 Cholelithiasis is commonly known as

   a. Disease of the liver.
   b. Disease of the colon.
   c. Gallstones.
   d. Pancreatic cancer.

9. LO 14.4 Necrotic tissue resulting from a loss of blood supply is known as

   a. Obstruction.
   b. Hemorrhage.
   c. Perforation.
   d. Gangrene.

10. LO 14.1 The gallbladder stores

    a. Calculus.
    b. Bile.
    c. Insulin.
    d. Blood.

Applying Your Knowledge

1. LO 14.1 What is the alimentary canal? List its components. _____

_____

2. LO 14.1 Explain the function of the tongue. _____

_____

3. LO 14.1 How many pairs of tonsils are there in the human body? Where are they located? _____

_____

4. LO 14.1 List four health conditions connected with poor oral hygiene. _____

_____

5. LO 14.1 Which is the largest gland in the body? Where is it located, and what is its function? _____

_____

6. LO 14.1 List five diagnostic lab tests that are used to identify problems with the liver or pancreas. _____

_____

7. LO 14.3/14.4/14.6 List four digestive conditions. _____

_____

8. LO 14.4 What is a hernia? List and explain several types. _____

_____

Using the techniques described in this chapter, carefully read through the case studies and determine the most accurate ICD-10-CM code(s) and external cause code(s), if appropriate, for each case study.

1. Carolina Montoya, a 17-year-old female, presents today complaining of a swollen spot on the roof of her mouth. Carolina is diagnosed with nasopalatine duct cyst.

   _____

2. Harris Parker, a 9-year-old male, is brought in by his parents. Harris is in obvious abdominal distress. Dr. Frazier diagnoses Harris with acute appendicitis with localized peritonitis.

   _____

3. Larry Tunney, a 27-year-old male, presents today with the complaint of loose and greasy stool and weight loss. Dr. Yahu diagnoses Larry with celiac disease.

   _____

4. Richard Nations, a 56-year-old male, comes in today complaining of decreased appetite and weight loss, nausea, and muscle aches and pains. After a thorough examination, Dr. Freed diagnoses Richard with acute hepatitis C.

   _____

5. Ed Peters, a 63-year-old male, presents today with fever and jaundice. Ed admits to drinking alcohol for decades. After testing, Dr. Fong diagnoses Ed with alcoholic cirrhosis of the liver with ascites.

   _____

6. June Callahan, a 34-year-old female, comes in today to see Dr. Jordan, complaining of small whitish-yellow spots on her tongue. Dr. Jordan diagnoses June with leukoplakia of the tongue.

   _____

7. Wanda Hanson, a 57-year-old female, presents today with abdominal pain and tenderness. After a thorough examination, Dr. Keels diagnoses Wanda with chronic proliferative peritonitis with diverticulosis of the jejunum.

   _____

8. Daniel Ackerman, a 46-year-old male, comes in today complaining of diarrhea and vomiting. Dan just finished radiation treatments for his hand malignancy. Dr. Ard diagnoses Dan with gastroenteritis due to radiation.

   _____

9. Alden Fallsman, a 38-year-old male, presents today with dull pain in his chest. After testing, Dr. Better diagnoses Alden with a diaphragmatic hernia with obstruction.

   _____

10. Anna Smokle, a 48-year-old female, comes in today to see Dr. Bradenton. Anna is complaining of abdominal pain and tenderness. Dr. Bradenton diagnoses her with chronic ischemic colitis.

    _____

11. Wallace Banardi, a 28-year-old male, was brought into the ED with apparent abdominal discomfort; a lump can be seen and felt near the navel. Dr. Phillips diagnoses Wallace with a strangulated parumbilical hernia.

    _____

12. Crystal Amera, a 22-year-old female, presents today with the complaint of intermittent high temperature with recurrent chills. After a thorough examination, Crystal is diagnosed with portal pyemia.

    _____

13. Fonda Purseman, a 63-year-old female, returns today to discuss the results of her tests. Dr. Faber diagnoses Fonda with an enterocolic fistula and recommends surgical repair.

    _____

14. Judah Westerman, a 72-year-old male, presents today with fecal incontinence (soiling) that resulted from his nontraumatic anal sphincter tear 1 year ago.

    _____

15. Harvey Liverpool, a 56-year-old male, comes in today with the complaint of long-lasting heartburn and pain under his breastbone. Harvey admits to taking aspirin several times a day for many years. Dr. Camut diagnoses Harvey with an ulcer of the esophagus due to ingestion of aspirin.

    _____

The following exercises provide practice in abstracting physicians' notes and learning to work with SOAP notes from our health care facility, *Taylor, Reader, & Associates*. These case studies (SOAP notes) are modeled on real patient encounters. Using the techniques described in this chapter, carefully read through the case studies and determine the most accurate ICD-10-CM code(s) and external cause code(s), if appropriate, for each case study.

TAYLOR, READER, & ASSOCIATES
A Complete Health Care Facility
975 CENTRAL AVENUE • SOMEWHERE, FL 32811 • 407-555-4321

PATIENT: GRISSOM, GISELLE
ACCOUNT/EHR #:   GRISGI001
DATE: 09/16/18

Attending Physician: Marcus R. Allen, MD

S: Patient is a 3-year-old female brought in by her mother with complaints of mouth pain, malaise, irritability, and a fever over the last week.

O: Gums are swollen and mucous membrane is extremely tender. Papulovesicular ulcers can be seen in the mouth and throat.

A: Herpetiformis stomatitis

P: Mother is instructed to rinse child's mouth with warm water tid. Topical anesthetic is prescribed for mouth pain from the ulcers prn.

Marcus R. Allen, MD

MRA/pw   D: 09/16/18 09:50:16   T: 09/16/18 12:55:01

Determine the most accurate ICD-10-CM code(s).

_____

_____

_____

TAYLOR, READER, & ASSOCIATES
A Complete Health Care Facility
975 CENTRAL AVENUE • SOMEWHERE, FL 32811 • 407-555-4321

PATIENT: BRUCKS, JEROME
ACCOUNT/EHR #:   BRUCJE001
DATE: 09/16/18

Attending Physician: Willard B. Reader, MD

Patient is a 53-year-old male diagnosed with continuing acid reflux. After examination last week, I sent him for a barium swallow fluoroscopy, esophageal pH probe, esophageal manometry, and esophagoscopy. He is here to discuss the results of those tests.

I explain that the test results indicate that he has gastroesophageal reflux (GERD). The first course of treatment is to adopt a low-fat, high-fiber diet. He needs to avoid caffeine, tobacco, and carbonated beverages from this point forward. In addition, food and drink should be stopped at least 2 hours before going to bed, and he should elevate his head 6 to 8 inches while in a supine position.

Patient was informed that surgery may be necessary if diet and positioning do not relieve symptoms.

_____

Willard B. Reader, MD

WBR/pw   D: 09/16/18 09:50:16   T: 09/16/18 12:55:01

Determine the most accurate ICD-10-CM code(s).

_____

_____

_____

TAYLOR, READER, & ASSOCIATES
A Complete Health Care Facility
975 CENTRAL AVENUE • SOMEWHERE, FL 32811 • 407-555-4321

PATIENT: CONQUER, TERESA
ACCOUNT/EHR #:   CONQTE001
DATE: 10/16/18

Attending Physician: Suzanne R. Taylor, MD

S: Teresa Conquer, a 43-year-old female, comes in with complaints of hematemesis and epigastric pain.

O: Fiberoptic endoscopy enabled visualization of esophageal tears.

A: Mallory-Weiss syndrome, confirmed.

P: I discussed the possibility of electrocoagulation therapy for hemostasis or surgery to suture the esophageal lacerations if the condition did not resolve itself.

Suzanne R. Taylor, MD

SRT/pw   D: 10/16/18 09:50:16   T: 10/18/18 12:55:01

Determine the most accurate ICD-10-CM code(s).

_____

_____

_____

TAYLOR, READER, & ASSOCIATES
A Complete Health Care Facility
975 CENTRAL AVENUE • SOMEWHERE, FL 32811 • 407-555-4321

PATIENT: TECHNIA, ISAAC
ACCOUNT/EHR #:   TECHIS001
DATE: 09/16/18

Attending Physician: Marcus R. Allen, MD

S: Patient is a 27-year-old male complaining of lower abdominal pain and diarrhea or constipation. Patient states these conditions seem to alternate. Abdominal distention is evident.

O: Complete history is obtained, including psychological profile. Sigmoidoscopy is completed.

A: Irritable bowel syndrome with diarrhea, confirmed.

P: Patient is advised to keep a food diary to identify trigger foods so they can be avoided to reduce symptoms. Next appointment should be made for 10 days to 2 weeks to evaluate progress.

_____

Marcus R. Allen, MD

MRA/pw   D: 09/16/18 09:50:16   T: 09/16/18 12:55:01

Determine the most accurate ICD-10-CM code(s).

_____

_____

_____

TAYLOR, READER, & ASSOCIATES
A Complete Health Care Facility
975 CENTRAL AVENUE • SOMEWHERE, FL 32811 • 407-555-4321

PATIENT: WILLOWS, WARREN
ACCOUNT/EHR #: WILLWA001
DATE: 09/16/18

Attending Physician: Willard B. Reader, MD

S: Patient is a 43-year-old male complaining of regular bouts of epigastric pain in the area of his belly button. He states that the pain seems to radiate toward his spine. However, last night the pain was severe, and he vomited most of the night.

O: Examination reveals crackles in lower lobe at the base of the lung, tachycardia, and a low-grade fever (101F). Lab results show increased serum lipase levels and increased polymorphonuclear leukocytes. Ultrasound shows enlarged pancreas.

A: Acute pancreatitis

P: Admit to hospital.

_____

Willard B. Reader, MD

WBR/pw   D: 09/16/18 09:50:16   T: 09/16/18 12:55:01

Determine the most accurate ICD-10-CM code(s).

_____

_____

_____

CODING DISEASES OF THE INTEGUMENTARY SYSTEM

15

Learning Outcomes *After completing this chapter, the student should be able to:*

LO 15.1 Identify the layers of skin and elements of the integumentary system.

LO 15.2 Apply the guidelines for reporting pressure ulcers.

LO 15.3 Distinguish the differences between types of lesions.

LO 15.4 Explain the various types of dermatitis and how to code each accurately.

LO 15.5 Interpret inclusive signs and symptoms of psoriasis.

LO 15.6 Abstract the notes to code disorders of skin appendages.

You may have heard someone refer to the human body as a *bag of bones*. This is not so far from the truth. The bag, so to speak, is the **skin,** which encases all of the anatomical elements that construct the body.

The integumentary system is more than just your skin, though. Your nails (fingers and toes) and your hair are also included, as well as sensory receptors, sebaceous (oil) glands, and sweat glands. Together, these additional components are known as *accessory structures* of the skin.

LO 15.1 The Integumentary System Anatomy

The Skin

The average person has roughly 2 square yards (5,184 inches) of skin surface area. As the largest organ in the human body, the skin does so much more than just keep all your internal organs covered. Each of its layers, the **epidermis** and the **dermis,** plays an important role in protecting the body, including:

- *Shielding internal organs:* The epidermis, dermis, and fatty tissue layers of the skin reduce internal injury.
- *Blocking the infiltration of pathogens and water:* The protective layers of the skin prevent viruses and bacteria from invading the internal organs and bloodstream and also prevent an overaccumulation of water—for example, while swimming.
- *Providing temperature control:* The body is better able to regulate its temperature thanks to the protective layer of the skin.

Key Terms

Blister
Bulla
Carbuncle
Cyst
Decubitus ulcer
Dermis
Epidermis
Furuncle
Gangrene
Hair
Hair follicle
Macule
Nevus
Nodule
Papule
Patch
Phalanges
Pressure ulcer
Pustule
Scale
Skin
Subcutaneous
Ulcer

- *Maintaining homeostasis:* The skin helps to maintain the equilibrium of the body's systems.
- *Accumulating vitamin D:* The energy of the UV light in sunlight is involved in the pathway that generates vitamin D, which is needed by the body to enable calcium absorption.
- *Sensing things through the tactile receptors:* The layers of the skin incorporate sensory receptors to enable the body to feel cold, pain, heat, and touch (feeling).

The epidermis, the outermost layer of the skin, is thin and made up of levels of epithelial cells. No blood vessels are present in this stratum of the skin, and it contains only a few nerve endings. However, there are special cells known as *melanocytes* in this top layer. Melanocytes create *melanin,* which determines skin color. For the most part, the color of the skin is determined by genetics—an individual's genes direct the melanin to produce more or less color. Melanin absorbs ultraviolet rays from sunlight, which can also influence the color, or pigment, of the skin. This is why sitting in the sun may cause light skin to tan—the melanin has absorbed more ultraviolet rays, becoming darker. In addition, the bright red color of blood will make light skin appear pinkish. When blood does not get the required amount of oxygen, its color will deepen, resulting in light skin appearing blue—a condition known as *cyanosis* (*cyan* = blue + *-osis* = condition). When there is an accumulation of bilirubin in the body, such as when the liver is malfunctioning, skin can appear yellowish—a condition known as *jaundice.* Some individuals lack melanin completely; this condition is known as *albinism.*

The dermis is a sturdy collagenous layer that connects the epidermis to the fatty tissue layer. Blood vessels, nerves, glands, hair follicles, and lymph channels are all located in this stratum of the skin. In Figure 15-1, you can see how all of the components of the integumentary system work together—the skin (epidermis and dermis)

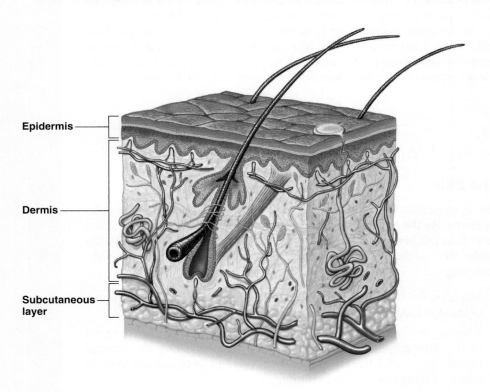

Epidermis

Dermis

Subcutaneous layer

FIGURE 15-1 The Layers of the Skin

Source: David Shier et al., HOLE'S HUMAN ANATOMY & PHYSIOLOGY, 12/e. © 2010 MHE. Figure 6.2a p. 172

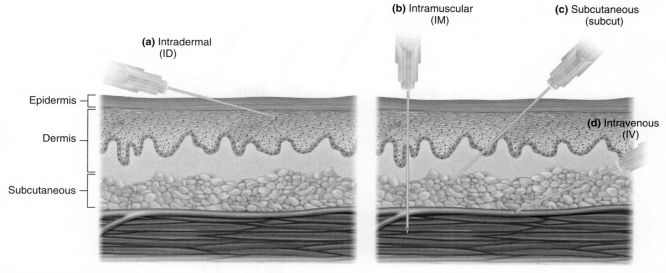

FIGURE 15-2 Injection Routes

Source: Booth et al., MA, 5e. Copyright © 2013 by McGraw-Hill. Figure 53-5, p. 1081

along with the accessory structures (hair, nails, glands, and sensory receptors). Notice how the line between the epidermis and the dermis has hills and ridges, known as *dermal papillae.* Fingerprints are formed by these genetically prompted elevations and valleys, which are then altered further during formation as a fetus presses against the wall of the uterus. This explains why no two people have the same fingerprints, not even identical twins.

Fastening the skin to the underlying elements of the anatomy is the fatty tissue, also known as the *hypodermis* (*hypo* = below + *dermis* = dermal) or the **subcutaneous** layer.

Some of these terms may sound familiar to you because we discussed them earlier when reviewing the various ways drugs can be administered into the body. In Figure 15-2, do you see how the needle illustrating an *intradermal* injection has its tip pointing into the dermis (*intra* = within + *dermal* = dermis)? The injection that is delivered *subcutaneously* has the tip of the needle all the way down into the fatty tissue layer. And the *intramuscular* (*intra* = within + *muscular* = muscle) injection leads down to the layer of muscle that lies below the fatty tissue layer.

subcutaneous
The layer beneath the dermis; also known as the *hypodermis.*

Hair

Hair is a pigmented (colored), hard keratin that grows from the **hair follicle**—the location of the hair root. As you can see in Figure 15-3, the follicle is embedded in the dermis and fatty tissue of the skin layers. As you probably know from your own body, hair may grow externally, such as on your scalp, as well as internally, such as inside the nasal or ear cavity. The hairs in the nose help to prevent certain particles from entering the respiratory system.

Hair growth begins at the base of the follicle as epidermal cells divide. The older cells then become keratinized and push outward. Stem cells continue this growth. Genetics determines the color of one's hair, just as it does with the skin.

Alopecia (hair loss or baldness) is reported with any one of many ICD-10-CM codes connected with the underlying cause, such as L64.0, Drug-induced androgenic alopecia, or A51.32, Secondary syphilitic alopecia.

A patient may be found to be suffering from pathologic compulsive hair-pulling, reported with code F63.3, Trichotillomania. Patients may also suffer from hirsutism (abnormal excessive hair), reported with code L68.0.

hair
A pigmented, cylindrical filament that grows out from the hair follicle within the epidermis.

hair follicle
A saclike bulb containing the hair root.

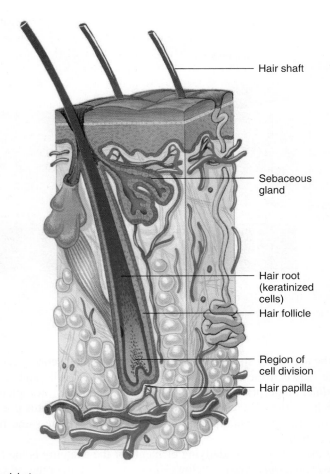

FIGURE 15-3 Hairs

Source: David Shier et al., HOLE'S HUMAN ANATOMY & PHYSIOLOGY, 12/e. © 2010 MHE. Figure 6.7a p. 178

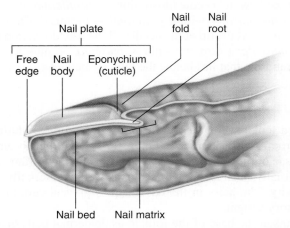

FIGURE 15-4 Anatomy of the Basic Parts of a Human Nail: nail plate, lunula, root, sinus, matrix, nail bed, hyponychium, free margin.

Source: Booth et al., MA, 5e. Copyright © 2013 by McGraw-Hill. Figure 23-4, p. 501

Nails

As you can see in Figure 15-4, there are several components of nails—those hard, protective layers at the ends of your **phalanges** (fingers and toes). The most well-known part of the nail is the *nail plate,* the main part of the nail, which lies upon a layer of skin (nail bed). At the point where the nail plate goes beneath the skin (*eponychium* = nail

phalanges
Fingers and toes.

fold + cuticle) of the finger (or toe) is the *lunula,* a white area shaped like a crescent moon (therefore, the term *lunula,* from *luna,* meaning moon). As the nail grows over the tip of the phalange, the area of epidermis beneath is called the *hyponychium.*

Physicians have known for centuries that the nails can communicate details about an individual's health and reveal early signs of some health care concerns. Some examples are:

- *Thickened nail plate* may reveal a fungal infection or impeded circulation to the phalanges.
- *Soft nail plate* may signify malnutrition, arthritis, or abnormalities in the endocrine system.
- *Longitudinal ridges* in the nail plate may indicate kidney failure, thyroid disease, or possibly malabsorption of minerals and vitamins.
- *Yellowed nail plate* may be a sign of diabetes mellitus, psoriasis, or the presence of fungus, or it may be drug-induced.
- *Spoon-shaped nail plate* may denote an iron deficiency or possible thyroid disease.

EXAMPLE

L60.2 Onychogryphosis
L60.5 Yellow nail syndrome

Glands

Three different types of glands are located within the skin:

- *Sebaceous glands* produce an oil-rich element, known as *sebum,* which lies on the outer surface of the epidermis and along the hair. The substance has a waterproofing effect. Individuals with oily skin may have overly active sebaceous glands.
- *Eccrine glands* are sweat glands that are responsible for maintaining proper body temperature by excreting sweat (water, salt, and wastes) via the pores in the skin. Production of more sweat is the reaction to cool an overheated body (see Figure 15-5).
- *Apocrine glands* releases out a discharge that is high in protein. Located in the axilla (armpits), anal, and genital areas, bacteria interact with the protein and create an odor.

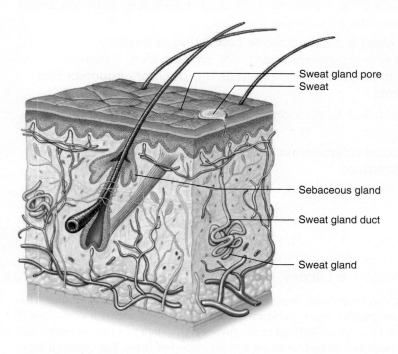

FIGURE 15-5 Sweat Glands

Source: Booth et al., MA, 5e. Copyright © 2013 by McGraw-Hill. Figure 23-1, p. 497

L74.512 Primary focal hyperhidrosis, palms

There is more about the endocrine system in Chapter 7 of this text.

Sensory Nerves

A part of the nervous system known as the *somatic* (relating to the body) *sensory system,* sensory nerve endings are located in the layers of the skin to provide sensory feedback—the sense of touch. These nerves enable you to feel pressure, pain, temperature (hot and cold), textures (rough and smooth), and more.

There is more about the nervous system in Chapter 9 of this text.

LET'S CODE IT! SCENARIO

Willow Washington is a 21-year-old female who came in to see Dr. Lappin with thickened, hardened skin and subcutaneous tissue on her forearms, bilaterally. Examination shows Addison's keloid present. She is given a referral to a plastic surgeon.

Let's Code It!

Dr. Lappin diagnosed Willow with *Addison's keloid* on both of her forearms. Let's begin by finding this key term in the Alphabetic Index:

Keloid, cheloid L91.0

Addison's L94.0

Let's find this code category in the Tabular List:

L94 Other localized connective tissue disorders

The terms here don't match exactly. Let's check a medical encyclopedia to find out exactly what an Addison's keloid is:

Addison's keloid is a skin disease consisting of patches of yellowish or ivory-colored hard, dry, smooth skin. It is more common in females. Also known as morphea or circumscribed scleroderma.

This helps a great deal. Read the complete code descriptions in this code category. Did you connect:

L94.0 Localized scleroderma [morphea] (Circumscribed scleroderma)

Fantastic!

pressure ulcer
An open wound or sore caused by pressure, infection, or inflammation.

decubitus ulcer
A skin lesion caused by continuous pressure on one spot, particularly on a bony prominence.

Conditions of the Skin

LO 15.2 Pressure Ulcers

A **pressure ulcer** can be created in an area of skin when tissue breaks down. Also known as a *bedsore, plaster ulcer, pressure sore,* or **decubitus ulcer,** it can occur if the patient is unable to move or shift his or her own weight, such as when an individual is confined to a wheelchair or bed, even for a short period of time. The constant pressure against the skin reduces the blood supply to that particular area, and the affected

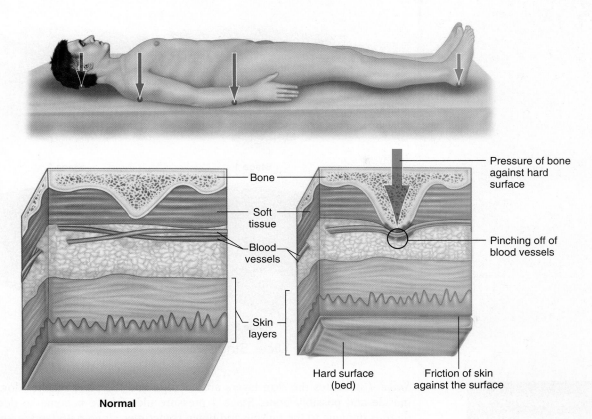

FIGURE 15-6 Etiology of Pressure Ulcers

tissue becomes necrotic (dies). You might have experienced this yourself with a pebble in your shoe or a simple fold of your sock within a tight shoe. The area where the pressure impacted your foot became more and more painful. If you took your shoe right off, you might have noticed a red area. If you waited a length of time before removing your shoe, you found a painful **blister**. The longer the pressure and irritation are maintained, the worse the damage to the skin (see Figure 15-6).

The National Pressure Ulcer Advisory Panel (NPUAP) defines a pressure ulcer as "a localized injury to the skin and/or underlying tissue, usually over a bony prominence, as a result of pressure, or pressure in combination with shear and/or friction."

As a professional coding specialist, you will need to know two factors to determine the correct codes for a diagnosed pressure ulcer:

- Anatomical location (where on the body the ulcer is).
- Depth of the lesion (also known as the *stage of ulcer*).

There are four stages of pressure ulcers (see Figure 15-7):

- *Stage 1* affects the epidermal layer and is recognized by persistent erythema (redness). A stage I pressure ulcer is visualized as a reddened area on the skin that, when pressed with the finger, is nonblanchable (does not turn white).
- *Stage 2* is a partial-thickness loss involving both the epidermis and the dermis; sometimes a fluid-filled blister is evident. A stage 2 pressure ulcer shows visible blisters or forms an open sore. The tissue surrounding the sore may be red and irritated like an abrasion, blister, or shallow crater with a red-pink wound bed.
- *Stage 3* pressure ulcer involves skin loss through and including the subcutaneous tissue. A stage 3 pressure ulcer looks like a crater with visible damage to the tissue below the skin. Full-thickness tissue loss may expose subcutaneous fatty tissue but not bone, tendon, or muscle.

blister
A bubble or sac formed on the surface of the skin, typically filled with a watery fluid or serum.

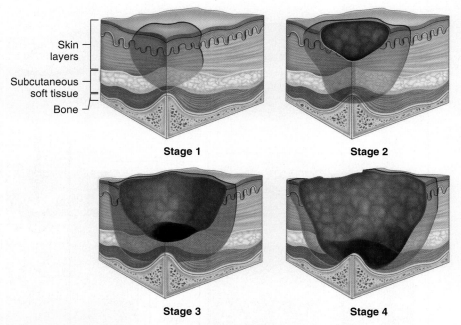

Skin layers
Subcutaneous soft tissue
Bone

Stage 1   Stage 2

Stage 3   Stage 4

FIGURE 15-7 Pressure Ulcer Stages

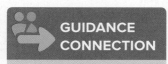

GUIDANCE CONNECTION

Review the ICD-10-CM Coding Guidelines, Section I.C.12, Chapter 12: **Diseases of the skin and subcutaneous tissue,** Subsection a, **Pressure ulcer stage codes**.

- *Stage 4* indicates the skin layers are necrotic and the ulcer reaches down into muscle and possibly bone. Stage 4 pressure ulcers have become so deep that there is damage to the muscle and bone, sometimes along with tendon and joint damage. While the depth of the ulcer varies on the basis of the anatomical site, there is full-thickness tissue loss with bone, tendon, or muscle exposed.

- An *unstageable ulcer* is *not* an unspecified stage. There are times when slough and eschar must be removed to reveal the base of the wound before the true depth, or stage, can be accurately determined. The lesion may be inaccessible—because it is covered by a wound dressing that has not been removed or by a sterile blister or because of some other documented reason.

ICD-10-CM has created combination codes, therefore requiring only one code to identify both the anatomical site and the stage of the ulcer.

EXAMPLE

The patient has a stage 3 pressure ulcer on his left hip.
    L89.223 Pressure ulcer of left hip, stage 3

Healing Pressure Ulcers

It is logical that a patient will be attended to by a health care professional during the time the pressure ulcer is healing. Typically, the documentation will identify the original stage and describe the ulcer as "healing." For example, "Harvey Rhoden was seen today by Dr. Steelman to follow up on his stage 2 pressure ulcer. Dr. Steelman documented that the ulcer is healing nicely." In this case, you would continue to code this as a stage 2 pressure ulcer.

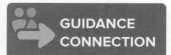

GUIDANCE CONNECTION

Review the ICD-10-CM Coding Guidelines, Section I.C.12, Chapter 12: **Diseases of the skin and subcutaneous tissue,** Subsection a(5), **Patients admitted with pressure ulcers documented as healing**.

Presence of Gangrene

Notice the *code first* notation beneath the code category L89, Pressure ulcer, to report the code for any gangrenous condition associated with the ulcer by using code I96,

Gangrene, not elsewhere classified (Gangrenous cellulitis). You are directed by this notation to list the gangrene code first, followed by the pressure ulcer code.

Did you notice that the code for gangrene is in the chapter of codes used to report diseases of the circulatory system? This makes sense because **gangrene** is necrosis, cell death and decay caused by insufficient blood supply to the affected cells. Remember that pressure ulcers are caused by the ongoing compression of the skin, often resulting in the prevention of blood flow into the area. Look again at Figure 15-6.

gangrene
Death and decay of tissue due to inadequate blood supply.

LET'S CODE IT! SCENARIO

After attempting to jump his motorcycle over five barrels and crashing on the other side, Sam ended up in the hospital for 6 weeks with a left, closed, transverse fractured femur, shaft; a right, closed oblique fractured femoral shaft; and three fractured ribs, left side. He was unable to move without extreme pain, so he lay in bed virtually motionless, except with help from the nurse. After several weeks, while changing the sheets, Nurse Beasley identified a pressure ulcer on each of his hips. Dr. Kennedy staged the ulcers bilaterally as stage 2 and ordered wound care immediately. While there, Dr. Kennedy also checked Sam's progress on the healing of his fractures.

Let's Code It!

Dr. Kennedy came in to stage and treat Sam's pressure ulcers: *bilateral hip pressure ulcers,* both documented as stage 2. Let's turn to the Alphabetic Index and find:

Ulcer, ulcerated, ulcerating, ulceration, ulcerative
Pressure L89.9-
Hip L89.2-

Perfect! Now let's turn to L89 in the Tabular List and read completely.

L89 Pressure Ulcer

Read the *Includes, code first,* and *Excludes2* notations. There is nothing here to direct you elsewhere, so continue reading and review *all* of the required fourth-character choices to determine the one that matches the physician's notes:

L89.2 Pressure ulcer of hip

This matches the notes, so you know you are in the right place. Next, you must determine the required fifth character for this ulcer code. Check the documentation; is the pressure ulcer on his right hip or left hip? Both, actually, so you will need two codes, one for each hip:

L89.21 Pressure ulcer of right hip
L89.22 Pressure ulcer of left hip

To identify the sixth characters, you will need to abstract from the documentation regarding the stage of each ulcer. The documentation states stage 2 for both.

L89.212 Pressure ulcer of right hip, stage 2
L89.222 Pressure ulcer of left hip, stage 2

These pressure ulcer codes will be reported first because the ulcers are the principal reason Dr. Kennedy came to see Sam for this encounter. Then follow these with the codes to report Sam's fractures, and you will have the diagnosis codes to report this encounter:

L89.212 Pressure ulcer of right hip, stage 2

L89.222 Pressure ulcer of left hip, stage 2

S72.325D Nondisplaced transverse fracture of shaft of left femur

S72.334D Nondisplaced oblique fracture of shaft of right femur

S22.42xD Multiple fractures of ribs, left side

LO 15.3 Lesions

Many people believe a lesion is a sore on the epidermis; however, lesions might also occur internally. Skin lesions are categorized as primary or secondary and are pathologically determined to be benign or malignant. Even though the majority of lesions are external, reporting them is not confined to the codes in the L00–L99 section, Diseases of the skin and subcutaneous tissue. Essentially, lesion codes are located throughout the code set; they are most often found in the section related to the anatomical location or by a specific term. Many skin lesions (see Figure 15-8) are identified by name or type, including:

- **Cyst:** a fluid-filled or gas-filled bubble in the skin.
- **Furuncle:** a staphylococcal infection in the subcutaneous tissue; commonly known as a *boil.*
- **Papule:** a raised lesion with a diameter of less than 5 mm.
- **Nodule:** a tissue mass or papule larger than 5 mm.
- **Macule:** a flat lesion with a different pigmentation (color) when compared with the surrounding skin. An *ephelidis* (freckle) is a small macule.
- **Nevus:** an abnormally pigmented area of skin. A birthmark is an example.
- **Patch:** a flat, small area of differently colored or textured skin; a large macule.
- **Bulla:** a large vesicle that is filled with fluid.
- **Pustule:** a swollen area of skin; a vesicle filled with pus.
- **Scale:** flaky exfoliated epidermis; a flake of skin.
- **Ulcer:** an erosion or loss of the full thickness of the epidermis.

EXAMPLE

L02.32 Furuncle of buttock

Let's turn to the Alphabetic Index and find the key term *lesion.* Review the terms shown in the indented list that follows, providing additional description for the type of lesion documented. For the most part, these lesions are directly described by their anatomical location, with no additional clinical terminology.

EXAMPLE

Lesion, aortic (valve) I35.9 (an internal lesion)

Lesion, lip K13.0 (an external lesion)

Lesion, basal ganglion G25.9 (an internal lesion)

Lesion, eyelid H00.03- (an external lesion)

Often, a skin lesion is diagnosed with a specific name or by type. Therefore, the most effective way to find the codes in the Alphabetic Index is to look up the exact

cyst
A fluid-filled or gas-filled bubble in the skin.

furuncle
A staphylococcal infection in the subcutaneous tissue; commonly known as a *boil.*

papule
A raised lesion with a diameter of less than 5 mm.

nodule
A tissue mass or papule larger than 5 mm.

macule
A flat lesion with a different pigmentation (color) when compared with the surrounding skin.

nevus
An abnormally pigmented area of skin. A birthmark is an example.

patch
A flat, small area of differently colored or textured skin; a large macule.

bulla
A large vesicle that is filled with fluid.

pustule
A swollen area of skin; a vesicle filled with pus.

scale
Flaky exfoliated epidermis; a flake of skin.

ulcer
An erosion or loss of the full thickness of the epidermis.

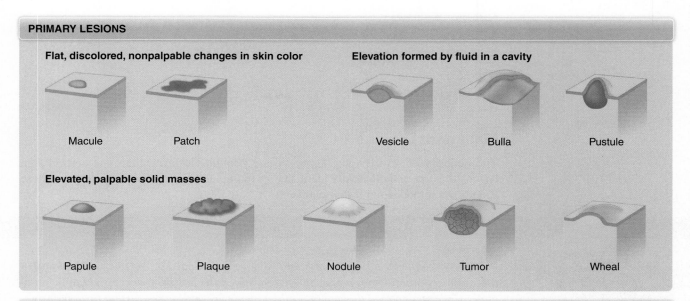

PRIMARY LESIONS

Flat, discolored, nonpalpable changes in skin color

Macule   Patch

Elevation formed by fluid in a cavity

Vesicle   Bulla   Pustule

Elevated, palpable solid masses

Papule   Plaque   Nodule   Tumor   Wheal

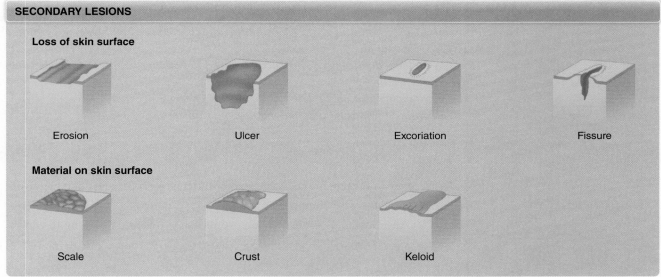

SECONDARY LESIONS

Loss of skin surface

Erosion   Ulcer   Excoriation   Fissure

Material on skin surface

Scale   Crust   Keloid

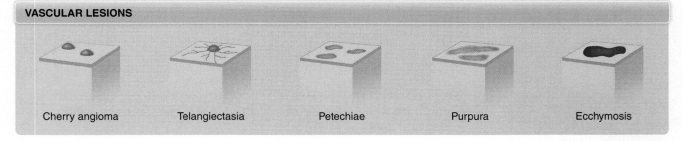

VASCULAR LESIONS

Cherry angioma   Telangiectasia   Petechiae   Purpura   Ecchymosis

FIGURE 15-8 Skin Lesions

Source: Booth et al., MA, 5e. Copyright © 2013 by McGraw-Hill. Figure 23-2, p. 498

term that the physician used in the diagnostic statement first, before trying to generalize by interpreting *lesion* and using that term. For example, **carbuncles** and furuncles, also known as *boils* (a type of pustule caused by an infection), are listed by the terms *carbuncle* and *furuncle,* rather than under the main term of *lesion,* with the fourth character identifying the anatomical location of the skin condition.

carbuncle
A painful, pus-filled boil due to infection of the epidermis and underlying tissues, often caused by staphylococcus.

Malignant Lesions

The majority of skin lesions diagnosed are benign. However, there are certain skin lesions that are pathologically identified as malignant. For more information on these lesions, refer to Chapter 9 in this text.

YOU CODE IT! CASE STUDY

Marlene Ingognetti, a 59-year-old female, comes in to see Dr. Wegner, complaining of an extremely painful spot on her thigh. She states she has been very tired lately, especially since she noticed this bump. Patient history reveals a preexistent furunculosis.

Examination shows deep follicular abscess of several follicles with several draining points. CBC shows an elevated white blood cell count. Wound culture identifies Staphylococcus aureus.

Area is cleaned thoroughly. Instructions given to patient to apply warm, wet compresses at home.

A: Carbuncle of the thigh, left

P: Rx for erythromycin, q8h and mupirocin ointment

You Code It!

Read Dr. Wegner's notes on his encounter with Marlene carefully, and code the visit.

Step 1: Read the case completely.

Step 2: Abstract the notes: Which key words can you identify relating to why Dr. Wegner cared for Marlene?

_____

Step 3: Query the provider, if necessary.

Step 4: Code the diagnosis or diagnoses.

_____

Step 5: Code the procedure(s): Office visit.

Step 6: Link the procedure codes to at least one diagnosis code to confirm medical necessity.

Step 7: Back code to double-check your choices.

Answer:

Did you determine the correct codes?

L02.436 Carbuncle of left lower limb

B95.61 Methicillin susceptible Staphylococcus aureus infection as the cause of diseases classified elsewhere

Good job!

LO 15.4 Dermatitis

Dermatitis is technically an inflammation of the skin (*derma* = skin + *-itis* = inflammation). However, it is not as simple as this; there are several types of dermatitis.

Atopic dermatitis (category L20) includes Besnier's prurigo, flexural eczema, infantile eczema, and intrinsic (allergic) eczema. Most often, this chronic inflammation affects infants (1 month to 1 year of age) with family histories of atopic conditions such as allergic rhinitis and bronchial asthma. Signs and symptoms include erythematous areas on extremely dry skin, appearing as lesions on the forehead, cheeks, arms, and legs. The pruritus nature of this condition results in scratching that induces scaling and edema.

Seborrheic dermatitis (category L21) includes seborrhea capitis and seborrheic infantile dermatitis, commonly affecting the scalp and face. Symptoms include itching, erythematous areas, and inflammation, characterized by lesions covered with brownish gray or yellow scales in areas in which sebaceous glands are plentiful.

Diaper dermatitis (category L22), commonly referred to as *diaper rash,* is caused by continuously wet skin. Often, this develops when diapers are not changed frequently enough to permit the area to dry out.

Allergic contact dermatitis (category L23) is the result of the skin touching a material or substance to which the patient is sensitive. In addition to erythematous areas, vesicles develop that itch, scale, and may ooze.

Irritant contact dermatitis (category L24) is caused by exposure of the skin to detergents, solvents, acids, or alkalis. Blisters and/or ulcerations may appear in the area that came in contact with the chemical.

Exfoliative dermatitis (category L26) is an acute and chronic inflammation with widespread erythema and scales. The loss of the stratum corneum (the outermost layer of the epidermis) is at the heart of this condition, along with hair loss, fever, and shivering.

Dermatitis due to substances taken internally (category L27) would include an inflammatory eruption of the epidermis in reaction to medications, drugs, ingested food, or other substances. It may be easy to think that this might be limited to a response only to oral medicines, but, technically, a drug injected, infused, or delivered via subcutaneous patch also places the pharmaceutical internally. Keep a watchful eye on the *use additional code* notations within this code category, which remind you to include an external cause code.

LO 15.5 Psoriasis

Identified by epidermal erythematous papules and plaques covered with silvery scales, psoriasis is a chronic illness. Exacerbations (flare-ups) can be treated to relieve the symptoms. Patients can inherit the tendency to develop psoriasis because it is genetically passed from parent to child. Its pruritic nature can sometimes result in pain along with itching in the areas covered with dry, cracked, encrusted lesions appearing on the scalp, chest, elbows, knees, shins, back, and buttocks. The silver scales may flake away easily or create a thickened cover over the lesion. There are several types of psoriasis, including the following:

Psoriasis vulgaris, also known as *nummular psoriasis* or *plaque psoriasis,* is the most common type of psoriasis. It usually causes dry, red skin lesions (plaques) covered with silvery scales. Reported with code L40.0.

Guttate psoriasis appears more often in young adults (under the age of 30) as well as children. Lesions covered by a fine scale will typically develop as small, teardrop-shaped sores on the scalp, arms, trunk, and legs. Reported with code L40.4.

Psoriatic arthritis mutilans presents with pain, edema, and/or loss of flexibility in at least one joint. When affecting the fingers or toes, the nails may show pitting or begin to separate from the nail bed. Reported with code L40.52.

Norman Waddell, a 39-year-old male, presents to Dr. Vendula with what he believes to be nonscarring male-pattern alopecia.

Examination reveals small patches of scalp, with some limited mild erythema.

"Exclamation point" hairs are located on the periphery with some indication of new patches and regrowth.

Explained to patient that complete regrowth is possible in this diagnosis.

Diagnosis: alopecia capitis

Treatment plan: intralesional corticosteroid injections followed by minoxidil applications.

You Code It!

Read Dr. Vendula's notes on his encounter with Norman carefully, and code the visit.

Step 1: Read the case completely.

Step 2: Abstract the notes: Which key words can you identify relating to why Dr. Vendula cared for Norman?

_____

Step 3: Query the provider, if necessary.

Step 4: Code the diagnosis or diagnoses.

_____

Step 5: Code the procedure(s): Office visit.

Step 6: Link the procedure codes to at least one diagnosis code to confirm medical necessity.

Step 7: Back code to double-check your choices.

Answer:

Did you determine the correct code?

L63.0 Alopecia (capitis) totalis

Good work!

LO 15.6 Disorders of Skin Appendages

Nail Disorders

The human body has 20 nails—10 fingernails and 10 toenails—and as with any other anatomical site, things can go wrong.

Onycholysis: This is a detachment of the nail from the bed of the nail. Onset occurs at either the distal or lateral attachment. Patients previously diagnosed with psoriasis or thyrotoxicosis are most often seen with this condition. Reported with code L60.1.

Beau's lines: These are deeply grooved, horizontal lines (from side to side) on either a fingernail or a toenail. Previous infection, injury, or other disruption to the nail fold, the location of nail formation, may be the cause. Reported with code L60.4.

Yellow nail syndrome: A thickened nail that has become yellowed is typically seen in patients previously diagnosed with systemic disease, such as lymphedema or bronchiectasis. This is reported with code L60.5.

Disorders of the Hair

For some patients, a bad hair day can be much more serious than a cowlick or frizz.

Alopecia mucinosa: This skin disorder may first be identified by erythematous plaqueing of the skin without any hair growth. The flat patches of hairlessness may occur on the scalp, face, or legs. Reported with code L65.2.

Trichorrhexis nodosa: Evidenced by a hair shaft defect that causes weak spots, this disorder results in hair that easily breaks. Most often, this condition is caused by environmental factors such as blow drying, permanent waves, or excessive chemical exposure. Reported with code L67.0.

Hirsutism: Women with this condition have excessive hair growth on anatomical sites where hair does not typically occur, such as the chest or chin. It is believed to be caused by an abnormal hormonal level, particularly male hormones such as testosterone. Reported with code L68.0.

Glandular Concerns

Eccrine Sweat Disorders (Code Category L74) As with any other anatomical site, the eccrine sweat glands can malfunction. One condition is known as *focal hyperhidrosis* (excessive sweating). This is reported with a specific character to identify the region of the body affected (i.e., axillae, face, palms, or soles). Primary hyperhidrosis is an idiopathic condition (no known etiology), whereas secondary focal hyperhidrosis (also known as *Frey's syndrome*) is often caused by damage to the parotid glands, resulting in excessive salivation. Hypohidrosis (code L74.4), also known as *anhidrosis,* is a condition in which the glands do not produce enough perspiration. This may lead to hyperthermia, heat stroke, or heat exhaustion.

Apocrine Sweat Disorders (Code Category L75) One of the challenges in dealing with an apocrine sweat disorder is the potential for embarrassment due to the increase in body odor. Natural odors can be a natural attraction between humans; however, when body oder is out of balance, this can cause both physiological and psychological problems. Bromhidrosis (foul-smelling perspiration, code L75.0) or chromhidrosis (pigmented perspiration, code L75.1) can be publicly humiliating to any adult.

Chapter Summary

With all the advertising about lotions to preserve youthful skin, shampoos and conditioners for soft hair, and manicures and pedicures for nails, you may forget that the elements of the integumentary system (skin, hair, nails) are not just cosmetic or decorative elements of our bodies. In addition, the glands embedded in the skin support the ongoing proper function of the body.

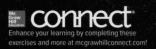

Using Terminology

Match each key term to the appropriate definition.

Part One

_____ **1.** LO 15.2 A bubble or sac formed on the surface of the skin, typically filled with a watery fluid or serum.

_____ **2.** LO 15.3 An erosion or loss of the full thickness of the epidermis.

_____ **3.** LO 15.2 Death and decay of tissue due to inadequate blood supply.

_____ **4.** LO 15.1 The layer beneath the dermis; also known as the *hypodermis.*

_____ **5.** LO 15.3 A painful, pus-filled boil due to infection of the epidermis and underlying tissues, often caused by staphylococcus.

_____ **6.** LO 15.2 A skin lesion caused by continuous pressure on one spot, particularly on a bony prominence.

_____ **7.** LO 15.1 A saclike bulb containing the hair root.

_____ **8.** LO 15.1 Fingers and toes.

_____ **9.** LO 15.1 A pigmented, cylindrical filament that grows out from the hair follicle within the epidermis.

_____ **10.** LO 15.1 The external layer of the skin, the majority of which is squamous cells.

_____ **11.** LO 15.1 The internal layer of the skin; the location of blood vessels, lymph vessels, hair follicles, sweat glands, and sebum.

_____ **12.** LO 15.3 A staphylococcal infection in the subcutaneous tissue; commonly known as a *boil.*

_____ **13.** LO 15.1 The external membranous covering of the body.

A. Blister
B. Carbuncle
C. Decubitus ulcer
D. Dermis
E. Epidermis
F. Furuncle
G. Gangrene
H. Hair
I. Hair follicle
J. Phalanges
K. Skin
L. Subcutaneous
M. Ulcer

Part Two

_____ **1.** LO 15.3 A large macule.

_____ **2.** LO 15.3 A raised lesion with a diameter of less than 5 mm.

_____ **3.** LO 15.3 An abnormally pigmented area of skin. A birthmark is an example.

_____ **4.** LO 15.3 A flat lesion with a different pigmentation (color) when compared with the surrounding skin.

_____ **5.** LO 15.3 A papule larger than 5 mm.

_____ **6.** LO 15.3 A fluid-filled or gas-filled bubble in the skin.

_____ **7.** LO 15.3 Flaky exfoliated epidermis.

_____ **8.** LO 15.3 A large vesicle that is filled with fluid.

_____ **9.** LO 15.3 A vesicle filled with pus.

A. Cyst
B. Papule
C. Nodule
D. Macule
E. Nevus
F. Patch
G. Bulla
H. Pustule
I. Scale

Checking Your Understanding

Choose the most appropriate answer for each of the following questions.

1. LO 15.1 The skin is responsible for all of the following roles *except*
   a. protecting internal organs.
   b. absorbing calcium.
   c. preventing invasion of pathogens.
   d. maintaining homeostasis.

2. LO 15.1 The layer below the dermis is called the
   a. fatty tissue.
   b. hypodermis.
   c. subcutaneous layer.
   d. all of these.

3. LO 15.1 The outermost layer of the skin is called the
   a. epidermis.
   b. dermis.
   c. fatty tissue.
   d. subcutaneous.

4. LO 15.1 Pathologic hair-pulling is known as
   a. trichotillomania.
   b. hirsutism.
   c. alopecia.
   d. cilia.

5. LO 15.2 The patient has been diagnosed with a stage 4 pressure ulcer of the left heel. What is the correct code?
   a. L97.419.
   b. L97.429.
   c. L89.613.
   d. L89.624.

6. LO 15.1/15.6 Apocrine glands may provide the material that results in
   a. oily hair.
   b. sweaty palms.
   c. body odor.
   d. baldness.

7. LO 15.3 A raised lesion with a diameter of less than 5 mm is a
   a. papule.
   b. furuncle.
   c. cyst.
   d. bulla.

8. LO 15.2 When skin layers are necrotic and erosion cuts down into the muscle, this is a _____ pressure ulcer.

    a. stage 1.
    b. stage 2.
    c. stage 3.
    d. stage 4.

9. LO 15.5 _____ appears as lesions covered by a fine scale which typically develop as small, teardrop-shaped sores on the scalp, arms, trunk, and legs.

    a. psoriasis vulgaris.
    b. psoriatic arthritis mutilans.
    c. plaque psoriasis.
    d. guttate psoriasis.

10. LO 15.2 The patient's right elbow has fluid-filled blisters with red surrounding tissue. This is a _____.

    a. stage 1 pressure ulcer.
    b. stage 2 pressure ulcer.
    c. stage 3 pressure ulcer.
    d. stage 4 pressure ulcer.

Applying Your Knowledge

1. LO 15.1 List the layers of the skin, and explain the purpose of the skin. _____

_____

2. LO 15.1 List the accessory structures of the integumentary system. _____

_____

3. LO 15.1 Explain how fingerprints are formed. _____

_____

4. LO 15.1 Explain the different types of glands that are located within the skin. What is the function of each? _____

_____

5. LO 15.1 Explain the role of the sensory nerves in relation to the integumentary system. _____

_____

6. LO 15.2 What are two factors a professional coding specialist needs to know in order to determine the correct code(s) for a diagnosed pressure ulcer? _____

_____

7. LO 15.2 List the stages of pressure ulcers, and explain how you differentiate among the stages. _____

_____

8. LO 15.3 List six types of skin lesions. _____

_____

9. LO 15.4 What is dermatitis? Give an example of a type of dermatitis. _____

_____

Using the techniques described in this chapter, carefully read through the case studies and determine the most accurate ICD-10-CM code(s) and external cause code(s), if appropriate, for each case study.

1. Linda Lagarde, a 56-year-old female, comes in today complaining of a red nose, which seems to her to be enlarged with the skin thicker than usual. After examination, Dr. Crawford notes enlarged pores and diagnoses Linda with rhinophyma.

   _____

2. Ned Goings, a 16-year-old male, is brought in today by his mother. Ned complains of small pustules on his shoulders and back. After an examination, Dr. Rabon diagnoses Ned with Bockhart's impetigo.

   _____

3. Tonya Pearson, an 82-year-old female, presents today with hypertrophy of her nails. After an examination, Dr. Peyton diagnoses Tonya with onychogryphosis, or ram's horn nails.

   _____

4. Frank Thompson, a 34-year-old male, comes in today with the complaint of red raised patches on his arms. They become sore and tender when he scratches or rubs the spots. After an examination and testing, Frank is diagnosed with dermatographic urticaria.

   _____

5. Martha Russell, a 48-year-old female, comes in today with the complaint of flaky skin and pimplelike sores along her hairline and behind her ears. After a thorough examination, Dr. Smyth diagnoses Martha with seborrheic dermatitis.

   _____

6. Sam Bridges, a 42-year-old male, presents today with patchy hair loss and dandruff. Dr. Kerr notes a circular-pattern hair loss with dandruff. Dr. Kerr diagnoses Sam with androgenic alopecia.

   _____

7. Thomas Floyd, a 25-year-old male, comes in today with a sore left toe. Tom states he does not remember hurting his toe, After Dr. Humbert examines Tom's toe and notes redness and warmth. Tom admits it's painful to touch. Dr. Humber diagnosed Tom with cellulitis of the left toe.

   _____

8. Jill Harman, a 32-year-old female, presents today with a blister on her left elbow. Her elbow is painful and warm to the touch. After an examination, Dr. Lane diagnoses Jill with a pressure ulcer of the elbow, stage 2.

_____

9. James Hamilton, a 55-year-old male, comes in today concerned that his fingernails have deep ruts running from side to side. After an examination, Dr. Cummings diagnoses James with Beau's lines.

_____

10. Sue Bridgeton, a 24-year-old female, comes in today complaining of red, tender skin and chills. Sue admits to sunbathing all day yesterday. After an examination, Dr. Dills diagnoses Sue with a first-degree sunburn.

_____

11. Jane Weir, a 16-year-old female, is brought in by her parents with the complaint of a sore just above her buttock. After an examination, Dr. Lewis notes a pus-filled cyst near the coccyx. Dr. Lewis diagnoses Jane with a pilonidal cyst.

_____

12. Julie McKinney, a 28-year-old female, presents today with the complaint of a rash that is prickly feeling. Julie states she was working in her yard and got hot but did not sweat. After an examination, Dr. Saul diagnosed Julie with miliaria profunda.

_____

13. Ann McCray, a 72-year-old female, complains of a deep sore on her right heel. After an examination, Dr. Miles notes that the subcutaneous tissue is visible, with necrosis. Dr. Miles diagnoses Ann with a decubitus ulcer of the heel, stage 3.

_____

14. Richard Golf, a 45-year-old male, presents today with a painful pus-filled lump on the nape of his neck. After an examination, Dr. Harris diagnoses Richard with a neck carbuncle.

_____

15. Robert Wilder, an 18-year-old male, presents today with fluid-filled blisters on his back. Robert states that the blisters are easily broken. After an examination and testing, Dr. Gardener diagnoses Robert with staphylococcal scalded skin syndrome with 14% exfoliation.

_____

The following exercises provide practice in abstracting physicians' notes and learning to work with SOAP notes from our health care facility, *Taylor, Reader, & Associates.* These case studies (SOAP notes) are modeled on real patient encounters. Using the techniques described in this chapter, carefully read through the case studies and determine the most accurate ICD-10-CM code(s) and external cause code(s), if appropriate, for each case study.

TAYLOR, READER, & ASSOCIATES
A Complete Health Care Facility
975 CENTRAL AVENUE • SOMEWHERE, FL 32811 • 407-555-4321

PATIENT: WATFORD, WAYNE
ACCOUNT/EHR #:   WATFWA001
DATE: 09/16/18

Attending Physician: Willard B. Reader, MD

Wayne Watford, a 65-year-old male, comes in today with a rash on the bottom of his feet. Patient admits that at times it's difficult to see and to empty his bladder.
VS normal; on visual foot examination rash has a cobblestone appearance. After a thorough examination and testing, Dr. Reader diagnoses Wayne with acquired keratoderma due to reactive arthritis of the foot joint (Reiter's disease).
Dr. Reader orders appropriate antibiotic therapy.

Willard B. Reader, MD

WBR/pw   D: 09/16/18 09:50:16   T: 09/16/18 12:55:01

Determine the most accurate ICD-10-CM code(s).

_____

_____

_____

TAYLOR, READER, & ASSOCIATES
A Complete Health Care Facility
975 CENTRAL AVENUE • SOMEWHERE, FL 32811 • 407-555-4321

PATIENT: BRILLION, ARTHUR
ACCOUNT/EHR #:   BRILAR001
DATE: 10/16/18

Attending Physician: Suzanne R. Taylor, MD

S: Arthur Brillion, a 39-year-old male, with advanced human immunodeficiency virus infection/AIDS, came into the emergency department with severe itching. He states this has been going on for 3 weeks, and it has been disturbing his sleep. On a scale of 1 to 10, he rates the itching as 10 of 10 in severity. Patient states he has not been compliant with his antiretroviral therapy. He is drinking excessively and taking diphenhydramine every 4 hours. This practice has apparently increased during the past few days. He admits to feeling depressed and often has thoughts of "ending it all"; however, he denies any active suicidal ideation. He has little support structure.

O: On examination, he is constantly scratching his skin. There is blood on his undershorts. His skin is extremely dry. Scattered brown patches are noted on his extremities. The scrotum appears lichenified. A skin scraping for scabies mite is performed and sent to the lab for analysis.

A: Scabies, HIV

P: Rx: Permethrin
    Follow-up appointment with personal physician

Suzanne R. Taylor, MD

SRT/pw   D: 10/16/18 09:50:16   T: 10/18/18 12:55:01

Determine the most accurate ICD-10-CM code(s).

_____

_____

_____

TAYLOR, READER, & ASSOCIATES
A Complete Health Care Facility
975 CENTRAL AVENUE • SOMEWHERE, FL 32811 • 407-555-4321

PATIENT: WAXMAN, LAWRENCE
ACCOUNT/EHR #: WAXMLAS001
DATE: 09/16/18

Attending Physician: Marcus R. Allen, MD

S: Lawrence Waxman, a 27-year-old male with recurrent herpes simplex labialis, comes in to see Dr. Allen after experiencing biannual, severe episodes, with a prodrome of tingling of his lip before the appearance of lesions. These episodes, typically lasting between 1 and 2 weeks, cause him discomfort. He believes that these episodes are interfering with his job performance and worries that people stare at his cold sores. He has no other medical problems, and would like some easy-to-follow recommendations to manage this chronic illness.

O: VS normal. On visual examination Dr. Allen documents a small blister/sore on the lower lip.

A: Recurrent herpes simplex labialis

P: 2 g of valacyclovir orally twice daily.

_____

Marcus R. Allen, MD

MRA/pw   D: 09/16/18 09:50:16   T: 09/16/18 12:55:01

Determine the most accurate ICD-10-CM code(s).

_____

_____

_____

TAYLOR, READER, & ASSOCIATES
A Complete Health Care Facility
975 CENTRAL AVENUE • SOMEWHERE, FL 32811 • 407-555-4321

PATIENT: COYLE, OLIVIA
ACCOUNT/EHR #:   COYLOL001
DATE: 09/16/18

Attending Physician: Willard B. Reader, MD

S: Olivia Coyle, a 54-year-old female, presents with an 8-month history of bilateral, painful erythematous lower legs. She states her legs feel "tight." HPI includes four hospital admissions for recurrent cellulitis of the legs. She reports improvement to her legs while hospitalized; however, the erythema returns soon after discharge.

O: On examination, both legs are affected from the knees downward; circumferentially and indurated, pitting +2.

A: Varix, lower extremities with edema

P: Compression therapy

_____

Willard B. Reader, MD

WBR/pw   D: 09/16/18 09:50:16   T: 09/16/18 12:55:01

Determine the most accurate ICD-10-CM code(s).

_____

_____

_____

TAYLOR, READER, & ASSOCIATES
A Complete Health Care Facility
975 CENTRAL AVENUE • SOMEWHERE, FL 32811 • 407-555-4321

PATIENT: MORRISON, JANELLE
ACCOUNT/EHR #:   MORRJA001
DATE: 09/16/18

Attending Physician: Marcus R. Allen, MD

Janelle Morrison, a 58-year-old female with a 5-month history of multiple ulcerations and abscesses involving both breasts came in to see Dr. Allen. Patient states the ulcerations began to appear after breast reduction surgery—performed because of pendulous breasts—at the surgical incision sites 3 weeks postoperatively. Her history is remarkable for treated hypertension and quiescent ulcerative colitis. The patient has had multiple admissions to plastic surgery for incision and drainage of breast abscesses and has had several short admissions to the infectious diseases service for treatment with intravenous antibiotics. Each admission led to temporary improvement in the ulcerations. Despite these hospital admissions for intravenous antibiotics and surgical debridement, the ulcerations have progressed. The patient had no history of ulcerations before the breast reduction surgery. Janelle is diagnosed with pyoderma gangrenosum. Dr. Allen prescribed oral prednisone.

Marcus R. Allen, MD

MRA/pw   D: 09/16/18 09:50:16   T: 09/16/18 12:55:01

Determine the most accurate ICD-10-CM code(s).

_____

_____

_____

CODING MUSCULAR CONDITIONS

16

As you lift your hand to turn a page in this book (whether paper or electronic), your muscles are controlling the bones of your arm and hand to make the motion. Raising your leg to take a step up on a staircase or to kick a ball is also a function of your muscles. And nodding your head up and down in agreement is, again, made possible by your muscles.

The human body has more than 600 muscles, ligaments, tendons, and connective tissues—the components of the muscular system. When muscle strength or action is abnormal, it can dramatically affect an individual's quality of life. Walking, talking, sitting, and turning your head are only a few of the uses of muscles, in conjunction with other anatomical sites. In your work as a professional coding specialist, it is important to abstract from the documentation details regarding the site of the disease or injury (the specific muscle) as well as the laterality (right side or left side), when applicable.

Key Terms

Articulation

Bursae

Dislocation

Involuntary

Ligament

Muscles

Myalgia

Point of insertion

Point of origin

Tendon

Voluntary

EXAMPLE

> M60.042 Infective myositis, left hand
> M62.221 Nontraumatic ischemic infarction of muscle, right shoulder

As you can see in Figure 16-1, the entire skeleton appears to be wrapped with muscles from top to bottom and all the way around. Each muscle has a specific function, and you will learn about most of them in this chapter.

LO 16.1 Types of Muscle Actions

There are two types of muscle action: voluntary and involuntary. Those muscles that function under voluntary control are moved when your brain tells them to move, as a conscious decision. You want to pick up a glass

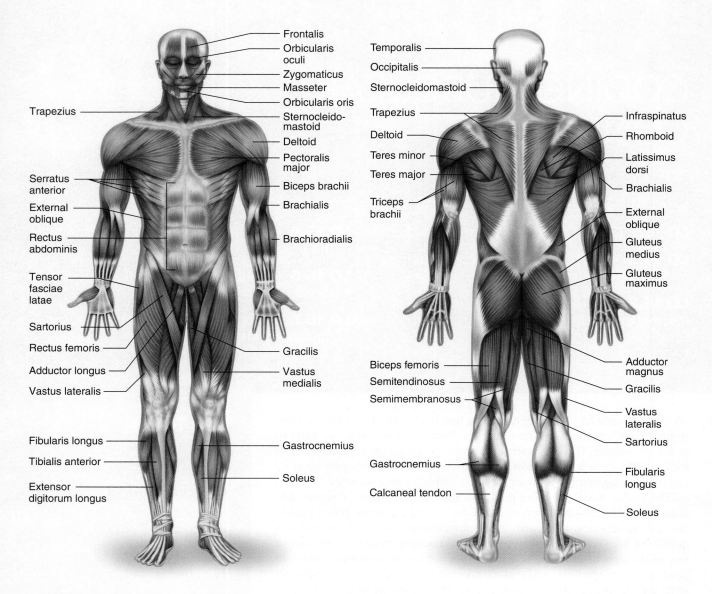

FIGURE 16-1 The Muscles of the Body

Source: David Shier et al., HOLE'S HUMAN ANATOMY & PHYSIOLOGY, 12/e. © 2010 MHE. Figure 9.23 and 9.24 p. 305–306

muscle
Tissue that contracts, causing an organ and/or other component of the body to move.

voluntary
With conscious purpose.

of water—that decision has your brain tell your **muscles** to move the bones in your arm and hand to pick up the glass. Skeletal muscles are **voluntary** muscles because they create the pulley system that enables you to move your bones where and when you choose.

When you make a conscious decision to move a part of your body, some muscle actions are identified by the way they move, or the action they provide:

- *Abductor muscle:* pulls away from the torso.
- *Adductor muscle:* pulls toward the torso.
- *Extensor muscle:* straightens an arm or leg.
- *Flexor muscle:* flexes a joint.
- *Levator muscle:* raises a body part.
- *Intrinsic muscle:* situated within a part.

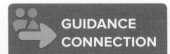

GUIDANCE CONNECTION

Review the ICD-10-CM Coding Guidelines, Section I.C.13, Chapter 13: **Diseases of the musculoskeletal system and connective tissue,** Subsection a, **Site and laterality.**

Involuntary muscles move in response to the autonomic nervous system. In other words, you do not have conscious control over these muscles. Cardiac muscles, the muscles around the heart, are an example of involuntary muscles. They beat continuously, as directed by your nervous system. This is a good thing. Can you imagine what would happen if you had to tell your heart to beat each and every beat? You would have difficulty doing much of anything else.

Tendons connect muscles to bone. A skeletal muscle always runs between a secure skeletal point on one side and a movable skeletal point at the other end. Skeletal muscles are referred to by these points: the **point of origin** (the secure side) and the **point of insertion** (the movable end). Sometimes, the muscle is named for these two points, such as the *sternocleidomastoid* muscle, whose origin is the sternum *(sterno-)* and the clavicle *(-cleido-)* and whose insertion point is the mastoid process *(-mastoid)*. This muscle is responsible for enabling the rotation and flexion of your head and neck.

LO 16.2 Joint-Related Components

Ligaments are bands of tissue that connect one bone to another and support the formation of the capsule (known as a *joint capsule*) within an **articulation** (joint).

Bursae are fluid-filled sacs located within spaces alongside joints between a tendon and certain bony prominences.

Muscles throughout the Body

Often, ICD-10-CM will require you to determine the specific name of the muscle affected (see Tables 16-1 to 16-5).

involuntary
Automatically; a systemic response.

tendon
An anatomical structure that connects a muscle to a bone.

point of origin
The secure side of the muscle.

point of insertion
The flexible or movable end of the muscle.

ligament
A band of connective tissues that bind the components of a joint and facilitate movement.

articulation
A joint.

bursa
A synovial-membrane-lined sac filled with fluid and located adjacent to an articulation.

TABLE 16-1 Muscles of the Head, Face, Neck, and Throat

Head Muscles (Figure 16-2)	
Auricularis muscle	Splenius capitis muscle
Masseter muscle	Temporalis muscle
Pterygoid muscle	Temporoparietalis muscle

(continued)

TABLE 16-1 (continued)

Facial Muscles	
Buccinator muscle	Levator labii superioris muscle
Corrugator supercilii muscle	Mentalis muscle
Depressor anguli oris muscle	Occipitofrontalis muscle
Depressor labii inferioris muscle	Orbicularis oris muscle
Depressor septi nasi muscle	Procerus muscle
Depressor supercilii muscle	Risorius muscle
Levator anguli oris muscle	Zygomaticus muscle
Levator labii superioris alaeque nasi muscle	

Neck Muscles, Right/Left (Figure 16-2)	
Anterior vertebral muscle	Scalene muscle
Arytenoid muscle	Splenius cervicis muscle
Cricothyroid muscle	Sternocleidomastoid muscle
Infrahyoid muscle	Suprahyoid muscle
Levator scapulae muscle	Thyroarytenoid muscle
Platysma muscle	

Tongue, Palate, Pharynx Muscles	
Chondroglossus muscle	Palatopharyngeal muscle
Genioglossus muscle	Pharyngeal constrictor muscle
Hyoglossus muscle	Salpingopharyngeus muscle
Levator veli palatine muscle	Styloglossus muscle
Longitudinal muscle, inferior	Stylopharyngeus muscle
Longitudinal muscle, superior	Tensor veli palatine muscle
Palatoglossal muscle	

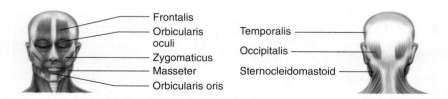

FIGURE 16-2 The Muscles of the Head and Neck

Source: David Shier et al., HOLE'S HUMAN ANATOMY & PHYSIOLOGY, 12/e. © 2010 MHE.
Figure 9.23 and 9.24 p. 305–306

TABLE 16-2 Muscles of the Optical System

Extraocular Muscles, Right/Left* (Figure 16-3)	
Oblique muscle, inferior	Levator palpebrae superioris
Oblique muscle, superior	Annulus of Zinn
Rectus muscle, inferior	Trochlea
Rectus muscle, lateral	Superior tarsus
Rectus muscle, medial	Sclera
Rectus muscle, superior	Optic nerve

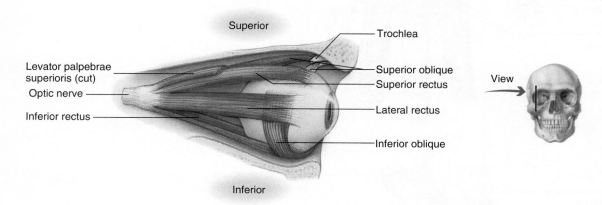

FIGURE 16-3 Muscles of the Eye

Source: Booth et al., MA, 5e. Copyright © 2013 by McGraw-Hill. Figure 35-5 (b), p. 675

TABLE 16-3 Muscles of the Shoulder, Arm, and Hand

Shoulder Muscles, Right/Left	
Deltoid muscle	Supraspinatus muscle
Infraspinatus muscle	Teres major muscle
Subscapularis muscle	Teres minor muscle
Upper Arm Muscles, Right/Left	
Biceps brachii	Coracrachialis muscle
Brachialis muscle	Triceps brachii muscle
Lower Arm and Wrist Muscles, Right/Left (Figure 16-4)	
Brachioradialis muscle	Flexor pollicis longus muscle
Extensor carpi radialis muscle	Palmaris longus muscle
Extensor carpi ulnaris muscle	Pronator quadratus muscle
Flexor carpi ulnaris muscle	Pronator teres muscle
Hand Muscles, Right/Left (Figure 16-4)	
Flexor pollicis brevis	Palmar interosseous muscle
Hypothenar muscle	Thenar muscle

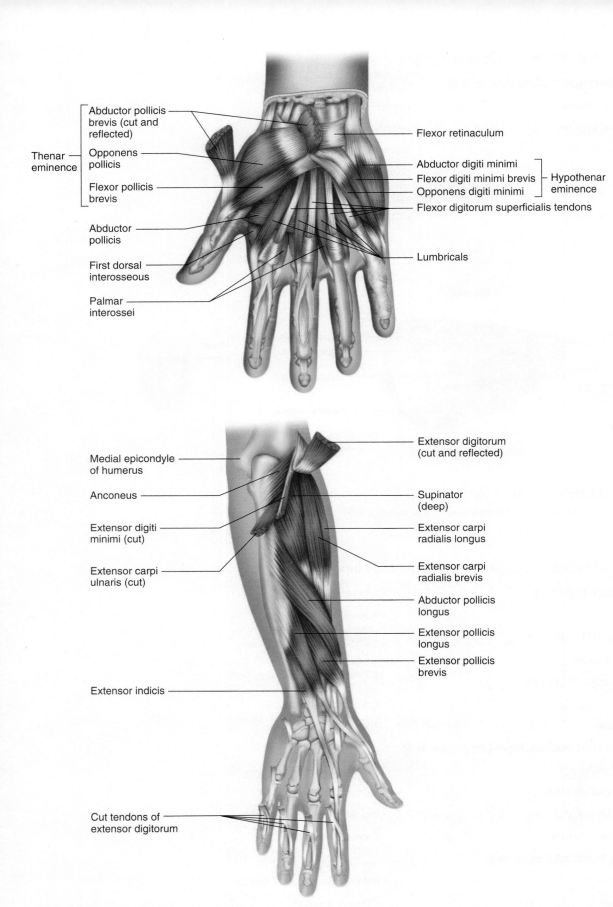

FIGURE 16-4 Muscles of the Arm

Source: Booth et al., MA, 5e. Copyright © 2013 by McGraw-Hill. Figure 25-8, p. 532

TABLE 16-4 Muscles of the Trunk through Hip

Trunk Muscles, Right/Left (Figure 16-5)	
Coccygeus muscle	Quadratus lumborum muscle
Erector spinae muscle	Rhomboid major muscle
Interspinalis muscle	Rhomboid minor muscle
Intertransversarius muscle	Serratus posterior muscle
Latissimus dorsi muscle	Transversospinalis muscle
Levator ani muscle	Trapezius muscle
Thorax Muscles, Right/Left (Figure 16-5)	
Intercostal muscle	Serratus anterior muscle
Levatores costarum muscle	Subclavius muscle
Pectoralis major muscle	Subcostal muscle
Pectoralis minor muscle	Tranversus thoracis muscle
Abdomen Muscles, Right/Left (Figure 16-5)	
Oblique muscle, external	Rectus abdominis muscle
Oblique muscle, internal	Transversus abdominis muscle
Pyramidalis muscle	
Perineum Muscles	
Bulbospongiosus muscle	Transverse perineal muscle, deep
Cremaster muscle	Transverse perineal muscle, superficial
Ischiocavernosus muscle	
Hip Muscles, Right/Left	
Gemellus muscle	Obturator muscle
Gluteus maximus muscle	Piriformis muscle
Gluteus medius muscle	Psoas muscle
Gluteus minimus muscle	Quadratus femoris muscle
Iliacus muscle	Tensor fasciae latae muscle

TABLE 16-5 Muscles of the Leg and Foot

Upper Leg Muscles, Right/Left (Figure 16-6)	
Adductor brevis muscle, right or left	Rectus femoris muscle
Adductor longus muscle, right or left	Sartorius muscle
Adductor magnus muscle, right or left	Semimembranosus muscle
Biceps femoris muscle	Semitendinosus muscle
Gracilis muscle	Vastus intermedius muscle
Pectineus muscle	Vastus lateralis muscle
Quadriceps (femoris)	Vastus medialis muscle

(continued)

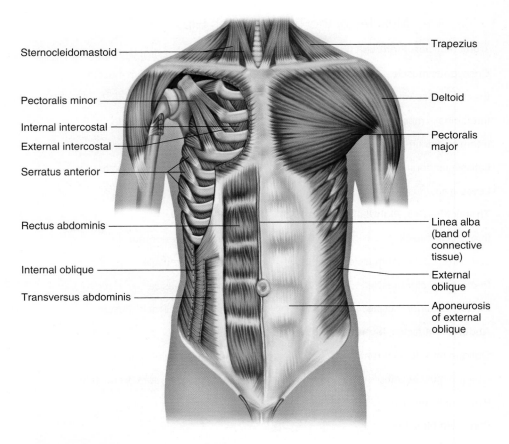

FIGURE 16-5 Muscles of the Torso

Source: David Shier et al., HOLE'S HUMAN ANATOMY & PHYSIOLOGY, 12/e. © 2010 MHE. Figure 9.28, p. 312

TABLE 16-5 *(continued)*

Lower Leg Muscles, Right/Left (Figure 16-6)	
Extensor digitorum longus muscle	Peroneus brevis muscle
Extensor hallucis longus muscle	Peroneus longus muscle
Fibularis brevis muscle	Popliteus muscle
Fibularis longus muscle	Soleus muscle
Flexor digitorum longus muscle	Tibialis muscle, anterior
Flexor hallucis longus muscle	Tibialis muscle, posterior
Gastrocnemius muscle	
Foot Muscles, Right/Left	
Abductor hallucis muscle	Flexor digitorum brevis muscle
Adductor hallucis muscle	Flexor hallucis brevis muscle
Extensor digitorum brevis muscle	Quadratus plantae muscle
Extensor hallucis brevis muscle	

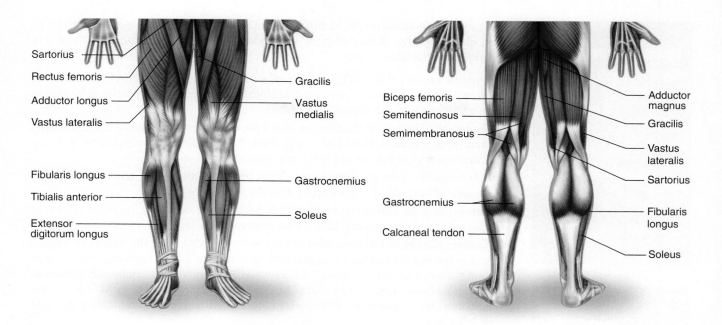

FIGURE 16-6 Muscles of the Leg

Source: David Shier et al., HOLE'S HUMAN ANATOMY & PHYSIOLOGY, 12/e. © 2010 MHE. Figure 9.23 and 9.24 p. 305–306

LO 16.3 Traumatic Injury to the Muscles

A muscle injury is most often the result of some type of trauma or overexertion during exercise or sports. Traumatic injuries to muscles may be described in a number of ways:

- *Strain* is a tearing of the fibers of the muscle involved, most often the result of overstretching the muscle during movement.
- *Sprain* is a partially torn or overstretched ligament.
- *Contusion* is usually the result of a minor trauma to a muscle, causing a bruise.
- *Tear* (muscle tear) is a separation within the muscle fibers. A bowstring tear, also known as a *bucket-handle tear,* occurs longitudinally in the meniscus.
- **Myalgia** is the medical term for muscle pain.
- *Rupture* is the tear in an organ or tissue.

myalgia
Pain in a muscle.

> **EXAMPLE**
>
> S53.21xA Traumatic rupture of right radial collateral ligament, initial encounter
> S76.122A Laceration of left quadriceps muscle, fascia, and tendon, initial encounter
> S83.211A Bucket-handle tear of medial meniscus, current injury, right knee, initial encounter

LO 16.4 Infection and Inflammation of the Muscles

Injuries are not the only concern that can affect an individual's musculoskeletal health. Diseases, infections, and other problems can occur. There are pathogens (bacteria, viruses, and fungi) that directly attack the muscles of the body.

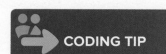 **CODING TIP**

Remember that whenever you are reporting an injury, you will also need to report external cause codes to explain how the patient got injured and identify the place of occurrence. To learn more, see the section "Reporting External Causes" later in this chapter. Also, many of the codes from ICD-10-CM Chapter 19, Injury, poisoning, and certain other consequences of external causes, require seventh characters for reporting the type of encounter.

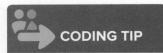
Myopathy:
myo = muscle + -pathy =
disease.
Arthropathy:
arthro = joint + -pathy =
disease.
Chondropathy: *chondro =*
cartilage + -pathy = disease.
Dorsopathy:
dorso = back + -pathy =
disease.
Spondylopathy: *spondylo =*
vertebra + -pathy = disease.

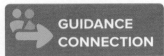
**GUIDANCE
CONNECTION**

Review the ICD-10-CM Coding Guidelines, Section I.C.13, Chapter 13: **Diseases of the musculoskeletal system and connective tissue,** Subsection b, **Acute traumatic versus chronic or recurrent musculoskeletal conditions,** in addition to Section I.C.19, Chapter 19: **Injury, poisoning, and certain other consequences of external causes,** Subsection b, **Coding of injuries.**

The physician's notes might identify the patient's condition as myopathy, arthropathy, chondropathy, dorsopathy, or spondylopathy. Some of these conditions are described in this list:

- *Myositis* identifies the inflammation of a muscle caused by a muscle strain. Code category M60, Myositis, requires additional characters with specific information about anatomical site and other details.
- *Tendonitis* is painful inflammation of a tendon, usually the result of a strain during exercise or sports. ICD-10-CM's Alphabetic Index includes a reference to "*see also* Enthesopathy" (a disorder of bone attachments [entheses]).
- *Fibromyositis* is the presence of tendonitis (inflammation of the tendon) along with myositis. Use code M79.7, Fibromyalgia (Fibromyositis).
- *Bursitis* is a painful inflammation of a bursa, most often the result of recurring trauma. Use code category M71, Other bursopathies.
- *Epicondylitis* is an inflammation of the elbow joint that typically begins as a small tear in the muscle and then is aggravated by activities. *Lateral epicondylitis* is commonly known as "tennis elbow," while *medial epicondylitis* is commonly known as "golfer's elbow," reported by codes M77.1, Lateral epicondylitis, or M77.0, Medial epicondylitis, respectively. Both codes require a fifth character to identify the right or left elbow.
- *Achilles tendon contracture* is a shortening of the tendo calcaneus (heel cord) that is caused by chronic poor posture, continual wearing of high-heeled shoes, or landing on the ball of the foot rather than the heel while jogging or is a manifestation of cerebral palsy or poliomyelitis. Use code M67.0, Short Achilles tendon (acquired), with a fifth character to identify the right or left ankle, or Q66.89, Other specified congenital deformities of feet.
- *Torticollis* is a condition in which the sternocleidomastoid muscles become spasmed (shortened), causing the head to bend to one side and the chin to the opposite side. This condition may be congenital or acquired. Use code M43.6, Torticollis, or Q68.0, Congenital (sternomastoid) torticollis.
- *Muscle spasms,* commonly known as *muscle cramps,* are involuntary twitches and are often caused by myositis or fibromyositis. Sometimes these spasms are caused by metabolic or mineral imbalances. Use code R25.2, Cramp and spasm.

LET'S CODE IT! SCENARIO

Everett Rotarine, a 43-year-old male, was having pain in his left thigh, which his orthopedist, Dr. Nixon, identified as excessive bone resorption, the osteoclastic phase of Paget's disease. X-rays and a urinalysis showing elevated levels of hydroxyproline confirmed the osteoclastic hyperactivity. Everett comes in today to discuss the test findings and treatment options.

Let's Code It!

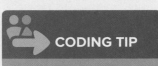
CODING TIP

Read carefully! Paget's disease and Paget-Schroetter syndrome may begin with the same name, but they are totally different conditions.

Dr. Nixon diagnosed Everett with *Paget's disease.* You may remember that this is an eponym and will be shown in the ICD-10-CM Alphabetic Index, so let's turn to find the suggested code. Find:

Paget's disease

Notice the long list of additional descriptors of this condition indented beneath this listing. Look at the scenario again.

Paget's disease

    Bone M88.9

        Femur M88.85-

Let's go to the Tabular List to check this code category. Find:

M88 Osteitis deformans (Paget's disease of bone)

Let's keep reading:

M88.8 Osteitis deformans of other bones

    M88.85 Osteitis deformans of thigh

        M88.852 Osteitis deformans of left thigh

Therefore, the most accurate code is:

M88.852 Osteitis deformans of left thigh

Good work!

LO 16.5 Diseases of the Muscles

Myasthenia gravis is a chronic autoimmune condition that causes muscle weakness, primarily in the face and neck, due to the immune system incorrectly attacking the muscle cells in the body. It may progress and involve additional weakness in the muscles of the extremities (arms and legs). Use code G70.00, Myasthenia gravis without (acute) exacerbation, or G70.01, Myasthenia gravis with (acute) exacerbation.

Duchenne's muscular dystrophy (DMD) is caused by a mutation of the DMD gene within the X chromosome, resulting in the body's inability to create the dystrophin protein within the muscles. Due to this, males are more likely to contract the condition because females have an additional X chromosome that may counteract the mutated gene, as long as the second X chromosome is not damaged as well. Initial signs and symptoms of DMD include leg muscle weakness followed by weakness of the shoulder muscles. DMD is most often diagnosed in early childhood and may be terminal by age 21 should the weakness spread to either heart or respiratory muscles. New trials using gene therapy are hopeful. Use code G71.0, Muscular dystrophy.

Rheumatoid arthritis (RA) is an autoimmune systemic inflammatory disease that affects joints as well as the surrounding muscles, tendons, and ligaments. Use code category M05, Rheumatoid arthritis with rheumatoid factor, or M06, Other rheumatoid arthritis.

Muscle tumors do not occur frequently and can often be malignant. Use code categories C49, Malignant neoplasm of other connective and soft tissue (including muscles, bursae, ligaments, and tendons); C79.89, Secondary malignant neoplasms of other specified sites; or D21, Other benign neoplasms of connective and other soft tissue (including muscles, bursae, ligaments, and tendons).

Congenital myopathies include minicore disease, nemaline myopathy, and fiber-type disproportion. One code, G71.2, reports several muscle abnormalities diagnosed in a neonate or infant. Most often, the infant will not meet normal developmental milestones, particularly those involving muscular actions, such as sitting up or rolling over. Such babies may also have problems feeding.

Paralytic syndromes are conditions in which muscle control is reduced or nonexistent. Cerebral palsy (code category G80), hemiplegia and hemiparesis (code category G81), and paraplegia (code category G82) are some of the conditions that may interfere with the activities of daily living.

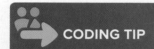

CODING TIP

Many people confuse RA (rheumatoid arthritis) with OA (osteoarthritis). RA is a condition that affects the muscles, joints, and/or connective tissue, whereas OA is the deterioration of cartilage within joints as well as spinal vertebrae.

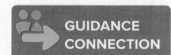

GUIDANCE CONNECTION

Review the ICD-10-CM Coding Guidelines, Section I.C.18, Chapter 18: **Symptoms, signs, and abnormal clinical and laboratory findings, not elsewhere classified,** Subsection f, **Functional quadriplegia.**

During marine boot camp training, Dr. Lake diagnosed Lawrence Allendale with a sprain of the lateral collateral ligament of the left knee after Lawrence landed the wrong way on his last parachute jump.

You Code It!

Go through the steps of coding, and determine the code or codes that should be reported for this encounter between Dr. Lake and Lawrence Allendale.

Step 1: Read the case completely.

Step 2: Abstract the notes: Which key words can you identify relating to why Dr. Lake cared for Lawrence?

_____

Step 3: Query the provider, if necessary.

Step 4: Code the diagnosis or diagnoses.

_____

Step 5: Code the procedure(s): Office visit, physical exam, x-ray.

Step 6: Link the procedure codes to at least one diagnosis code to confirm medical necessity.

Step 7: Back code to double-check your choices.

Answer:

Did you determine the correct codes to be:

S83.422A Sprain of lateral collateral ligament of left knee, initial encounter

V97.22xA Parachutist injured on landing, initial encounter

Y99.1 Military activity

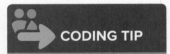

CODING TIP

An external cause code can *never* be a first-listed code, and it can *never* be the only code reported. External cause codes are reported secondary to the codes that report the injury itself.

LO 16.6 Reporting External Causes

When a patient has been injured traumatically, telling the whole story means that you also need to report codes that explain:

- *Cause of the injury,* such as a car accident or a fall off a ladder.
- *Place of the occurrence,* such as the park or the kitchen.
- *Activity during the occurrence,* such as playing basketball or gardening.
- *Patient's status,* such as paid employment, on-duty military, or leisure activity.

That's a lot of information. However, think of how important these details are to the reimbursement process, as well as to research studies. When you report that the patient's status was "civilian activity done for income or pay," it will be clear that this is a workers' compensation case and not a claim to be sent to the patient's health insurance carrier. If the cause of the injury was "driver of pickup truck or van injured in collision with heavy transport vehicle or bus in nontraffic accident," this information may direct the claim to the auto insurance company (not the health insurance carrier), and there may be the possibility that the information can support any legal action. Including a code to report a "fall into swimming pool" may help with getting improved fencing and saving others.

To begin the process of determining the appropriate external cause codes for a specific encounter, you will start in the Alphabetic Index. However, these codes have a separate index. You will not use the *Alphabetic Index to Diseases,* which you have been using in previous chapters and cases. Instead, you will use the *Alphabetic Index to External Causes,* often located after the *Alphabetic Index to Diseases,* after the *Table of Drugs and Chemicals,* and before the *Tabular List.*

Cause of the Injury Code

When a part of the body meets with an external object that results in injury, you must explain what that external object or force was, along with the code or codes for the injury itself. The cause may be anything from being stepped on by a cow (W55.29x-) to falling from scaffolding (W12.xxx-) to the forced landing of a (hot air) balloon injuring the occupant (V96.02x-). Domestic violence, child abuse, and elder abuse are considered assault and may be the cause of a physical injury (code category Y07). Whatever it may have been, you need to determine from the documentation what it was that caused the fracture, **dislocation,** sprain, or strain and report it with the appropriate code or codes.

Place of the Occurrence Code

Where was the patient when he or she was injured? Code category Y92, Place of occurrence of the external cause, provides you with many options so you can report, for example, that the swimming pool at which the patient slipped and tore his deltoid muscle was at a single-family (private) house, a mobile home, a boarding house, a nursing home, or another noninstitutional or institutional location. The codes are quite specific, so you need to ensure that your physicians understand the need to be equally specific in their documentation.

Activity Code

Code category Y93, Activity codes, provides you with many activities from which to choose to identify what exactly the patient was doing when he or she became injured. Dancing, yoga, gymnastics, trampolining, cheerleading . . . each has its own code, and this is just one subcategory!

Patient's Status

This sounds a bit obscure, certainly. What was the patient's status at the time the injury occurred? There are four options within code category Y99, External cause status:

- *Civilian activity done for income or pay*—in other words, on the job for pay or other compensation, excluding on-duty military or volunteers.
- *Military activity,* excluding off-duty status at the time.
- *Volunteer activity.*
- *Other external cause status,* which includes leisure activities, student activities, and working on a hobby.

As we discussed earlier in this section, this detail is important to the entire process, including reimbursement as well as continuity of care.

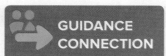

GUIDANCE CONNECTION

Review the ICD-10-CM Coding Guidelines, Section I.C.20, Chapter 20: **External causes of morbidity,** Subsection a, **General external cause coding guidelines**.

dislocation
The movement of a muscle away from its normal position.

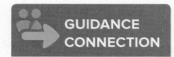

GUIDANCE CONNECTION

Review the ICD-10-CM Coding Guidelines, Section I.C.20, Chapter 20: **External causes of morbidity,** Subsection c, **Activity code**.

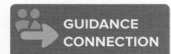

GUIDANCE CONNECTION

Review the ICD-10-CM Coding Guidelines, Section I.C.20, Chapter 20: **External causes of morbidity,** Subsection b, **Place of occurrence guideline**.

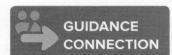

GUIDANCE CONNECTION

Review the ICD-10-CM Coding Guidelines, Section I.C.20, Chapter 20: **External causes of morbidity,** Subsection k, **External cause status**.

LET'S CODE IT! SCENARIO

Annette Pringle, a 27-year-old female, was learning to rock climb at her gym. As she was scaling the wall, her foot slipped and Annette grabbed on with her right hand, pulling something in her shoulder. The severe pain caused her to stop by her physician's office on her way home. Dr. Vega took x-rays and determined that she had an inferior dislocation of the humerus, right side. Dr. Vega put Annette's arm into a sling and gave her a prescription for a pain reliever.

Dr. Vega diagnosed Annette with an *inferior dislocation of the humerus, right side.* Turn to the Alphabetic Index and look up *dislocation, humerus.* Read down the list and see:

Dislocation, humerus, proximal end—*see* Dislocation, shoulder

Even though Dr. Vega's notes didn't specify proximal, that was necessary to get to inferior—anatomically:

Dislocation, shoulder
Humerus
Inferior S43.03-

Perfect! Now, turn to the Tabular List and confirm the code. Start reading at:

S43 Dislocation and sprain of joints and ligaments of shoulder girdle

There is a *code also* note reminding you to also report a code for any associated open wound. Annette does not have an open wound, so this does not apply. There is also an *Excludes2* note that mentions a strain of muscle, fascia, and tendon of the shoulder and upper arm (S46.-). However, Annette dislocated her humerus, so you can keep reading down the column to review the fourth-character and fifth-character options and determine which matches Dr. Vega's documentation:

S43.0 Subluxation and dislocation of shoulder joint

S43.03 Inferior subluxation and dislocation of humerus

Go back to Dr. Vega's notes and see that this matches exactly. Terrific! Now a sixth character is required. Review the options, check the documentation again, and determine:

S43.034- Inferior dislocation of right humerus

Fantastic! A seventh character is required to explain where in the treatment path this encounter is. You can see the options direction under the code category S43. This is the first time that Dr. Vega is treating Annette's dislocation. Great! This leads you to the complete, most accurate code to report Annette's injury:

S43.034A Inferior dislocation of right humerus, initial encounter

This code tells the whole story about Annette's specific injury.

Now you need to find the external cause code(s) to explain how Annette's injury happened. Turn to the external cause code Alphabetic Index. *Climb*—no; *exercise*—no; *fall*—possibly. None of these listings really describe how Annette got hurt. Actually, she was involved in an "activity," so let's take a look:

Activity (involving) (of victim at time of event) Y93.9

Keep reading down the long indented list below until you get to:

Climbing NEC Y93.39
Mountain Y93.31
Rock Y93.31
Wall climbing Y93.31

Perfect! That is exactly what she was doing. Let's take a look in the Tabular List:

Y93 Activity codes
Y93.3 Activities involving climbing, rappelling, and jumping off

The Excludes note lists activities not related to Annette's injury, so keep reading down the list:

Y93.31 Activity, mountain climbing, rock climbing and wall climbing

A code is needed to report the place of occurrence. Where was Annette when she got injured? At her gym.

Y92 Place of occurrence of the external cause

Y92.39 Other specific sports and athletic area as the place of occurrence of the external cause (Gymnasium)

One more thing: What was Annette's status, which you can describe using the codes within Y99, External cause status? The wall climbing was a leisure activity for Annette, so you will report:

Y99.8 Other external cause status (hobby not done for income)

Now you have all of the codes you need to tell the *whole story* about Annette's injury and why Dr. Vega treated her:

S43.034A Inferior dislocation of right humerus, initial encounter

Y93.31 Activity, mountain climbing, rock climbing and wall climbing

Y92.39 Other specific sports and athletic area as the place of occurrence of the external cause (Gymnasium)

Y99.8 Other external cause status (hobby not done for income)

Good work!

YOU CODE IT! CASE STUDY

After completing a full course of radiation treatments for a malignant tumor, Tarlissa Montgomery started having trouble with her back. Dr. Panocchi diagnosed her with scoliosis of the thoracic region as a result of the radiation.

You Code It!

Go through the steps of coding, and determine the code or codes that should be reported for this encounter between Dr. Panocchi and Tarlissa.

Step 1:   Read the case completely.

Step 2:   Abstract the notes: Which key words can you identify relating to why Dr. Panocchi cared for Tarlissa?

_____

Step 3:   Query the provider, if necessary.

Step 4:   Code the diagnosis or diagnoses.

_____

Step 5:   Code the procedure(s): Office visit.

Step 6:   Link the procedure codes to at least one diagnosis code to confirm medical necessity.

Step 7:   Back code to double-check your choices.

Answer:

Did you determine the correct codes to be:

M41.54 Other secondary scoliosis, thoracic region

Y84.2 Radiological procedure and radiotherapy as the cause of abnormal reaction of the patient, or of later complication, without mention of misadventure at the time of the procedure.

CODING TIP

Why is Tarlissa's condition coded as *secondary scoliosis* and not:

M41.24 Other idiopathic scoliosis, thoracic region

Idiopathic means with no known cause. But the notes *do* state a cause of her scoliosis—the radiation. So this cannot be correct.

What about this code:

Q67.5 Congenital scoliosis

Congenital means present at birth. But Tarlissa was not born with scoliosis—it developed as a result of her having radiation treatments.

Secondary means that something else (other than nature or something unknown) caused this condition. In this case, the radiation caused the scoliosis. The radiation came first, and the scoliosis came second.

TABLE 16-6 Interesting Facts about Human Muscles

Longest muscle = **Sartorious** (thigh) muscle
Smallest muscle = **Stapedius** (in the ear)
Largest muscle = **Gluteus maximus** (buttocks)
Strongest muscle = **Masseter** (chewing)
Busiest muscles = Eye muscles
Goosebump muscles = Tiny muscles in the hair root
Smiling requires 17 facial muscles.
Frowns require 42 facial muscles.

Chapter Summary

The entire body is wrapped from head to toe and all the way around by muscles: voluntary muscles that assist movement of the skeleton, and involuntary muscles that are controlled by the nervous system. Each muscle has its specific function and they are all susceptible to injury, inflammation, and disease. For some interesting facts about muscles, see Table 16-6.

CHAPTER **16** REVIEW
Coding Muscular Conditions

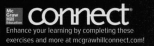
Enhance your learning by completing these
exercises and more at mcgrawhillconnect.com!

Using Terminology

Match each key term to the appropriate definition.

Part One

_____ **1.** LO 16.6 The displacement of a limb, bone, or organ from its customary position.

_____ **2.** LO 16.1 The secure side of the muscle.

_____ **3.** LO 16.2 A synovial-membrane-lined sac filled with fluid and located adjacent to an articulation.

_____ **4.** LO 16.1 An anatomical structure that connects a muscle to a bone.

_____ **5.** LO 16.1 The specific anatomical location of the disease or injury.

_____ **6.** LO 16.2 A band of connective tissues that bind the components of a joint and facilitate movement.

_____ **7.** LO 16.1 Automatically; a systemic response.

_____ **8.** LO 16.1 Tissue that contracts, causing an organ and/or other component of the body to move.

_____ **9.** LO 16.2 A joint.

_____**10.** LO 16.1 The flexible or movable end of the muscle.

_____**11.** LO 16.1 The right or left side of anatomical sites that have locations on both sides of the body.

_____**12.** LO 16.3 Pain in a muscle.

_____**13.** LO 16.1 With conscious purpose.

A. Articulation
B. Bursae
C. Dislocation
D. Involuntary
E. Laterality
F. Ligament
G. Muscles
H. Myalgia
I. Point of insertion
J. Point of origin
K. Site
L. Tendon
M. Voluntary

Part Two

_____ **1.** LO 16.6 Masseter (chewing).

_____ **2.** LO 16.6 Stapedius (in the ear).

_____ **3.** LO 16.6 Tiny muscles in the hair root.

_____ **4.** LO 16.6 Requires 42 facial muscles.

_____ **5.** LO 16.6 Eye muscles.

_____ **6.** LO 16.6 Sartorious (thigh) muscle.

_____ **7.** LO 16.6 Gluteus maximus (buttocks).

_____ **8.** LO 16.6 Requires 17 facial muscles.

A. Longest muscle
B. Smallest muscle
C. Largest muscle
D. Strongest muscle
E. Busiest muscles
F. Goosebump muscles
G. Smiling
H. Frowning

Part Three

_____**1.** LO 16.1 Raises a body part.

_____**2.** LO 16.1 Pulls toward the torso.

_____**3.** LO 16.1 By contracting, this muscle straightens an arm or leg.

_____**4.** LO 16.1 Pulls away from the torso.

_____**5.** LO 16.1 Flexes a joint.

_____**6.** LO 16.1 Situated within a part.

A. Abductor muscle
B. Adductor muscle
C. Extensor muscle
D. Flexor muscle
E. Levator muscle
F. Intrinsic muscle

Checking Your Understanding

Choose the most appropriate answer for each of the following questions.

1. LO 16.1 Tissue that contracts, causing an organ and/or other component of the body to move, is known as

   a. tendons.
   b. ligaments.
   c. muscles.
   d. articulation.

2. LO 16.1 The two types of muscle action are

   a. tendon and ligament.
   b. voluntary and involuntary.
   c. sprain and strain.
   d. site and laterality.

3. LO 16.1 A _____ connects a muscle to a bone.

   a. ligament.
   b. cartilage.
   c. bursa.
   d. tendon.

4. LO 16.2 A synovial-membrane-lined sac filled with fluid and located adjacent to an articulation is known as a

   a. ligament.
   b. cartilage.
   c. bursa.
   d. tendon.

5. LO 16.3 The patient was diagnosed with back strain, subsequent encounter. What is the correct code?

   a. S39.002A.
   b. S39.012D.
   c. S39.022D.
   d. S39.092S.

6. LO 16.3 The patient was diagnosed with a laceration of right thumb with damage to nail, initial encounter. What is the correct code?

   a. S61.111A.
   b. S61.111D.
   c. S61.121A.
   d. S61.021D.

7. LO 16.4 The medical term *chondropathy* means

   a. muscle disease.
   b. joint disease.
   c. cartilage disease.
   d. back disease.

8. LO 16.4 _____ is an inflammation of the elbow joint that typically begins as a small tear in the muscle and then is aggravated by activities.

   a. myositis.
   b. tendonitis.
   c. fibromyositis.
   d. epicondylitis.

9. LO 16.5 _____ is an autoimmune systemic inflammatory disease that affects joints as well as the surrounding muscles, tendons, and ligaments.

   a. myasthenia gravis.
   b. duchenne's muscular dystrophy.
   c. rheumatoid arthritis.
   d. nemaline myopathy.

10. LO 16.6 An external cause code can be

    a. reported as the primary code.
    b. the only code.
    c. reported secondary to the injury itself.
    d. does not need to be reported.

Applying Your Knowledge

1. LO 16.1 Explain the types of muscle action. _____

   _____

2. LO 16.1 Differentiate between point of origin and point of insertion of a muscle. _____

   _____

3. LO 16.1/16.2 Differentiate between tendons, ligaments, and bursae. _____

   _____

4. LO 16.2 List four shoulder muscles. _____

   _____

5. LO 16.2 List three thorax muscles. _____

   _____

6. LO 16.3/16.4 Explain the difference between a pathologic muscle disorder and a traumatic injury to a muscle. _____

_____

7. LO 16.4 List four types of inflammatory conditions of the muscles, tendons, and bursae. _____

_____

8. LO 16.5 List three diseases of the muscles. _____

_____

9. LO 16.6 What are external cause codes? Why are they important to the reimbursement process? _____

_____

Using the techniques described in this chapter, carefully read through the case studies and determine the most accurate ICD-10-CM code(s) and external cause code(s), if appropriate, for each case study.

1. Larry Williams, a 14-year-old male, was playing flag football without a helmet with friends in his backyard. Larry was hit on the head when the football was thrown for a pass. After the game, he complained of a headache and was brought to see Dr. Anderson by his mother. After an examination, Dr. Anderson diagnosed Larry with a bruised scalp.

   _____

2. Angela Cummings, a 32-year-old female, participated in rhythmic gymnastics yesterday at the local gym. She woke up this morning and her left ankle was stiff and achy. After an examination, Dr. Jefferson diagnosed Angela with Achilles tendinitis.

   _____

3. Steve Russell, a 56-year-old male, presents today with the complaint that his right eyelid is drooping and he gets tired easily, but the fatigue is better after he rests for a period of time. Dr. Walters completes the appropriate tests and performs a thorough examination. Steve is diagnosed with myasthenia gravis.

   _____

4. Jill Tolland, a 28-year-old female, comes in today with the complaint of a sore right forearm. Jill was working in her home garden this morning and stumbled over her dog; she broke the fall with her right arm. After an examination, Dr. Coleman diagnoses Jill with a laceration with splinter in the flexor carpi ulnaris (FCU) muscle; no inflammation is noted.

   _____

5. Kenny Burkley, a 36-year-old male, presents today with left knee pain and swelling, which started yesterday. He stated it was painful to get out of his car today. Kenny can't remember any recent activity that could have caused the injury. After clinical testing, Dr. Case diagnoses Kenny with a tear of his left lateral meniscus, bucket-handle, current.

   _____

6. Karen Pullman, a 58-year-old female, comes in today to see Dr. Cobb with the complaint that her left elbow is stiff, is painful, and feels warm. Karen doesn't remember hitting her elbow on anything. After an examination, Dr. Cobb diagnoses Karen with olecranon bursitis of the elbow.

   _____

7. Charles Corley, a 16-year-old male, presents today with the complaint of pain in his right thigh. Charles admits to participating in a wrestling match this morning

during his physical education class at his high school. After an examination, Dr. Cockrell diagnoses Charles with a quadriceps strain.

_____

8. Doretta Carson, a 57-year-old female, comes in today with widespread aching, tiredness, and a tingling sensation, as well as some muscle twitching. After Dr. Foster completes clinical testing, Doretta is diagnosed with fibromyalgia.

_____

9. Robert Foulkes, a 42-year-old male, presents today with pain on the inside of his left elbow, with a tingling in his little finger. Robert is an avid golfer. After testing, Robert is diagnosed with golfer's elbow.

_____

10. Erin Molnar, a 64-year-old female, comes in today to see Dr. Smyth. Erin complains that her head is tilting without her doing it. She also admits to neck spasms, and it seems to her that it is worse after she has taken her afternoon walk. After a thorough examination and testing, Dr. Smyth diagnoses Erin with spasmodic torticollis.

_____

11. Jody Bayer, a 6-year-old female, is brought in today by her parents. Jody has not felt like playing the last few days and has had a poor appetite. Her mother noticed Jody limping yesterday, and her right ankle seems swollen and painful. This morning Jody said her ankle was stiff, but it is feeling better now. After an MRI and clinical testing, Jody is diagnosed with juvenile rheumatoid arthritis of the ankle.

_____

12. Leonard Tate, a 3-month-old male, was brought in today by his parents for a well-baby check. Dr. White notes proximal muscle weakness, "floppy" and hypotonic, with a slender physique. After appropriate testing, Leonard is diagnosed with congenital nemaline myopathy (NM).

_____

13. Doris Tatham, a 62-year-old female, comes in today with ulceration on her right external ear that does not seem to heal. Doris also states it periodically bleeds. After visual examination, Dr. Swift notes hard, raised edges. After Dr. Swift completes the appropriate tests, Doris is diagnosed with a primary carcinoma of the external ear cartilage.

_____

14. Edward Swayze, an 8-month-old male, is brought in by his parents with concerns of Ed's body movement, which seems somewhat involuntary at times. Dr. Michaels notes that Ed is having difficulty maintaining posture/balance while sitting. The doctor also notes that reaching for objects seems to be challenging for Ed. After a thorough examination and clinical testing, Ed is diagnosed with dyskinetic cerebral palsy.

_____

15. Anthony Washington, a 9-month-old male, is brought in by his parents. Anthony's eyelids are drooping and his legs seem weak. Dr. Gilyard completes the appropriate clinical tests and notes respiration difficulty, joint contractures with limited range of movement, and scoliosis. Anthony is diagnosed with Duchenne's muscular dystrophy.

YOU CODE IT! Application
Chapter 16: Coding Muscular Conditions

The following exercises provide practice in abstracting physicians' notes and learning to work with SOAP notes from our health care facility, *Taylor, Reader, & Associates*. These case studies (SOAP notes) are modeled on real patient encounters. Using the techniques described in this chapter, carefully read through the case studies and determine the most accurate ICD-10-CM code(s) and external cause code(s), if appropriate, for each case study.

TAYLOR, READER, & ASSOCIATES
A Complete Health Care Facility
975 CENTRAL AVENUE • SOMEWHERE, FL 32811 • 407-555-4321

PATIENT: CASSIDY, MONOLA
ACCOUNT/EHR #:   CASSMO001
DATE: 07/16/18

Attending Physician: Benjamin T. Cypress, MD

S: Monola Cassidy, a 27-year-old female, came to see Dr. Cypress complaining of double vision.

O: On exam, the left eye is found to be higher on the alternate-cover test. This leads Dr. Cypress to believe that, possibly, the weak depressor muscles (the superior oblique and the inferior rectus muscles) in the left eye or the weak elevators (the superior rectus and the inferior oblique muscles) in the right eye are involved.

The diplopia (double vision) is identified as worse in her right vision. The left superior oblique and the right superior rectus muscles are both intorters (inward rotators).
On the left head tilt, she states her vision is worse, involving the left eye intorters and the right eye extorters. This points to a malfunction of the left superior oblique muscle.

A: Paralysis of the superior oblique muscle

P: Recommend surgical correction

Benjamin T. Cypress MD

BTC/pw   D: 07/16/18 09:50:16   T: 07/18/18 12:55:01

Determine the most accurate ICD-10-CM code(s).

_____

_____

_____

TAYLOR, READER, & ASSOCIATES
A Complete Health Care Facility
975 CENTRAL AVENUE • SOMEWHERE, FL 32811 • 407-555-4321

PATIENT: BROWNE, LAKEESHA
ACCOUNT/EHR #:   BROWLA001
DATE: 07/16/18

Attending Physician: Suzanne R. Taylor, MD

S: Lakeesha Browne, a 13-year-old female, came in to see Dr. Taylor with complaints of dysphagia (difficulty swallowing) and occasional problems speaking. She complains of dyspnea (shortness of breath) and finds it painful to raise her arms over her head. In the last couple of days, she states that climbing stairs and even getting up from a chair are painful and challenging.

O: ROM indicates weakness in the proximal muscles, specifically shoulders and hips. Both MRI and electromyography indicate polymyositis with myopathy. This was confirmed by autoimmune antibody testing.

A: Polymyositis with myopathy

P: Rx: Prednisone
    Rx: Methotrexate

___

Suzanne R. Taylor, MD

SRT/pw   D: 08/11/18 09:50:16   T: 08/13/18 12:55:01

Determine the most accurate ICD-10-CM code(s).

_____

_____

_____

TAYLOR, READER, & ASSOCIATES
A Complete Health Care Facility
975 CENTRAL AVENUE • SOMEWHERE, FL 32811 • 407-555-4321

PATIENT: TRAVIS, NATALIE
ACCOUNT/EHR #:   TRAVNA001
DATE: 07/16/18

Attending Physician: Willard B. Reader, MD

S: Natalie Travis, a 12-year-old female, was brought in by her father to see Dr. Reader. She had just returned from a school hiking trip in the mountains when her parents noticed a problem with her right shoulder. The patient states that her shoulder started bothering her early Sunday morning but by the time she arrived home Sunday evening, it was worse. Her mother called a nurse hotline and the nurse suggested an anti-inflammatory, so the parents gave her 250 mg of Tylenol. All other body and organ systems are fine.

The patient is right-handed and noticed, upon waking this morning, that she could not move her arm properly. She also noticed tingling in her hand, particularly her fingers, and later weakness in the right hand flexion. She denies any fall or accident during the trip.

O: Exam revealed some muscle wasting, observed around the right scapula. Movements of the elbow and wrist were both within normal range. However, abduction of her right arm was difficult. She denies being able to extend the arm without support, and she required movement of her entire upper arm to accomplish abduction of this arm.

Additional specific history about activities during the trip revealed that throughout the weekend, she carried a heavy backpack. The left strap had broken, so the entire weight was supported by her right shoulder and arm, creating a traction-countertraction force centered on the axilla and neck area, which produced a stretching force. She stated that each day she carried this on her right shoulder for as long as 10 or 12 hours.

A: Dislocation of the inferior acromioclavicular joint

P: Sling
   Rest and Ice packs
   Rx: Nonsteroidal anti-inflammatory

_____

Willard B. Reader, MD

WBR/pw   D: 08/21/18 09:50:16   T: 08/23/18 12:55:01

Determine the most accurate ICD-10-CM code(s).

_____

_____

_____

TAYLOR, READER, & ASSOCIATES
A Complete Health Care Facility
975 CENTRAL AVENUE • SOMEWHERE, FL 32811 • 407-555-4321

PATIENT: CALAHAN, YANCY
ACCOUNT/EHR #:   CALAYA001
DATE: 07/16/18

Attending Physician: Benjamin T. Cypress, MD

Yancy Calahan, a 59-year-old male, came to see Dr. Cypress with pain, swelling, and erythema in his left foot and ankle. He stated that he was diagnosed with open-angle glaucoma and prescribed acetazolamide (a diuretic) by Dr. Eli, his ophthalmologist. He stated he never mentioned he was using a topical lotion of urea (a diuretic) prescribed by his dermatologist to hydrate his dry skin. Yancy stated he didn't think a lotion would count when asked about current medications.

    Dr. Cypress realized the combination of the two diuretics lowered his serum uric acid too quickly, causing drug-induced gout.

Benjamin T. Cypress MD

BTC/pw   D: 07/16/18 09:50:16   T: 07/18/18 12:55:01

Determine the most accurate ICD-10-CM code(s).

_____

_____

_____

TAYLOR, READER, & ASSOCIATES
A Complete Health Care Facility
975 CENTRAL AVENUE • SOMEWHERE, FL 32811 • 407-555-4321

PATIENT: WOLFE, REGINALD
ACCOUNT/EHR #:   WOLFRE001
DATE: 07/16/18

Attending Physician: Suzanne R. Taylor, MD

S: Reginald Wolfe, a 57-year-old male, came in to see Dr. Taylor with complaints of seeing double, with one image on top of another. He denied any excessive alcohol consumption or use of recreational drugs. He has a history of Graves' disease.

O: Dr. Taylor determines that the muscles involved must be either the weak elevators of the right eye (right superior rectus and right inferior oblique muscles) or the weak depressors of the left eye (the left superior oblique and left inferior rectus muscles). On exam, the patient states the double imaging is worse in his right eye and is more severe on right head tilt. This directs Dr. Taylor to conclude that the right superior rectus is the problem, malfunctioning, with probable paralysis of this muscle.

A: Vertical diplopia caused by Graves' disease

P: Prisms and orthoptics, therapy
    If patient doesn't respond to therapy, then surgery and occlusion options will be explored.

_____

Suzanne R. Taylor, MD

SRT/pw   D: 08/11/18 09:50:16   T: 08/13/18 12:55:01

Determine the most accurate ICD-10-CM code(s).

_____

_____

_____

CODING SKELETAL CONDITIONS

Learning Outcomes *After completing this chapter, the student should be able to:*

LO 17.1 Identify the components of the axial skeletal system.

LO 17.2 Identify the components of the appendicular skeletal system.

LO 17.3 Enumerate the types of fractures.

LO 17.4 Differentiate between pathologic and traumatic fractures.

LO 17.5 Identify the possible sequelae of fractured bones.

LO 17.6 Recognize the use of seventh characters and what they report.

Key Terms

Appendicular skeleton

Articulation (joint)

Axial skeleton

Bony thorax

Cancellous

Cranium

Diaphysis

Epiphysis

Fracture

Intervertebral disc

Laterality

Malunion

Nonunion

Osseous

Site

Skull

Sutures

Tuberosity

Vertebra

The skeleton of the human body (see Figure 17-1) provides the structure for both form and function. The 206 bones in the adult body comprise a framework hinged together at the **articulations** (joints) that is stabilized by muscles and connective tissues.

In your job as a professional coding specialist, it is important to abstract from the documentation details regarding the **site** of the disease or injury (the specific bone) as well as the **laterality** (right side or left side), when applicable.

Bones are made of two types of **osseous** tissue. Compacted tissue is hard and designed to withstand impact, while spongy (**cancellous**) formation of bone is lacy, with more spaces. Even though bone is dense, it can still be damaged by disease, such as osteoporosis, or trauma, such as a fall.

Categories of Bones

The various bones of the human skeleton are generally categorized by their shape. For example, the parietal bone of the skull is referred to as a *flat bone* due to its flat shape, similar to the scapula—also a flat bone. The ethmoid bone and the vertebrae are examples of irregular-shaped bones. The clavicle and the tibia are examples of long bones, while the carpals (bones in the hand) are examples of short bones. The medical term for the shaft of a long bone is **diaphysis,** and each end is known as an **epiphysis.**

Many joints and junctures in the skeleton are named for the two bones that meet at that point. For example, the temporomandibular joint is the juncture between the temporal bone of the skull and the mandible (lower part of the jaw).

EXAMPLE

S03.0xxA Dislocation of jaw (temporomandibular (joint)), initial encounter

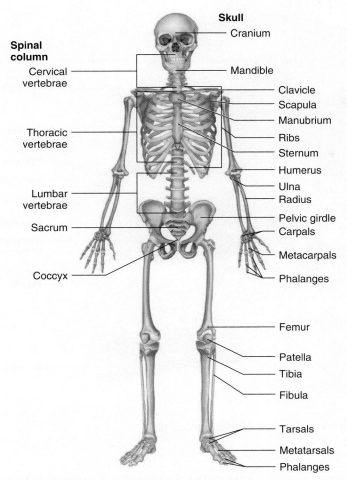

Spinal column
- Cervical vertebrae
- Thoracic vertebrae
- Lumbar vertebrae
- Sacrum
- Coccyx

Skull
- Cranium
- Mandible

- Clavicle
- Scapula
- Manubrium
- Ribs
- Sternum
- Humerus
- Ulna
- Radius
- Pelvic girdle
- Carpals
- Metacarpals
- Phalanges

- Femur
- Patella
- Tibia
- Fibula

- Tarsals
- Metatarsals
- Phalanges

FIGURE 17-1 The Bones of the Human Skeleton

LO 17.1 The Axial Skeleton

Of the 206 bones in the body, 80 make up the **axial skeleton** and are responsible for structure and support of the central segments of the body: the head (the **skull**), spine (the vertebral column), and rib cage (the **bony thorax**).

The Skull

While it appears quite compact and simple, the skull is actually one of the most complex structures of the human skeleton (see Figure 17-2). Technically, the skull is a combination of 22 bones: 8 **cranium** and 14 facial bones.

The cranium, which most people refer to as the *skull,* is made up of eight bones:

- Parietal: 1 right and 1 left
- Temporal: 1 right and 1 left
- Frontal
- Occipital
- Sphenoid
- Ethmoid

The visible lines where each of these bones are fused together to create the cranium are called **sutures.** Think of them as the seams of the skull. The sphenoid and temporal bones together form the base of the skull, also known as the *skull floor.* The frontal

---

articulation
A joint.

site
The specific anatomical location of the disease or injury.

laterality
The right or left side of anatomical sites that have locations on both sides of the body; e.g., right arm or left arm.

osseous
Bony-like substance.

cancellous
Latticelike shaped bone; also known as *spongy bone.*

diaphysis
Shaft of a long bone.

epiphysis
The end of a long bone, either the distal or proximal end.

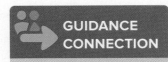

GUIDANCE CONNECTION

Review the ICD-10-CM Coding Guidelines, Section I.C.13, Chapter 13: **Diseases of the Musculoskeletal System and Connective Tissue,** Subsection a, **Site and laterality**.

axial skeleton
The bones that construct the central segment of the body.

skull
The bones that protect the head and create the face.

bony thorax
The rib cage.

cranium
Bones that comprise the skull segments that cover the brain.

sutures
The junctures of the parts of the cranium and skull.

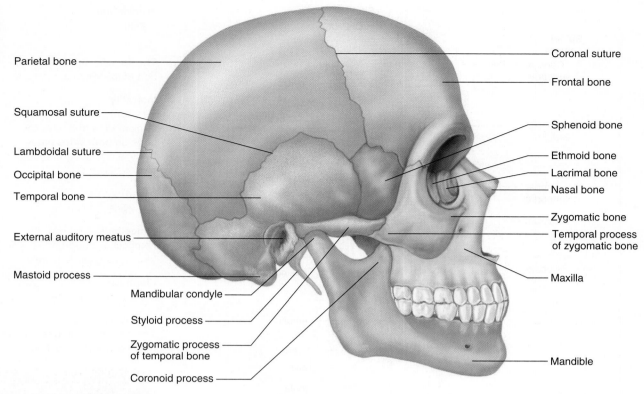

FIGURE 17-2 Bones of the Skull

Source: David Shier et al., HOLE'S HUMAN ANATOMY & PHYSIOLOGY, 12/e. © 2010 MHE. Figure 7.19, pg. 210

and parietal bones create the vault of the skull dome and are primarily responsible for protecting the brain.

In addition to protecting the brain, the skull is a point of attachment for the muscles of the head and neck. A point of attachment of muscle or ligament to any bone is known as a **tuberosity.**

The facial bones form the foundation for a person's face. These bones are created with openings to support the sense organs (your eyes [sight], your nose [smell], and your ears [hearing]), as well as with entrance points for air and food (the mouth).

There are 14 facial bones (see Figure 17-3):

- *Mandible,* also known as the lower jawbone, is hinged to the skull at the tempero-mandibular joint. The mandible itself is identified in several sections: The *condylar* process is the rounded portion of the mandible that fits into the temporal bone to create the hinge; the *coronoid* process is anterior to the condylar; the *ramus* (a term that means branch) is the portion of the mandible that comes vertically down from the hinge; the *angle* is the curve of the jaw line; and the *body* is the portion of the mandible that forms what we commonly call the chin. In the center of the chin is the mandible's *symphysis*—a juncture of two bones that have fused together.
- *Maxillary,* the bone that forms the upper jaw and central portion of the facial skeleton, is actually identified as a pair of bones: one right and one left.
- *Zygomatic bones* are also known as the *cheekbones:* one right and one left.
- *Nasal bones* are two bones fused together that form the bridge of the nose. Even though you have one bridge, these bones are still referred to as a pair: one right and one left.
- *Lacrimal bones* lie between the eye and the nose, alongside the nose: one right and one left.

tuberosity

A rounded nodule at the end of a bone where a muscle or ligament attaches.

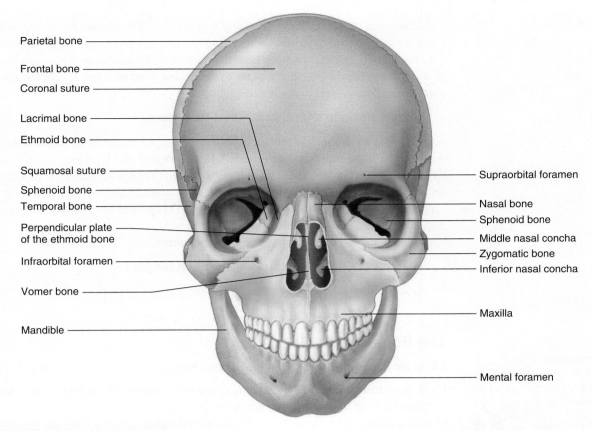

FIGURE 17-3 The Facial Bones

Source: David Shier et al., HOLE'S HUMAN ANATOMY & PHYSIOLOGY, 12/e. © 2010 MHE. Figure 7.17, p. 209

- *Palatine bones* form the roof of the mouth and walls of the nasal cavity. Again, even though they are fused, they are referred to as a pair: one right and one left.
- *Vomer* is a bone that is part of the nasal septum.
- *Inferior nasal conchae* form part of the lateral walls of the nasal cavity, one right and one left.

LET'S CODE IT! SCENARIO

Aurora Gendori, a 33-year-old female, came to see Dr. Jackson, complaining of pain and stiffness in her lower jaw. Upon examination, Dr. Jackson noted swelling and erythema at the temporomandibular joint. Dr. Jackson diagnosed Aurora with arthralgia of temporomandibular joint, right side.

Let's Code It!

Dr. Jackson diagnosed Aurora with *arthralgia of temporomandibular joint*. In the Alphabetic Index, find:

Arthralgia –

        Temporomandibular M26.62

Let's turn to the Tabular List and locate the beginning of the code category:

M26 Dentofacial anomalies (including malocclusion)

Beginning at the code category was a good idea. There is an *Excludes1* notation. Read it carefully and determine whether any of this guidance is applicable to this specific encounter. There is nothing here that relates to Aurora's condition, so review all of the choices for the fourth character to determine what matches Dr. Jackson's documentation about Aurora's diagnosis:

M26.6 Temporomandibular joint disorders

There is an *Excludes2* notation with two temporomandibular conditions listed. Again, read it carefully and determine whether any of this guidance is applicable to this specific encounter. There is nothing here that relates to Aurora's condition, so review all of the choices for the fourth character to determine what matches Dr. Jackson's documentation about Aurora's diagnosis. This part of the coding process is very important to determining the correct code to report.

Review the list of fifth characters. The documentation will bring you to:

M26.62 Arthralgia of temporomandibular joint

Good job!

The Bones of the Ear

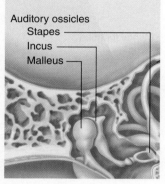

Auditory ossicles
Stapes
Incus
Malleus

FIGURE 17-4 The Bones of the Ear

Source: Booth et al., MA, 5e. Copyright © 2013 by McGraw-Hill. Figure 35-7, p. 679

There are three bones located in the ear (see Figure 17-4), all in the middle section:

- *Malleus* resembles a mallet (hammer) and is responsible for transferring vibrations (sounds) from the eardrum to the incus.
- *Incus,* shaped like an anvil, continues the vibrations relayed from the malleus and forwards these sounds to the stapes.
- *Stapes* resembles a stirrup and is the innermost bone of the ear, responsible for transferring the sounds to the inner ear.

More details about the ear are discussed in Chapter 11, Diseases of the Auditory System (Ears).

The Hyoid Bone

The hyoid bone is a small bone that sits in the ligaments of the neck just below the mandible. Although it is not connected with any other bone, it is considered an associated bone of the skull and is a part of the axial skeleton. The hyoid also serves as an attachment for the muscles that enable swallowing.

The Spine

From the neck, where the *atlas* (C1—the first cervical vertebra) articulates with the skull, and all the way down the column to the *coccyx,* the spine is a long stack of individual bones called **vertebrae,** separated by **intervertebral discs.**

vertebra
A bone that is a part of the construction of the spinal column.

intervertebral disc
A fibrocartilage segment that lies between vertebrae of the spinal column and provides cushioning and support.

Vertebrae An individual vertebra is more than just a bone—it is actually a complex segment of the anatomical structure. In each of the sections of the vertebral column, the size and shape of the vertebrae change. The cervical, thoracic, and lumbar vertebrae are shaped slightly differently as the bones reconfigure on the basis of their position in the column and the support that is necessary. The cervical vertebrae are the smallest of all, and the lumbar vertebrae are the largest. The various aspects of all the vertebrae, however, are the same. As you can see in Figure 17-5, the vertebral body protects the spinal cord anteriorly, while the spinous process and pedicle protect it posteriorly.

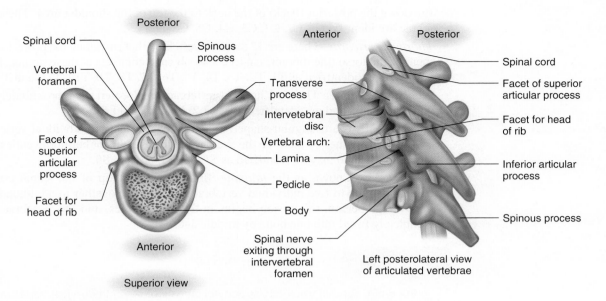

FIGURE 17-5 The Aspects of the Vertebrae

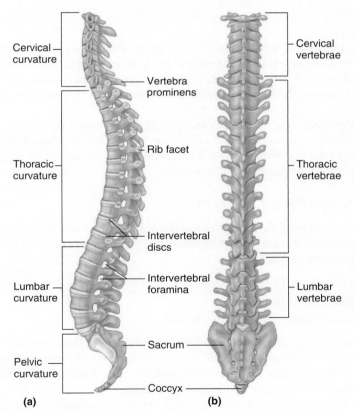

FIGURE 17-6 The Spinal Column

Source: David Shier et al., HOLE'S HUMAN ANATOMY & PHYSIOLOGY, 12/e. © 2010 MHE. Figure 7.32, p. 219

Vertebrae are identified by their location and position in each section of the spinal column (see Figure 17-6):

- *Cervical vertebrae:* There are seven cervical vertebrae—beginning with the atlas (the first cervical vertebra) followed by the axis (the second cervical vertebra)—that run down the posterior (back) of the neck to the top of the shoulder area. These vertebrae are identified as C1, C2, C3, C4, C5, C6, and C7.

- *Thoracic vertebrae:* There are 12 thoracic vertebrae that run along the posterior segment of the torso (the thoracic cavity). The rib cage connects at these points. These vertebrae are identified as T1, T2, T3, T4, T5, T6, T7, T8, T9, T10, T11, and T12.
- *Lumbar vertebrae:* The five lumbar vertebrae are located at approximately the waist/hips area and are identified as L1, L2, L3, L4, and L5.
- *Sacrum:* This is a triangular-shaped bone that begins as five individual vertebrae, which fuse together by the time the average person is in his or her midtwenties. The sacrum vertebrae may be identified as S1, S2, S3, S4, and S5.
- *Coccyx:* Also known as the *tailbone,* this bottommost tip of the spinal column begins as three to five individual vertebrae, which fuse together in adulthood. For the average person, this fusion begins in the midtwenties, and the vertebrae have completely fused into one bone by middle age.

EXAMPLE

> S12.64xA Type III traumatic spondylolisthesis of seventh cervical vertebra, initial encounter for closed fracture
>
> S32.032A Unstable burst fracture of third lumbar vertebra, initial encounter for closed fracture

Intervertebral Discs The bones of the spinal column do not actually rest upon each other. In between every two vertebrae is an intervertebral disc—a cushion made of fibrocartilage. The outermost layer of the disc is called the *annulus fibrosus,* while the center of the disc is the *nucleus pulposus,* a soft gelatinous core consisting of about 75% water.

One of the things that influences the loss of height that older people experience is the diminishing amount of water inside the intervertebral discs, which results in compression of the vertebral column. This reduced cushioning can be painful and can provide opportunity for damage to the bone.

The Rib Cage (Bony Thorax)

The skeletal structure of the torso is called the *thoracic cage* and is designed to protect the internal organs (the heart, lungs, thymus, etc.). This portion of the skeleton consists of three sections (see Figure 17-7):

- Thoracic vertebrae: T1–T12
- Ribs, also known as the *costae*
- Sternum, commonly called the *breastbone*

The 12 pairs of ribs attach to each of the 12 thoracic vertebrae and curve around to the front (anterior) to form a cage. The first seven pairs of ribs (counting from the neck down, ribs 1–7) are called the *vertebrosternal ribs* (also known as the *true ribs*) and attach directly to the sternum via the *costal cartilage.*

The next three pairs (ribs 8–10) are called the *vertebrochondral ribs,* or *false ribs.* These bones attach to costal cartilage that connects them to the sternum.

The final two pairs of ribs (ribs 11 and 12) are called *floating ribs* because these lower ribs do not connect to the sternum as do the first 10 ribs.

The sternum is referred to in three sections:

- *Manubrium:* the triangular top section of the sternum, closest to the neck.
- *Body:* The long flat bone of the sternum that runs down the center of the chest.
- *Xiphoid process:* The taillike structure extending from the bottom of the sternum body.

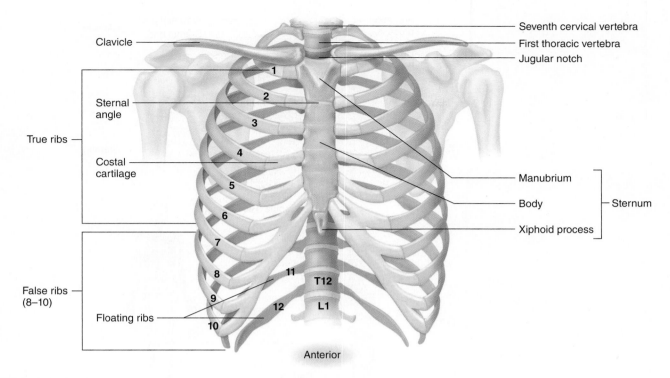

FIGURE 17-7 The Rib Cage

Source: Rod Seeley et al., SEELEY'S ANATOMY & PHYSIOLOGY, 12/e. © 2010 MHE. Figure 6.21, p. 129

EXAMPLE

S22.21xB Fracture of manubrium, initial encounter for open fracture
S22.31xA Fracture of one rib, right side, initial encounter for closed fracture

LO 17.2 The Appendicular Skeleton

Attached to the central section of the skeleton (the axial skeleton) are the bones that construct the arms and the legs (appendages to the body)—the **appendicular skeleton.** The 126 bones that make up the appendicular skeleton in an adult include the pectoral girdles and the upper limbs, as well as the pelvic girdle and the lower limbs.

appendicular skeleton
The bones that construct the upper and lower extremities.

The Pectoral Girdle

When you really look at the construction of the human skeleton, you can see how each upper limb (arm) attaches to each pectoral girdle (see Figure 17-8), commonly known as the *shoulder.* The two parts of each pectoral girdle are:

- *Scapula:* This is the triangular-shaped bone that sits across from your acromioclavicular joint (arm socket) along your posterior (back) to form your medial border (shoulder blade). The coracoid process is a bone that extends over the acromioclavicular joint. The glenoid cavity sits below it and secures the superior end (the head) of the humerus (upper arm bone).

- *Clavicle:* This bone, commonly called the *collarbone,* runs from your acromioclavicular joint (arm socket) across the anterior (front) and connects to the manubrium of the sternum.

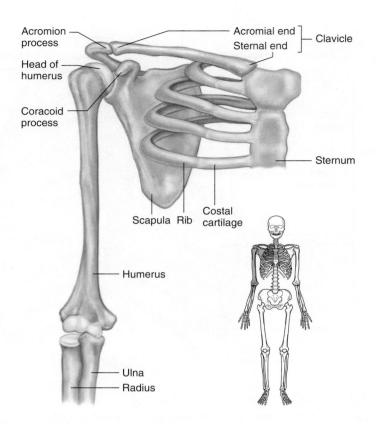

FIGURE 17-8 The Pectoral Girdle

Source: David Shier et al., HOLE'S HUMAN ANATOMY & PHYSIOLOGY, 12/e. © 2010 MHE. Figure 7.40, p. 227

EXAMPLE

S42.015B   Posterior displaced fracture of sternal end of left clavicle, initial encounter for open fracture

S42.144A   Nondisplaced fracture of glenoid cavity of scapula, right shoulder, initial encounter for closed fracture

The Upper Limb

Also known as the *upper extremity* or *upper arm,* the upper limb is made up of these bones:

Humerus: The head (upper end or proximal end) of the humerus, the long bone of the upper arm, fits into the glenoid cavity like a ball and socket (see Figure 17-9). The distal or inferior end of the humerus connects to the elbow joint. The parts of the humerus are:

- *Upper end* (proximal end—closest to the pectoral girdle).
- *Greater tubercle* (attachment spot for the supraspinatus, infraspinatus, and teres minor muscles).
- *Anatomical neck.*
- *Lesser tubercle* (attachment spot for the subscapularis muscle).
- *Surgical neck.*
- *Shaft:*
    - Deltoid tuberosity (attachment spot for the deltoid muscle).

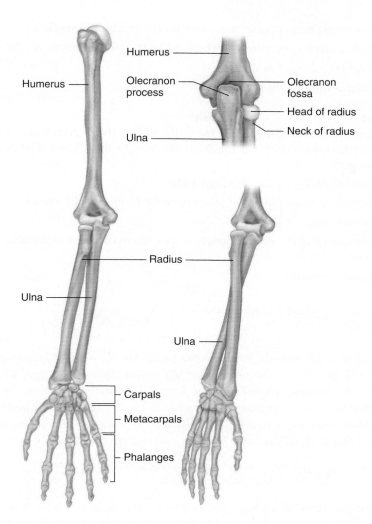

FIGURE 17-9 Bones of the Arm

Source: David Shier et al., HOLE'S HUMAN ANATOMY & PHYSIOLOGY, 12/e. © 2010 McGraw-Hill Education. Figure 7.42, pg. 228

- *Distal end:*
  - Coronoid fossa
  - Olecranon fossa
  - Lateral epicondyle
  - Medial epicondyle
  - Capitulum
  - Trochlea

Elbow joint: This two-part connector acts like a hinge to permit flexibility and mobility between the humerus and the lower arm.

Lower arm (forearm): The segment of the upper limb between the elbow and the wrist consists of two parallel long bones:

- *Ulna:* The proximal (superior) tip, called the *olecranon,* is also known as the tip of the elbow. The end of the bone fits into the olecranon fossa, an indentation in the distal end of the humerus, to enable the function of the elbow joint. The parts of the ulna are:
  - *Olecranon process* (at the proximal end; attachment spot for the triceps brachii muscle).
  - *Trochlear notch.*

- *Coronoid process* (attachment spot for the brachialis muscle).
- *Radial notch* (juncture spot where the head of the radius meets the ulna).
- *Shaft* (also known as diaphysis).
- *Head of ulna* (at the distal end).
- *Styloid process.*

- *Radius:* The head of the radius meets the ulna at the proximal end at the radial notch (the radius does not reach all the way to the elbow). The parts of the radius are:
  - *Head of radius* (at the proximal end).
  - *Radial tuberosity* (point of attachment for biceps brachii muscle).
  - *Radial shaft.*
  - *Ulna notch of the radius* (juncture spot where the head of the ulna meets the radius).
  - *Styloid process.*

YOU CODE IT! CASE STUDY

Belinda Baron, a 23-year-old female, came to see Dr. Herre for a follow-up to check the healing of her Colles' fracture of her left radius. Four weeks ago, Belinda was running for the bus and tripped over the foot of someone standing on the sidewalk. She stretched her arm out in front of her to break her fall, and this resulted in a radial fracture. After exam and x-ray, Dr. Herre stated the fracture was healing nicely. She stated that Belinda could probably have the cast removed in about 2 weeks.

You Code It!

Go through the steps of coding, and determine the code or codes that should be reported for this encounter between Dr. Herre and Belinda. Code for the injury only, not the external cause.

Step 1: Read the case completely.

Step 2: Abstract the notes: Which key words can you identify relating to why Dr. Herre cared for Belinda?

_____

Step 3: Query the provider, if necessary.

Step 4: Code the diagnosis or diagnoses.

_____

Step 5: Code the procedure(s): Office visit.

Step 6: Link the procedure codes to at least one diagnosis code to confirm medical necessity.

Step 7: Back code to double-check your choices.

Answer:

Did you determine the correct code to be:

S52.532D Colles' fracture of left radius, subsequent encounter for fracture with routine healing

The wrist and hand: At the distal end of the radius and ulna is a collection of eight irregular-shaped carpal bones that form the carpus (wrist) (see Figure 17-10):

- Navicular (scaphoid).
- Lunate (semilunar) bone.
- Triquetral (cuneiform) bone.
- Pisiform.
- Trapezium bone (larger multangular).
- Trapezoid bone (smaller multangular).
- Capitate bone (os magnum).
- Hamate (inciform) bone.

Like a collection of small rocks, these eight bones cluster as a juncture between the forearm (the ulna and radius) and the metacarpal bones (the hand). The five metacarpal bones are categorized as long bones, with the main sections of each metacarpal called the *shaft, the proximal base* (the end closest to the wrist), and the *neck* (the distal end that meets the phalange [the finger]). These bones are numbered, beginning with the base of the thumb as number 1.

Each of the phalanges (except the thumb) has three bones—the proximal (closest to the hand), the middle, and the distal (the tip of the finger)—and the thumb has two (proximal and distal) for a total of 14 bones. The fingers are identified as the thumb, second digit (index finger), third digit (middle finger), fourth digit (ring finger), and fifth digit (pinkie).

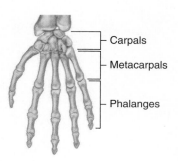

FIGURE 17-10 Bones of the Hand

Source: David Shier et al., HOLE'S HUMAN ANATOMY & PHYSIOLOGY, 12/e. © 2010 MHE. Figure 7.42, p. 228

EXAMPLE

S62.012A Displaced fracture of distal pole of navicular (scaphoid) bone of left wrist, initial encounter for closed fracture

S62.312A Displaced fracture of base of third metacarpal bone, right hand, initial encounter for closed fracture

The Pelvic Girdle

The ilium, the ischium, and the pubis fuse together to form the os coxae (hip bone). The right and left ossa coxae (plural of *os coxae*) make up the pelvic girdle. The two ossa coxae meet at the pubic symphysis at the anterior and on either side of the sacrum at the posterior (see Figure 17-11).

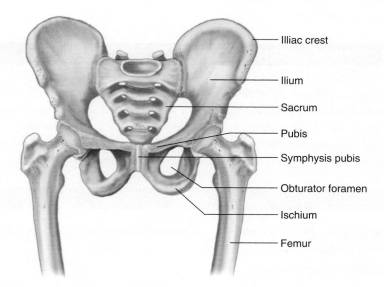

FIGURE 17-11 The Pelvic Girdle and Lower Extremity

Source: Booth et al., MA, 5e. Copyright © 2013 by McGraw-Hill. Figure 24-11(a), p. 519

The Lower Limb

Also known as the lower extremity, the lower limb consists of these bones:

Femur (the thigh bone) is the longest and heaviest bone in the body. The proximal end (head) sits in the acetabulum of the os coxae like a ball and socket (see Figure 17-11), and its distal end is at the knee joint. The segments of the femur are:

- *Epiphysis* (head—proximal end).
- *Neck.*
- *Greater trochanter* (point of attachment for gluteus medius and gluteus minimus muscles).
- *Lesser trochanter* (point of attachment for psoas major and iliacus muscles).
- *Gluteal tuberosity.*
- *Linea aspera.*
- *Shaft* (also known as *diaphysis*).
- *Lateral epicondyle.*
- *Medial epicondyle.*
- *Medial condyle.*
- *Lateral condyle.*
- *Intercondylar fossa.*
- *Patellar surface.*

Patella, also known as the *kneecap,* is a large sesamoid bone positioned to protect the knee joint, where the femur meets the tibia.

Tibia (the shinbone) is a large medial bone of the leg. The segments of the tibia are:

- *Intercondylar eminence* (proximal surface).
- *Lateral condyle.*
- *Medial condyle.*
- *Tibial tuberosity.*
- *Anterior crest.*
- *Shaft* (also known as *diaphysis*).
- *Medial malleolus.*

Fibula is a slender long bone that sits parallel to the tibia. It does not connect to the knee joint but does provide stabilization for the ankle. The segments of the fibula are:

- *Head* (proximal end).
- *Shaft* (also known as *diaphysis*).
- *Lateral malleolus.*

LET'S CODE IT! SCENARIO

Calvin Clyde, a 16-year-old male, was tackled during a football game with his friends at the park. His left leg twisted when he fell to the ground, and he was brought to the emergency room by his father. Dr. Baker looked at the x-rays and determined that Calvin had a closed oblique nondisplaced fracture of the fibular shaft of his left leg. A thigh-to-toe cast was applied, and Calvin was sent home.

Let's Code It!

Dr. Baker diagnosed Calvin with *a closed oblique nondisplaced fracture of the fibular shaft.* In the Alphabetic Index, find:

Fracture, traumatic –

Fibula (shaft) (styloid) S82.40-

Let's turn to the Tabular List and locate the beginning of the code category:

S82 Fracture of lower leg, including ankle

It was a good idea to begin at the code category. There is a note, as well as *Includes, Excludes1,* and *Excludes2* notations, plus a long list of seventh characters from which to choose. Read all this carefully and determine whether any of this guidance is applicable to this specific encounter. Except for the seventh-character list, there is nothing here to direct you elsewhere, so review all of the choices for the fourth character to find what matches Dr. Baker's documentation about Calvin's diagnosis.

S82.4 Fracture of shaft of fibula

Review the list of fifth characters. You can see the piece of information you need next is the specific type of fracture. The documentation will bring you to:

S82.43 Oblique fracture of shaft of fibula

Great! To determine which sixth character is correct, you must determine two more pieces of information: whether the fracture is displaced or nondisplaced and which leg (right or left) was injured. These details will lead you to:

S82.435- Nondisplaced oblique fracture of shaft of left fibula

One more character, the seventh character, must be determined. Do you remember that you saw the list of characters available to use back at the top of code category S82? Turn there now and review the choices carefully. Did you determine the correct code for this diagnosis to be:

S82.435A Nondisplaced oblique fracture of shaft of left fibula, initial encounter for closed fracture

Good job! Of course, you will also need to determine the external cause codes:

Y93.61 Activity, American tackle football

Y92.830 Public park as the place of occurrence of the external cause

Y99.8 Other external cause status

The Ankle and Foot

The distal ends of the tibia and fibula, the medial malleolus and the lateral malleolus, respectively, meet at the tarsus (ankle). This joint is made up of seven bones (see Figure 17-12):

Talus: This bone distributes the weight of the body from the tibia and transmits it toward the phalanges (toes), helping to stabilize the ankle.

Calcaneus: When standing, most of the body's weight is transmitted from the tibia to the talus to the calcaneus (the heel bone), the largest tarsal bone.

Cuboid: This irregular-shaped bone at the base of the ankle on the outside (pinkie-toe side of the foot) contributes to balance.

Navicular: Similar to the cuboid bone, this irregular-shaped bone sits on the internal side (the great-toe side of the foot).

Cuneiform bones: These three small bones align along the base of the metatarsal bones of the foot. These are:

- Lateral cuneiform bone
- Intermediate cuneiform bone
- Medial cuneiform bone

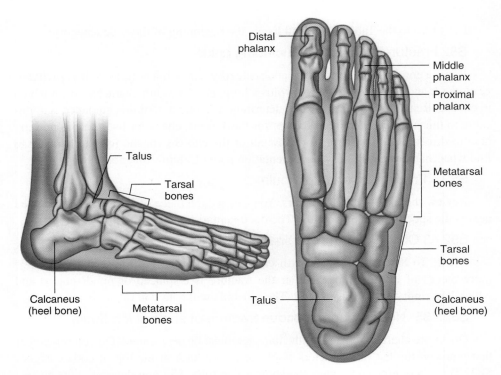

FIGURE 17-12 Bones of the Ankle and Foot

Five metatarsal bones sit side-by-side to form the metatarsus (see Figure 17-12). Just like the metacarpal bones of the hand, the metatarsals are numbered 1 through 5 beginning with the great toe as number 1. The phalanges of the foot (the toes), like the phalanges of the hand (the fingers), are made up of three bones each (except for the great toe): proximal, middle, and distal segments. The toes are referred to by number as well, with the great toe first, followed by the second digit, third digit, fourth digit, and the fifth toe (the pinkie toe).

> ### EXAMPLE
>
> Q66.0 Congenital talipes equinovarus
> S92.212A Displaced fracture of cuboid bone of left foot, initial encounter for closed fracture

LO 17.3 Fractured Bones

Both bone and cartilage can break—that is, become fractured. **Fractures** can be the result of trauma, such as a fall or car accident, or they can be the result of a pathologic condition (underlying disease), such as osteoporosis, that causes the bone to weaken so much that it breaks. This is important information for you to abstract from the physician's documentation because traumatic fractures and pathologic fractures are coded differently. Actually, they have separate listings in the Alphabetic Index: Fracture, pathological, and Fracture, traumatic.

When a fracture of a bone occurs, the coder must identify the segment of the bone that was affected. For example: The sternal end of the clavicle is called this because it is the end that connects to the sternum (ICD-10-CM code S42.011, Anterior displaced fracture of sternal end of right clavicle). The acromial or lateral end of the clavicle connects to the acromioclavicular joint (ICD-10-CM code S42.031, Displaced fracture of lateral end of right clavicle).

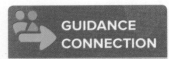

GUIDANCE CONNECTION

Review the ICD-10-CM Coding Guidelines, Section I.C.13, Chapter 13: **Diseases of the musculoskeletal system and connective tissue,** Subsection b, **Acute traumatic versus chronic or recurrent musculoskeletal conditions,** in addition to Section I.C.19, Chapter 19: **Injury, poisoning, and certain other consequences of external causes,** Subsection b, **Coding of injuries.**

fracture
Broken cartilage or bone.

Types of Fractures

One of the first factors needed for accurate coding of a fracture is whether the fracture is *open* or *closed* (see Figure 17-13).

An open fractured bone is found in conjunction with an open wound through which the bone may or may not extend. A closed, or simple, fracture has no accompanying wound and remains within the confines of the body. Some types of fractures are explained in the following paragraphs.

Avulsion fractures happen when a tiny bone piece breaks off at the point where a ligament or tendon attaches to the bone. This is an occurrence of a piece of bone that has broken away at a tubercle. When the fracture is not displaced, treatment is similar to that for a soft tissue injury. In severe cases, surgery may be required to realign and stabilize an affected growth plate.

Burst fractures occur when a vertebra has been crushed in all directions. This fracture may be described as stable or unstable. Imaging (x-rays, CT scan, or MRI), as well as physical and neurologic exams, typically will support a diagnosis. Stable burst fractures may be treated with a molded turtle shell brace or a body cast. If neurologic damage is identified, then the fracture is considered unstable and will require surgery. An anterior or posterior approach may be used to insert internal fixation, a bone graft, and/or fusion. The specific bone affected will determine the code.

Comminuted fracture identifies the breaking of the bone into several pieces. A closed reduction may be required prior to immobilization by cast or splint. Internal fixation may be necessary to correct an impacted fracture with an open reduction.

Depressed fracture indicates that the bone has been displaced inward.

Fatigue fractures occur most often in the second or third metatarsal shaft and are typically the result of continuous weight-bearing activities such as long-distance running, ballet dancing, or sports. An example is M48.4-, Fatigue fracture of vertebra. Additional names for this type of fracture include march fracture, Deutschlander's disease, and stress fracture— reported from subcategory M84.3-, Stress fracture (fatigue fracture) (march fracture).

Fissured (linear) fracture is a break that runs along the length of a long bone.

Greenstick fracture is one in which the fracture exists on one side of the bone while the other side is not broken but bent. Example: S42.311A Greenstick fracture of shaft of humerus, right arm, initial encounter for closed fracture.

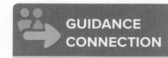

GUIDANCE CONNECTION

Review the ICD-10-CM Coding Guidelines, Section I.C.19, Chapter 19: **Injury, poisoning, and certain other consequences of external causes,** Subsection c, **Coding of traumatic fractures,** as well as Section I.C.20, Chapter 20: **External causes of morbidity,** Subsection a, **General external cause coding guidelines**.

CODING TIP

Open fractures may also be documented as infected, missile, puncture, compound, or with a foreign body.

Closed fractures may also be documented as comminuted, depressed, elevated, fissured, greenstick, impacted, linear, simple, slipped epiphysis, or spiral.

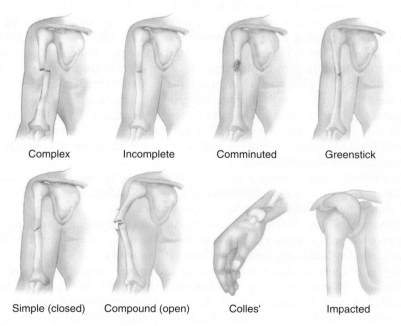
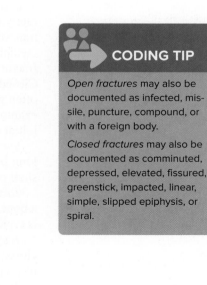

| Complex | Incomplete | Comminuted | Greenstick |

| Simple (closed) | Compound (open) | Colles' | Impacted |

FIGURE 17-13 Types of Fractures

Impacted fracture occurs when a fragment from the broken bone embeds itself into the body of another.

Infected fracture documents that there is presence of an infection at the fracture site. This often will require additional codes to report the underlying bacterium or virus, as well as the infection itself.

Lateral mass fracture of the atlas (C1), as the name implies, involves the lateral masses. These are the sturdiest sections of the C1 vertebra and include a superior facet and an inferior facet. This fracture occurs at the point where the spine meets the base of the cranium. A stable fracture means the transverse ligament is still intact, and a cervical collar or cervicothoracic brace is the first course of treatment. For unstable fractures, cranial traction will support a reduction of the displaced bone. After time, a halo vest can be used. Fusion of C1–C3 may be required for more severe subluxation. Use code S12.040, Displaced lateral mass fracture of first cervical vertebra, or S12.041, Non-displaced lateral mass fracture of first cervical vertebra.

Maisonneuve's fracture is a spiral fracture of the proximal portion of the fibula. This type of fracture includes a disruption of ligaments. Stable fractures can be treated with a long leg cast. Internal fixation may be required in more severe cases.

Oblique fracture is a fracture line that runs at an angle to the axis of the bone. Casting is the typical first course of treatment. In severe cases, an open reduction and possibly internal fixation will be used. Repair to surrounding ligaments may be required as well.

Periosteal fractures occur below the periosteum (membrane covering the bone surface) and are usually not displaced.

Pilon fracture is an oblique, comminuted fracture of the distal tibia. Treatment may begin with stabilization, using external traction to permit the soft tissue injuries to heal prior to surgical intervention. Open reduction with internal fixation, as well as external fixation and percutaneous plating, may be used once the soft tissue has recovered.

Puncture fracture can identify that a puncture from outside the body penetrated to cause the fracture or that the broken bone has punctured the skin after the fracture occurred. Example: S91.231B Puncture wound without foreign body of right great toe with damage to nail, initial encounter for open fracture.

Segmental fracture is similar to the comminuted fracture; however, the broken pieces of the bone separate. Internal fixation with open reduction is used to prevent misalignment of the bone fragments. In some cases, bone cement is included in the repair. Some surgical procedures also include attachment of external fixation.

Salter-Harris physeal fracture is a fracture of the epiphyseal plate (a thin layer of bone; a growth plate, an area near the end of a long bone that contains growing tissue, also known as the *physis*), and it is commonly found in children. ICD-10-CM separately codes four of the nine types of Salter-Harris fracture: Salter-Harris type I is a transverse fracture of the growth plate; type II is a fracture of the growth plate and the metaphysis; type III is a fracture of the growth plate and the epiphysis; and type IV is a fracture line that travels through all three: the growth plate, metaphysis, and epiphysis. Closed reductions and traction can be used for less severe cases. Types III and IV more often will require surgical intervention using open reduction and internal fixation. For example: S79.011A Salter-Harris type I physeal fracture of upper end of right femur, initial encounter for closed fracture.

Spiral fracture happens when a twisting force causes the bone to break around a long bone in a spiral direction. Example: S52.244A Nondisplaced spiral fracture of shaft of ulna, right arm, initial encounter for closed fracture.

Torus fracture is also known as a *buckle fracture;* it is a compression of one side of a bone's protrusion, also known as the *torus,* while the other side is bent. This fracture is typically nondisplaced and, therefore, is correctable with a cast or splint.

Transverse fracture is a fracture line that runs across the bone; it may be an open or closed fracture. An open reduction with internal fixation may be required if the bone has separated. A closed reduction might alternatively be employed. Casting is typical.

Transcondylar fracture is a fracture that runs through a condyle (a rounded knob-like prominence at the end of a bone). Such fractures are categorized as flexion or extension fractures. Treatment can begin with immobilization for nondisplaced injury. However, treatment for this type of fracture can be difficult due to the break's location and the lack of bone available for successful union. Example: S42.431A Displaced fracture (avulsion) of lateral epicondyle of right humerus, initial encounter for closed fracture.

Wedge compression fracture occurs when only the anterior portion of a vertebra is crushed, which causes the vertebra to take on a wedge shape. Vertebroplasty will stabilize the fracture and prevent further damage. Example: A wedge compression fracture of L3 would be reported with code S32.030A, Wedge compression fracture of third lumbar vertebra, initial encounter for closed fracture.

Skull Fracture A skull fracture will first be qualified by which area is injured, such as the vault of the skull (frontal or parietal bone—code S02.0xxA) or the base of the skull (sphenoid or temporal bone—code S02.19xA). *Note:* A second code would report any intracranial injury, if applicable.

Fractures of the skull are characterized differently than others throughout the body and include the following:

- *Basal skull fracture* is a break in the floor of the skull.
- *Blowout fracture* indicates a break in the floor of the orbit that is typically caused by a severe blow to the eye.
- *Depressed skull fracture* identifies an inward displacement of one of the bones of the skull.
- *Stellate fracture* is one with a clear central point of the fracture and with break lines radiating from this central spot.

Maxillary Fracture Facial trauma might result in a LeFort fracture, which is a bilateral maxillary fracture with involvement of the surrounding bone, including the zygomatic bones. Such fractures are identified by type: A LeFort I fracture (code S02.411-) is a downward horizontal facial fracture and typically involves the maxillary alveolar rim and inferior nasal aperture. A LeFort II fracture (code S02.412-) is more triangular, involving the inferior orbital rim, the nasal bridge, and the frontal processes of the maxilla. A LeFort III fracture (code S02.413-) is a transverse fracture, sometimes referred to as a *craniofacial dissociation*. This fracture involves the zygomatic arch, the nasal bridge, and the upper maxilla and extends along the orbit floor (posteriorly).

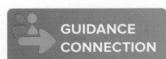

GUIDANCE CONNECTION

Review the ICD-10-CM Coding Guidelines, Section I.C.19, Chapter 19: **Injury, poisoning, and certain other consequences of external causes,** Subsection c, **Coding traumatic fractures.**

EXAMPLE

S02.402A Zygomatic fracture, unspecified, initial encounter for closed fracture

S02.413D LeFort III fracture, subsequent encounter for fracture with routine healing

LO 17.4 Pathophysiological Fractures and Conditions

Some conditions may affect any part of the skeletal system and therefore require that the specific anatomical location be documented. Diseases and other conditions can create problems with the bones and may be caused by a congenital malformation, pathology, or a traumatic event. As always, these are important details for coders to know.

Developmental dysplasia of the hip (DDH), also known as *congenital hip dysplasia,* is most common in a baby born breech, a large neonate, or a multiparity baby. DDH is a condition in which the head of the femur is displaced from the acetabulum. Treatments include a splint-brace or harness, a night splint, or bilateral traction. Use code Q65.89, Other specified congenital deformities of hip (congenital acetabular dysplasia).

GUIDANCE CONNECTION

Review the ICD-10-CM Coding Guidelines, Section I.C.13, Chapter 13: **Diseases of the musculoskeletal system and connective tissue,** Subsection c, **Coding of pathologic fractures.**

Ectromelia or *hemimelia* can occur in either the upper or lower limb. Ectromelia is the congenital absence or imperfection of one or more limbs. Hemimelia is a congenital abnormality affecting only the distal segment of either the upper or lower limb. A surgical knee mobilization is one of several potential treatment options. This condition is reported with code Q73.8, Other reduction defects of unspecified limb (ectromelia of limb NOS) (hemimelia of limb NOS).

Genu recurvatum, the backward curving of the knee joint, as well as other bowing of the long bones of the leg, may be treated with braces, casting, and/or orthotics. Congenital genu recurvatum is reported with code Q68.2, Congenital deformity of knee. When this condition is the sequela (late effect) of rickets, it is reported with M21.26-, Flexion deformity, knee, followed by code E64.3, Sequela of rickets.

Gout, also known as *gouty arthritis,* is the result of the buildup of uric acid in the body. Caused by either a malfunction that produces too much uric acid or an anomaly that makes it difficult for the body to get rid of uric acid, the specific underlying cause is still unknown. Gout presents in the joints, most often a toe, knee, or ankle, and begins with a throbbing or extreme pain in the middle of the night. The joint will be tender, warm to the touch, and erythematous (red). The most common treatment is a prescription for NSAIDs (nonsteroidal anti-inflammatory drugs). In ICD-10-CM, gout is reported from code category M1A, Chronic Gout, with additional characters required to report the underlying cause (i.e., drug-induced, idiopathic, etc.) as well as the specific anatomical location (i.e., ankle, elbow, foot, etc.).

Klippel-Feil syndrome is a condition characterized by the development of a short, wide neck due to either an abnormal number of cervical vertebrae or fused hemivertebrae (the incomplete development of one side of a vertebra). Surgery to relieve craniocervical instability, cervical instability, and/or pressure on the spinal cord may be necessary. Use code Q76.1, Klippel-Feil syndrome (cervical fusion syndrome).

Kyphosis is a bending forward of the vertebral column, most often at the thoracic vertebrae. This condition may be congenital or may be caused by poor posture or other spinal disorder. Kyphosis used to be commonly referred to as "dowager's hump." A brace and exercise are often the first course of treatment. Spinal arthrodesis may relieve symptoms, and surgery may be done when neurologic function is impaired. This condition is reported with code M40.04, Postural kyphosis, thoracic region. However, multiple codes are available for kyphosis determined by section of the spine as well as underlying cause.

Osteoarthritis is a chronic degeneration of the articular cartilage simultaneous with the formation of bone spurs on the underlying bone within a joint. The cause of the osteoarthritis might be an idiomatic condition (such as code M17.11, Unilateral primary osteoarthritis, right knee); secondary to another underlying condition (such as code M18.52, Other unilateral secondary osteoarthritis of first carpometacarpal joint, left hand); or posttraumatic (such as code M19.172, Post-traumatic osteoarthritis, left ankle and foot). Treatments typically begin with NSAIDs and/or corticosteroid injections. In some cases, a brace or crutches may be helpful.

Osteochondrosis, also known as *osteochondropathy* or *Osgood-Schlatter disease,* is a painful separation of the epiphysis of the tibial tubercle from the tibial shaft. This condition most often affects preteen and early teenage boys after a traumatic event. Treatments include immobilization of the knee and rest. In severe cases, surgical repair may be required. One code example is M93.1, Kienbock's disease of adults (adult osteochondrosis of carpal lunates).

Osteoitis deformans, also known as *Paget's disease,* may cause severe and chronic pain as well as impaired movement due to abnormal bone growth on the spinal cord. The preferred first phase of treatment is pharmaceutical. Report this from code category M88, Osteitis deformans (Paget's disease of bone), with additional characters to report the specific bone affected as well as laterality.

Osteoporosis is a disease that is believed to be the manifestation of slowing bone formation that occurs simultaneously with an increase in the body's reabsorption of bone. One exception is *posttraumatic osteoporosis,* also known as *Sudeck's atrophy.*

The existence of osteoporosis increases the patient's susceptibility to fractures. The presence of a pathologic fracture will change the code determination in ICD-10-CM. Code category M80 reports osteoporosis with a current pathologic fracture, while code category M81 reports osteoporosis without a current pathologic fracture.

Spina bifida is a condition in which the bony encasement of the spinal cord fails to close. Surgical repair is done as soon as possible in an effort to reduce serious handicaps. There have been some successful cases of in utero surgical repair. This condition is reported from code category Q05, Spina bifida, with an additional character to identify the specific area of the spine that is affected.

Type III traumatic spondylolisthesis of the axis (C2) is a displacement of the vertebra anteriorly over the vertebra below it. An open reduction of the C2 vertebra followed by a posterior spinal fusion with a pedicle lag screw is used to repair the injury. Report this with code M43.12, Spondylolisthesis, cervical region.

GUIDANCE CONNECTION

Review the ICD-10-CM Coding Guidelines, Section I.C.13, Chapter 13: **Diseases of the musculoskeletal system and connective tissue,** Subsection d, **Osteoporosis.**

LO 17.5 Sequelae (Late Effects) of Fractures

Once a bone has been given the opportunity to heal, it may not heal properly. The most common types of late effects of fractures are **malunion** and **nonunion.** A malunion (*mal* = bad + *union* = together) of a fractured bone means that the pieces of the bone healed back together but not in an effective way. Unfortunately, the most common treatment for a malunion is for the physician to rebreak the bone and set it again, hoping that it will heal properly the second time. When the parts of a broken bone do not heal back together at all, despite the proper treatment and time allotment, this is known as a nonunion (*non* = not + *union* = together).

In ICD-10-CM's Alphabetic Index, when you look up *Fracture, malunion,* you will see the notation "*See* Fracture, by site." When you look up *Fracture, nonunion,* you will see the notation "*See* Nonunion, fracture." At *Nonunion, fracture,* the notation states, "*See* Fracture, by site."

malunion
A fractured bone that did not heal correctly; healing of bone that was not in proper position or alignment.

nonunion
A fractured bone that did not heal back together; no mending or joining together of the broken segments.

LO 17.6 Seventh Character

Surely, you remember from Chapter 3 of this textbook that some ICD-10-CM codes require a seventh character. Different subsections use this position—the seventh character—to add various types of information. The choices will be listed at the top of the code category and are used for all codes within that category. With this in mind, you must always check the top of the code category for this information.

Within the ICD-10-CM chapter on diseases of the musculoskeletal system and connective tissue, the appropriate seventh character is to be added to each code:

A initial encounter for fracture

D subsequent encounter for fracture with routine healing

G subsequent encounter for fracture with delayed healing

K subsequent encounter for fracture with nonunion

P subsequent encounter for fracture with malunion

S sequela

When you are reporting an injury to an anatomical site within the muscular or skeletal systems, you will find variations to this list. Within the chapter on injury, poisoning, and certain other consequences of external causes, you will see:

The appropriate 7th character is to be added to each code:

A initial encounter

D subsequent encounter

S sequela

GUIDELINE CONNECTION

Review the ICD-10-CM Coding Guidelines, Section I.C.20, Chapter 20: **External causes of morbidity,** Subsection i, **Sequelae (late effects) of external cause guidelines.**

or

A initial encounter for closed fracture

D subsequent encounter for fracture with routine healing

G subsequent encounter for fracture with delayed healing

K subsequent encounter for fracture with nonunion

P subsequent encounter for fracture with malunion

S sequela

or

A initial encounter for closed fracture

B initial encounter for open fracture type I or II; initial encounter for open fracture NOS

C initial encounter for open fracture type IIIA, IIIB, or IIIC

D subsequent encounter for closed fracture with routine healing

E subsequent encounter for open fracture type I or II with routine healing

F subsequent encounter for open fracture type IIIA, IIIB, or IIIC with routine healing

G subsequent encounter for closed fracture with delayed healing

H subsequent encounter for open fracture type I or II with delayed healing

J subsequent encounter for open fracture type IIIA, IIIB, or IIIC with delayed healing

K subsequent encounter for closed fracture with nonunion

M subsequent encounter for open fracture type I or II with nonunion

N subsequent encounter for open fracture type IIIA, IIIB, or IIIC with nonunion

P subsequent encounter for closed fracture with malunion

Q subsequent encounter for open fracture type I or II with malunion

E subsequent encounter for open fracture type IIIA, IIIB, or IIIC with malunion

S sequela

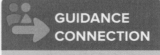

GUIDANCE CONNECTION

Review the ICD-10-CM Coding Guidelines, Section I.A, **Conventions for the ICD-10-CM,** Subsection 5, **7th characters**.

The Tabular List contains all the details you need. All you have to do is read the choices and determine which is the most accurate, as per the physician's documentation.

LET'S CODE IT! SCENARIO

Walter Robinson came to see Dr. Santos with complaints of sudden-onset, severe low back pain. He states that the pain is in the left side of his buttocks, his left leg, and sometimes his left foot. At times, he states that his leg seems weak as well. Dr. Santos takes a complete patient history, including specific times and actions that intensify the pain. Then x-rays, followed by an MRI, are taken of Walter's spine, showing a herniated (intervertebral) disc at L3–L4.

Dr. Santos diagnosed Walter with a *herniated (intervertebral) disc.* Turn to the Alphabetic Index, look up *herniated,* and read down the list to find *disc.* Hmmm. It is not there. Try looking for *intervertebral.* Look down and see:

Hernia, hernia

    Intervertebral cartilage or disc—*see* Displacement, intervertebral disc

OK, let's turn to that in the Alphabetic Index:

Displacement, displaced

    Intervertebral disc NEC

        Lumbar region M51.26

You might ask, How do we know that it is the lumbar region? Look back at Dr. Santos's notes. He wrote that the herniated disk is at L3–L4. The "L" means the lumbar vertebrae, and the notation L3–L4 indicates that the affected intervertebral disc is between the third and fourth lumbar vertebrae. Now turn to the Tabular List and confirm the code.

Start reading at:

M51 Thoracic, thoracolumbar, and lumbosacral intervertebral disc disorders

There is an *Excludes2* note that mentions disorders of the cervical and sacral discs. However, Walter's lumbar disc is what is dislocated, so you can keep reading down the column to review the fourth-character and fifth-character options and determine which matches Dr. Santos's documentation:

M51.2 Other thoracic, thoracolumbar, and lumbosacral intervertebral disc displacement

M51.26 Other intervertebral disc displacement, lumbar region

Go back to Dr. Santos's notes and see that while this doesn't match exactly, it does tell the story of why Dr. Santos cared for Walter. Terrific!

This code tells the whole story about Walter's specific injury. Now ask yourself, Do I need to find the external cause code(s) to explain how Walter's injury happened? No. A herniated disc is not necessarily the result of a traumatic event. Therefore, there is no need to report any external cause.

Good work!

YOU CODE IT! CASE STUDY

Felicia LaMasters, an 83-year-old female, was brought into the ED last night and admitted into the hospital with a fracture of her right shoulder. She was dancing and when she kicked out her foot, she slipped and landed on her shoulder. Felicia stated she was diagnosed with age-related osteoporosis 5 years ago. Dr. Rambeau diagnosed her with a pathologic fracture of the right shoulder.

Go through the steps of coding, and determine the code or codes that should be reported for this encounter between Dr. Rambeau and Felicia.

Step 1: Read the case completely.

Step 2: Abstract the notes: Which key words can you identify relating to why Dr. Rambeau cared for Felicia?

_____

Step 3: Query the provider, if necessary.

Step 4: Code the diagnosis or diagnoses.

_____

Step 5: Code the procedure(s): Admission into the hospital.

Step 6: Link the procedure codes to at least one diagnosis code to confirm medical necessity.

Step 7: Back code to double-check your choices.

Answer:

Did you determine the correct code to be:

M80.011A Age-related osteoporosis with current pathological fracture, right shoulder, initial encounter for fracture

Good job!!!

Chapter Summary

The 206 bones of the adult human skeleton provide the foundational structure for the components of the body. These bones protect internal organs as well as enable certain functions. Each bone is categorized by its shape: long bones, flat bones, short bones, irregularly shaped bones, and sesamoid bones. Any of these bones can be afflicted by malformation during gestation (congenital conditions), disease (pathologic conditions), or injury (traumatic conditions).

CHAPTER **17** REVIEW
Coding Skeletal Conditions

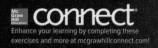
Enhance your learning by completing these
exercises and more at mcgrawhillconnect.com!

Using Terminology

Match each key term to the appropriate definition.

Part One

_____ **1.** LO 17.1 The end of a long bone, either the distal or proximal end.

_____ **2.** LO 17.1 Bones that comprise the skull segments that cover the brain.

_____ **3.** LO 17.1 A fibrocartilage segment that lies between vertebrae of the spinal column and provides cushioning and support.

_____ **4.** LO 17.1 A bone that is a part of the construction of the spinal column.

_____ **5.** LO 17.1 The bones that construct the central segment of the body.

_____ **6.** LO 17.2 The bones that construct the upper and lower extremities.

_____ **7.** LO 17.1 A joint.

_____ **8.** LO 17.1 The rib cage.

_____ **9.** LO 17.1 The bones that protect the head and create the face.

_____ **10.** LO 17.1 Shaft of a long bone.

A. Appendicular skeleton
B. Articulation
C. Axial skeleton
D. Bony thorax
E. Cranium
F. Diaphysis
G. Epiphysis
H. Intervertebral disc
 I. Skull
 J. Vertebra

Part Two

_____ **1.** LO 17.1 Latticelike shaped bone; also known as *spongy bone*.

_____ **2.** LO 17.3 Broken cartilage or bone.

_____ **3.** LO 17.1 The right or left side of anatomical sites that have locations on both sides of the body.

_____ **4.** LO 17.1 Bonylike substance.

_____ **5.** LO 17.1 A rounded nodule at the end of a bone where a muscle or ligament attaches.

_____ **6.** LO 17.1 The specific anatomical location of the disease or injury.

_____ **7.** LO 17.5 A fractured bone that did not heal back together; no mending or joining together of the broken segments.

_____ **8.** LO 17.1 The junctures of the parts of the cranium and skull.

_____ **9.** LO 17.5 A fractured bone that did not heal correctly; healing of bone that was not in proper position or alignment.

A. Cancellous
B. Fracture
C. Laterality
D. Malunion
E. Nonunion
F. Osseous
G. Site
H. Sutures
 I. Tuberosity

Checking Your Understanding

Choose the most appropriate answer for each of the following questions.

1. LO 17.1 _____ is the shaft of a long bone.

   a. Epiphysis.

   b. Diaphysis.

   c. Cranium.

   d. Bony thorax.

2. LO 17.1 A rounded nodule at the end of a bone where a muscle or ligament attaches is referred to as

  a. Sutures.
  b. Osseous.
  c. Tuberosity.
  d. Cancellous.

3. LO 17.1 C1 is the first

  a. Thoracic vertebra.
  b. Lumbar vertebra.
  c. Sacrum vertebra.
  d. Cervical vertebra.

4. LO 17.1 Which of the following is part of the sternum?

  a. Scapula.
  b. Xiphoid process.
  c. Incus.
  d. Occipital.

5. LO 17.2 The pelvic girdle includes which of the following?

  a. Scapula.
  b. Clavicle.
  c. Humerus.
  d. Os coxae.

6. LO 17.3 The term *greenstick fracture* refers to

  a. A break that runs along the length of a long bone.
  b. A fracture existing on one side of the bone while the other side is not broken but bent.
  c. A bone that has been displaced inward.
  d. A bone that has been broken into several pieces.

7. LO 17.3 If the physician's notes do not specify the fracture as open or closed, you must code it as

  a. Open.
  b. Closed.
  c. Unspecified.
  d. Not otherwise specified.

8. LO 17.6 The seventh character "G" represents which of the following?

  a. Initial encounter for fracture.
  b. Subsequent encounter for fracture with routine healing.
  c. Subsequent encounter for fracture with delayed healing.
  d. Subsequent encounter for fracture with nonunion.

9. LO 17.6 Which seventh character represents an initial encounter for a fracture?

  a. K.
  b. P.
  c. D.
  d. A.

10. LO 17.6 How many bones are there in the adult human skeleton?

    a. 106.

    b. 206.

    c. 250.

    d. 275.

Applying Your Knowledge

1. LO 17.1 What consitutes the axial skeleton, and what is this skeleton's function? _____

_____

2. LO 17.2 What constitutes the appendicular skeleton? _____

_____

3. LO 17.1 How are bones categorized? Include examples. _____

_____

4. LO 17.1 List four categories of bones. _____

_____

5. LO 17.1 List the bones of the ear. _____

_____

6. LO 17.1 The spinal column is divided into sections. What are these sections, how many vertebrae are in each section, and how are the vertebrae identified? _____

_____

7. LO 17.2 List the parts of the pectoral girdle. _____

_____

8. LO 17.2 Describe the parts of the pelvic girdle. _____

_____

9. LO 17.3 Explain the difference between a fracture and a dislocation. _____

_____

10. LO 17.3 List five alternate terms for an open fracture. _____

_____

11. LO 17.3/17.4 Explain the difference between a traumatic fracture and a pathologic fracture. Why is it important to know the difference? _____

_____

12. LO 17.3 List four different types of fractures. _____

_____

13. LO 17.5 List two terms that would indicate a late effect of an earlier fracture. _____

_____

14. LO 17.4 List four pathophysiologic bone disorders or conditions. _____

_____

YOU CODE IT! Practice

Chapter 17: Coding Skeletal Conditions

Using the techniques described in this chapter, carefully read through the case studies and determine the most accurate ICD-10-CM code(s) and external cause code(s), if appropriate, for each case study.

1. Norman Wilhelm, a 64-year-old male, was returning home from a business trip. The train pulled into the train station and came to a stop; as Norman was stepping off the train the car suddenly jerked forward. Norman fell, injuring his right leg, and was taken to the nearest ER, where he was diagnosed with a torus fracture of the proximal end of both the tibia and fibula.

   _____

2. Isis Graham, a 5-year-old female, fell from the monkey bars at the playground 5 weeks ago and was diagnosed with a nondisplaced shaft fracture of her left clavicle. Isis is brought in today by her parents with the complaint that Isis's left shoulder is still painful. After an x-ray, Dr. Govan notes a malunion of the fracture.

   _____

3. Ivan Scotto, a 19-year-old male, dove into a lake while swimming with his friends and hit the bottom. Dr. Polarris diagnosed him with a Jefferson fracture (C1 vertebra fracture) with C1 spinal cord injury.

   _____

4. Sylvia York, a 43-year-old female, was driving down Main Street when her car was struck by another car. Sylvia suffered a comminuted shaft fracture of her left humerus.

   _____

5. Janine Samuels, a 22-year-old female, enjoys boxing as a recreational sport. Three weeks ago, while boxing, Janine was struck by her opponent on the side of the head and suffered a dislocated jaw. Janine presents today complaining it's difficult to chew. After an examination, Dr. Floyd notes her jaw is healing within normal expectations.

   _____

6. Walter Baumann, a 62-year-old male, has been a Shriner for many years. Walter was given the privilege of riding the elephant in the annual circus parade at the local stadium. Halfway around, he fell off the animal. Walter complained of right side pain and was taken to the ER, where he was diagnosed with four fractured ribs, right side.

   _____

7. Francine Baumann, a 58-year-old female, was trying to help her husband, Walter (the previous case study), after he fell from the elephant. The elephant stepped on her left foot and caused displaced fractures of the fourth and fifth metatarsal bones.

   _____

8. Lee Rogers, a 39-year-old male, was in astronaut training when he hit his head in the weightlessness simulator at the space center. He was unconscious for 15 minutes. Dr. Sousman determined Lee had a fractured parietal bone.

_____

9. Bennett Bernardo, a 47-year-old male, has been morbidly obese for over a decade. Six weeks ago, Dr. Jaffe diagnosed him with a stress fracture of the metatarsals of the right foot. Bennett presents today with the complaint of continued pain in his right foot. After an x-ray, Dr. Jaffe notes a malunion of the right metatarsal fracture.

_____

10. Colleen O'Donnell, a 33-year-old female, presents today with severe pain in her left arm. Colleen lives in an apartment, and while showering this morning she slipped and fell in her bathtub. Dr. Holder takes an x-ray and diagnoses Colleen with a fractured left radius with ulna, distal end, and a posterior dislocation of the radial head of the left elbow.

_____

11. Elaine Gregory, a 79-year-old female, was diagnosed 4 weeks ago with a pathologic fracture of the right humerus due to postmenopausal osteoporosis. Elaine presents today for a follow-up visit. After an examination, Dr. Spaulding notes that the fracture is slow (delayed) healing.

_____

12. Three weeks ago, Robert Emory, a 15-year-old male, was riding his nonmotorized scooter down a hill, hit a bump, and fell off his scooter. Robert was diagnosed with a dislocated medial meniscus, complex, of his left knee. Robert presents today for a follow-up visit, and Dr. Kennedy notes the tear is healing within normal range.

_____

13. Clayton Harrison, a 25-year-old male, had the weekend off and decided to go hang gliding at the beach. Clayton lost control of his hang glider and was forced to land, injuring his hip. He was diagnosed with a fractured acetabulum, medial wall.

_____

14. Everett Callman, a 33-year-old male, was diagnosed 5 weeks ago with a pathologic fracture of the vertebrae due to a metastatic carcinoma of the bone from the right lung, upper lobe. Everett presents today with continued back pain. After an x-ray, Dr. Douglas notes a slow/delayed healing process.

_____

15. Olivia Campbell, a 13-year-old female, was jumping rope in her front yard and stepped off the curb the wrong way and hurt her left ankle. X-rays confirmed Dr. Conner's diagnosis of a nondisplaced trimalleolar fracture.

_____

The following exercises provides practice in abstracting physicians' notes and learning to work with SOAP notes from our health care facility, *Taylor, Reader, & Associates.* These case studies (SOAP notes) are modeled on real patient encounters. Using the techniques described in this chapter, carefully read through the case studies and determine the most accurate ICD-10-CM code(s) and external cause code(s), if appropriate, for each case study.

TAYLOR, READER, & ASSOCIATES
A Complete Health Care Facility
975 CENTRAL AVENUE • SOMEWHERE, FL 32811 • 407-555-4321

PATIENT: FRACMAN, GERALD
ACCOUNT/EHR #:   FRACGE001
DATE: 04/25/18

Attending Physician: Willard B. Reader, MD

S: Patient is a 29-year-old male who states he was driving home from a business trip in a company car when his car was struck from behind by another car. He was driving on the interstate highway near his office. Patient is complaining of severe neck pain and difficulty turning his head.

O: PE reveals tightness upon palpitation of ligaments in neck and shoulders, most pronounced C3 to C4. X-rays are taken of head and neck, including the cervical vertebrae. Radiologic review denies any fracture.

A: Dislocation of fourth cervical vertebra

P: 1. Cervical collar to be worn during all waking hours
   2. Rx Vicodin (hydrocodone) 500 mg po prn
   3. 1,000 mg aspirin qid
   4. Pt to return in 2 weeks for follow-up

Willard B. Reader, MD

WBR/pw   D: 04/25/18 09:50:16   T: 04/30/18 12:55:01

Determine the most accurate ICD-10-CM code(s).

_____

_____

_____

TAYLOR, READER, & ASSOCIATES
A Complete Health Care Facility
975 CENTRAL AVENUE • SOMEWHERE, FL 32811 • 407-555-4321

PATIENT: WHITMAN, ELOISE
ACCOUNT/EHR #: WHITEL01
DATE: 09/16/18

Attending Physician: Suzanne R. Taylor, MD

S: This new Pt is a 31-year-old female who was involved in an accident when the motorcycle she was driving was struck by a car on a street near her house. Eloise admits to riding motorcycles for recreation. She is complaining about some neck pain. She has tingling into her hand and her feet. She states that her left arm hurts when she tries to pull it overhead. A friend apparently told her that she should likely see a spine doctor, but somehow she came to see me first. PMH is remarkable for kidney trouble. Past bronchoscopy, laparoscopy, and kidney stone surgery, otherwise noncontributory as per the medical history form completed by the patient and reviewed at this visit.

O: Ht 5′5″ Wt. 179 lb. R 16. Pt presented in a sling. She was told to use it by the same friend. She states if she does not use it, her arm does not feel any different, so I had her remove it. On exam, the left shoulder demonstrates full passive motion. She has normal strength testing. She has no deformity. She has some tenderness over the trapezial area. The reflexes are brisk and symmetric. X-rays of her chest 2 views and C spine AP/LAT are relatively benign, as are complete x-rays of the shoulder.

A: Anterior displaced type II dens fracture of the second cervical vertebra, and an anterior dislocation of the proximal end of the left humerus.

P: 1. Rx Naprosyn
    2. Referral to PT
    3. Referral to orthopedist

Suzanne Taylor, MD

SRT/mg   D: 9/16/18 09:50:16   T: 9/18/18 12:55:01

Determine the most accurate ICD-10-CM code(s).

_____

_____

_____

TAYLOR, READER, & ASSOCIATES
A Complete Health Care Facility
975 CENTRAL AVENUE • SOMEWHERE, FL 32811 • 407-555-4321

PATIENT: BRADLEY, JOE
ACCOUNT/EHR #:   BRADJO001
DATE: 09/20/18

Attending Physician: Willard B. Reader, MD

S: Pt is a 42-year-old male who was working in his machine shop at his home garage 5 weeks ago and hit his hand on the wall by accident, resulting in a fracture of the proximal phalanx, ring finger, left hand. He presents today with significant pain in his left ring finger.

O: Ht 5′9″ Wt. 163 lb. R 16. X-ray of the left ring finger confirmed a malunion of the fracture.

A: Malunion fracture of left ring finger proximal phalanx, subsequent encounter

P: Refer to orthopedic specialist

Willard Reader, MD

WBR/mg   D: 09/20/18 09:50:16   T: 09/22/18 12:55:01

Determine the most accurate ICD-10-CM code(s).

_____

_____

_____

TAYLOR, READER, & ASSOCIATES
A Complete Health Care Facility
975 CENTRAL AVENUE • SOMEWHERE, FL 32811 • 407-555-4321

PATIENT: ALLISON, JOANNA
ACCOUNT/EHR #:   ALLIJO01
DATE: 09/16/18

Attending Physician: Suzanne R. Taylor, MD

S: Pt is a 23-year-old female who fell from the porch in front of her house and hurt her back while pruning tree limbs. She states that the pain is mostly in her lower back. She denies any personal history of back problems. She states she had trouble sitting up and finds slight relief when lying flat. She claims she cannot bend over at all because the pain is too severe.

O: Ht 5'7" Wt. 129 lb. R 16. X-rays of back, L1–L5 A/P and lateral. Films confirm a nondisplaced wedge compression fracture of L1 and L2 vertebral bodies. Patient is placed into a back brace and told to get bed rest.

A: Nondisplaced wedge compression fractures L1–L2

P: 1. Rx Tylenol with codeine for pain, as directed
   2. Referral to PT
   3. Referral to orthopedist

Suzanne R. Taylor, MD

SRT/pw   D: 9/16/18 09:50:16   T: 9/18/18 12:55:01

Determine the most accurate ICD-10-CM code(s).

_____

_____

_____

TAYLOR, READER, & ASSOCIATES
A Complete Health Care Facility
975 CENTRAL AVENUE • SOMEWHERE, FL 32811 • 407-555-4321

PATIENT: CONTINALE, THEODORE
ACCOUNT/EHR #:   CONTTH001
DATE: 02/11/18

Attending Physician: Willard B. Reader, MD

S: Pt is a 50-year-old male who fell down the icy front steps of his house. He hit his head on the concrete step and sustained a head injury but did not lose consciousness. He also noted that his right ankle swelled up and was so painful he could not put his weight on it.

O: Ht 5′11″ Wt. 187 lb. R 20. T 98.6. BP 130/95 Patient sent to radiology for x-rays of right ankle—A/P/L views as well as the skull. Physical examination HEENT: Pt denies any problems with vision, PERLA. X-rays indicate a closed trimalleolar fracture of the medial and lateral malleolus with anterior lip of tibia involvement. No fracture of skull revealed.

A: Displaced fracture of trimalleolar with involvement of the medial and lateral malleolus and anterior lip of tibia; mild brain concussion.

P: 1. Pt to return 3 weeks.
     2. Rx Tylenol with codeine for pain.
     3. Patient sent to casting room for short leg cast. Triped cane provided for walking.

Willard B. Reader, MD

WBR/pw   D: 08/11/18 09:50:16   T: 08/13/18 12:55:01

Determine the most accurate ICD-10-CM code(s).

_____

_____

_____

18 CODING DISEASES OF THE URINARY SYSTEM

Learning Outcomes *After completing this chapter, the student should be able to:*

LO 18.1 Identify the components of the urinary system.

LO 18.2 Explain the signs and symptoms of urologic malfunction.

LO 18.3 Explain the stages of chronic kidney disease.

LO 18.4 Determine how to code chronic kidney disease when found with other conditions.

LO 18.5 Report infections in urinary organs correctly.

LO 18.6 Report conditions affecting the prostate accurately.

Key Terms

Anemic

Benign prostatic hyperplasia (BPH)

Bladder cancer

Chronic kidney disease (CKD)

Glomerular filtration rate (GFR)

Kidney

Prostatitis

Urea

Ureter

Urethra

Urinary bladder

Urinary system

Urinary tract infection (UTI)

The components of the **urinary system** (see Figure 18-1) are the same in both men and women. This organ system is responsible for removing waste products (known as **urea**) that are left behind by protein (food), excessive water, disproportionate amounts of electrolytes, and other nitrogenous compounds from the blood and the body. A failure to eliminate these

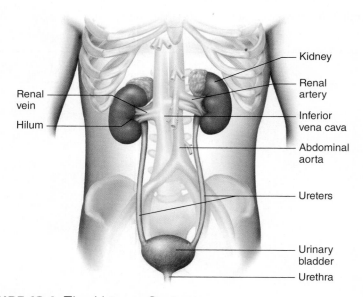

Renal vein

Hilum

Kidney

Renal artery

Inferior vena cava

Abdominal aorta

Ureters

Urinary bladder

Urethra

FIGURE 18-1 The Urinary System

Source: David Shier et al., HOLE'S HUMAN ANATOMY & PHYSIOLOGY, 12/e. © 2010 MHE. Figure 20.1, p. 776

wastes from the body in a timely fashion may actually result in the body poisoning itself. The organ components of the urinary system include:

- *Kidney* (right and left), each leading to a
- *Ureter* (right and left), each leading to the
- *Urinary bladder,* which then passes urine through the
- *Urethra,* to travel outside the body.

LO 18.1 The Urinary System

The Kidneys

The **kidneys** are responsible for the production and elimination of urine, thereby maintaining homeostasis (sustaining equilibrium by fine-tuning physiological processes) (see Figure 18-2). These organs detoxify the blood by eliminating wastes, regulating fluid volume, and balancing the concentration of electrolytes in body fluids. As the waste products are collected, the kidneys create urine using glomerular filtration (filtering the blood as it flows through the kidneys), tubular reabsorption, and tubular secretion. The urine, carrying that waste, is transported via the ureters to the bladder.

The renal arteries subdivide into five smaller arteries that supply blood to various areas of each kidney. Renal veins also branch out and ultimately deliver blood into the inferior vena cava.

EXAMPLE

N00.0 Acute nephritic syndrome with minor glomerular abnormality

N17.0 Acute kidney failure with tubular necrosis

The Ureters

The **ureters** are tubelike structures whose purpose is to transport urine, processed by the kidney and ready for elimination, to the urinary bladder. Each kidney has its own ureter (see Figure 18-2). Even though there is no sphincter between the ureter and the urinary bladder, the position and angle of the attachment between the two creates a mucosal fold that functions in a similar fashion to control the flow. A sphincter is a circular muscle that can open to permit the passage of fluid or other material and close to prevent transit.

EXAMPLE

N20.1 Calculus of ureter

N28.86 Ureteritis cystica

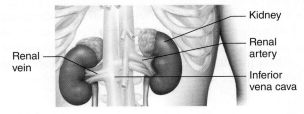

FIGURE 18-2 The Kidneys

Source: David Shier et al., HOLE'S HUMAN ANATOMY & PHYSIOLOGY, 12/e. © 2010 MHE. Figure 20.1, p. 776

urinary system
The organ system responsible for removing waste products that are left behind by protein, excessive water, disproportionate amounts of electrolytes, and other nitrogenous compounds from the blood and the body.

urea
A compound that results from the breakdown of proteins and is excreted in urine.

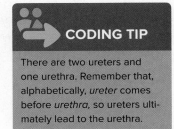

CODING TIP

There are two ureters and one urethra. Remember that, alphabetically, *ureter* comes before *urethra,* so ureters ultimately lead to the urethra.

kidney
A bean-shaped organ that filters blood and excretes urine.

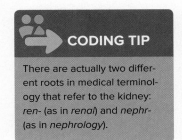

CODING TIP

There are actually two different roots in medical terminology that refer to the kidney: *ren-* (as in *renal*) and *nephr-* (as in *nephrology*).

ureter
A long tubular passageway for urine traveling from the kidney to the urinary bladder.

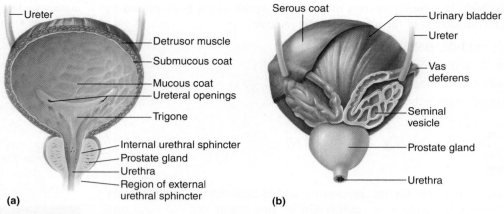

FIGURE 18-3 The Urinary Bladder

Source: David Shier et al., HOLE'S HUMAN ANATOMY & PHYSIOLOGY, 12/e. © 2010 MHE. Figure 20.29, p. 800

The Urinary Bladder

urinary bladder
A hollow organ that collects and temporarily stores urine.

The **urinary bladder** is a sac constructed of muscles, located anteroinferior (in front and below) to the peritoneal cavity (see Figure 18-3). The primary sectors of the urinary bladder include:

Fundus: the large, curved superior aspect of the bladder. The medical term *fundus* actually means the segment of an organ furthermost from its orifice.
Apex: the anterosuperior area.
Body: the posteroinferior area and the location of the points of attachment for the ureters, known as the *ureteral orifices.*
Neck: the inferior region of the bladder and the location of the urethral orifice.

Note: The area known as the *renal trigone* includes the three orifices (two ureteral and one urethral).

EXAMPLE

N30.30 Trigonitis without hematuria
N32.0 Bladder-neck obstruction

The Urethra

urethra
A tubular structure that carries urine from the urinary bladder to the outside of the body

The tubular structure leading from the urinary bladder is called the **urethra,** and it transports urine from the bladder to the outside of the body (see Figure 18-4). There are sphincters at each end of the urethra—the superior end *(internal urethral sphincter)* and the inferior end *(external urethral sphincter)*—that contract (close) to stop the outflow or relax to permit the expulsion of urine (known as *micturition*). When an individual cannot control these sphincters, due to malfunction or age-related issues, this can result in a condition known as *enuresis* (urinary incontinence). Kegel exercises, a method of strengthening the pelvic-floor muscles (those that support the bladder and bowel, as well as the uterus in females), may enable a patient to prevent—or at least reduce—urinary incontinence. *Note:* Physicians warn about performing Kegel exercises with a full bladder or while in the process of micturition.

EXAMPLE

N36.41 Hypermobility of urethra
N39.3 Stress incontinence (female)(male)

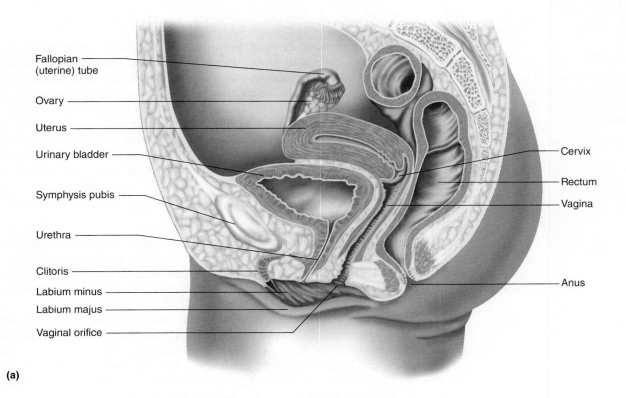

(a)

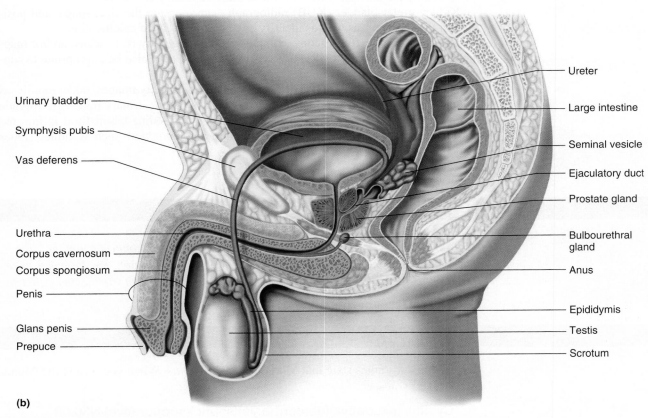

(b)

FIGURE 18-4 The Urethra: (a) in the female anatomy, (b) in the male anatomy

Source: David Shier et al., HOLE'S HUMAN ANATOMY & PHYSIOLOGY, 12/e. © 2010 MHE. Figure 20.28a and 20.28b, p. 799

LO 18.2 Renal and Urologic Malfunctions

As with many body systems, diseases and illnesses, congenital anomalies, medications, and pathogens can cause havoc within the urinary system. These problems may require straightforward treatments, such as using antibiotics for a **urinary tract infection (UTI),** or more complex treatments, such as dialysis or transplantation.

Renal malfunction affects every organ and body system, so physical examination may alert the physician to a concern in this area. The skin's color and texture can change, periorbital edema can modify vision, or the patient may develop difficulty with muscle function, including gait and posture. Mental status can also be influenced. Electrolyte imbalance can alter hypertension levels, while metabolic acidosis can result in hyperventilation.

Diagnostic Tools

A patient history of hypertension, diabetes mellitus, and/or bladder infections may also be indicative of urinary system conditions. Genetic predispositions can be identified with family histories that include glomerulonephritis or polycystic kidney disease. Nephrotoxicity can be caused by the patient's abuse of antibiotics or analgesics.

Blood tests can measure the levels of uric acid, creatinine, and blood urea nitrogen (BUN), providing insight into kidney function. Of course, urinalysis can add data about pH as well as clarity, color, and odor of the specimen. Measurement of urine output may require 24-hour specimen collection. Checking levels of antidiuretic hormone (ADH), produced by the pituitary gland, and/or levels of aldosterone, a hormone produced by the adrenal cortex, may also indicate kidney concerns.

Kidney-ureter-bladder (KUB) radiography can measure the size, shape, and position of these organs, as well as identify any possible areas of calcification.

Ultrasonography, fluoroscopy, computerized tomography (CT) scans, and/or magnetic resonance imaging (MRI) of the urinary system may also be appropriate to support the confirmation of a diagnosis.

An intravenous pyelogram (IVP) records a series of x-ray images, taken rapidly, as contrast material injected intravenously passes through the urinary tract. A retrograde pyelogram also uses contrast material; however, this iodine-based fluid is injected through the ureters to investigate a suspicion of an obstruction, such as kidney stones (calculi).

LET'S CODE IT! SCENARIO

Marla Nichols, a 25-year-old female, just returned from her honeymoon in the islands. She is feeling a burning sensation and some pain on urination, so she came to see Dr. Tomlinson. After exam and urinalysis, Marla was diagnosed with acute cystitis due to E. coli.

Let's Code It!

Dr. Tomlinson's notes state that Marla has *acute cystitis.* When you turn to the Alphabetic Index, you see:

Cystitis (exudative)(hemorrhagic)(septic)(suppurative) N30.00

When you turn to the Tabular List, you confirm:

N30 Cystitis

Take a second to read the *use additional code* and *Excludes1* notations carefully. Do you know what the infectious agent is, so you can code it? Yes, you do. Dr. Tomlinson included this detail *(E. coli)* in his notes. And Marla does not have prostatocystitis. Great! But first, we must determine the code for the cystitis. Did you find:

N30.0 Acute cystitis

There is an *Excludes1* notation listing two diagnoses. Take a minute to review them and determine whether either one applies to Marla's condition. No, neither of them do, so continue down and review all of the fifth-character choices. Which matches Dr. Tomlinson's notes?

N30.00 Acute cystitis without hematuria

Wait, you are not done yet. You still need to report the infectious agent. The *use additional code* notation referred you to code range B95–B97. Let's turn to B95 in the Tabular List. Review all of the code descriptions in this subsection. Did you find:

B96.20 *Escherichia coli [E. coli]* as the cause of diseases classified elsewhere

That's good. However, you need more information to determine the accurate fifth character. Did you realize there was more than one type of *E. coli?* Hmm. Even though you have documentation that the infectious agent is *E. coli*, it is not enough information. For this exercise, you will need to report the unspecified version. Once you get on the job, you will need to double-check the pathology report to be more specific.

N30.00 Acute cystitis without hematuria
B96.20 *Escherichia coli [E. coli]* as the cause of diseases classified elsewhere

LO 18.3 Chronic Kidney Disease

The kidneys are so important to the extraction of waste within the body. Therefore, when one or both malfunction, toxicity can form and the patient can become very ill. Chronic kidney disease (CKD) can be caused by disease, trauma, or an adverse reaction to medication.

In the section about the kidneys, you learned that glomerular filtration is an important process in removing wastes (creatinine) from the blood as it flows through the kidneys. The **glomerular filtration rate (GFR)** is measured by blood tests to check the creatinine level. When kidney function is not at an optimum level, creatinine continues to amass in the blood because it is not being removed as necessary. The National Kidney Foundation identifies a normal GFR range as 90–120 mL/min. GFR decreases with age, so geriatric patients are likely to have lower levels. Actually, a 90-year-old patient may have kidney function at 50% solely due to age-related changes.

Monthly tests would be performed to identify a chronic condition. **Chronic kidney disease (CKD)** may be indicated by the lab results:

glomerular filtration rate (GFR)
The measurement of kidney function; used to determine the stage of kidney disease. GFR is calculated by the physician using the results of a creatinine test in a formula with the patient's gender, age, race, and other factors; normal GFR is 90 and above.

chronic kidney disease (CKD)
Ongoing malfunction of one or both kidneys.

- *Normal GFR:* Kidney damage may exist even with a normal GFR—CKD stage 1, code N18.1.
- *GFR between 60 – 89:* CKD stage 2 (mild renal disease), code N18.2.
- *GFR between 30 – 59:* CKD stage 3 (moderate renal disease), code N18.3.
- *GFR between 15 – 29:* CKD stage 4 (severe renal disease), code N18.4.
- *GFR below 15:* CKD stage 5, code N18.5.
- *End-stage renal disease (ESRD):* CKD stage 5 requiring ongoing dialysis or transplantation, code N18.6.

LeMander Jones, a 35-year-old male, was tested as part of his annual physical. He came in today with his wife to get his test results. Dr. Pundar diagnosed him with moderate chronic kidney disease. She sat and discussed treatment options with LeMander and his wife.

You Code It!

Go through the steps of coding, and determine the code or codes that should be reported for this encounter between Dr. Pundar and LeMander Jones.

Step 1: Read the case completely.

Step 2: Abstract the notes: Which key words can you identify relating to why Dr. Pundar cared for LeMander?

_____

Step 3: Query the provider, if necessary.

Step 4: Code the diagnosis or diagnoses.

_____

Step 5: Code the procedure(s): Office visit.

Step 6: Link the procedure codes to at least one diagnosis code to confirm medical necessity.

Step 7: Back code to double-check your choices.

Answer:

Did you determine the correct code to be:

N18.3 Chronic kidney disease, stage 3 (moderate)

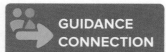

GUIDANCE CONNECTION

Review the ICD-10-CM Coding Guidelines, Section I.C.14, Chapter 14: **Diseases of the genitourinary system,** Sub-sections: a(1), **Stages of chronic kidney diseases (CKD);** a(2), **Hypertensive chronic kidney disease;** and a(3), **Chronic kidney disease with other conditions.**

LO 18.4 CKD with Other Conditions

CKD can be caused by hypertension, diabetic neuropathy (diabetes mellitus), untreated obstruction such as renal calculi (kidney stones), or a congenital anomaly such as polycystic kidneys. CKD progresses slowly; therefore, early diagnosis and treatment provide the best prognosis.

Hypertensive Chronic Kidney Disease When a patient is documented to have both hypertension and CKD, you are to assume that there is a cause-and-effect relationship between the two conditions. The physician does not have to specifically state that one caused the other in the documentation. Report this with a code from category:

I12 Hypertensive chronic kidney disease

Diabetes with Renal Manifestations A patient who has been diagnosed with diabetes may develop problems with his or her kidneys, such as chronic kidney disease, diabetic nephropathy, or Kimmelstiel-Wilson syndrome. When this is documented, regardless of the specific reason for the encounter, you will report a code from one of the following code categories, depending upon the type of diabetes mellitus:

E08.2 Diabetes mellitus due to underlying condition with kidney complications

E09.2 Drug or chemical induced diabetes mellitus with kidney complications

E10.2 Type 1 diabetes mellitus with kidney complications

E11.2 Type 2 diabetes mellitus with kidney complications

E13.2 Other specified diabetes mellitus with kidney complications

In all of these code categories, if the patient's kidney complication is CKD, you will need to report an additional code to identify the stage of the disease. You will see the *use additional code* notation.

LET'S CODE IT! SCENARIO

Eliott Impale, a 19-year-old male, was diagnosed with type 1 diabetes mellitus when he was 8 years old. He has been lax about testing his glucose and giving himself his insulin shots because he has been so busy with his courses and activities at Hillgraw University. After a complete HPI and exam, Dr. Kalmari performed a glucose test and a urinalysis. The results showed the early signs of type 1 diabetic nephrosis.

Let's Code It!

Dr. Kalmari's notes state that Eliott has *type 1 diabetic nephrosis*. When you turn to the Alphabetic Index, you see:

Diabetes, diabetic (mellitus)(sugar) E11.9

The word *nephrosis* is not there, but "kidney complications" is shown, suggesting code E11.29. Let's take a look in the Tabular List:

E11 Type 2 diabetes mellitus

Oh, wait a minute. This code category is for type 2 diabetes. Dr. Kalmari's notes document that Eliott has type 1 diabetes. Turn the pages and review this whole section to see if you can determine a more accurate code category. Did you find:

E10 Type 1 diabetes mellitus

There is an *Includes* note as well as an *Excludes1* notation listing several diagnoses. Take a minute to review them and determine whether any apply to Eliott's condition. No, none of them do, so continue down and review all of the fourth-character choices. Which matches Dr. Kalmari's notes?

E10.2 Type 1 diabetes mellitus with kidney complications

You remember that *nephrosis* is an abnormal condition of the kidney. Review the three potential fifth-character options. Which do you believe most accurately reports Eliott's condition?

E10.2 Type 1 diabetes mellitus with diabetic nephropathy

Nephropathy (*nephro* = kidney + *-pathy* = disease) means the same as *nephrosis,* so you have found the correct code. Good job!

Anemia in CKD The malfunction of the kidneys as they attempt to filter out the impurities in the body may trigger an **anemic** condition in the body. This condition can leave the patient weak, fatigued, and potentially short of breath because there is less oxygen carried through the bloodstream to the cells. When the patient is documented with these two conditions, you will need to:

- *Code first* the underlying chronic kidney disease (CKD) (N18.-).
- Follow this with code D63.1, Anemia in chronic kidney disease.

Dialysis There are two types of dialysis that may be used to treat a patient with renal malfunction: peritoneal dialysis and hemodialysis.

Peritoneal dialysis infuses a dialysate solution into the peritoneal cavity. Subsequently, the solution passes through the peritoneal membrane (which lines the abdominal cavity), collecting waste. The solution is then drained and thereby removes the waste.

Hemodialysis draws blood out of the body via an intravenous tube and passes the blood through a machine that removes waste products and returns clean blood to the body via a second intravenous connection.

When the patient is preparing for the dialysis treatments, you will need to know which type of dialysis the patient will be receiving:

Z49.01 Encounter for fitting and adjustment of extracorporeal dialysis catheter

or

Z49.02 Encounter for fitting and adjustment of peritoneal dialysis catheter

Plus, note the reminder directly beneath the code category:

Code also associated end stage renal disease (N18.6)

Within the first few weeks after beginning the series of dialysis treatments, the physician will want to have the patient come in for an efficiency or adequacy test. The purpose of the test is to measure the exchanges to ensure that the treatments are removing enough urea. The test results enable the health care professionals to adjust the dose, or amount, of the dialysis in each treatment. To report the reason for the encounter, report one of these codes:

Z49.31 Encounter for adequacy testing for hemodialysis

or

Z49.32 Encounter for adequacy testing for peritoneal dialysis

Most patients will need to receive dialysis several times each week, usually until a transplant is available. For each of these encounters, the diagnosis codes to report will include:

Z99.2 Dependence on renal dialysis (hemodialysis status)(peritoneal dialysis status)(presence of arteriovenous shunt for dialysis)

Sadly, some patients cannot deal with an ongoing need for treatment and may not come in for their sessions. As you learned, this can have a negative impact on their health, and it must be documented. The diagnosis codes to report will include:

Z91.15 Patient's noncompliance with renal dialysis

Transplantation At the point when the kidney is so severely damaged that it cannot be rehabilitated, a transplant may be the solution to improve the patient's health and possibly save his or her life. A patient receiving a transplant must deal with the challenge of needing lifelong medication, as well as follow-up care. However, great success has been achieved in increasing transplant patients' quality of life. Of course, there is always the possibility that the patient's body might reject the new organ, but the greatest roadblock for these patients is the long wait for a donor:

Z76.82 Awaiting organ transplant status

Of course, a donor is needed. With kidney transplants, the donor may be either a live individual or a cadaver. If a live donor, the individual will need this diagnosis code to support medical necessity for the preoperative testing, the procedure itself to remove the donated organ, and the postoperative care:

Z52.4 Kidney donor

Organ transplantation is an incredible health care procedural accomplishment, giving thousands of individuals with previously terminal conditions a second chance to live a normal and productive life. Patients who have received an organ transplant will typically need to take antirejection medication and receive regular checkups. Therefore, after the transplant has taken place, the patient's posttransplant status may need to be reported:

Z94.0 Kidney transplant status

Transplanting an organ from one person into another person is not always a perfect cure. There may be several issues that may require additional treatment. In some cases, the transplant does not eliminate all of the kidney disease. One kidney may have a milder case of CKD and not need transplantation, whereas the other kidney does. Therefore, it is acceptable to report both posttransplant status and current CKD in the same patient at the same time when the physician documents both conditions concurrently.

When a transplanted organ begins to show signs of rejection, failure, infection, or other complication, this will need to be treated and, in some cases, the transplanted organ will need to be removed.

T86.11 Kidney transplant rejection

T86.12 Kidney transplant failure

T86.13 Kidney transplant infection (use additional code to report specific infection)

T86.19 Other complication of kidney transplant

Z98.85 Transplanted organ removal status

Acute Renal Failure

Acute renal failure (ARF) is a sudden malfunction of the kidney often caused by an obstruction, circulatory problem, or possible renal parenchymal disease. This condition is often reversible with medical treatment.

The most typical cause of ARF in critically ill patients, and the cause of approximately 75% of all cases of ARF, is a condition known as *acute tubular necrosis (ATN),* also called *acute tubulointerstitial nephritis (ATIN)*—code N10. Nephrotoxic injury, such as that caused by the ingestion of certain chemicals, can cause ATN but is reversible when diagnosed and treated early. Ischemic ATN may be the result of an injury to the glomerular epithelial cells causing cellular collapse or injury to the vascular endothelium, resulting in cellular swelling and therefore obstruction.

Report this condition with a code from category N17, Acute kidney failure, with an additional character to identify accompanying tubular necrosis, acute cortical necrosis, or medullary necrosis.

Treatment typically includes the provision of diuretics and fluids to flush the system. Electrolyte and fluid balances must be maintained to avoid fluid overload. Some cases require peritoneal dialysis.

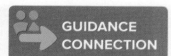

GUIDANCE CONNECTION

Review the ICD-10-CM Coding Guidelines, Section I.C.14, Chapter 14: **Diseases of the genitourinary system,** Subsection a(2), **Chronic kidney disease and kidney transplant status.**

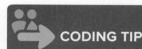

CODING TIP

Code category T86, Complications of transplanted organs and tissue, has a *use additional code* notation to remind you to also report any other transplant complications, such as:

Graft-versus-host disease (D89.81-)
Malignancy associated with organ transplant (C80.2-)
Post-transplant lymphoproliferative disorders (PTLD) (D47.Z1)

Frieda Wolf, a 79-year-old female, has been having problems with her kidneys for a while, with two kidney infections over the last 5 years. Dr. Plettenberg diagnosed her with acute renal insufficiency.

You Code It!

Go through the steps of coding, and determine the code or codes that should be reported for this encounter between Dr. Plettenberg and Frieda Wolf.

Step 1: Read the case completely.

Step 2: Abstract the notes: Which key words can you identify relating to why Dr. Plettenberg cared for Frieda?

_____

Step 3: Query the provider, if necessary.

Step 4: Code the diagnosis or diagnoses.

_____

Step 5: Code the procedure(s): Office visit.

Step 6: Link the procedure codes to at least one diagnosis code to confirm medical necessity.

Step 7: Back code to double-check your choices.

Answer:

Did you determine the correct code to be:

N28.9 Disorder of kidney and ureter, unspecified (renal insufficiency (acute))

CODING TIP

Infections can occur commonly, particularly in an organ system that is open to the outside of the body. Conditions such as a kidney infection, cystitis (bladder infection), or a urinary tract infection (UTI) are certainly not exotic infectious conditions. In these cases, you will need to:

- *Use additional code* to identify organism.

You may have to check the pathology report to determine what the organism is if it is not specified in the physician's notes.

LO 18.5 Urinary Tract Infection

Cystitis and urethritis are both lower urinary tract infections (UTIs), which are often resolved easily with treatment. Ten times more women than men are affected by one of these conditions. In the elderly, a weakening of the bladder muscles may create a foundation for bladder infections (cystitis). Children with a confirmed UTI should be examined for a urinary tract abnormality. This condition would not only predispose them to UTI but may also present a greater likelihood for renal damage in the future. Report this with a code from category N30, Cystitis, with an additional character to report specifics.

Most UTIs are caused by a Gram-negative enteric bacterium. The pathology report will identify which one. This is important to know because there is a *use additional code* notation to identify the infectious agent. Additionally, a urinary catheter, a neurogenic (neuromuscular dysfunction) bladder, or a fistula between the intestine and the bladder might cause a UTI. Medicare may consider a UTI caused by a urinary catheter to be a nonreimbursable hospital-acquired condition (HAC).

Urinalysis of a clean-catch midstream void will confirm this diagnosis and will provide the specific name of the pathogen for coding.

Renal Calculi

Renal calculi, commonly known as *kidney stones*, might actually form anywhere within the urinary system; however, formation in the renal pelvis or the calyces of the kidneys is most common. While the precise cause of these uncomfortable formations is not known, decreased urine production, infection, urinary stasis, and metabolic conditions, such as gout, are considered predispositions. Code category N20, Calculus of kidney and ureter; N21, Calculus of lower urinary tract; or N22, Calculus of urinary tract in diseases classified elsewhere, would be appropriate for reporting this diagnosis.

When the individual stones are small, hydration is prescribed to enable natural passage of the calculi. Larger stones may need to be removed surgically, most often using a cystoscope or using lithotripsy to break up the larger pieces to permit natural passage.

YOU CODE IT! CASE STUDY

Jamal Brady, a 49-year-old male, was in so much pain that he was doubled over. He went to the emergency department at the hospital near his house. Dr. Baldwin took an x-ray and determined that Jamal had nephrolithiasis. She discussed treatment options with him.

You Code It!

Go through the steps of coding, and determine the code or codes that should be reported for this encounter between Dr. Baldwin and Jamal Brady.

Step 1: Read the case completely.

Step 2: Abstract the notes: Which key words can you identify relating to why Dr. Baldwin cared for Jamal?

_____

Step 3: Query the provider, if necessary.

Step 4: Code the diagnosis or diagnoses.

_____

Step 5: Code the procedure(s): Office visit.

Step 6: Link the procedure codes to at least one diagnosis code to confirm medical necessity.

Step 7: Back code to double-check your choices.

Answer:

Did you determine the correct code to be:

N20.0 Calculus of kidney (Nephrolithiasis)

LO 18.6 Conditions Affecting the Prostate

Prostatitis

In men, the prostate is a gland that sits inferior to the urinary bladder. It is shaped like a chestnut and wraps around the urethra as the urethra descends from the bladder to the outside of the body. Due to the proximity of the prostate to the urethra and

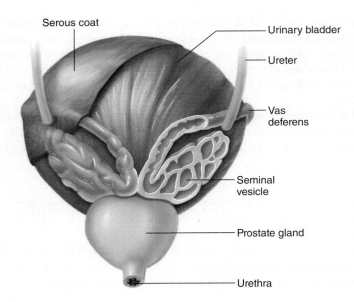

The Prostate diagram with labels: Serous coat, Urinary bladder, Ureter, Vas deferens, Seminal vesicle, Prostate gland, Urethra

FIGURE 18-5 The Prostate

Source: Booth et al., MA, 5e. Copyright © 2013 by McGraw-Hill. Figure 31-6 (b), p. 616

prostatitis
Inflammation of the prostate.

bladder (see Figure 18-5), the most common underlying condition promoting UTI is **prostatitis.** *E. coli* is the pathogen causing approximately 80% of these cases. A urine culture of specimens collected using a four-step process known as the *Meares and Stamey technique* provides the best data for a confirmed diagnosis. Antibiotics are the standard-of-care treatment. Code category N41, Inflammatory diseases of the prostate, requires a fourth character to identify whether the inflammation is acute, chronic, an abscess, or another issue.

Benign Prostatic Hyperplasia

benign prostatic hyperplasia (BPH)
Enlarged prostate that results in depressing the urethra.

bladder cancer
Malignancy of the urinary bladder.

Benign prostatic hyperplasia (BPH), also known as *benign prostatic hypertrophy,* most often diagnosed in men over 50 years of age, is a condition in which the prostate enlarges and results in depressing the urethra. This interferes with the flow of urine from the bladder to the outside. Code category N40, Enlarged prostate, with a fourth character would be used to report this condition. BPH can also result in urine retention, severe hematuria (blood in urine), or hydronephrosis. Treatments for this condition range from massage and sitz baths to suprapubic (transvesical) resection or retropubic (extravesical) resection.

Malignant Neoplasm of the Bladder

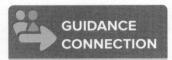

GUIDANCE CONNECTION

Review the ICD-10-CM Coding Guidelines, Section I.C.2, Chapter 2: **Neoplasms**.

Malignant neoplasm of the bladder, commonly known as **bladder cancer,** is the fourth most frequently diagnosed cancer in men and the eighth most frequent in women. While various types of malignant cells can invade this organ, transitional cell carcinoma is seen most often and develops in the lining of the urinary bladder. This would be reported with a code from category C67, Malignant neoplasm of the bladder, with an additional character to report the specific location of the tumor (trigone, dome, etc.). The definitive test to confirm this condition is a cystoscopy with biopsy.

YOU CODE IT! CASE STUDY

Allen Wallace contracted syphilis of his kidney, and now Dr. Lawson determines that an anterior urethral stricture has developed as a result.

Go through the steps of coding, and determine the code or codes that should be reported for this encounter between Dr. Lawson and Allen Wallace.

Step 1:   Read the case completely.

Step 2:   Abstract the notes: Which key words can you identify relating to why Dr. Lawson cared for Allen?

_____

Step 3:   Query the provider, if necessary.

Step 4:   Code the diagnosis or diagnoses.

_____

Step 5:   Code the procedure(s): Office visit.

Step 6:   Link the procedure codes to at least one diagnosis code to confirm medical necessity.

Step 7:   Back code to double-check your choices.

Answer:

Did you determine the correct codes to be:

N35.114 Post-infective anterior urethral stricture, not elsewhere classified

A52.75 Syphilis of kidney and ureter

Chapter Summary

The urinary system is designed to remove the urea from the blood, manufacture urine, and perform waste removal by eliminating the urine. It supports many of the other body systems by ensuring fluid balance and eliminating waste products to avoid toxicity. Understanding the components of this system and their functions will help you correctly interpret the documentation to determine the most accurate code or codes. Some conditions affecting organs in the urinary system are the manifestations of other diseases, such as hypertension or diabetes, whereas others may be the result of an infectious organism. Coders must read carefully (as always) to determine the correct coding process.

CHAPTER **18** REVIEW
Coding Diseases of the Urinary System

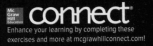

Enhance your learning by completing these
exercises and more at mcgrawhillconnect.com!

Using Terminology

Match each key term to the appropriate definition.

_____ **1.** LO 18.1 The organ system responsible for removing waste products that are left behind by protein, excessive water, disproportionate amounts of electrolytes, and other nitrogenous compounds from the blood and the body.

_____ **2.** LO 18.2/18.5 Inflammation of any part of the urinary tract: kidney, ureter, bladder, or urethra.

_____ **3.** LO 18.1 A long tubular passageway for urine traveling from the kidney to the urinary bladder.

_____ **4.** LO 18.6 Enlarged prostate that results in depressing the urethra.

_____ **5.** LO 18.3 Ongoing malfunction of one or both kidneys.

_____ **6.** LO 18.1 A hollow organ that collects and temporarily stores urine.

_____ **7.** LO 18.3 Glomerular filtration rate, the measurement of kidney function; used to determine the stage of kidney disease.

_____ **8.** LO 18.6 Inflammation of the prostate.

_____ **9.** LO 18.1 A bean-shaped organ that filters blood and excretes urine.

_____ **10.** LO 18.6 Malignancy of the urinary bladder.

_____ **11.** LO 18.1 A compound that results from the breakdown of proteins and is excreted in urine.

_____ **12.** LO 18.4 Suffering from a low red blood cell count.

_____ **13.** LO 18.1 A tubular structure that carries urine from the urinary bladder to the outside of the body.

A. Anemic

B. Benign prostatic hyperplasia (BPH)

C. Bladder cancer

D. Chronic kidney disease (CKD)

E. GFR

F. Kidney

G. Prostatitis

H. Urea

I. Ureter

J. Urethra

K. Urinary bladder

L. Urinary system

M. Urinary tract infection (UTI)

Checking Your Understanding

Choose the most appropriate answer for each of the following questions.

1. LO 18.1 All of the following are part of the urinary system *except*

    a. kidney.

    b. ureter.

    c. urethra.

    d. pyelogram.

2. LO 18.1 The kidneys are responsible for the production of

    a. urine.

    b. bile.

    c. insulin.

    d. HTP.

3. LO 18.1 The _____ is a sac constructed of muscles, located anteroinferior to the peritoneal cavity.

    a. ureter.

    b. urethra.

    c. urinary bladder.

    d. prostate.

4. LO 18.2 Which of the following is a diagnostic tool used to diagnose kidney disease?

    a. UTI.

    b. KUB.

    c. BPH.

    d. CKD.

5. LO 18.3 CKD stage 3 (moderate renal disease) would be coded with which of the following ICD-10-CM codes?

    a. N18.1.

    b. N18.2.

    c. N18.3.

    d. N18.4.

6. LO 18.3 GFR below 15 is stage _____ CKD and would be coded _____.

    a. 2, N18.2.

    b. 3, N18.3.

    c. 4, N18.4.

    d. 5, N18.5.

7. LO 18.4 When a patient is diagnosed with anemia in CKD, how would you code the encounter?

    a. code CKD.

    b. code anemia.

    c. code CKD and then anemia.

    d. code anemia first and then CKD.

8. LO 18.5 Another term for renal calculi is

    a. cystitis.

    b. kidney stones.

    c. urethritis.

    d. gallstones.

9. LO 18.1/18.2 The patient is diagnosed with acute medullary necrosis. Which ICD-10-CM code should be used?

    a. N17.0.

    b. N17.1.

    c. N17.2.

    d. N17.9.

10. LO 18.1 Inability to eliminate waste products from the body may result in

    a. toxicity.

    b. hypertension.

    c. diabetes mellitus.

    d. bladder infections.

Applying Your Knowledge

1. LO 18.1 What is the responsibility of the urinary system, and what are some of the conditions that can affect the organs of this system? _____

_____

2. LO 18.1 List the components of the urinary system. _____

_____

3. LO 18.2 List four diagnostic tools used in diagnosing kidney disease. _____

_____

4. LO 18.3 What is chronic kidney disease, and what are the stages of CKD? _____

_____

5. LO 18.4 Explain the two types of dialysis. _____

_____

6. LO 18.5 What are UTIs? What causes most UTIs? Why is it important for a coder to know this? _____

_____

7. LO 18.1 List the primary sectors of the urinary bladder. _____

_____

8. LO 18.6 What is BPH, and what code category represents BPH? _____

_____

9. LO 18.6 What are the treatments for BPH? _____

_____

10. LO 18.6 Discuss malignant neoplasm of the bladder, including frequency of this disease in our population, and state which code category represents bladder cancer. _____

_____

YOU CODE IT! Practice

Chapter 18: Coding Diseases of the Urinary System

Using the techniques described in this chapter, carefully read through the case studies and determine the most accurate ICD-10-CM code(s) and external cause code(s), if appropriate, for each case study.

1. Anca Neagu, a 42-year-old female, comes in today with the complaint of light pink urine and low-volume output. After the appropriate tests and a thorough examination, Dr. Kline diagnoses Anca with acute nephrotic syndrome with focal and segmental glomerular lesions.

   _____

2. Larry Kota, a 6-month-old male, is brought in today by his parents. Larry's parents are concerned because his urine has a bad smell, he cries when he urinates, and he has a low-grade fever. After thorough examination and clinical testing, Larry is diagnosed with vesicoureteral reflux with reflux nephropathy without hydroureter, bilateral.

   _____

3. Rebekah Oxendine, a 27-year-old female, comes in today complaining of a burning sensation during urination. After a urinalysis, Dr. Franklin diagnoses Rebekah with a UTI due to streptococcus, group B.

   _____

4. Albert Tisdale, a 52-year-old male, comes in today with cloudy urine and believes he has another UTI. After the appropriate tests, Albert is diagnosed with acute prostatitis due to _E. coli._

   _____

5. Lula Thompson, a 43-year-old female, presents today with urine leakage. Lula states that when she sneezes, coughs, or laughs, she has urine leakage, which is becoming uncomfortable. Patient denies overactive bladder issues. After a thorough examination, Dr. Odom diagnoses Lula with stress incontinence.

   _____

6. Mark Windham, a 66-year-old male, comes in today with the complaint that he is having difficulty voiding (straining). When he does void, the stream is light, but he feels like his bladder is empty afterward. Mark denies urgency and incontinence. After the appropriate tests are completed, Mark is diagnosed with an enlarged prostate with LUTS.

   _____

7. Melinda Gibbs, a 33-year-old female, presents today with severe pain around her ribs and hips. After clinical testing, Melinda is diagnosed with hydronephrosis with ureteral obstruction due to calculus.

_____

8. Maurice Pare, an 18-year-old male, presents today with pink urine. Dr. Parham notes this is the second time in 6 months that Maurice has experienced hematuria. Dr. Parham diagnoses Maurice with recurrent hematuria.

_____

9. Alice Kirby, a 54-year-old female, has been a patient of Dr. Hanson for over 10 years. Alice has a history of hypertension and presents today with shortness of breath and fatigue. After a thorough examination and the appropriate clinical tests, Alice is diagnosed with mild chronic kidney disease due to hypertension.

_____

10. Chris Lee, a 58-year-old male, was diagnosed with type 2 diabetes mellitus 5 years ago. Chris has been having difficulty with recent high blood pressure. Urinalysis results were positive for proteinuria, and Dr. Knox noted some uremic frost on the skin. After the appropriate clinical tests were completed, Dr. Knox diagnosed Chris with moderate chronic kidney disease.

_____

11. Carol McCord, a 12-year-old female, is brought in by her mother for her annual physical. Dr. Parker has been Carol's pediatrician since she was 4 years old. Dr. Parker completes the appropriate examination and notes that a renal ultrasound confirms a small left kidney. The patient is asymptomatic at this time.

_____

12. Matthew Carter, a 65-year-old male, has been in moderate chronic kidney failure for several years due to hypertension. Today he presents with weight loss and vomiting. After the appropriate clinical tests are completed, Matthew is diagnosed with end-stage renal disease requiring regular hemodialysis.

_____

13. Carmilla Spann, a 72-year-old female, was diagnosed with mild chronic kidney disease 2 years ago. She presents today with the complaint of feeling weak and short of breath. After a thorough examination, Carmilla is diagnosed with anemia due to CKD.

_____

14. Ben Morin, a 7-year-old male, is brought in by his parents today with the complaint of fever. His mother admits that lately he has been unable to make it to the bathroom in time, which causes him to wet his pants. Dr. Bricker has been Ben's pediatrician since birth. After an examination, Ben is diagnosed with trigonitis due to *Staphylococcus aureus* (MSSA).

_____

15. Karen Ford, a 26-year-old female, gave vaginal birth 12 hours ago. She is now having difficulty emptying her bladder and feels the urgency to void. When she is able to urinate, the stream is weak, with terminal dribbling. Dr. Haywood completes the appropriate tests and diagnoses Karen with a posttraumatic urethral stricture due to childbirth.

_____

The following exercises provide practice in abstracting physicians' notes and learning to work with SOAP notes from our health care facility, *Taylor, Reader, & Associates*. These case studies (SOAP notes) are modeled on real patient encounters. Using the techniques described in this chapter, carefully read through the case studies and determine the most accurate ICD-10-CM code(s) and external cause code(s), if appropriate, for each case study.

TAYLOR, READER, & ASSOCIATES
A Complete Health Care Facility
975 CENTRAL AVENUE • SOMEWHERE, FL 32811 • 407-555-4321

PATIENT: MEETZE, ANN
ACCOUNT/EHR #:   MEETAN01
DATE: 10/17/18

Attending Physician: Willard B. Reader, MD

S: Ann Meetze, a 68-year-old female, was diagnosed with end-stage renal disease requiring regular dialysis maintenance 8 months ago. Ann presents today with shortness of breath, nausea, hiccups, and overall weakness. Ann admits to noncompliance with her dialysis plan.

O: Ht 5'3" Wt. 115 lb. P 85. R 26. BP 145/92. HEENT: unremarkable. Serum creatinine of 1.7 mg/dL, GFR 14 mL/min/1.73 m, hemaglobin 6.4, edema pitting 2+.

A: End-stage renal disease with regular dialysis, noncompliance; anemia due to ESRD

P: Admit to inpatient with immediate hemodialysis session and transfusion

---

Willard B. Reader, MD

WBR/pw   D: 10/17/18 09:50:16   T: 10/19/18 12:55:01

Determine the most accurate ICD-10-CM code(s).

_____

_____

_____

TAYLOR, READER, & ASSOCIATES
A Complete Health Care Facility
975 CENTRAL AVENUE • SOMEWHERE, FL 32811 • 407-555-4321

PATIENT: MCMILLIAN, SCOTT
ACCOUNT/EHR #:   MCMISC001
DATE: 10/17/18

Attending Physician: Suzanne R. Taylor, MD

S: Scott McMillian, a 57-year-old male, comes in today with frequent painful urination and feeling the need to void without being able to do so. Scott smoked cigarettes for 10+ years but has been smoke-free for 1.5 years.

O: Ht 6′ 1″ Wt. 225 lb. P 80. R 19. BP 135/72. HEENT: unremarkable, oxygen saturation 100% in RA. Afebrile. Skin: warm and well perfused with no rash. Back exam: no deformities or defects. Neuro exam: normal tone and strength. Urinalysis is positive for hematuria. Cystoscopy results positive for bladder carcinoma.

A: Bladder cancer, anterior wall, primary.

P: Transurethral resection—discuss TUR option with patient. Scott will think about it and will return in 1 week.

_____

Suzanne R. Taylor, MD

SRT/pw   D: 10/17/18 09:50:16   T: 10/18/18 12:55:01

Determine the most accurate ICD-10-CM code(s).

_____

_____

_____

TAYLOR, READER, & ASSOCIATES
A Complete Health Care Facility
975 CENTRAL AVENUE • SOMEWHERE, FL 32811 • 407-555-4321

PATIENT: HAMILTON, JENNIFER
ACCOUNT/EHR #:   HAMIJE001
DATE: 10/17/18

Attending Physician: Suzanne R. Taylor, MD

S: Jennifer Hamilton, a 49-year-old female, comes in today with concerns about urinating during the night. She states that recently she has had interrupted sleep because of being awakened with an urgency to void. The past 2–3 nights she has gotten up to void at least three times each night, and she is becoming tired. Jennifer also admits that during the day she has to urinate a good bit and yesterday she counted voiding 10 times within a 24-hour period. She states that her fluid intake has not changed and she is not on any medications. Jennifer denies any incontinence at this time.

O: Ht 5′5″ Wt. 125 lb. P 76. R 17. BP 132/83. HEENT: unremarkable, oxygen saturation 100% in RA. Afebrile. Patient history is noncontributory. Abdomen: flat, soft, nontender. Back exam: no deformities or cutaneous defect. Neuro exam: normal tone, strength, and activity. Finger stick shows glucose levels within normal range. UA is negative for hematuria and infection. Cystourethroscopy ruled out any tumors and kidney stones. Patient denies any pain association with micturition.

A: Detrusor muscle hyperactivity

P: Rx: Darifenacin
   Restrict fluid intake

___

Suzanne R. Taylor, MD

SRT/pw   D: 10/17/18 09:50:16   T: 10/18/18 12:55:01

Determine the most accurate ICD-10-CM code(s).

___

___

___

TAYLOR, READER, & ASSOCIATES
A Complete Health Care Facility
975 CENTRAL AVENUE • SOMEWHERE, FL 32811 • 407-555-4321

PATIENT: PARRISH, DOROTHY
ACCOUNT/EHR #:   PARRDO001
DATE: 10/17/18

Attending Physician: John S. Warwick, MD

Dorothy Parrish, an 83-year-old female, was diagnosed with end-stage renal disease requiring regular dialysis last month and presents today for adequacy testing for peritoneal dialysis.

John S. Warwick, MD

JSW/pw   D: 10/16/18 09:50:16   T: 10/18/18 12:55:01

Determine the most accurate ICD-10-CM code(s).

_____

_____

_____

TAYLOR, READER, & ASSOCIATES
A Complete Health Care Facility
975 CENTRAL AVENUE • SOMEWHERE, FL 32811 • 407-555-4321

PATIENT: GERSHMAN, ALLEN
ACCOUNT/EHR #: GERSAL001
DATE: 10/17/18

Attending Physician: Willard B. Reader, MD

S: Allen Gershman, a 48-year-old male, presents today with the complaint of painful urination with frequency and urgency. Allen also admits to nocturia and perineal pain.

O: Ht 5′9″ Wt. 168 lb. P 68. R 18. HEENT: unremarkable, oxygen saturation 100% in RA. Neuro exam: normal tone, strength, and activity. Skin: warm and well perfused with no rash. No hepatosplenomegaly. Needle biopsy confirmed granulomatous prostatitis; culture confirmed *H. pylori*.

A: Granulomatous prostatitis due to *Helicobacter pylori*

P: Rx. Esomeprazole 20 mg bid. for 7 days, followed by 40 mg od. to complete an 8-week course
Sitz bath
Massage

Willard B. Reader, MD

WBR/pw   D: 10/17/18 09:50:16   T: 10/19/18 12:55:01

Determine the most accurate ICD-10-CM code(s).

_____

_____

_____

CODING FOR OBSTETRICS AND GYNECOLOGY

19

Learning Outcomes *After completing this chapter, the student should be able to:*

LO 19.1 Identify the components of the female genital system.

LO 19.2 Explain the stages of reproduction.

LO 19.3 Apply guidelines for coding routine obstetrics care.

LO 19.4 Determine the correct codes for reporting complications of pregnancy.

LO 19.5 Correctly report labor and delivery encounters.

LO 19.6 Enumerate the most common gynecologic diseases.

Females of all ages may go to the **gynecologist (GYN)** for specialized health care. Sometimes, the physician is referred to as an *OB/GYN,* an abbreviation for the dual specialization of **obstetrics (OB),** which focuses on care during pregnancy and the **puerperium,** and gynecology.

LO 19.1 The Female Genital System

The Breast

Across the top of the chest, laterally from the midline where the sternum lies, are fleshy mammary glands, commonly referred to as the **breasts** (see Figure 19-1). The main area of the breast, known as the *body,* sits atop the pectoralis major muscle and is filled with ligaments that suspend the skin. A secondary area, known as the *axillary tail,* reaches out toward the axilla (armpit). The nipple protrudes from the center of the areola, the circle of differently pigmented (colored) skin.

In addition to the ligaments, within the body of the breast are adipose tissues, connective tissues, and a system of ducts that branch through and connect at the nipple. Each of these ducts, called *lactiferous ducts,* branches off one of the mammary gland's 15 to 20 lobes, each of which contains secretory alveoli—the center of milk production. Just inside the nipple is an area called the *lactiferous sinus*—a cavity that stores milk awaiting release.

EXAMPLE

N61 Inflammatory disorders of breast
N64.3 Galactorrhea not associated with childbirth

Key Terms

Abortion

Breasts

Cervix

Clitoris

Endometrium

Fallopian tubes

Gestation

Gynecologist

Labium majus

Labium minus

Mons pubis

Obstetrics

Ovaries

Prenatal

Puerperium

Uterus

Vagina

Vulva

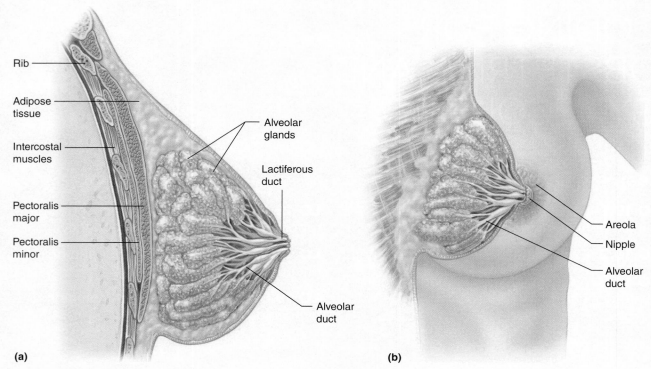

FIGURE 19-1 Female Breast

Source: David Shier et al., HOLE'S HUMAN ANATOMY & PHYSIOLOGY, 12/e. © 2010 MHE. Figure 22.34, p. 862

gynecologist
A physician specializing in the care of the female genital tract.

obstetrics
A health care specialty focusing on the care of women during pregnancy and the puerperium.

puerperium
The time period from the end of labor until the uterus returns to normal size, typically 3 to 6 weeks.

breasts
Two mammary glands that extend from the chest in women after puberty.

ovaries
Bilateral oval-shaped glands that produce female hormones and oocytes (eggs).

fallopian tubes
A pair of tubular structures that reach from the ovaries to the uterus.

Internal Female Genitalia

Internally, a woman's reproductive tract consists of the **ovaries;** the **fallopian tubes;** the **uterus,** lined with the **endometrium;** the **cervix;** and the **vagina** (see Figure 19-2).

Ovaries (oophors), encapsulated within the tunica albuginea, are situated laterally within the pelvic cavity (one on each side) and house approximately 400,000 oocytes (eggs). Midway through menstruation, the process of ovulation occurs, ejecting eggs from the ovary. Some will travel into the *infundibulum* (the funnel-shaped end of the fallopian tube), while others will fall into the pelvic cavity and disintegrate.

Fallopian tubes (or *oviducts*) are pathways, one on each side of the pelvic cavity, for oocytes to move from the ovaries into the uterus. It may take 3 or 4 days for the oocytes to travel the 4-inch length of the tube—from infundibulum to uterus. Collectively, the ovaries and the fallopian tubes are known as the *uteral adnexa.*

The *uterus* is an oval-shaped organ that has three areas: the fundus, the body, and the cervix. The fundus is the large, curved area at the superior aspect between the attachment points of the right and left fallopian tubes. The central portion of the uterus is referred to as the *body,* and the inferior aspect of the uterus is the cervix, which leads down into the vaginal canal.

The innermost lining of the uterus—the *endometrium*—will cradle and support an oocyte that has been fertilized. If an oocyte is not fertilized by a sperm, this lining will release and empty through the vagina (menstruation). The middle layer of the wall of the uterus—the *myometrium*—is composed of smooth muscle, while the outer layer of this wall—the *perimetrium*—is a continuation of the broad ligament that wings out through the pelvic cavity.

> ## EXAMPLE
>
> N70.02 Acute oophoritis
> N70.11 Chronic salpingitis

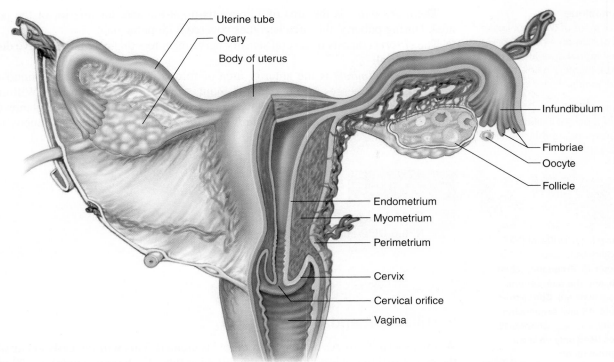

FIGURE 19-2 Female Pelvis

Source: David Shier et al., HOLE'S HUMAN ANATOMY & PHYSIOLOGY, 12/e. © 2010 MHE. Figure 22.27, pg. 853

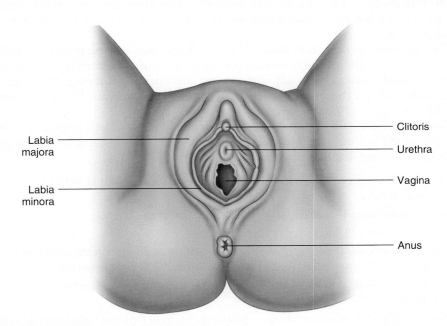

FIGURE 19-3 External Female Genitals

External Female Genitalia

Collectively, the external genitalia of the female are known as the **vulva** (see Figure 19-3). It comprises the **mons pubis,** the **clitoris,** the **labium minus** (plural *labia minora*), and the **labium majus** (plural *labia majora*). The vaginal opening is in the approximate center of this area.

uterus
A hollow, pear-shaped organ in the lower abdominal cavity of the female body; responsible for menstruation and for the housing of a fetus during pregnancy.

endometrium
The mucosal lining of the uterus.

cervix
A necklike structure connecting from the lower part of the uterus to the vagina.

vagina
A passageway extending from the cervix of the uterus to the vulva and the outside of the body.

vulva
The external genital organs of a woman.

mons pubis
A plot of adipose (fatty) tissue that lies over the juncture of the two pubic bones in women.

clitoris
An erectile mass of tissue, the primary site of female sexual arousal, at the superior, anterior aspect of the vulva.

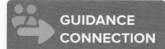

GUIDANCE CONNECTION

Review the ICD-10-CM Coding Guidelines, Section I.C.15, Chapter 15: **Pregnancy, childbirth, and the puerperium,** Subsections a(1), **Codes from chapter 15 and sequencing priority,** and a(2), **Chapter 15 codes used only on the maternal record.**

gestation
The length of time for the complete development of a baby from conception to birth; on average, 40 weeks.

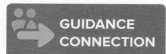

GUIDANCE CONNECTION

Review the ICD-10-CM Coding Guidelines, Section I.C.15, Chapter 15: **Pregnancy, childbirth, and the puerperium,** Subsections a(3), **Final character for trimester;** a(4), **Selection of trimester for inpatient admissions that encompass more than one trimester;** a(5), **Unspecified trimester;** and b(3), **When no delivery occurs.**

The *mons pubis* is the area of adipose tissue at the anterior inferior of the pelvic area. During puberty, this area becomes covered with pubic hair.

The *clitoris* consists of several sensory nerve receptors that become sensitive during sexual arousal.

The *labium minus* is the anterior area of folded skin that creates the hood over the clitoris and merges into the labium majus toward the posterior area. Within the *labia majora,* at the entrance to the vaginal orifice, are small, pea-size glands (one on each side) called *Bartholin glands* that lubricate the vagina with mucus upon sexual arousal.

EXAMPLE

N75.1 Abscess of Bartholin's gland
N76.6 Ulceration of vulva

LO 19.2 Reproduction

Fertilization and Gestation

When a sperm fertilizes an oocyte, a zygote is created. This will typically occur while the egg is still in the last portion of the fallopian tube. Each oocyte (egg) has 23 chromosomes, and each sperm contains 23 chromosomes (in the nucleus in the head of the sperm). When they combine during fertilization, the zygote then has the complete set of 46 chromosomes. This may be confirmed by a pregnancy test; the medical necessity for this visit is reported with a code such as Z32.01, Encounter for pregnancy tests, result positive.

The *embryonic period,* from weeks 2 through 8 after fertilization, is the time during which external structures and internal organs begin to form. Additionally, the placenta, umbilical cord, amnion, yolk sac, and chorion are established during this time. At week 8, the embryo, about 1 inch in length, is considered a fetus, and all organ systems are in place.

Gestation, the length of the pregnancy, is measured in trimesters, beginning on the first day of the last menstrual period (LMP). For coding purposes, ICD-10-CM provides the following definitions:

- *First trimester:* from the first day of the last menstrual period (LMP) to less than 14 weeks 0 days.
- *Second trimester:* 14 weeks 0 days to less than 28 weeks 0 days.
- *Third trimester:* 28 weeks 0 days until delivery.
- *Preterm (premature) neonate:* one with a gestation of 28 completed weeks or more but less than 37 completed weeks (between 196 and 258 completed days).
- *Postterm neonate:* one with over 40 completed weeks up to 42 completed weeks of gestation.
- *Prolonged gestation of a neonate:* a gestational period that has lasted over 42 completed weeks (294 days or more).

Weeks of Gestation

Cases in which a complication has been identified require additional specificity, beyond the current trimester of the pregnancy, and you will need to report the specific number of weeks of gestation. Code category Z3A, Weeks of gestation, provides you with codes that specify the individual week, from 8 weeks to 42 weeks gestation. In addition, codes are available for less than 8 weeks and greater than 42 weeks.

Ingrid went into labor and ultimately delivered the baby. She and her husband were very concerned because she was only at 33 weeks:

O60.14X0 Preterm labor third trimester with preterm delivery third trimester, single gestation

Z3A.33 33 weeks gestation of pregnancy

LO 19.3 Routine Obstetrics Care

Prenatal Visits

A woman often has three items noted in her chart: *gravida (G)* reports how many times the woman has been pregnant; *para,* or *parity (P)* reports how many babies this woman has given birth to (after 20 weeks of gestation); and *abortus (A)* identifies how many pregnancies did not come to term or make it past the 20th week. Gravida and para may be noted using an abbreviation, such as G2 P1.

G1 P1 tells you that the woman has been pregnant once and given birth once.

G1 P2 tells you that the woman has been pregnant once and given birth twice—twins!

G2 P1 tells you that the woman has been pregnant twice and given birth once. If she is pregnant now, this is her second pregnancy; if she is not pregnant now, she may have had a miscarriage in the past.

Normal Pregnancy Routine outpatient **prenatal** checkups are very important to the health and well-being of both the mother and the baby. For a healthy pregnant woman, the visits are typically scheduled at specific points throughout the pregnancy, as determined by the number of weeks of gestation.

When coding routine visits, with the patient having no complications, you will choose from the available Z codes. Remember that you will use a Z code when the patient is not encountering the health care provider because of any current illness or injury. A healthy, pregnant woman has neither a current illness nor a current injury.

prenatal
Prior to birth; also referred to as *antenatal.*

> **Z34.01 Encounter for supervision of normal first pregnancy, first trimester**
>
> **Z34.82 Encounter for supervision of other normal pregnancy, second trimester**

As you can see, you will need to determine which code to use on the basis of the physician's notes on the woman's gravida.

High-Risk Pregnancy In cases where the pregnancy is considered to be medically high-risk, you will use a code from category O09, Supervision of high-risk pregnancy, for the routine visit.

You will determine the fourth digit for the O09 code according to the reason stated in the physician's notes that the pregnancy is considered high-risk. The reason might be a history of infertility (O09.0-), a very young mother (O09.61-), an older mother (O09.51-), or another issue.

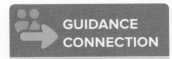

GUIDANCE CONNECTION

Review the ICD-10-CM Coding Guidelines, Section I.C.15, Chapter 15: **Pregnancy, childbirth, and the puerperium,** Subsection b(1), **Routine outpatient prenatal visits.**

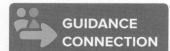

GUIDANCE CONNECTION

Review the ICD-10-CM Coding Guidelines, Section I.C.15, Chapter 15: **Pregnancy, childbirth, and the puerperium,** Subsection b(2), **Prenatal outpatient visits for high-risk patients.**

The fifth or sixth character is used to report which trimester the patient is in at the encounter.

EXAMPLE

O09.211 Supervision of pregnancy with history of pre-term labor, first trimester

O09.32 Supervision of pregnancy with insufficient antenatal care, second trimester

Incidental Pregnant State You may be in an office when a pregnant woman comes in for services or treatment from a physician for a reason that has nothing to do with her pregnancy at all. Even though the actual treatment or service is not related to her pregnancy, the fact that she is pregnant will affect the way the doctor treats her condition. Therefore, you must always include code Z33.1, Pregnant state, incidental, to indicate the pregnancy. It will never be a first-listed code.

EXAMPLE

Sue Ellen is 15 weeks pregnant and works at a bank. As she was walking to her car, she slipped and fractured her toe. Dr. Galliano prescribed one pain medication rather than another because Sue was pregnant. He also took extra precautions while x-raying her foot. You will report:

S92.424A Nondisplaced fracture of distal phalanx of right great toe, initial encounter

Z33.1 Pregnant state, incidental

YOU CODE IT! CASE STUDY

Marlene Scoda, a 31-year-old female, G1 P0, came to see Dr. Goebe for her routine 20-week prenatal checkup. Dr. Goebe noted that Marlene's blood pressure was elevated and told her to come back in 10 days for a recheck.

You Code It!

Go through the steps of coding, and determine the code or codes that should be reported for this encounter between Dr. Goebe and Marlene Scoda.

Step 1: Read the case completely.

Step 2: Abstract the notes: Which key words can you identify relating to why Dr. Goebe cared for Marlene?

_____

Step 3: Query the provider, if necessary.

Step 4: Code the diagnosis or diagnoses.

_____

Step 5: Code the procedure(s): Office visit.

Step 6: Link the procedure codes to at least one diagnosis code to confirm medical necessity.

Step 7: Back code to double-check your choices.

Answer:

Did you determine the correct codes to be:

Z34.02 Encounter for supervision of normal first pregnancy, second trimester

R03.0 Elevated blood pressure reading, without diagnosis of hypertension

Good job!

LO 19.4 Pregnancies with Complications

A complication of pregnancy is considered to be any condition or illness that may:

- Threaten the pregnant state, such as an ectopic pregnancy or an abortion.
- Affect or threaten the health of the woman, such as hemorrhage or vomiting.
- Influence the manner in which the woman will be treated, such as preexisting cardiovascular disease or chromosomal abnormality in the fetus.

A complication may be something as common as mild hyperemesis gravidarum (code O21.0), commonly known as *morning sickness,* or something of concern, such as a kidney infection (e.g., O23.03, Infections of kidney in pregnancy, third trimester).

YOU CODE IT! CASE STUDY

Beatrice Bradley, a 25-year-old female, G2 P1, is 17 weeks pregnant. Dr. Calibre is meeting with her to discuss her lab test results, which indicate that Beatrice has anemia. Dr. Calibre is concerned about how the anemia will affect her pregnancy.

You Code It!

Go through the steps of coding, and determine the code or codes that should be reported for this encounter between Dr. Calibre and Beatrice Bradley.

Step 1: Read the case completely.

Step 2: Abstract the notes: Which key words can you identify relating to why Dr. Calibre cared for Beatrice?

_____

Step 3: Query the provider, if necessary.

Step 4: Code the diagnosis or diagnoses.

_____

Step 5: Code the procedure(s): Office visit.

Step 6: Link the procedure codes to at least one diagnosis code to confirm medical necessity.

Step 7: Back code to double-check your choices.

Answer:

Did you determine the correct code to be:

O99.012 Anemia complicating pregnancy, second trimester

Good work!

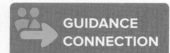

GUIDANCE CONNECTION

Review the ICD-10-CM Coding Guidelines, Section I.C.15, Chapter 15: **Pregnancy, childbirth, and the puerperium,** Subsections c, **Pre-existing conditions versus conditions due to the pregnancy;** d, **Pre-existing hypertension in pregnancy;** and g, **Diabetes mellitus in pregnancy.**

Preexisting Conditions Affecting Pregnancy

Some diseases and illnesses are coded differently when the only thing that has changed is that the woman is now pregnant. Such cases most often involve conditions, such as diabetes mellitus or hypertension, which are systemic (involving the whole body) and, therefore, will complicate the pregnancy, childbirth, or puerperium:

O10.01- Pre-existing hypertension complicating pregnancy

O11- Pre-existing hypertension with pre-eclampsia

O24 .01- Pre-existing diabetes mellitus, type 1, in pregnancy

O24.11- Pre-existing diabetes mellitus, type 2, in pregnancy

O24.81- Other pre-existing diabetes mellitus in pregnancy

O98.7 HIV complicating pregnancy, childbirth, and the puerperium

Gestational Conditions

Other conditions solely related to pregnancy may make caring for a woman and her unborn baby more challenging. Gestational conditions develop as a result of any of the many changes a woman's body goes through and are typically transient, meaning they are expected to go away once the pregnancy is complete.

O13- Gestational [pregnancy-induced] hypertension without significant proteinuria

O22.43 Hemorrhoids in pregnancy, third trimester

O24.4- Gestational diabetes mellitus

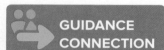

GUIDANCE CONNECTION

Review the ICD-10-CM Coding Guidelines, Section I.C.15, Chapter 15: **Pregnancy, childbirth, and the puerperium,** Subsection i, **Gestational (pregnancy-induced) diabetes.**

Multiple Gestations

Code category O30 provides you with the code options available to report a multiple gestation. In addition to determining the number of fetuses from the documentation, you will also need to determine:

- The number of placenta (monochorionic, dichorionic, or more).
- The number of amniotic sacs (monoamniotic, diamniotic, or more).
- The specific trimester the gestation is in during this encounter.

EXAMPLE

O30.032 Twin pregnancy, monochorionic/diamniotic, second trimester
O30.111 Triplet pregnancy with two or more monochorionic fetuses, first trimester

Fetal Abnormalities

When a woman is pregnant, all care for both her and the baby is provided to the woman herself. Therefore, if there is a change to the treatment or care plan of the mother that is prompted by an issue with the fetus, it must be documented and reported. This may be necessary to support medical necessity for admission to the hospital, for example. Code categories O35, Maternal care for known or suspected fetal abnormality and damage, and O36, Maternal care for other fetal problems, provide you with the options.

EXAMPLE

Code O36.593-, Maternal care for other known or suspected poor fetal growth, third trimester, might result in the mother being referred to a nutritionist for a special diet.

> Code O35.3XX-, Maternal care for (suspected) damage to fetus from viral disease in mother, may require special laboratory tests or an amniocentesis.
>
> *Note:* The seventh character reports which fetus is, or may be, damaged or abnormal. The number 0 (zero) is used for a single gestation, the number 1 for the first of a multiple gestation, the number 2 for the second fetus, and so on.

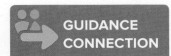

GUIDANCE CONNECTION

Review the ICD-10-CM Coding Guidelines, Section I.C.15, Chapter 15: **Pregnancy, childbirth, and the puerperium,** Subsection e, **Fetal conditions affecting the management of the mother.**

Seventh Character

You may have noticed that many of these codes require a seventh character. If the pregnancy is a single gestation, you will report a zero (0). However, when there is more than one fetus, you will need to determine, from the documentation, which specific fetus is having the problem described by the code. For example:

> O64.2xx3 Obstructed labor due to face presentation, fetus 3
>
> O69.1xx2 Labor and delivery complicated by cord around neck, with compression, fetus 2

LO 19.5 Labor and Delivery

The time has come for the baby to make its way into the world (see Figure 19-4). When the event goes picture-perfectly, requiring minimal or very little assistance from the obstetrician, everything is simpler, including the coding. On the mother's chart, every encounter that results in the birth of a baby requires at least two codes:

- The delivery itself.
- The outcome of that delivery—number of babies, alive or not (Z37.-).

Additional codes may be required if there are any complications.

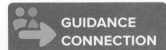

GUIDANCE CONNECTION

Review the ICD-10-CM Coding Guidelines, Section I.C.15, Chapter 15: **Pregnancy, childbirth, and the puerperium,** Subsection a(6), **7th character for fetus identification.**

Normal Delivery

When the baby is coming by the old-fashioned route—spontaneous, full-term, vaginal, live-born, single infant—and there are *no current* complications or issues related to the pregnancy, your principal diagnostic code will be:

> O80 Encounter for full-term uncomplicated delivery

Antepartum conditions may have been a concern; however, in order to use code O80, they must have been resolved prior to the big event.

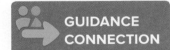

GUIDANCE CONNECTION

Review the ICD-10-CM Coding Guidelines, Section I.C.15, Chapter 15: **Pregnancy, childbirth, and the puerperium,** Subsections b(4), **When a delivery occurs,** and n, **Normal delivery, code O80.**

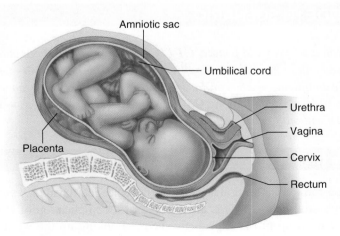

FIGURE 19-4 The Fetus

Source: Deborah Roiger, ANATOMY & PHYSIOLOGY: FOUNDATIONS FOR THE HEALTH PROFESSIONS, 1/e. © 2013 McGraw-Hill Education. Figure 16.20, pg. 619

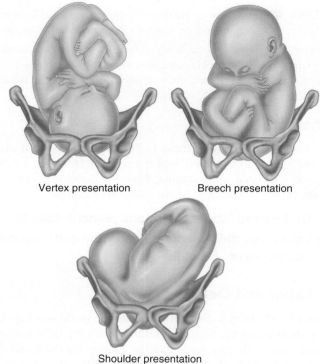

Vertex presentation

Breech presentation

Shoulder presentation

FIGURE 19-5 Birth Presentations

Special Circumstances Related to Delivery

The process of labor and the ultimate delivery of the baby are a natural and joyous occasion. Of course, things don't always happen as they should. There may be an issue that requires ongoing observation, admission into the hospital, or some other factor requiring a change to the original delivery plan (see Figure 19-5). For example:

- O64.1xx- Obstructed labor due to breech presentation
- O60.14xx- Preterm labor third trimester with preterm delivery third trimester
- O69.0xx- Labor and delivery complicated by prolapse of cord

LET'S CODE IT! SCENARIO

Wanda Taylor, a 33-year-old female, G1 P0, is in the birthing room and in full labor, ready to give birth to her baby vaginally. All of a sudden, Dr. Beyers tells her to stop pushing. The umbilical cord has prolapsed, and they cannot seem to move it. Dr. Beyers immediately orders Wanda into the OR, where he performs a c-section. Wanda's baby girl was born without further incident.

Let's Code It!

Dr. Beyers performed a c-section because the umbilical cord had *prolapsed,* endangering the baby's well-being. This is an example of a complication of childbirth. How should you look it up in the Alphabetic Index? Looking up the word *complication* won't work, so let's take a look at the key diagnostic words, the reason *why* Dr. Beyers performed the c-section (the procedure)—*prolapsed umbilical cord.*

> Prolapse, prolapsed
>> Umbilical cord
>>> Complicating delivery O69.0

Let's check this out in the Tabular List. You find:

O69 Labor and delivery complicated by umbilical cord complications

There is a notation about the seventh character required. First, you must determine the first six characters, so continue reading down. The code suggested by the Alphabetic Index is the first one:

O69.0xx- Labor and delivery complicated by prolapse of cord

Notice that the code requires a seventh character. Go back up to the list shown directly below the O69. Which is the most accurate seventh character? A single baby was delivered:

O69.0xx0 Labor and delivery complicated by prolapse of cord, single gestation

Good job! You will also need to report an outcome-of-delivery code. Keep reading to learn all about this.

Outcome of Delivery

As stated earlier in this chapter, *every* time a patient gives birth during an encounter, you have to code the birth process (the delivery code) *and* you have to report the result of that birth process (the outcome-of-delivery code).

The very last code on the mother's chart that will have anything to do with the baby is a code chosen from the Z37, Outcome of delivery, category. The fourth character for the code is determined by two elements:

1. How many babies were born during this delivery.
2. Live-born, stillborn (dead), or, if a multiple birth, a combination.

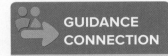

GUIDANCE CONNECTION

Review the ICD-10-CM Coding Guidelines, Section I.C.15, Chapter 15: **Pregnancy, childbirth, and the puerperium,** Subsection b(5), **Outcome of delivery.**

LET'S CODE IT! SCENARIO

Paula Burke, a 31-year-old female, had some third-trimester bleeding, so she went to her doctor. Dr. Briscoe performed a pelvic examination and was concerned. A transvaginal ultrasound scan confirmed that she was suffering from total placenta previa. Because she is in her 36th week, Dr. Briscoe arranged to do a c-section immediately. Paula's baby girl was born without further incident.

Let's Code It!

Dr. Briscoe performed a c-section on Paula because she had *total placenta previa with bleeding.* Go to the Alphabetic Index and look up:

> Placenta, placental—*see* Pregnancy, complicated by (care of) (management affected by), specified condition

So let's turn to:

> Pregnancy
>> Complicated by
>>> Placenta previa O44.1-

In the Tabular List, you confirm it is an appropriate code. Start reading at:

O44 Placenta previa

There are no notations or directives, so keep reading down the column to determine the most accurate fourth character:

O44.0- Placenta previa specified as without hemorrhage

O44.1- Placenta previa with hemorrhage

Be certain not to go too fast, or you might miss that the first code, O44.0, states "without hemorrhage." Paula was hemorrhaging (bleeding). This makes O44.1 more accurate.

Now, you need to determine the required fifth character. As with all codes in this chapter of ICD-10-CM, you will need to determine, from the documentation, which trimester Paula was in at this encounter. Dr. Briscoe stated, "some third-trimester bleeding."

Put it all together and your code for this encounter is:

O44.13 Placenta previa with hemorrhage, third trimester

That's good. But coding for the encounter with Paula is not complete.

Paula is in only her 36th week of gestation. Therefore, you need to include this detail. Turn to the Alphabetic Index, and look up *weeks*—nothing there. Try *gestation*—not there, either. Let's turn to:

Pregnancy
>**Weeks of gestation**
>>**36 weeks Z3A.36**

Turn to the Tabular List to confirm, as is required by the Official Guidelines:

Z3A Weeks of gestation
>**Z3A.36 36 weeks gestation**

Terrific! You need one more code, to report the outcome of delivery. Paula had one live-born baby.

Z37 Outcome of delivery

There are no notations or directives, so read down the column to determine the required fourth character that will accurately report Paula's outcome of delivery:

Z37.0 Outcome of delivery, single live birth

Excellent!

O44.13 Placenta previa with hemorrhage, third trimester
Z3A.36 36 weeks gestation
Z37.0 Outcome of delivery, single live birth

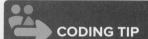

CODING TIP

The last code on the mother's chart regarding the baby is a code from category Z37, Outcome of delivery. Once the baby is born, he or she will get his or her own chart. The first code on the baby's chart is a code from category Z38, Place of birth/type of delivery. Chapter 20 in this text has more information about coding for the baby's medical record.

YOU CODE IT! CASE STUDY

Mark drove his wife, Abigail Horton, a 21-year-old female, to the hospital. She had gone into labor, but she was only at 35 weeks gestation. Dr. Arthur assisted in the delivery of her twin girls. However, there was a problem, and one of the twins was stillborn.

Review Dr. Arthur's notes on this encounter with Abigail and the birth process, and determine the most accurate codes.

Step 1: Read the case completely.

Step 2: Abstract the notes: Which key words can you identify relating to why Dr. Arthur cared for Abigail?

_____

Step 3: Query the provider, if necessary.

Step 4: Code the diagnosis or diagnoses.

_____

Step 5: Code the procedure(s): Delivery.

Step 6: Link the procedure codes to at least one diagnosis code to confirm medical necessity.

Step 7: Back code to double-check your choices.

Answer:

Did you determine the correct codes to be:

O60.14x1 Preterm labor third trimester with preterm delivery third trimester, fetus 1

O60.14x2 Preterm labor third trimester with preterm delivery third trimester, fetus 2

Z3A.35 35 weeks gestation

Z37.3 Outcome of delivery, twins, one liveborn and one stillborn

Good job!

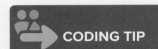

CODING TIP

Preterm labor is defined as the spontaneous onset of labor before 37 completed weeks of gestation.

Postpartum and Peripartum Conditions

After the birth, the woman's body continues to go through changes. In some cases, treatment of an antepartum condition extends into the postpartum period. On other occasions, health care concerns develop during or after delivery. The _postpartum_ period begins at delivery and extends for 6 weeks. The _peripartum_ period runs from the beginning of the last month of pregnancy and ends 5 months after delivery.

Routine postpartum care, just like routine prenatal care, is reported with a Z code:

Z39 Encounter for maternal postpartum care and examination

Z39.0 Encounter for care and examination of mother immediately after delivery

Z39.1 Encounter for care and examination of lactating mother

Z39.2 Encounter for routine postpartum follow-up

Whenever the health care concern arises—even if the diagnosis falls outside the 6-week period—if the physician's notes document that it is a postpartum complication, or pregnancy-related, you are to code it as a postpartum condition.

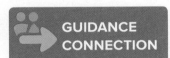

GUIDANCE CONNECTION

Review the ICD-10-CM Coding Guidelines, Section I.C.15, Chapter 15: **Pregnancy, childbirth, and the puerperium**, Subsection o, **The peripartum and postpartum periods.**

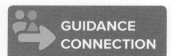

GUIDANCE CONNECTION

Review the ICD-10-CM Coding Guidelines, Section I.C.15, Chapter 15: **Pregnancy, childbirth, and the puerperium,** Subsection p, **Code O94, sequelae of complications of pregnancy, childbirth, and the puerperium.**

Sequelae (Late Effects) of Obstetric Complications

Late effects of obstetric complications, as identified by the attending physician in his or her notes, are coded the same way as all other sequelae. The late effect code—O94, Sequelae of complication of pregnancy, childbirth, and the puerperium—is added when a condition begins during pregnancy but requires continued treatment. The code is placed after the code describing the actual health condition. Notice the notation beneath this code:

Code first condition resulting from (sequela) of complication of pregnancy, childbirth, and the puerperium

YOU CODE IT! CASE STUDY

Wilma Launde, a 25-year-old female, gave birth, vaginally, to a beautiful baby girl 3 weeks ago. She comes today to see Dr. Valeen because of feelings of fatigue. After exam and blood tests, Dr. Valeen diagnoses her with postpartum cervical infection caused by Enterococcus.

You Code It!

Go through the steps of coding, and determine the code or codes that should be reported for this encounter between Dr. Valeen and Wilma Launde.

Step 1: Read the case completely.

Step 2: Abstract the notes: Which key words can you identify relating to why Dr. Valeen cared for Wilma?

_____

Step 3: Query the provider, if necessary.

Step 4: Code the diagnosis or diagnoses.

_____

Step 5: Code the procedure(s): Office visit.

Step 6: Link the procedure codes to at least one diagnosis code to confirm medical necessity.

Step 7: Back code to double-check your choices.

Answer:

Did you determine the correct codes to be:

O86.11 Cervicitis following delivery

B95.2 Enterococcus as the cause of diseases classified elsewhere

O94 Sequela of complication of pregnancy, childbirth, and the puerperium

Abortive Outcomes

abortion
The end of a pregnancy prior to or subsequent to the death of a fetus.

The term **abortion** should not automatically start a political or religious discussion. Abortions can be spontaneous (caused by a biological or natural trigger) or be induced (initiated by an artificial or therapeutic source). What is commonly known as a *miscarriage* is clinically known as an *abortion*.

Many different situations can result in the loss of the fetus:

O00 Ectopic pregnancy

O01 Hydatiform mole

O02 Other abnormal products of conception

O03 Spontaneous abortion

O04 Complications following (induced) termination of pregnancy

O07 Failed attempted termination of pregnancy

EXAMPLE

Elyse, a 20-year-old female who was 10 weeks pregnant, was reading a text message while driving her SUV in slow traffic and didn't notice that the car in front of her had stopped. She hit it. The steering wheel struck and severely bruised her abdomen. This trauma caused her to hemorrhage, resulting in a complete miscarriage. You would report codes:

O03.6 Delayed or excessive hemorrhage following complete or unspecified spontaneous abortion

V47.51xA Driver of sport utility vehicle injured in collision with fixed or stationary object in traffic accident

GUIDANCE CONNECTION

Review the ICD-10-CM Coding Guidelines, Section I.C.15, Chapter 15: **Pregnancy, childbirth, and the puerperium,** Subsection q, **Termination of pregnancy and spontaneous abortions.**

Routine Encounters

Most women understand the importance of getting their annual well-woman examination. It may take place at the office of a specialized OB/GYN or be performed by a family or general practitioner. Typically, the visit includes a routine physical exam, pelvic exam, and breast exam. Often, the visit also includes a Papanicolaou *cervical* smear, better known as a *Pap smear*. The encounter is coded:

Z01.411 Encounter for routine gynecological examination (general) (routine) with abnormal findings

or

Z01.419 Encounter for routine gynecological examination (general) (routine) without abnormal findings

These codes include a *cervical* Pap smear. However, when a *vaginal* Pap smear (which is different from a *cervical* Pap smear and must be specified in the documentation) is included in the visit, add a second code:

Z12.72 Encounter for screening for malignant neoplasm of vagina (vaginal pap smear)

Procreative Management

A woman may want to see her doctor regarding her desire to have children now or in the future. Code category Z31, Encounter for procreative management, is used only for testing conducted with anticipation of procreation (having children). Code subcategory Z31.6, Encounter for general counseling and advice on procreation, will provide you with a few fifth-character options to include additional details.

Perhaps a patient comes in for a test to determine whether or not she is a carrier of a genetic disease before getting pregnant. Most often, such a woman wants to be aware of the possibilities of passing inherited diseases, such as sickle cell anemia or Tay-Sachs, to her baby. The code or codes to report her encounter would be:

Z31.430 Encounter of female for testing for genetic diseases carrier status for procreative management

and/or

Z31.438 Encounter for other genetic testing of female for procreative management

Code Z31.5, Encounter for genetic counseling, would be used after a genetic test has been done and shown positive results.

With good news so far, our female patient may come in next time for fertility testing or, perhaps, a pregnancy test:

Z31.41 Encounter for fertility testing

Z32.00 Encounter for pregnancy test, result unknown

Z32.01 Encounter for pregnancy test, result positive

Z32.02 Encounter for pregnancy test, result negative

LET'S CODE IT! SCENARIO

Greta Ronstand, a 29-year-old female, came to see Dr. Cousins to have an intrauterine device (IUD) inserted. She and her husband, Trent, want to wait a while before having children.

Let's Code It!

Greta came to get an *IUD*. The purpose of this visit is to prevent Greta from getting pregnant, also termed *contraception*. Let's go to the Alphabetic Index and look up *contraception*. Look down the list indented under *contraception,* and you see *device.* However, none of the terms indented under *device* seems to really match Dr. Cousins's notes. This is the first encounter relating to contraception, so perhaps "initial prescription" would be a place to begin.

Contraception, contraceptive
  Device
    Initial prescription Z30.014

Turn to the Tabular List, and confirm that this is the best, most accurate code:

Z30 Encounter for contraceptive management

There are no notations or directives, so continue reading down the column to determine the most accurate required fourth character:

Z30.014 Encounter for initial prescription of intrauterine contraceptive device

Be sure to read further down the column to determine whether any other code descriptions may be more accurate than this description. Sometimes, the Alphabetic Index gets us to only the best subsection of the Tabular List.

Z30.430 Encounter for insertion of intrauterine contraceptive device

There it is! Good job!

LO 19.6 Other Gynecologic Conditions

Concerns and disorders relating to other aspects of the female anatomy are not always related to pregnancy. Let's investigate some of the most common problems affecting women and how to report them.

Endometriosis

Endometriosis (code category N80) is an inflammation or swelling of the tissue that lines the uterus. The condition is estimated to affect 2% to 10% of women of childbearing age in the United States. Although the disorder is identified as being within the uterus, endometriosis can be observed in a woman's ovary, cul-de-sac, uterosacral ligaments, broad ligaments, fallopian tube, uterovesical fold, round ligament, vermiform appendix, vagina, and/or rectovaginal septum. This means that a diagnosis of endometriosis is not sufficient to determine the most accurate code. You have to know the specific site of the condition.

Uterine Fibroids

Also known as *uterine leiomyoma* or *uterine fibromyoma, uterine fibroids* (code category D25, Leiomyoma of uterus) are tumors located in the female reproductive system. Only about one-third of women with these tumors are actually diagnosed. Uterine fibroids are not related to cancer, do not increase the patient's risk of developing cancer later, and are found to be benign 99% of the time.

Pelvic Pain

Female pelvic and perineal pain (code R10.2) may be related to a specific genital organ or an area around a genital organ or may be psychological in nature. The physician may be able to diagnose a particular cause, such as sexual intercourse or menstruation, or the source of the pain may remain unknown.

Sexually Transmitted Diseases

Age, employment status, income level, gender, number of sexual encounters . . . nothing shields anyone from getting a sexually transmitted disease (STD) other than taking proper precautions during sex. This is true for all types of sexual encounters in which bodily fluids are exchanged—not just intercourse. The paragraphs below present an overview of the STDs considered the most common by the Centers for Disease Control (CDC).

Bacterial Vaginosis *Bacterial vaginosis (BV)*—the most common vaginal infection in women 16 to 45 years of age, often affecting pregnant women—is caused by an overgrowth of bacteria. Symptoms include odor, itching, burning, pain, and/or a discharge. Code N76.0, Acute vaginitis, would be reported, along with a second code to identify the infectious agent.

Chlamydia Caused by a bacterium *(Chlamydia trachomatis), chlamydia* can result in infertility or other irreversible damage to a woman's reproductive organs. The symptoms are mild or absent, so most women don't know they have a problem unless their partner is diagnosed. Chlamydia can cause a penile discharge in men. It is the most commonly reported bacterial STD in the United States, according to the CDC. In ICD-10-CM, code A55, Chlamydial lymphogranuloma (venereum), is reported for chlamydia that is transmitted by sexual contact. *Note:* Do not confuse this with A70, Chlamydia psittaci infections; A74.0, Chlamydial conjunctivitis; A74.81, Chlamydial peritonitis; A74.89, Other chlamydial diseases; or A74.9, Chlamydial infection unspecified, all of which are reported when chlamydia causes another disease.

Genital Herpes *Genital herpes* is caused by one of the herpes simplex viruses: type 1 (HSV-1) or type 2 (HSV-2). In this STD, one or more blisters may appear on or in the genital or rectal area. Once the blister bursts, it can take several weeks for the ulcer to heal. The virus will remain in the body indefinitely, even though no more breakouts may be experienced, because there is no cure. Treatment can reduce the number of outbreaks and diminish the opportunity of transmission to a partner. To code from category A60, Anogenital herpesviral [herpes simplex] infections, you must know the specific anatomical site, such as penis or cervix, to determine the additional characters required.

Gonorrhea *Gonorrhea,* a bacterial STD, can develop in the reproductive organs of men (urethra) and women (cervix, uterus, fallopian tubes, and urethra), in addition to the mouth, throat, eyes, and anus. Symptoms in men include a burning sensation during urination, a penile discharge (white, yellow, or green), and/or swelling or pain in the testes. Women typically do not experience any symptoms. You will report this diagnosis from ICD-10-CM code category A54, Gonococcal infection, which requires identification of the specific anatomical site of the infection to determine additional characters.

Human Immunodeficiency Virus Both types of *human immunodeficiency virus (HIV)*—HIV-1 and HIV-2—destroy cells within the body that are responsible for helping fight disease (those that are part of the immune system). Soon after the initial infection, some individuals may suffer flu-like symptoms, while others will have no symptoms at all and feel fine. Current medications can help individuals continue to feel well and decrease their ability to transmit the disease. HIV, especially untreated HIV, has known manifestations, including cardiovascular, renal, and liver disease. In the late stages of the disease, when the patient's immune system is quite damaged, acquired immune deficiency syndrome (AIDS) may develop. Currently, there is no cure for HIV or AIDS. You will report a confirmed diagnosis of HIV with code B20, HIV, when the patient has, or has had, manifestations or code Z21 when the patient is asymptomatic.

Human Papillomavirus There are over 40 different types of *human papillomavirus (HPV)* that can infect the genital regions, mouth, and/or throat of both men and women. This infection will not cause any signs or symptoms; however, it is known to contribute to the development of genital warts as well as cervical cancer (in women). A connection has also been made between HPV and malignancies in the penis, anus, vulva, vagina, and oropharynx. A patient getting a test to screen for HPV will be reported with code Z11.51, Encounter for screening for human papillomavirus (HPV). Reporting for a female patient with a positive test result will come from R87.8, Other abnormal findings in specimens from female genital organs. Additional characters are required based on the anatomical location (cervix or vagina) and on whether the patient is identified as high-risk or low-risk. Male and female patients would both be reported with a code from R85.8, Other abnormal findings in specimens from digestive organs and abdominal cavity, for HPV-positive results in the anus. A confirmed diagnosis for either a male or female patient would be reported with A63.0, Anogenital (venereal) warts due to (human) papillomavirus (HPV).

Pelvic Inflammatory Disease *Pelvic inflammatory disease (PID)* is often a complication of previous chlamydial, gonococceal, or other STD infection, occurring when the bacterium moves from the vagina into a woman's uterus or fallopian tubes. It causes lower abdominal pain. Serious consequences of untreated PID include chronic pelvic pain, formation of abscesses, ectopic pregnancy, and possible infertility. Use code A56.11, Chlamydial female pelvic inflammatory disease, or A54.24, Gonococcal female pelvic inflammatory disease, when sexually transmitted, or use code N73, Other female pelvic inflammatory diseases, or N74, Female pelvic inflammatory disorders in diseases classified elsewhere.

Syphilis In its early stages, *syphilis,* caused by a bacterium *(Treponema pallidum),* is easy to cure. Signs and symptoms include a rash, particularly on the palmar and plantar surfaces, as well as a small, round, painless sore on the genitals, anus, or mouth. However, these symptoms mimic many other diseases, often resulting in delayed diagnosis. Code category A50, Congenital syphilis; A51, Early syphilis; A52, Late syphilis; or A53, Other and unspecified syphilis, would be reported when this condition is sexually transmitted.

Trichomoniasis *Trichomoniasis (trich), a protozoan parasitic (Trichomonas vaginalis) STD*, is more common in older women than in men. Most individuals do not know they are infected because only approximately 30% develop any symptoms, such as a genital discharge. While the condition is curable, a person who has trich and goes without treatment increases his or her risk of getting human immunodeficiency virus (HIV). Trich, when present in a pregnant woman, can cause premature delivery of low-birth-weight neonates. Code category A59, Trichomoniasis, requires additional characters to identify the specific anatomical site of the infection.

YOU CODE IT! CASE STUDY

Alicia Claire, a 27-year-old female, came to see Dr. Leistner with complaints of feeling bloated. She stated that she has felt this way for over a month and cannot connect it to anything she has been eating. After taking a complete history, doing an exam, and performing an ultrasound, Dr. Leistner explained that Alicia had a simple cyst on her right ovary.

You Code It!

Go through the steps of coding, and determine the code or codes that should be reported for this encounter between Dr. Leistner and Alicia Claire.

Step 1: Read the case completely.

Step 2: Abstract the notes: Which key words can you identify relating to why Dr. Leistner cared for Alicia?

_____

Step 3: Query the provider, if necessary.

Step 4: Code the diagnosis or diagnoses.

_____

Step 5: Code the procedure(s): Office visit, ultrasound.

Step 6: Link the procedure codes to at least one diagnosis code to confirm medical necessity.

Step 7: Back code to double-check your choices.

Answer:

Did you determine the correct code to be:

N83.29 Other ovarian cysts (simple cyst of ovary)

You are really getting to be a great coder!

Chapter Summary

The anatomical sites included in the female genital system are the definition of the phrase "private places." These organs have important functions and are susceptible to disease and injury, as with other body systems. Female anatomy includes many organs and anatomical sites that can be subject to health concerns. Well-woman exams and preventive tests should be annual events in every woman's life. Each time, a medical necessity for the visit must be documented. Remember that staying healthy or catching illness or disease early is a medical necessity.

CHAPTER 19 REVIEW
Coding for Obstetrics and Gynecology

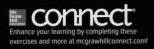

Enhance your learning by completing these
exercises and more at mcgrawhillconnect.com!

Using Terminology

Match each key term to the appropriate definition.

Part One

_____ **1.** LO 19.1 One of a pair of liplike folds of skin surrounding the opening of the vagina.

_____ **2.** LO 19.1 An erectile mass of tissue, the primary site of female sexual arousal, at the superior, anterior aspect of the vulva.

_____ **3.** LO 19.1 A pair of tubular structures that reach from the ovaries to the uterus.

_____ **4.** LO 19.1 One of a set of two thin, liplike folds of skin on either side of the vaginal opening to the outside; located inside the labium majus.

_____ **5.** LO 19.1 A plot of adipose (fatty) tissue that lies over the juncture of the two pubic bones in women.

_____ **6.** LO 19.1 A hollow, pear-shaped organ in the lower abdominal cavity of the female body; responsible for menstruation and for the housing of a fetus during pregnancy.

_____ **7.** LO 19.1 The mucosal lining of the uterus.

_____ **8.** LO 19.1 Bilateral oval-shaped glands that produce female hormones and oocytes.

_____ **9.** LO 19.1 A necklike structure connecting from the lower part of the uterus to the vagina.

_____ **10.** LO 19.1 The external genital organs of a woman.

_____ **11.** LO 19.1 Two mammary glands that extend from the chest in women after puberty.

_____ **12.** LO 19.1 A passageway extending from the cervix of the uterus to the vulva and the outside of the body.

A. Breasts
B. Cervix
C. Clitoris
D. Labium majus
E. Labium minus
F. Endometrium
G. Fallopian tubes
H. Mons pubis
I. Ovaries
J. Uterus
K. Vagina
L. Vulva

Part Two

_____ **1.** LO 19.1 A health care specialty focusing on the care of women during pregnancy and the puerperium.

_____ **2.** LO 19.1 A physician specializing in the care of the female genital tract.

_____ **3.** LO 19.2 The length of time for the complete development of a baby from conception to birth; on average, 40 weeks.

_____ **4.** LO 19.1 The time period from the end of labor until the uterus returns to normal size, typically 3 to 6 weeks.

_____ **5.** LO 19.3 Prior to birth; also referred to as _antenatal._

_____ **6.** LO 19.5 The end of a pregnancy prior to or subsequent to the death of a fetus.

A. Abortion
B. Gestation
C. Gynecologist
D. Obstetrics
E. Prenatal
F. Puerperium

Checking Your Understanding

Choose the most appropriate answer for each of the following questions.

1. LO 19.3 A woman noted to be G2 P2 has given birth
   a. once.
   b. never.
   c. twice.
   d. four times.

2. LO 19.3 You would use code Z33.1 for a pregnant woman who came to see the doctor for
   a. a broken leg.
   b. a regular first-pregnancy checkup.
   c. a regular third-pregnancy checkup.
   d. a regular pregnancy checkup for a woman 37 years old.

3. LO 19.2 A normal gestation lasts
   a. 35–38 weeks.
   b. 34–37 weeks.
   c. 41–42 weeks.
   d. 38–40 weeks.

4. LO 19.3 A pregnancy would be considered high-risk for all of the following reasons *except*
   a. a history of infertility.
   b. a woman who will be 35 or older at delivery.
   c. a normal first pregnancy.
   d. a woman who will be younger than 16 at delivery.

5. LO 19.4 A condition is considered a complication of pregnancy when
   a. the condition existed before the pregnancy.
   b. the condition threatens the health of the woman.
   c. the condition is antepartum.
   d. the condition is postpartum.

6. LO 19.4 A new diagnosis of hypertension in a pregnant woman is coded as
   a. essential hypertension.
   b. family history of hypertension.
   c. gestational hypertension.
   d. malignant hypertension.

7. LO 19.5 The encounter at which a woman gives birth will always have at least
   a. two codes.
   b. one code.
   c. four codes.
   d. three codes.

8. LO 19.5 An abortion can be

    a. spontaneous.

    b. induced.

    c. biologically triggered.

    d. all of these.

9. LO 19.5 When are sequelae of complications of pregnancy, childbirth, and the puerperium coded with O94?

    a. always.

    b. when the original problem was obstetrical.

    c. never.

    d. only when the woman is over 35.

10. LO 19.3 If a patient comes for a routine prenatal checkup and is found to have a complication of pregnancy, you must code

    a. the complication only.

    b. high-risk pregnancy.

    c. the complication first and then the routine visit.

    d. the routine visit first and then the complication.

Applying Your Knowledge

1. LO 19.1 List the internal female genitalia. _____

_____

2. LO 19.1 List the external female genitalia. _____

_____

3. LO 19.2 Explain the stages of reproduction. _____

_____

4. LO 19.4 List three preexisting conditions affecting pregnancy. _____

_____

5. LO 19.5 List two different birth presentations. _____

_____

6. LO 19.6 List four sexually transmitted diseases (STDs). _____

_____

Using the techniques described in this chapter, carefully read through the case studies and determine the most accurate ICD-10-CM code(s) and external cause code(s), if appropriate, for each case study.

1. Beryl Bornstein, a 27-year-old female, is hospitalized at 9 months pregnant in prolonged labor, G2 P1. Beryl has a short, stocky physique with a slightly abnormal gait. Dr. Terrence diagnoses Beryl with obstructed labor due to a generally contracted pelvis. Dr. Terrence assisted with the vaginal delivery of her baby girl today.

   _____

2. Evelyn Morris, a 31-year-old female, is 5 months pregnant. Evelyn has a high blood glucose level of 126 mg/dL and is diagnosed with gestational diabetes. Her diabetes is being controlled with insulin, long term.

   _____

3. Sara-Lynn Shevlin, a 12-year-old female, was riding her brother's bicycle in the front yard of her house. When she tried to get off the bicycle, she fell onto the cross bar. Dr. Oreta diagnosed her with a hematoma of the vulva.

   _____

4. Jaquinta Singer, a 24-year-old female, is in labor in a supine position when she suddenly goes into bradycardia, begins sweating, and is dizzy. The nurse shifted her weight by placing a wedge under her right hip and elevated her legs. Dr. Payton was notified and assisted Jaquinta in a vaginal birth of a beautiful 7-pound baby boy an hour later. Dr. Payton diagnosed Jaquinta with maternal hypotension syndrome.

   _____

5. Marlena Ray, an 18-year-old female, is in labor and shows signs of sluggish uterine contractions. Dr. Billing diagnoses primary uterine inertia and assists as Marlena gives birth to a healthy baby girl.

   _____

6. Dayle Willey, a 48-year-old female, presents today with the complaint that almost every time she sneezes or coughs, she leaks urine. Dr. Dominguez diagnoses her with stress incontinence.

   _____

7. Dr. Reynosa admitted Charlene Clement, a 22-year-old female, to the hospital after determining that her baby (single fetus) was "large-for-dates." The 9-pound 7-ounce boy was delivered 2 hours later.

   _____

8. Grace Martinez, a 23-year-old female, headed toward the hospital when she was 39 weeks pregnant and had labor pains. Once there, Dr. Stromm determined she was in false labor and sent her home.

   _____

9. Lena Harrison, a 36-year-old female, was admitted to the hospital in labor. Dr. Gentile performed an episiotomy during labor. However, Lena suffered a fourth-degree perineal laceration while giving birth to her twin daughters 1 hour later.

   _____

10. Juana Culpepper, a 26-year-old female, comes in today concerned because her right breast is swollen, tender, and warm to the touch. She admits it burns when breast-feeding her son, who was born 2 weeks earlier. Dr. Pullman diagnoses Juana with right breast abscess, associated with the puerperium.

    _____

11. Valentina Porado, a 32-year-old female, presents today with a painful lump in her vagina. Dr. McIntosh examines her and diagnoses a cyst of a Bartholin's gland.

    _____

12. Kimberly Sanchez, a 26-year-old female, presents today 13 weeks pregnant. Kim has been vomiting so much that she now suffers from dehydration. Dr. Sherman diagnoses her with hyperemesis gravidarum and admits her to the hospital for rehydration.

    _____

13. Loree Allendale, a 16-year-old female, is brought in today by her mother because Loree discovered a discharge from her right nipple. Dr. Livingston examines Loree and notes a cloudy white discharge. Loree admits that she was wearing a rough-textured shirt without a bra. Dr. Livingston diagnoses her with nipple discharge due to clothing irritation.

    _____

14. Sasha Silverheels, a 20-year-old female, is 19 weeks pregnant and comes to see Dr. Gaines for a regular checkup because she has a bicornuate uterus.

    _____

15. Dorothy Marin, a 35-year-old female, presents today with fever, pelvic tenderness, low abdominal pain, and irregular periods. After a gynecologic examination, culture, and ultrasound, Dr. Norris diagnoses Dorothy with chlamydial pelvic inflammatory disease.

    _____

The following exercises provide practice in abstracting physicians' notes and learning to work with SOAP notes from our health care facility, *Taylor, Reader, & Associates*. These case studies (SOAP notes) are modeled on real patient encounters. Using the techniques described in this chapter, carefully read through the case studies and determine the most accurate ICD-10-CM code(s) and external cause code(s), if appropriate, for each case study.

TAYLOR, READER, & ASSOCIATES
A Complete Health Care Facility
975 CENTRAL AVENUE • SOMEWHERE, FL 32811 • 407-555-4321

PATIENT: SCOTT, ANNA
ACCOUNT/EHR #:   SCOTAN001
DATE: 9/17/18

Attending Physician: Suzanne R. Taylor, MD

S: Anna Scott, a 29-year-old female, presents today with vaginal bleed and abdominal pain. Anna is 8 weeks pregnant.

O: Ht 5′ 3″ Wt. 135 lb. T 98.7. R18. P 75. Oxygen saturation 100% in RA. HEENT unremarkable; neck supple; chest clear; abdomen tender. Transvaginal ultrasonography confirms an abdominal ectopic pregnancy with salpingitis. Patient is currently stable. I discussed the option of possible surgical intervention if miscarriage is not complete.

A: Abdominal ectopic pregnancy with salpingitis.

P: Patient would like to discuss any options with her husband and will contact us tomorrow. Surgical intervention if necessary.

Suzanne R. Taylor, MD

SRT/pw   D: 9/17/18 09:50:16   T: 9/18/18 12:55:01

Determine the most accurate ICD-10-CM code(s).

_____

_____

_____

TAYLOR, READER, & ASSOCIATES
A Complete Health Care Facility
975 CENTRAL AVENUE • SOMEWHERE, FL 32811 • 407-555-4321

PATIENT: MCDOUGAN, ZENA
ACCOUNT/EHR #:   MCDOZE001
DATE: 9/17/18

Attending Physician: John S. Warwick, MD

S: Zena McDougan is a 22-year-old female, 26.5 weeks pregnant with her first pregnancy. Presents today for a regular checkup. Zena states everything is going well, no complaints.

O: OB ultrasound reveals: A single fetus is seen in the breech presentation with limb motion and heart motion visualized. No organ abnormalities are seen. The placenta lies posteriorly and is grade 1. The amount of amniotic fluid is within normal limits.

The estimated menstrual age based on:
BPD of 6.4 cm = 25.5 weeks   FL of 5.1 cm = 27.0 weeks
AC of 21.9 cm = 26.0 weeks   HC of 25.1 cm = 26.5 weeks
Average = 26.3 weeks

The ratios of: Normal Ratios
FL to BPD = 79% (79% +/− 8)
FL to AC = 23% (22% +/− 2)
HC to AC = 1.15% (1.13 +/− 0.9)

Estimate fetal weight is 1,000 grams.

The cephalic index = 70% (70–80).

Normal-appearing intrauterine pregnancy estimated to be 26.3 weeks menstrual age. No fetal abnormalities are identified. The fetus is currently in the breech presentation.

A: Normal supervision of first pregnancy

P: Continue to supervision

_____

John S. Warwick, MD

JSW/pw   D: 9/16/18 09:50:16   T: 9/18/18 12:55:01

Determine the most accurate ICD-10-CM code(s).

_____

_____

_____

TAYLOR, READER, & ASSOCIATES
A Complete Health Care Facility
975 CENTRAL AVENUE • SOMEWHERE, FL 32811 • 407-555-4321

PATIENT: OSGOOD, BENITA
ACCOUNT/EHR #:   OSGOBE001
DATE: 9/17/18

Attending Physician: Suzanne R. Taylor, MD

S: Benita Osgood, a 29-year-old female, G1 P0, presents at term with regular uterine contractions. The patient's antepartum course has been uncomplicated to date. Sonogram and amniocentesis were normal. GBS culture was negative.

O: Ht 5′ 6″ Wt. 137 lb. T 98.4. P 82. R 20. BP 118/84. Oxygen saturation 100% in RA; FHR 130s. Location LLQ; HEENT unremarkable; neck supple; chest clear; abdomen guarded, soft. Contractions: Q3–4 minutes, 45–50 second duration; membrane ruptured @ 21:45 with clear fluid; vaginal discharge: show; vaginal exam: 3 cm dilated, Eff 80%, Sta 2; fetal status: reassuring.

A: Term pregnancy, in spontaneous delivery, uncomplicated

P: Normal spontaneous delivery

Suzanne R. Taylor, MD

SRT/pw D: 9/17/18 09:50:16 T: 9/18/18 12:55:01

Determine the most accurate ICD-10-CM code(s).

_____

_____

_____

TAYLOR, READER, & ASSOCIATES
A Complete Health Care Facility
975 CENTRAL AVENUE • SOMEWHERE, FL 32811 • 407-555-4321

PATIENT: CABOT, OLIVIA
ACCOUNT/EHR #: CABOOL01
DATE: 9/17/18

Operative Report

Preoperative DX:	1. First trimester missed abortion; 2. Undesired fertility
Postoperative DX:	Same
Operation:	1. Dilation and curettage with suction; 2. Laparoscopic bilateral tubal ligation using Kleppinger bipolar cautery
Surgeon:	Rodney L. Cohen, MD
Assistant:	None
Anesthesia:	General endotracheal anesthesia
Findings:	Pt had products of conception at the time of dilation and curettage. She also had normal-appearing uterus, ovaries, fallopian tubes, and liver edge.
Specimens:	Products of conception to pathology
Disposition:	To PACU in stable condition

Procedure: The patient was taken to the operating room, and she was placed in the dorsal supine position. General endotracheal anesthesia was administered without difficulty. The patient was placed in dorsal lithotomy position. She was prepped and draped in the normal sterile fashion. A red rubber tip catheter was placed gently to drain the patient's bladder. A weighted speculum was placed in the posterior vagina and Deaver retractor anteriorly. A single-tooth tenaculum was placed in the anterior cervix for retraction. The uterus sounded to 9 cm. The cervix was dilated with Hanks dilators to 25 French. This sufficiently passed a #7 suction curet. The suction curet was inserted without incident, and the products of conception were gently suctioned out. Good uterine cry was noted with a serrated curet. No further products were noted on suctioning. At this point, a Hulka tenaculum was placed in the cervix for retraction. The other instruments were removed.

Attention was then turned to the patient's abdomen. A small vertical intraumbilical incision was made with the knife. A Veress needle was placed through that incision. Confirmation of placement into the abdominal cavity was made with instillation of normal saline without return and a positive handing drop test. The abdomen was then insufflated with sufficient carbon dioxide gas to cause abdominal tympany. The Veress needle was removed and a 5-mm trocar was placed in the same incision. Confirmation of placement into the abdominal cavity was made with placement of the laparoscopic camera. Another trocar site was placed two fingerbreadths above the pubic symphysis in the midline under direct visualization. The above noted intrapelvic and intraabdominal findings were seen. The patient was placed in steep trendelenburg. The fallopian tubes were identified and followed out to the fimbriated ends. They were then cauterized four times on either side. At this point, all instruments were removed from the patient's abdomen. This was done under direct visualization during the insufflation. The skin incisions were reapproximated with 4-0 Vicryl suture. The Hulka tenaculum was removed without incident.

(Continued)

The patient was placed back in the dorsal supine position. Anesthesia was withdrawn without difficulty. The patient was taken to the PACU in stable condition. All sponge, instrument, and needle counts were correct in the operating room.

_____

Rodney L. Cohen, MD

RLC/pw   D: 9/17/18 09:50:16   T: 9/19/18 12:55:01

Determine the most accurate ICD-10-CM code(s).

_____

_____

_____

TAYLOR, READER, & ASSOCIATES
A Complete Health Care Facility
975 CENTRAL AVENUE • SOMEWHERE, FL 32811 • 407-555-4321

PATIENT: GEORGE, ALEXANDRA
ACCOUNT/EHR #:   GEORAL001
DATE: 9/17/18

Attending Physician: Willard B. Reader, MD

S: Alexandra George, a 23-year-old female, is 34 weeks pregnant. Presents today with the complaint of continuous contractions and a slight bloody vaginal discharge.

O: Ht 5′ 2″ Wt. 115 lb. T 97.8. P 78. R 17. BP 122/76. Oxygen saturation 100% in RA. HEENT unremarkable; neck supple; chest clear; abdomen guarded; contractions rapid. OB ultrasound reveals a single fetus with heart and limb motion visualized. No fetal abnormalities are seen; however, there is evidence of class 1 placental abruption. The amount of amniotic fluid is within normal limits.

A: Abruptio placentae, neither mother nor fetus are in any distress.

P: Hospitalizing until a change in condition or fetal maturity, whichever comes first.

_____

Willard B. Reader, MD

WBR/pw   D: 9/17/18 09:50:16   T: 9/19/18 12:55:01

Determine the most accurate ICD-10-CM code(s).

_____

_____

_____

CODING CONGENITAL AND PEDIATRIC CONDITIONS

20

Learning Outcomes *After completing this chapter, the student should be able to:*

LO 20.1 Correctly code the infant's birth.

LO 20.2 Apply guidelines for well-baby encounters.

LO 20.3 Code clinically significant conditions accurately.

LO 20.4 Identify the mother's conditions affecting the infant.

LO 20.5 Apply guidelines for coding genetic conditions.

LO 20.6 Distinguish between genetic conditions and congenital malformations.

Key Terms

Anomaly

Apgar

Clinically significant

Congenital

Deformity

Genetic abnormality

Low birth weight (LBW)

Malformation

Morbidity

Mortality

Neonate

Perinatal

Prematurity

Most of the time, the arrival of a baby is a joyous occasion. It is always a wondrous event. A **neonate** is the focal point of so much attention. Every year more than 4 million babies are born—about seven babies every minute—in the United States. According to the Centers for Disease Control and Prevention (CDC), approximately 3% of these babies are born with some type of birth defect.

An assessment of the baby's health begins almost immediately after delivery. Through gestational assessment the baby's physical maturity is determined, the neuromuscular maturity is established, and an **Apgar** test is usually performed. The Apgar test, devised by Virginia Apgar in 1952, provides the doctor and health care team with a quick health assessment of the infant. The test is performed at 1 minute and then again at 5 minutes after the baby is born. If the score is low, the physician may decide to do the test again at 10 minutes. Table 20-1 shows you what an Apgar score indicates about a neonate.

Once the baby is born, the baby gets his or her own chart. From that point forward, anything having to do with the baby is coded for the baby and stays off the mother's chart.

LO 20.1 Coding the Birth

You may remember from our chapter on pregnancy and childbirth that the very last code directly relating to the baby that is placed on the mother's chart is a code from category Z37, Outcome of delivery. The *very first code on the baby's chart* will be from code category Z38, Liveborn infants according to place of birth and type of birth. This Z code is used to report that a newborn baby has arrived, and it is always the principal (first-listed) code. A code from this category can be used only once, for the date of birth.

neonate
An infant from birth to 1 month of age.

apgar
Assessment of a neonate's condition on the basis of five factors: muscle tone, heart rate, reflex response, skin color, and breathing.

TABLE 20-1 Apgar Scoring for Newborns

Score	Interpretation
0–3	Baby needs immediate lifesaving procedures
4–6	Baby needs some assistance; requires careful monitoring
7–10	Normal

LET'S CODE IT! SCENARIO

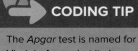

CODING TIP

The *Apgar* test is named for Virginia Apgar, but it also has come to stand for the following:

*A*ctivity (muscle tone)
*P*ulse rate (heart rate)
*G*rimace (reflex response)
*A*ppearance (skin color)
*R*espiratory (breathing effort)

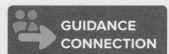

GUIDANCE CONNECTION

Review the ICD-10-CM Coding Guidelines, Section I.C.16, Chapter 16: **Certain conditions originating in the perinatal period,** Subsection a, **General perinatal rules,** for more input.

Richard Harold was born via vaginal delivery in the Carrolton Birthing Center at 10:58 a.m. on September 1. He weighed 8 pounds 5 ounces and was 21 inches long, with Apgar scores of 9 and 9. Dr. Smith, a pediatrician, performed a comprehensive examination immediately following Richard's birth. Baby Ricky was sent home at 6:30 p.m. in the care of his mother, Katherine.

Let's Code It!

Ricky was just born, and this is his first health care chart. As you learned, his very first code must be from the Z38 range. As with all other cases, begin in the Alphabetic Index. What should you look up? *Birth* would be a logical choice. However, when you turn to this term in the Alphabetic Index, you are going to see a long list of adjectives, none of which apply to Ricky, or any other baby being born without a problem. As you look down the list, you may notice this item:

Birth
   Infant—*see* Newborn

OK, you have nothing to lose. Let's go look up the term *newborn*.

Newborn (infant)(liveborn)(singleton) Z38.2

Check Dr. Smith's notes. It is documented that Ricky was a *single, liveborn* baby.
   Let's go to the Tabular List and look at our choices. Begin with:

Z38 Liveborn infants according to place of birth and type of delivery

As you read down, you can see that code Z38.2 reports *Single liveborn infant, unspecified as to place of birth.* The documentation clearly indicates where Ricky was born—in the Carrolton Birthing Center (not a part of a hospital). So this code is not accurate. Keep reading. The answer from the documentation will bring you to the correct code:

Z38.1 Single liveborn infant, born outside the hospital

Good work!

LO 20.2 Routine Well-Baby Checkups

Once released from the hospital, all children should have regularly scheduled checkups with their pediatrician or family physician (see Figure 20-1). Typically, these visits involve the physician communicating with the parent about any behaviors and/or concerns. A physical exam is performed, including auscultation (listening to the baby's heartbeats and sounds, respirations, and intestinal sounds), palpation, percussion, and a routine ophthalmic exam, and vital signs are recorded.

These encounters, just like adult physicals and other checkups, are scheduled by the age of the child: 2 to 4 days, 1 month, 2 months, 4 months, 6 months, 9 months, 1 year, 15 months, 18 months, 2 years, 2.5 years, 3 years, and then annually. The age of the child also influences which codes are reported for the well-baby encounter:

Z00.110 Health examination for newborn under 8 days old

Z00.111 Health examination for newborn 8 to 28 days old

Z00.121 Encounter for routine child health examination with abnormal findings Use additional code to identify abnormal findings

Z00.129 Encounter for routine child health examination without abnormal findings

LO 20.3 Clinically Significant Conditions

The guidelines state that you must code all clinically significant conditions noted on the baby's chart during the standard newborn examination. You may be concerned about how you, as a coder, can determine what is **clinically significant** and what is not. Good news! It is not your decision to make. Only the physician can determine and document this. However, you must ensure that the documentation gives you the diagnostic conditions that support any of the following:

- *Therapeutic treatments performed:* For example, perhaps the baby is placed on a respirator.
- *Diagnostic procedures done:* For example, perhaps additional and specific blood tests are performed on the baby.
- *Keeping the baby in the hospital longer than usual:* Perhaps the physician is concerned about an issue so he or she does not discharge the baby yet.
- *Increased monitoring or nursing care:* Perhaps the physician orders 24-hour private-duty nursing care for continuous monitoring.
- *Any implication that the child will need health care services in the future* as a result of a condition, sign, or symptom that can be identified now: Perhaps there is evidence that there may be brain damage as a result of the birth process; however, this cannot be confirmed until the child is about 2 years old.

When a congenital or **perinatal** condition has been resolved and no longer has an impact on the child's health and well-being, you will need to assign a code from the range Z85–Z87, Personal history of . . . .

LO 20.4 Maternal Conditions Affecting the Infant

When the physician's notes specify that a mother's illness, injury, or condition had a direct impact on the baby's health, you will include a code on the baby's chart from the subsection code range P00–P04, Newborn affected by maternal factors and by complications of pregnancy, labor, and delivery.

Conditions in the mother, such as nutrition, smoking, high blood pressure, the presence of certain infections, or an abnormal uterus or cervix, can increase the possibilities that the baby might be born **prematurely** and/or with a **low birth weight (LBW)**. A mother's heart, kidney, and/or lung problems might also affect the baby's health.

While the reasons are not completely understood by physicians, a woman may experience spontaneous *p*remature *r*upture *o*f the *m*embranes (PROM), which results

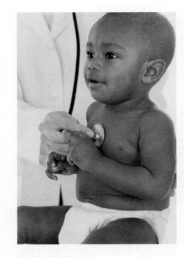

FIGURE 20-1 Well-Baby Checkup

© Corbis Images/JupiterImages

clinically significant
Signs, symptoms, and/or conditions present at birth that may impact the child's future health status.

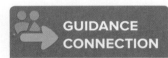

GUIDANCE CONNECTION

Review the ICD-10-CM Coding Guidelines, Section I.C.16, Chapter 16: **Certain conditions originating in the perinatal period,** Subsections a(6), **Code all clinically significant conditions,** and c, **Coding additional perinatal diagnoses,** for more input.

perinatal
The time period from before birth to the 28th day after birth.

prematurity
Birth occurring prior to the completion of 37 weeks gestation.

low birth weight (LBW)
A baby born weighing less than 5 pounds 8 ounces, or 2,500 grams.

in spontaneous preterm labor. There is virtually nothing that can be done to prevent the situation that so often leads to the birth of a premature, LBW baby.

A preterm (premature) neonate is one who has been in gestation for at least 28 completed weeks but less than 37 completed weeks (or between 196 and 258 completed days). While the baby's chart will almost always include a notation of the number of weeks gestation at birth, you are permitted to code "prematurity" only when it is specifically documented by the physician.

A weight of less than 2,500 grams at birth is also an indicator of prematurity. When a fetus has not had the prescribed length of time to grow, the neonate can be susceptible to certain health concerns, realized in the near or distant future.

Premature, LBW babies are more likely to be at risk for developing certain conditions now and later in life. Incomplete growth of the fetus's central nervous system can result in feeding difficulties for the neonate/infant, recurrent apnea, and/or poor vasomotor control. Testing for neonatal hyperbilirubinemia, especially when jaundice is visible, can indicate that the liver did not develop sufficiently to create and excrete bilirubin (a yellowish component of bile, which is made by the liver). This is why it is so important that the documentation and the coding accurately report the baby's situation from the beginning. Some of the most common conditions include:

- Breathing problems, including respiratory distress syndrome (RDS).
- Periventricular and/or intraventricular hemorrhage (bleeding in the brain).
- Patent ductus arteriosus (PDA), a dangerous heart problem.
- Necrotizing enterocolitis (NEC), an intestinal problem that leads to difficulties in feeding.
- Retinopathy of prematurity (ROP).
- Low body temperature (caused by a lack of body fat used by newborns to maintain normal body temperature), which promotes slow growth, breathing problems, and other complications.
- Apnea, an interruption in breathing.
- Jaundice, a result of incomplete liver development.
- Anemia.
- Bronchopulmonary dysplasia, also known as *chronic lung disease.*
- Infections, due to the inability of immature immune systems to fight off bacteria and viruses.

Respiratory distress syndrome (RDS) is the leading cause of **mortality** and **morbidity** of premature neonates. The immature lungs have an insufficient quantity of surfactant—the secretion within the lungs that supports the alveoli and keeps them from collapsing. Maternal diabetes and neonatal asphyxia are known contributing factors. RDS causes hypoxia, which can then lead to pulmonary ischemia, pulmonary capillary damage, and fluid leaking inappropriately into the alveoli. Cyanosis, increased respiratory effort, anoxia, and acidosis are signs and complications. Report a diagnosis of RDS with code P22.0, Respiratory distress syndrome of newborn.

You will find the codes needed to report an infant's prematurity and/or LBW, as well as long gestation and high birth weight, as documented in the physician's notes, within code categories:

P05 Disorders of newborn related to slow fetal growth and fetal malnutrition

P07 Disorders of newborn related to short gestation and low birth weight, not elsewhere classified

P08 Disorders of newborn related to long gestation and high birth weight

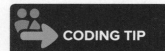

CODING TIP

Usually, the physician will write the baby's birth weight in grams. However, you should learn how to convert from pounds and ounces to grams:

1 ounce = 28.375 grams
1 pound = 16 ounces = 454 grams
1 gram = 0.0022 pound

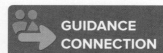

CODING TIP

Codes from category P05 and category P07 may not be reported on the same claim at the same time.

mortality
Death.

morbidity
Unhealthy.

GUIDANCE CONNECTION

Review the ICD-10-CM Coding Guidelines, Section I.C.16, Chapter 16: **Certain conditions originating in the perinatal period**, Subsections d, **Prematurity and fetal growth retardation**, and e, **Low birth weight and immaturity status**, for more input.

Michael Young was born today at 27 weeks 2 days gestation by cesarean section at Barton Hospital. He weighed 945 grams at birth, and his lungs are immature. Dr. Forsyth admits Michael into the neonatal intensive care unit (NICU) with a diagnosis of extreme immaturity.

You Code It!

Read through Dr. Forsyth's notes on Michael Young, and determine the correct diagnosis code or codes.

Step 1: Read the case completely.

Step 2: Abstract the notes: Which key words can you identify relating to why Dr. Forsyth cared for Michael?

_____

Step 3: Query the provider, if necessary.

Step 4: Code the diagnosis or diagnoses.

_____

Step 5: Code the procedure(s): Birth.

Step 6: Link the procedure codes to at least one diagnosis code to confirm medical necessity.

Step 7: Back code to double-check your choices.

Answer:

Did you determine the correct codes?

Z38.01 Single liveborn, born in hospital, delivered by Cesarean

P07.03 Extremely low birth weight newborn, 750–999 grams

P07.26 Extreme immaturity of newborn, gestational age 27 completed weeks

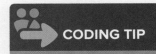

CODING TIP

See the notation beneath code category P07:

Note: When both birth weight and gestational age of the newborn are available both should be coded with birth weight sequenced before gestational age.

Suzette Collier was born, full term, vaginally at Barton Hospital. Her mother has been an alcoholic for many years and would not stop drinking during the pregnancy. Suzette weighed only 1,575 grams, small for a full-term neonate. After testing, she was diagnosed at birth with fetal alcohol syndrome and admitted into the NICU.

You Code It!

Read the notes on Suzette, and determine the most accurate diagnosis code(s).

Step 1: Read the case completely.

Step 2: Abstract the notes: Which key words can you identify relating to why Suzette was cared for?

_____

Step 3: Query the provider, if necessary.

Step 4: Code the diagnosis or diagnoses.

Step 5: Code the procedure(s): Birth.

Step 6: Link the procedure codes to at least one diagnosis code to confirm medical necessity.

Step 7: Back code to double-check your choices.

Answer:

Did you determine the correct codes?

Z38.00 Single liveborn infant, delivered vaginally

P05.16 Newborn small for gestational age, 1500–1749 grams

Q86.0 Fetal alcohol syndrome (dysmorphic)

Terrific!

Perinatal Sepsis

Many things are dealt with differently when they exist in a newborn rather than an adult. A diagnosis of sepsis is one such instance. Let's say that Dr. Frances diagnoses Judy, a 15-day-old newborn, with sepsis due to *E. coli.* When you look *sepsis* up in the Alphabetic Index, read carefully. You will see:

Sepsis (generalized) (unspecified organism) A41.9

There is a long list of descriptors indented beneath this. It seems that you don't have any additional information, so let's turn to the Tabular List to check:

A41 Other sepsis

This certainly matches, doesn't it? Professional coding specialists need to be very careful, so read the *code first, Excludes1,* and *Excludes2* notations, as you always do, to be certain. Listed under the *Excludes1* notations, you see:

Neonatal (P36-)

This is exactly why these notes are there—to help you if you land in the wrong place. So turn to P36 in the Tabular List to double check:

P36 Bacterial sepsis of newborn

Read the *includes* and the *use additional code(s)* notations carefully. OK, it seems you are in the correct location this time. You need a fourth character, so read down the column. The best choice is:

P36.4 Sepsis of newborn due to *Escherichia coli*

LO 20.5 Genetics

Genetics is the study of diseases passed from parent to child, a process known as *hereditary transmission.* There are more than 1,000 diseases that might be inherited. A genetic disorder may be *dominant*—the result of one defective gene in a pair—or it may be *recessive*—the result of both alleles being defective. Some examples of dominant genetic disorders are *familial hypercholesterolemia* (code E87.8) and *familial retinoblastoma* (code C69.2-). Examples of recessive genetic disorders include *cystic fibrosis* (code E84.9) and *Gaucher's disease* (code E75.22). Certain diseases that have

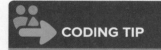

CODING TIP

Remember, if the physician does not specify the organism in his or her notes, you will need to check the pathology report to determine the correct code or codes.

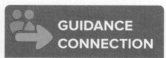

GUIDANCE CONNECTION

Review the ICD-10-CM Coding Guidelines, Section I.C.16, Chapter 16: **Certain conditions originating in the perinatal period,** Subsection f, **Bacterial sepsis of newborn,** for more input.

been correlated to genetics cause accelerated aging, such as *Hutchinson-Gilford progeria* (code E34.8), an inherited endocrine disorder.

If the patient is diagnosed with a specific genetic condition, you will need to report the code for the confirmed diagnosis. However, there are times when the patient does not exhibit any signs or symptoms of the condition. In these cases, it may be important to document the *family history* of the condition to support more frequent screenings or other preventive or early detection services, such as *family history of alcohol abuse and dependence,* reported with code Z81.1.

LO 20.6 Genetic Conditions versus Congenital Malformation

The term **congenital anomaly** means an abnormality present at birth and therefore refers to any variation from the norm for a neonate. The abnormality may be genetic in nature or may be a malformation that occurred during gestation. A genetic condition may indicate that a chromosomal alteration has been inherited—passed down from parent to child via chromosomal and cell structures. Or the condition may be a congenital malformation, or damage to a chromosome during formation. A congenital **malformation** means that something went awry during the gestational process. Such alterations can occur spontaneously or can be an adverse reaction to a pathogen, drug, radiation, or chemical.

congenital
A condition existing at the time of birth.

anomaly
An abnormal, or unexpected, condition.

malformation
An irregular structural development.

EXAMPLE

Q91.2 Trisomy 18, translocation
Q93.3 Deletion of short arm of chromosome 4

Inherited Conditions Your blue eyes or brown hair are the product of genetics—qualities in the chromosomes you received from your father and mother. Sadly, a genetic abnormality will negatively affect the health of a child. An inherited mutation in the DNA causes a permanent alteration that will affect each and every cell as it multiplies during the maturation of the zygote to embryo to fetus to neonate. There is also a strong probability that this person will pass this condition along to his or her children.

Congenital Malformations A congenital malformation, also known as a *birth defect,* is a permanent physical defect—the incomplete development of an anatomical structure—that is identified in a neonate. It may be the effect of a genetic mutation, or it may have been caused by a prenatal event. The fetal development of many organs, including the brain, heart, lungs, liver, bones, and/or intestinal tract, may have been altered by alcohol or drugs used by the mother at a particular point during gestation, by exposure to an environmental factor, or by an injury sustained during delivery.

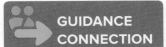

GUIDANCE CONNECTION

Review the ICD-10-CM Coding Guidelines, Section I.C.17, Chapter 17: **Congenital malformations, deformations, and chromosomal abnormalities,** for more input.

EXAMPLE

Q14.1 Congenital malformation of retina
Q64.4 Malformation of urachus

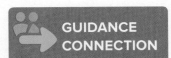

GUIDANCE CONNECTION

Review the ICD-10-CM Coding Guidelines, Section I.C.17, Chapter 17: **Congenital malformations, deformations, and chromosomal abnormalities,** for more input.

Testing Health care research has found ways to identify the presence or the likelihood of genetic disorders and congenital anomalies.

Genetic testing can be performed prior to fertilization so the potential parents can gain insights on the possibility of passing along certain diseases to their future children.

A family tree analysis, called a *pedigree,* is a diagram of the individual's family that includes diseases and causes of death. A geneticist (a physician specializing in the study of genetics) can use this diagram to identify *inheritance patterns* and probabilities. In addition, a blood test known as a *karyotype* can be used. During this test, multiple staining techniques can illuminate each chromosomal band to enable visualization of a mutation.

Prenatal blood and DNA tests can currently detect more than 600 genetic disorders prior to the baby's birth. This information can allow parents to make informed decisions and to become prepared emotionally, intellectually, and financially for the birth of a child with a genetic disorder. In addition, the physician can make certain appropriate arrangements, such as method of delivery and timing of delivery, that may reduce the severity or impact of the condition.

Amniocentesis is the process of collecting a sample of amniotic fluid via needle aspiration from a pregnant uterus. *Chorionic villus sampling* is the process of obtaining tissues from the placenta for prenatal testing by passing a catheter through the vagina and threading it up to the placenta.

Genetic tests are not limited to potential or impending parents. Adults can use this information, as well. For example, many women are tested for the BRCA1 or BRCA2 gene that identifies a potential for the development of breast and/or ovarian cancer.

EXAMPLE

Z14.1 Cystic fibrosis carrier
Z15.01 Genetic susceptibility to malignant neoplasm of breast

Gene Therapy Researchers continue to experiment with gene therapy to prevent or treat these types of diseases. The goal is to find a safe and effective way to correct a malfunctioning gene. Methods currently being investigated include:

- Placing a normal gene into the genome in a nonspecific place so it can provide the correct function of the nonfunctional gene.
- Using homologous recombination to remove the abnormal gene and replace it with a normal gene.
- Using selected reverse mutation to actually repair the gene so it will function properly.

In such cases, the term *placed* or *inserted* does not mean the same as it typically does in the context of other health care procedures. One method is to put the therapeutic gene into a carrier molecule, known as a *vector,* which is a genetically altered virus. Nonviral methods include the injection of the therapeutic gene directly into its target cell. However, this can be accomplished only with a limited number of tissue types. Studies are being conducted on the effectiveness of using an artificial liposome and/or certain chemicals to achieve the successful delivery of the therapeutic gene.

Genetic Disorders

Chromosomal Abnormalities

Down syndrome (trisomy 21) is a spontaneous **genetic abnormality** and is not inherited. Manifestations include mental retardation, unusual facial features including slanted eyes (see Figure 20-2) and protruding tongue, and congenital heart defects, as well as respiratory and related complications. *Mosaicism* is possible in a child with Down syndrome. This is the occurrence of cells with two different genetic makeups

genetic abnormality
An error in a gene (chromosome) that affects development during gestation; also known as a *chromosomal abnormality.*

within one person. The possibility of having a child with Down syndrome increases with the age of the mother at the time of delivery. Treatment of manifestations can improve the patient's quality of life and extend the life span. Use code category Q90, Down syndrome (trisomy 21), with an additional character to report non-mosaicism, mosaicism, or translocation. An additional code to identify specific physical and intellectual disabilities is required.

Klinefelter's syndrome is a genetic abnormality that results in the inclusion of an extra X chromosome in a male child. Testicular changes occur at puberty, including eventual infertility due to the deterioration of the testicles. In addition, gynecomastia may develop, learning disabilities may become apparent, facial hair may be sparse, and reduced libido causing impotence will become evident. There is a mosaic form of Klinefelter's. Report this syndrome with a code from category Q98, Other sex chromosome abnormalities, male phenotype, not elsewhere classified.

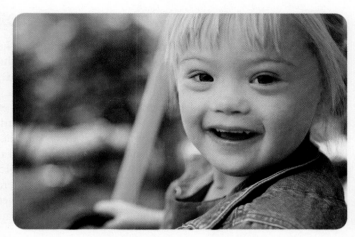

FIGURE 20-2 A Child with Down Syndrome

© Rhea Anna/Aurora/Getty Images

Autosomal Recessive Inherited Diseases

Cystic fibrosis is seen most often in Caucasian children and rarely seen in black or Asian populations. This disease causes chronic pulmonary disease and deficient exocrine pancreatic function, development of thickened mucus that can block bile flow from the liver, and other manifestations. Use code category E84, Cystic fibrosis, with an additional character to identify manifestations.

Tay-Sachs disease (Tay-Sachs amaurotic familial idiocy) is an inherited disease that results in the child's death before the age of 4. Symptoms include increasing deterioration of motor skills and mental acuity, identifiable in the infant at 6 to 10 months of age. Genetic tests can screen potential parents. Report this disease with code E75.02, Tay-Sachs disease.

Phenylketonuria (PKU) is a genetic disorder that causes a gradual deterioration of the patient's mental faculties, often discernable by 1 year of age. Many hospitals perform a simple blood test for PKU as a part of the birth evaluation. This condition can be treated with a semisynthetic diet. Outcomes improve with early detection. Report PKU with code E70.0, Classical phenylketonuria, or E70.1, Other hyperphenylalaninemias (maternal).

Sickle cell anemia is an inherited hemolytic anemia that develops as the result of a defective hemoglobin molecule that causes the red blood cells to be misshapen. This half-moon- (sickle-) shaped cell (instead of the rounded, button shape) interferes with circulation and manifests itself as fatigue, dyspnea, and swollen joints. Pharmaceutical treatments can reduce ill health. Sickle cell disorders are grouped into code category D57, Sickle-cell disorders. You will need additional characters to identify the specific type of sickle cell, possibly requiring a pathology report at some point, and to identify whether the patient is having a crisis at this time or not. For example: D57.20 Sickle-cell/Hb-C disease without crisis.

Multifactorial Abnormalities

Cleft lip and cleft palate are malformations of the upper lip and/or palate that occur during the first 2 months of gestation. This **deformity** may be seen unilaterally or bilaterally (medial is rare) and may extend into the nasal cavity and/or the maxilla (upper jaw). Use code categories Q35, Cleft palate (additional character to identify hard palate, soft palate, etc.); Q36, Cleft lip (additional character to specify laterality); and Q37, Cleft palate with cleft lip (additional character to specify laterality).

deformity
A size or shape (structural design) that deviates from that which is considered normal.

X-Linked Inherited Diseases

Hemophilia is an inherited hemostatic disorder that causes difficulty with the occurrence of coagulation. The abnormal bleeding can be problematic, especially after an injury or surgical procedure. On occasion, spontaneous bleeding may occur, causing damage to the brain, nerves, or muscle function, depending upon the location of the hemorrhage. Treatment can extend life expectancy. Report code D66, Hereditary factor VIII deficiency (hemophilia NOS).

Fragile X syndrome is the most frequently diagnosed underlying cause of inherited mental retardation, and it affects both males and females. An accurate pedigree would be important in predicting the likelihood of this condition because probabilities increase with each generation. Males display profound mental retardation, while females may or may not reveal this dysfunction. Use code Q99.2, Fragile X chromosome, to report this condition.

Congenital Malformations

Spina bifida is a condition that results from an incomplete closure of the vertebral column, the spinal cord, or both. Presented often by a hole in the skin covering the area of the spine, it is an abnormality in the development of the central nervous system. In the 1990s, researchers discovered that folic acid (a B vitamin), when taken before and during the first trimester of pregnancy, could actually prevent some cerebral and spinal birth defects. In 1996, the U.S. Food and Drug Administration ordered that folic acid be added into breads, cereals, and other grain products. The number of cases of spina bifida dropped from 2,490 in 1995–1996 to 1,640 in 1999–2000. Spina bifida is sometimes accompanied by hydrocephalus. Code category Q05, Spina bifida (aperta) (cystica), requires an additional character to report the location on the spine (cervical, thoracic, lumbar, sacral), as well as to report the presence or absence of hydrocephalus. *Spina bifida occulta* is reported with Q76.0. This version of spina bifida is evidenced by a tiny gap between vertebrae with no involvement of the nervous system. It can be seen only on an x-ray of the affected area and generally has no signs or symptoms.

Congenital hernia can occur in several locations in the body, just as with adult hernias. The difference with reporting such conditions is the specification in the documentation that the hernia is congenital. Some of the codes include Q79.0, Congenital diaphragmatic hernia; Q40.1, Congenital hiatus hernia; and Q79.51, Congenital hernia of bladder.

Congenital heart defects have been determined by the CDC to affect close to 400,000 babies born in the United States each year. They are the most common type of congenital anomaly and one of the most common causes of death in infants. Research has proved a strong connection between cigarette smoking, especially during the first trimester of gestation, and neonates with pulmonary valve stenosis and type 2 atrial septal defects, among other congenital heart malformations. Code from categories Q20, Congenital malformations of cardiac chambers and connections; Q21, Congenital malformations of cardiac septa; Q23, Congenital malformations of aortic and mitral valves; and Q24, Other congenital malformations of heart. Additional characters are required to provide specific details, such as Q21.1, Atrial septal defect, and Q22.1, Congenital pulmonary valve stenosis.

Fetal (Prenatal) Surgery

Starting in 1981, physicians have found several methods enabling treatment of certain congenital conditions while the fetus is still in utero, thus diminishing the impact of the condition after birth and improving health outcomes throughout the baby's lifetime. The surgery can be performed using an open approach, in which an incision is made, the amniotic fluid is drained, the procedure is performed, and the amniotic fluid is replaced. A minimally invasive endoscopic procedure, known as *fetoscopic* surgery, is similar to other laparoscopic surgeries using tiny incisions guided by sonography.

Closure of neural tube defects, congenital diaphragmatic hernias, spina bifida, fetal bladder obstructions, congenital heart defects, and some other conditions can be eligible for this prenatal repair.

LET'S CODE IT! SCENARIO

Heather Lombardi brought her 45-day-old daughter, Tabitha, to Dr. Abuin for her routine health check. During the examination, Heather related that Tabitha's head accidentally was banged into the table and she was worried about neurologic problems. Dr. Abuin checked her head and found no bruise or laceration. To calm Heather, he took Tabitha down the hall to have a special neurologic screening for traumatic brain injury. Fortunately, the scan was negative.

Let's Code It!

What key words in the notes provide you with the information you need to report this encounter? Why did Dr. Abuin care for Tabitha? Tabitha was brought in for her "routine health check"—her regular well-baby visit. What will you look up in the Alphabetic Index? *Routine?* Nothing there. *Well-baby?* Nothing there. Try a term that is not technically a diagnosis: *examination.* Take a look and find:

Examination (for)(following)(general)(of) (routine) Z00.00

Read down the long list of additional descriptors and find:

Child (over 28 days old) Z00.129

That sounds accurate. So let's turn to the Tabular List and check it out:

Z00 Encounter for general examination without complaint, suspected or reported diagnosis

There are no notations or directives, so read down the column to determine the most accurate fourth character:

Z00.12 Encounter for routine child health examination

Read the notations beneath this code. First, notice that it states "Health check (routine) for child over 28 days old." How old is Tabitha? She is 45 days, so this is the correct code. Carefully read the *Excludes1* notation, and ask yourself: Does this apply to Dr. Abuin's caring for Tabitha during this encounter? No, it doesn't. Read down to review the sixth-character choices. The notes state that he did a neurologic screening because of the bang to her head. You will need to check the documentation for the results of this screening so you can report "abnormal findings" or not. The documentation states that "the scan was negative," so you will report:

Z00.129 Encounter for routine child health examination without abnormal findings.

You still need to report the neurologic screening. Go back to the Alphabetic Index, and look up:

Screening (for) Z13.9

Neurological condition Z13.89

That's really the only suggested code, so let's take a look at it in the Tabular List:

Z13 Encounter for screening for other diseases and disorders

Go back to the notes and see that Dr. Abuin wrote "neurologic screening for traumatic brain injury." Therefore, you know that Z13.850, Encounter for screening for traumatic brain injury, is accurate and matches what Dr. Abuin wrote in the notes.

One more code—remember, you need to report a code for the bang on the head because this led Dr. Abuin to do the screening. Check the notes and see that Dr. Abuin found no bruises or lacerations and that Heather did not report any other signs or symptoms, such as vomiting or seizure. The bang on the head will have to be reported with an external cause code because it is an external factor that explains why Dr. Abuin screened Tabitha for a TBI. Check the External Causes Code Alphabetic Index and look up *strike, striking,* because Tabitha's head struck the table (furniture). Code W22.03 is suggested. Let's check the Tabular List:

W22 Striking against or struck by other objects

W22.03x- Walked into furniture

This cannot be accurate because Tabitha is only 45 days old and she cannot walk yet. Review all of the other codes in this subsection to determine the code that will report what happened:

W22.8xxA Striking against or struck by other objects, initial encounter

So for Tabitha's visit to Dr. Abuin, you have three codes to report:

Z00.129 Encounter for routine child health examination without abnormal findings

Z13.850 Encounter for screening for traumatic brain injury

W22.8xxA Striking against or struck by other objects, initial encounter

Chapter Summary

Babies are precious and should always be treated with tender loving care. From the moment they are born, babies receive a special version of health care services created especially for them, due to their size and growth patterns. The guidelines for coding the reasons for these services are very specific. Congenital anomalies, whether inherited or caused by an interaction with a chemical, drug, or other environmental factor during gestation, can have a lifelong effect on the child as well as the family. Congenital deficits can cause a minor inconvenience, present a challenge, require years of health care treatments, or result in premature death.

CHAPTER 20 REVIEW
Coding Congenital and Pediatric Conditions

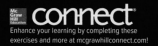
Enhance your learning by completing these
exercises and more at mcgrawhillconnect.com!

Using Terminology

Match each key term to the appropriate definition.

Part One

_____ **1.** LO 20.6 An abnormal, or unexpected, condition.

_____ **2.** LO 20.6 A condition existing at the time of birth.

_____ **3.** LO 20.1 Assessment of a neonate's condition on the basis of five factors: muscle tone, heart rate, reflex response, skin color, and breathing.

_____ **4.** LO 20.4 A baby born weighing less than 5 pounds 8 ounces, or 2,500 grams.

_____ **5.** LO 20.4 Unhealthy, diseased.

_____ **6.** LO 20.1 An infant from birth to 1 month of age.

_____ **7.** LO 20.3 The time period from before birth to the 28th day after birth.

_____ **8.** LO 20.4 Birth occurring prior to the completion of 37 weeks gestation.

_____ **9.** LO 20.3 Signs, symptoms, and/or conditions present at birth that may impact the child's future health status.

_____ **10.** LO 20.4 Death.

A. Anomaly
B. Apgar
C. Clinically significant
D. Congenital
E. Low birth weight (LBW)
F. Morbidity
G. Mortality
H. Neonate
I. Perinatal
J. Prematurity

Checking Your Understanding

Choose the most appropriate answer for each of the following questions.

1. LO 20.1 The first code on the baby's chart is

  a. place of birth, type of birth.
  b. vaginal delivery, cesarean delivery.
  c. type of delivery, outcome of delivery.
  d. birth weight, weeks of gestation.

2. LO 20.6 A congenital malformation is also known as a(n)

  a. inherited condition.
  b. birth defect.
  c. breech birth.
  d. pediatric factor.

3. LO 20.3 The perinatal period runs

  a. from the time of conception to birth.
  b. from before birth to the 28th day after birth.
  c. from birth to 60 days after birth.
  d. from birth to 24 months of age.

4. LO 20.4 The infant is considered premature when born prior to

  a. 40 weeks of gestation.
  b. 30 weeks of gestation.
  c. 37 weeks of gestation.
  d. 28 weeks of gestation.

5. LO 20.4 A baby born weighing less than 2,500 grams is termed

   a. normal birth weight.
   b. light for dates.
   c. slow fetal growth.
   d. low birth weight.

6. LO 20.2 A routine well-baby checkup is coded as a(n)

   a. part of the delivery supervision.
   b. Z code for health supervision.
   c. congenital observation.
   d. observation and evaluation.

7. LO 20.1 Apgar is a(n)

   a. congenital anomaly.
   b. type of birth.
   c. maternal condition that affects a neonate.
   d. assessment performed on a newborn.

8. LO 20.3 When a congenital condition has been resolved, it is coded

   a. with a personal history code.
   b. with a family history code.
   c. never again.
   d. only if the baby was premature.

9. LO 20.4 _____ is the leading cause of mortality and morbidity of a premature neonate.

   a. down syndrome.
   b. respiratory distress syndrome (RDS).
   c. cystic fibrosis.
   d. phenylketonuria (PKU).

10. LO 20.4 A neonate has been diagnosed with sepsis due to *Staphylococcus aureus*. Which code should be used to report this?

   a. B95.61.
   b. A41.01.
   c. P36.8.
   d. P36.2.

Applying Your Knowledge

1. LO 20.1 What does Apgar stand for? _____

   _____

2. LO 20.1 Explain coding the birth, including what code category goes on the mother's chart (and its sequence) and what code category goes on the newborn's chart, including its sequence and how many times this code can be reported. _____

   _____

3. LO 20.2 Explain routine well-baby checkups. What does the exam include? What is the encounter schedule, and what determines this schedule? _____

   _____

4. LO 20.3 What is the coder's responsibility concerning the coding of clinically significant conditions for a newborn? _____

   _____

5. LO 20.6 When the documentation states that the condition is congenital, what does that mean? _____

   _____

6. LO 20.6 Explain the differences between genetic conditions and congenital malformations. _____

   _____

7. LO 20.6 List four categories of genetic disorders. _____

   _____

YOU CODE IT! Practice

Chapter 20: Coding Congenital and Pediatric Conditions

Using the techniques described in this chapter, carefully read through the case studies and determine the most accurate ICD-10-CM code(s) and external cause code(s), if appropriate, for each *newborn's/child's* case study.

1. Dee Dee Meyerson, a 32-year-old female, is at 40 weeks gestation and is admitted with labor in progress. The baby is found to have the umbilical cord wrapped tightly around its neck. Baby girl Meyerson is quickly delivered vaginally, resuscitated because of moderate asphyxia, and given oxygen in the NICU for the first 40 minutes of life. There are no further complications. Mother and baby are discharged on the second day postpartum.

   _____

2. Juan Haverty, a 6-month-old male, is brought in today by his mother for a routine well-baby checkup and is diagnosed with a congenital anomaly of the left middle ear, which is causing sensorineural hearing loss on that side; the right ear test reveals hearing within normal range for age.

   _____

3. Raul Torres, a 7-month-old male, was born with penoscrotal hypospadias. He is brought in to the Barton Ambulatory Center today for the first stage of the surgical correction that requires transplantation of the prepuce, but no skin flap.

   _____

4. Stephen Cheng, a 3-month-old male, was born with bilateral hydrocele. He also has reducible inguinal hernias on both sides. The condition has become troublesome, so the parents and Dr. Jamerson, his pediatrician, have decided that surgical correction is warranted. The Chengs bring Stephen to Barton Ambulatory Center today for the surgery.

   _____

5. Dr. Dennis, a neonatologist, was called in to treat Diana Norman, a spontaneously delivered newborn who was born in this hospital 1 hour ago and was diagnosed with respiratory failure and erythroblastosis fetalis due to Rh antibodies. Dr. Dennis transferred Diana into the NICU.

   _____

6. Judson Jacoby, a 6-month-old male, was born with cryptorchism, abdominal. His testes have not descended. Judson is brought in today by his parents, and Dr. Kilroy performs an orchiopexy.

   _____

7. Carter Webster III, a 2-month-old male, was born with talipes equinovarus and was treated by manipulation and short leg casting. His parents brought him to see Dr. Baumgartner, his regular pediatrician, today for a foot and ankle manipulation and replacement of the plaster cast.

   _____

8. Lorena Yankowsky, a 3-week-old female, was born with spina bifida of the thoracic region with hydrocephalus. She is brought to the office today by her parents to see Dr. Fleming, her pediatrician, to check her status.

_____

9. Paulette Seriphina is in her late third trimester and sustains a complicated fracture of the skull during an automobile accident. As a direct result of her injuries, she goes into labor, and when she reaches the hospital, Josiah Seriphina, a baby boy, is delivered. Because of his early delivery due to his mother's injury, Josiah suffers respiratory distress type I syndrome. Code Josiah's chart.

_____

10. Caitlyn Katzman was born prematurely in her father's car on the way to the hospital. She was born at 31 completed weeks of gestation, and her birth weight was measured at the hospital at 610 grams. Dr. Flannery, the on-call pediatrician, assessed Caitlyn as extremely immature and admitted her to the hospital.

_____

11. Hannah Sue Langdon was born full-term, delivered by cesarean, in Barton Hospital on Saturday, May 29, at 2:55 p.m. (today). Mother and baby are doing fine.

_____

12. Annabelle Darlington, a 25-day-old female, was a full-term baby weighing just 1,200 grams at birth. Dr. Schweitzer, the hospital pediatrician, sees her today for her well-baby weight checkup. Annabelle is doing well and gaining weight.

_____

13. Denise Van Hooten, a 33-year-old female, was admitted to the labor and delivery room of the Barton Birthing Center. She gave birth to Craig Stanford Van Hooten, 2,750 grams, at 41 weeks gestation. Denise took baby Craig home a few hours later. Code Craig's chart.

_____

14. Oscar Franklin, Jr., a 9-day-old male, was born full-term, thought to be healthy, and discharged on the second day postpartum. His sister, Elizabeth, 5 years old, just came down with rubella. Oscar is brought in today by his mother to see Dr. Belkin, his pediatrician. After a thorough examination, Oscar is diagnosed with congenital rubella pneumonitis.

_____

15. Marian Abernathy went into labor, and her husband, Roger, was driving her to the hospital when they got caught in a traffic jam. Marian gave birth in the car, and Roger cut the umbilical cord with his utility knife, kept in the trunk. Upon arrival at the hospital, Dr. Peterson performed a complete newborn examination and diagnosed the baby with tetanus neonatorum, caused by the use of the nonsterile instrument during delivery.

_____

The following exercises provide practice in abstracting physicians' notes and learning to work with SOAP notes from our health care facility, *Taylor, Reader, & Associates.* These case studies (SOAP notes) are modeled on real patient encounters. Using the techniques described in this chapter, carefully read through the case studies and determine the most accurate ICD-10-CM code(s) and external cause code(s), if appropriate, for each *newborn's/child's* case study.

TAYLOR, READER, & ASSOCIATES
A Complete Health Care Facility
975 CENTRAL AVENUE • SOMEWHERE, FL 32811 • 407-555-4321

PATIENT: HENNY, SOPHIA
ACCOUNT/EHR #:   HENNSO01
DATE: 9/17/18

Attending Physician: Pravdah H. Jeppard, MD

S: The patient is a female, gestational age 38 weeks 4 days, born vaginally in this facility, 09/17/16, 02:35:12.

O: Neonate was of a single birth, BWT 2,859 grams, without significant OR procedures, with a normal newborn diagnosis. 19″ long. Head circumference: 32 cm. Amniotic fluid: Clear. Cord: 3 vessels. Evidence of a benign tumor of blood vessels due to malformed angioblastic tissues (vascular hamartomas) at right groin. Appears pale, poor skin turgor, mucousy, and transitional stool.

Apgar score: 1 min = 9; 5 min = 9. Heart rate: >100; respiratory effort: good; muscle tone: active; response to catheter in nostril: cough; color: body pink, extremities blue.

Maternal History: 33 years old, G1, blood type O+; spontaneous labor, 17 h 21 min, epidural anesthesia. HIV tested during pregnancy: neg.

Administrations: Hepatitis B, Peds, Vaccine (Recomb) 5 mcg/0.5 mL, given: 9/17/16
Newborn hearing screening: passed.

A: Portwine nevus, congenital

P: Follow-up in office 2 days

Pravdah H. Jeppard, MD

PHJ/mg   D: 09/17/18 03:50:16   T: 09/18/18 12:55:01

Determine the most accurate ICD-10-CM code(s).

_____

_____

_____

TAYLOR, READER, & ASSOCIATES
A Complete Health Care Facility
975 CENTRAL AVENUE • SOMEWHERE, FL 32811 • 407-555-4321

PATIENT: WILLIS, ERIK
ACCOUNT/EHR #:   WILLER001
DATE: 09/17/18

Attending Physician: Pravdah H. Jeppard, MD

S: Pt is a 3-day-old male who comes in for his first office visit after birth. He was a full-term infant, vaginally delivered. Mother provides prenatal history, family history including the paternal Rh factor, and information regarding inherited red cell defects.

O: Wt. 5 lb 7 oz. T 98.6. Skin has yellowish coloration, including sclerae. Tests, including direct and indirect bilirubin levels, reveal Gram-negative bacterial infection and serum bilirubin levels at 7 mg/dL. Blood tests are also performed to test infant and mother both for blood group incompatibilities, hemoglobin level, direct Coombs' test, and hematocrit.

A: Hyperbilirubinemia, due to Gram-negative bacterial infection

P: 1. Rx albumin administration (1 g/kg of 25% salt-poor albumin)
   2. Rx antibiotics for infection
   3. Follow-up appointment in 3 days

_____

Pravdah H. Jeppard, MD

PHJ/mg   D: 09/17/18 09:50:16   T: 09/18/18 12:55:01

Determine the most accurate ICD-10-CM code(s).

_____

_____

_____

TAYLOR, READER, & ASSOCIATES
A Complete Health Care Facility
975 CENTRAL AVENUE • SOMEWHERE, FL 32811 • 407-555-4321

PATIENT: TOBIAS, TRISTA
ACCOUNT/EHR #:   TOBITR001
DATE: 09/17/18

Attending Physician: Pravdah H. Jeppard, MD

S: This is an 18-month-old female who is brought into the emergency department by her mother in a carriage. Upon arrival, child is sleeping. Skin is hot to touch. She is irritable initially upon awakening but then lethargic. Occasional whimper. Mother reports loose yellow stool. Also reports child has been coughing and vomiting over the past 6 days. Child was seen in clinic for an ear infection and has been on amoxicillin 125 mg/5 mL for 3 days.

Allergies: NKA (no known allergies).

O: W 30 lb. T 104.3. AR 158. R 60. BP 103/58. Pulse Ox 99%. Abdomen is distended. Tachypenic. Lungs clear. Eyes clear, pupils reactive. No eye contact is made. CBC, CMET, BCx1, CXR ordered. Growth/Development: WNL (within normal limits).

A: Hypokalemia, fever

P: Admit to hospital pediatrics unit

_____

Pravdah H. Jeppard, MD

PHJ/mg   D: 09/17/18 09:50:16   T: 09/18/18 12:55:01

Determine the most accurate ICD-10-CM code(s).

_____

_____

_____

TAYLOR, READER, & ASSOCIATES
A Complete Health Care Facility
975 CENTRAL AVENUE • SOMEWHERE, FL 32811 • 407-555-4321

PATIENT: BELGUM, ALLEN
ACCOUNT/EHR #: BELGAL001
DATE: 09/17/18

Attending Physician: Pravdah H. Jeppard, MD

Consultant: Vivian D. Pixar, MD

Reason for Consultation: Screening for retinopathy of prematurity

S: The patient was born on 08/15/16, with a birth weight of 2,620 grams, gestational age of 36 weeks; given oxygen in NICU for the first 60 minutes of life. Child discharged third day postpartum with oxygen saturation of 98%.

O: Retinal follow-up examination this date shows normal external exam, well-dilated pupils. Indirect exam shows clear media, normal optic nerves both eyes, with normal right retinal vessel extension to the periphery without evidence of retinopathy. Left retinal vessel extension shows a faint demarcation line at the junction between the vascularized and avascular border.

A: Prematurity retinopathy, stage 1, left eye

P: Follow-up 1 week

_____

Vivian D. Pixar, MD

VDP/mg   D: 09/17/18 09:50:16   T: 09/18/18 12:55:01

Determine the most accurate ICD-10-CM code(s).

_____

_____

_____

TAYLOR, READER, & ASSOCIATES
A Complete Health Care Facility
975 CENTRAL AVENUE • SOMEWHERE, FL 32811 • 407-555-4321

PATIENT: EDWARDS, MANUEL

ACCOUNT/EHR #:   EDWAMA001

DATE: 10/10/18

PREOP DIAGNOSIS: Hypoxic ischemic encephalopathy (HIE); feeding problems

POSTOP DIAGNOSIS: Same

OPERATION: Gastrostomy

SURGEON: Robert R. Singer, MD

ANESTHESIOLOGIST: John Katzman, MD

INDICATIONS FOR OPERATION: This is a neonatal patient who weighs approximately 2,200 grams. The child has severe hypoxic ischemic encephalopathy, cannot be fed without an NG tube. The child had an upper GI which shows minimal reflux. The child was brought to the operation room at this time for a gastrostomy.

PROCEDURE: The patient was placed in the supine position under general endotracheal anesthesia, and the abdomen was prepped and draped in the usual sterile manner. A midline upper abdominal incision was made. The abdomen was entered. The stomach was grasped with a Babcock clamp and brought up to the wound. Two concentric purse strings of 3-0 silk were placed. A 12 Malecot catheter was placed in the stomach through a stab wound in the center of the purse string. The two purse strings were tied consecutively, and the stomach was packed to the GE tube. The Malecot catheter was brought out through a separate stab wound in the left upper quadrant. The stomach was sutured to the abdominal wall using 3-0 chromic. A suture was placed on the outside to secure the gastrostomy tube and prevent it from being dislodged. The midline incision was closed with interrupted 3-0 silk. The skin was closed with 5-0 plain subcuticular stitches. A Steri-strip dressing and Telfa were placed at the GE tube site. The patient tolerated the procedure well and was taken back to the neonatal unit in fair condition.

Robert R. Singer, MD

RRS/mg   D: 10/10/18 09:50:16   T: 10/13/18 12:55:01

Determine the most accurate ICD-10-CM code(s).

_____

_____

_____

CODING INJURIES, POISONINGS, AND CERTAIN OTHER CONSEQUENCES OF EXTERNAL CAUSES

21

Learning Outcomes
After completing this chapter, the student should be able to:

LO 21.1 Identify the various types of traumatic wounds.

LO 21.2 Apply guidelines for coding burns.

LO 21.3 Distinguish between an adverse effect and a poisoning.

LO 21.4 Demonstrate coding protocols for reporting abuse and neglect.

LO 21.5 Accurately report complications of care.

LO 21.6 Confirm the use of external cause codes.

You have already learned about certain injuries that can occur, such as pressure ulcers (Chapter 15), muscle sprains (Chapter 16), and fractures (Chapter 17). Now, in this chapter, you will review details and directions for reporting some other injuries and types of harm. The term *injury* refers to traumatic damage to some aspect of the body, virtually always caused by a fall, crash, weapon, or some other external cause. The damage may be minor (superficial) or be life-threatening; may occur during time at work or while playing; may be the result of an automobile accident or a fight; or may occur during an indoor or outdoor activity.

LO 21.1 Traumatic Wounds

Lacerations (Superficial Wounds)

Each one of us has had a laceration at some time or another. Perhaps a paper cut or a cut from a knife while chopping vegetables, this smooth slit or opening in the epidermal layer is typically superficial and does not bleed. A **laceration**, also caused by a sharp object, is generally a ragged wound (see Figure 21-1). Unlike a superficial cut, a laceration is deeper, damaging the dermal layer of the skin. It penetrates the blood vessels, resulting in bleeding. These more severe injuries may also be vulnerable to infection and pain. Depending upon the specific object or event that caused the laceration, the physician may order an x-ray to determine whether any foreign bodies, such as shards of glass or splinters from wood, are lodged within the wound.

Key Terms
Abuse
Adverse effect
Avulsion
Burn
Chemicals
Corrosion
Drugs
Extent
First degree
Intent
Interaction
Laceration
Physicians' Desk Reference (PDR)
Poisoned
Rule of nines
Second degree
Severity
Site
Therapeutic
Third degree
Toxic effect
Underdosing

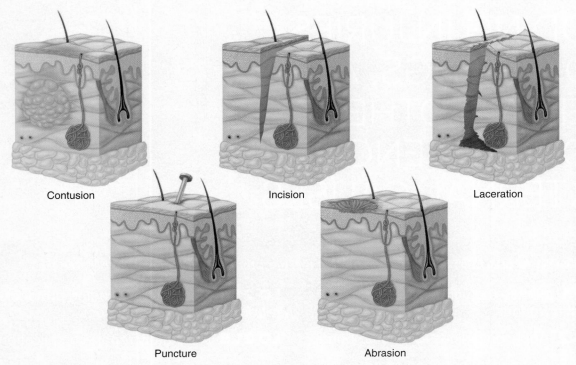

Contusion

Incision

Laceration

Puncture

Abrasion

FIGURE 21-1 Different Types of Wounds, Including Lacerations and Puncture Wounds

Source: Booth et al., MA, 5e. Copyright © 2013 by McGraw-Hill. Figure 57-7, p. 1191

CODING TIP

The Tabular List categorizes the codes used to report injuries first by anatomical site (the location of the injury) and then by the specific injury (contusion, insect bite, etc.).

laceration
Damage to the epidermal and dermal layers of the skin made by a sharp object.

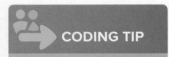

CODING TIP

A *gash* is a lay term used to indicate a large, very deep laceration.

avulsion
Injury in which layers of skin are traumatically torn away from the body.

Contusions and Hematomas

A *contusion,* commonly known as a *bruise* or "black-and-blue mark," is an injury to the body that typically does not break the skin but does damage to the underlying blood vessels. The bleeding in the dermal layer is seen only through the epidermis as a dark color. As the contusion heals, the colors change until the collected blood is dissipated and everything has healed. When the bleeding coagulates into a blood clot, this is called a *hematoma.* The seriousness of these injuries largely depends on the anatomical site where the bleeding and/or clot is located. A contusion or hematoma on the leg or arm is typically a minor event that rarely requires a physician's skill, whereas a contusion to the brain or a subdural hematoma could be life-threatening.

Puncture Wounds

When a pointed, narrow object enters deeply into the visceral (inside) aspects of the body, the injury is known as a *puncture wound* (see Figure 21-1). A carpenter's nail, a knife, scissors, and a fishhook are just a few items that can cause an injury of this nature. Due to the characteristics of this type of wound, infection and internal damage are possible. The physician may check for dirt, debris, or foreign objects within the wound, as well as order blood tests to check for a pathogen that might cause an infection. Stitches and possible surgery may be required, depending upon the specific depth and location of the injury.

Avulsions

The medical term **avulsion** describes a situation in which all layers of the skin (epidermis and dermis) are forcibly torn away from the body, typically a surface trauma. Due to the pulling off of the dermal layers, the underlying structures, including adipose, muscles, tendons, and bone, become open to the outside. Rock climbers may suffer "flappers," an avulsion of the fingertip pad. When this occurs to a fingernail or toenail, it is known as a *nail avulsion*—the nail plate is torn off the nail bed. Unlike the case with avulsions at other anatomical sites, in nail avulsions the nail is not reattached. Instead, the fingertip and nail bed are covered to protect the area until the keratin has formed a new nail.

Animal, Insect, or Human Bites

Animal bites and human bites can be a particular concern due to the potential spread of bacteria and viruses via saliva transference. Insects may transmit their own fluids and sometimes venom.

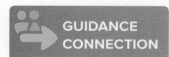

GUIDANCE CONNECTION

Review the ICD-10-CM Coding Guidelines, Section I.C.19, Chapter 19: **Injury, poisoning, and certain other consequences of external causes,** Subsection a, **Application of 7th characters in chapter 19,** for more input.

LET'S CODE IT! SCENARIO

Ciara Rollins, a 9-year-old female, was hiking in a public park with her Girl Scout troop when they came to a clearing and she saw a foal and its mother. She reached out her left hand to pet the foal, and the mother horse bit her thumb. Her leader took her to the emergency room. After examination and some tests, Dr. Ravenna cleaned the wound, applied a sterile dressing, and gave Ciara an antibiotic.

Let's Code It!

Dr. Ravenna's notes state that Ciara had been bitten on the thumb by a horse. When you turn to the Alphabetic Index, you see:

> **Bite**
>> **Thumb S61.05**

Remember the Coding Tip from the beginning of this chapter? These codes are first categorized by the anatomical site and then by the specific injury.

When you turn to the Tabular List, you confirm:

S61 Open wound of wrist, hand and fingers

Before you continue reading, be certain to pay attention to the notations here. There is a *code also* if a wound infection is documented; there is an *Excludes1* notation with two diagnoses that do not relate to Ciara's case; and there are options for the required seventh character. You will need to come back to this after you determine the correct code. So keep reading to determine the correct fourth character:

S61.0 Open wound of thumb without damage to nail

There is another *Excludes1* notation. Has Dr. Ravenna documented that the nail was also damaged? No. So continue reading to determine the correct fifth character:

S61.05 Open bite of thumb without damage to nail

There is another detail you need to abstract from the documentation: Ciara's right or left thumb?

S61.052- Open bite of left thumb without damage to nail

Now you need to determine the correct seventh character. Go back to the beginning of this code category and review your choices.

S61.052A Open bite of left thumb without damage to nail, initial encounter

Perfect! Yet you have not explained the whole story about why Dr. Ravenna cared for Ciara. This code states she was bitten on the left thumb, but not by whom or what.

To report how Ciara got bitten and by what, you will need external cause codes. Turn to the Alphabetic Index to External Causes and look up:

> **Bite**
>
>> **Horse W55.11**

Turn in the Tabular List to:

> **W55 Contact with other mammals**

Of course, you are going to read this code's *Excludes1* notation carefully. None of the exclusions apply to this case. And there are your options for the seventh character. But, first, read down to determine the correct fourth, fifth, and sixth characters:

> **W55.1 Contact with horse**
>
> **W55.11x Bitten by horse**

And now, go back up for the seventh character:

> **W55.11xA Bitten by horse, initial encounter**

Terrific! You will also need to determine the codes to report the place of occurrence, activity, and the external cause status. Try this on your own. Did you determine that the codes are:

> **Y92.830 Public park as the place of occurrence of the external cause**
>
> **Y93.01 Activity, walking, marching and hiking**
>
> **Y99.8 Other external cause status**

You are really getting to be a great coder!

Foreign Bodies

Sometimes items get into the body that should not be there. Anything that is not anatomical is considered a foreign body—a splinter, a chard of glass, or gravel from a road. Foreign bodies often occur in children—for example, a jelly bean up the nose (code T17.1xxA) or a nickel down the throat. Actually, coins are the most common objects swallowed by children.

burn
Injury by heat or fire.

corrosion
A burn caused by a chemical; chemical destruction of the skin.

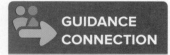

GUIDANCE CONNECTION

Review the ICD-10-CM Coding Guidelines, Section I.C.19, Chapter 19: **Injury, poisoning, and certain other consequences of external causes,** Subsection d, **Coding of burns and corrosions,** for more input.

LO 21.2 Burns

A patient can sustain a **burn** or **corrosion** to any part of the body in many different ways. It can be the result of the skin coming near or in actual contact with a flame, such as a candle or the flame on a gas stove. A burn can happen when contact is made with a hot object, such as a hot plate or curling iron. Chemicals, such as lye or acid, can cause a corrosion upon contact with a person's skin. As a professional coding specialist, you may need to code the diagnosis of a burn or corrosion.

When a patient has suffered a burn, you have to *S/S.E.E.* the burn in order to code it correctly. This acronym can help you remember the details you need, the minimum number of codes you need, and the order in which to report those codes. You need at least three codes to properly report the diagnosis of a burn:

First-listed code(s): S/S = *s*ite and *s*everity (from categories T20–T25).
Next-listed code: E = *e*xtent (from code category T31).
Last-listed code(s): E = *e*xternal cause code(s).

Let's look at these components and what they mean.

Site

Your first-listed code or codes will be combination codes that report both the **site** and **severity** of the injury. *Site* refers to the anatomical site that is affected by the burn. When you look at the descriptions for the codes in range T20–T28, you see that each code category is first defined by a general part or section of the human body:

> T20 Burn and corrosion of head, face, and neck
>
> T21 Burn and corrosion of trunk
>
> T22 Burn and corrosion of shoulder and upper limb, except wrist and hand
>
> T23 Burn and corrosion of wrist and hand
>
> T24 Burn and corrosion of lower limb, except ankle and foot
>
> T25 Burn and corrosion of ankle and foot
>
> T26 Burn and corrosion confined to eye and adnexa
>
> T27 Burn and corrosion of respiratory tract
>
> T28 Burn and corrosion of other internal organs

EXAMPLE

Hope Rockfield suffered a burn to her left thigh. Lower limb is the general anatomical site, and knee is the specific site of the burn.

Severity

The fourth character for each category (except categories T26–T28) identifies the severity. Using the layers of the skin, the severity of a burn is identified by degree (see Figure 21-2):

- *First-degree burns* are evident by erythema (redness of the epidural layer).
- *Second-degree burns* are identified by fluid-filled blisters in addition to the erythema.
- *Third-degree burns* have damage evident in the epidermis, dermis, and fatty tissue layers and can involve the muscles and nerves below.
- *Deep third-degree burned* skin will show necrosis (death of the tissue) and at times may result in the loss (amputation) of a body part.

site
The location on or in the human body; the anatomical part.

severity
The level of seriousness.

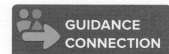

GUIDANCE CONNECTION

Review the ICD-10-CM Coding Guidelines, Section I.C.19, Chapter 19: **Injury, poisoning, and certain other consequences of external causes,** Subsections d(2), **Burns of the same local site,** and d(5), **Assign separate codes for each burn site,** for more input.

first degree
Redness of the epidermis (skin).

second degree
Blisters on the skin; involvement of the epidermis and the dermis layers.

third degree
Destruction of all layers of the skin, with possible involvement of the subcutaneous fat, muscle, and bone.

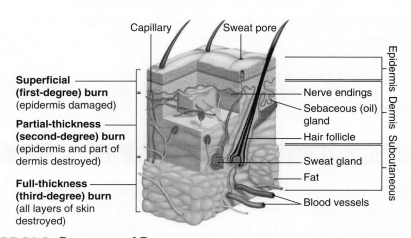

FIGURE 21-2 Degrees of Burns

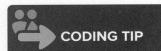
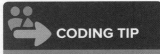
The fourth characters available in this section give you the ability to report the documented severity of the burn or corrosion:

> .0 Unspecified degree
> .1 Erythema (first degree)
> .2 Blisters, epidermal loss (second degree)
> .3 Full-thickness skin loss (third degree NOS)
> .4 Corrosion of unspecified degree
> .5 Corrosion of first degree
> .6 Corrosion of second degree
> .7 Corrosion of the third degree

Specific Site

The fifth character gives you the opportunity to report additional details regarding the anatomical site of the burn. Of course, these details will change in accordance with the anatomical region of the code category. Let's take a look at samples from code category T23, Burn and corrosion of wrist and hand:

> T23.-1 Burn . . . of thumb (nail)
> T23.-2 Burn . . . of single finger (nail) except thumb
> T23.-3 Burn . . . of multiple fingers (nail), not including thumb
> T23.-4 Burn . . . of multiple fingers (nail), including thumb
> T23.-5 Burn . . . of palm
> T23.-6 Burn . . . of back of hand
> T23.-7 Burn . . . of wrist
> T23.-9 Burn . . . of multiple sites of wrist and hand

EXAMPLE

Dwayne was talking to his buddy and stepped back, hitting the back of his right calf on the hot tailpipe of his motorcycle. The doctor at the emergency room documented second-degree burns.

The first three characters = T24 *Burn and corrosion of lower limb, except ankle and foot.*

The fourth character = T24.2 *Burn of second degree of lower limb, except ankle and foot.*

The fifth character = T24.23 *Burn of second degree of lower leg.*

The sixth character = T24.231 *Burn of second degree of right lower leg.*

The seventh character = T24.231A *Burn of second degree of right lower leg, initial encounter.*

And there you have the complete code to report Dwayne's injury. Of course, as you remember from Chapter 16, you will also need to report an external cause code to explain how Dwayne's leg became burned.

LET'S CODE IT! SCENARIO

Julian Ingles, a 15-year-old male, was working on a school project in the basement and accidentally released the hot glue gun onto the palm of his left hand. Dr. Tremont treated him for third-degree burns of the palm of his hand.

Julian was diagnosed with *third-degree burns of the palm.* Let's turn to the Alphabetic Index and look up *burns:*

Burn

palm(s) T23.059

Turn to the Tabular List, and read:

T23 Burn and corrosion of wrist and hand

Notice the available seventh-character options listed directly beneath this code. You will need that information later. First, you need to determine the other characters, so read through your choices for the fourth character:

T23.3 Burn of third degree of wrist and hand

That is much more specific and accurate. Now you have to review the fifth-character choices for code T23.3. Did you notice that there is a character to specify that the burn was on his palm?

T23.35 Burn of third degree of palm

The choices for the sixth character clearly identify which palm:

T23.352 Burn of third degree of left palm

One more character—remember, the options for the seventh character for this code are shown directly beneath the three-character code category. Is this the first time Dr. Tremont is seeing Julian for this burn? Yes:

T23.352A Burn of third degree of left palm, initial encounter

This code tells the complete story, doesn't it? Of course, you will need to also report the external cause code, as you learned in Chapter 16.

Multiple Sites Fall into the Same Code Category

When various sites fall into the same code category (the first three characters of the code), you will report all of these sites with just one code. If the burns are of different severity, use the fourth character that reports the most severe burn (determined by severity), the highest degree.

Then identify that more than one specific site has been burned by using the fifth character that reports "multiple sites," such as T25.19-, Burn of first degree of multiple sites of ankle and foot.

LET'S CODE IT! SCENARIO

Frank opened the cover of the bar-b-que to see how the coals were doing. He decided to add some lighter fluid to hurry it along, and flames roared up into his face. Therese, his wife, rushed him to the emergency department. After an exam, Dr. O'Toole diagnosed Frank with a third-degree burn on his chin and second-degree burns on his nose and cheek.

Let's begin by abstracting Frank's condition. He has:

> Third degree burn on his chin
>
> Second degree burn on his nose
>
> Second degree burn on his cheek

In the Alphabetic Index, turn to the term *burn*. You will notice that the long, long list of terms indented beneath this main term all identify anatomical sites, the location on the body that has been burned. Find the suggested codes for all three of Frank's burns:

Burn, chin, third-degree T20.33

Burn, nose, second-degree T20.24

Burn, cheek, second-degree T20.26

Notice that the code category T20 is the same for all three sites: chin, nose, and cheek. Therefore, you use only one code to report these burn sites. Turn to code T20 in the Tabular List:

T20 Burn and corrosion of head, face, and neck

Read carefully the *Excludes2* listed diagnoses. None of them apply to Frank's condition. Remember that your seventh-character options are listed here, as well, for later.

Go ahead and read down the column to review all of the choices for the required fourth character. Now you need to determine which fourth character to use. The burn on his chin is a third-degree burn (fourth character 3) but the burns on his nose and cheek are only second-degree burns (fourth character 2). Should you report both? The guidelines direct you to report only one code, with the fourth character that reports the *most severe* of all the burns, so you need to use the fourth character of 3:

T20.3 Burn of third degree of head, face, and neck

Notice that the *use additional external cause code* notation is here to remind you that you need to do this next, after you determine all of the appropriate codes to report the injury itself.

Review the fifth-character options in this subcategory:

> The fifth character 3 reports his chin was burned.
>
> The fifth character 4 reports his nose was burned.
>
> The fifth character 6 reports his cheek was burned.

Again, the guidelines tell you that you must combine all of these into one accurate code. Take a look at the fifth character 9 that reports multiple sites of face, head, and neck. Perfect!

Put it all together and get the most accurate code that tells the whole story:

T20.39x- Burn of third degree of multiple sites of head, face, and neck

Look back up to the beginning of the code category to review your options for the seventh character. This is the first time Dr. O'Toole is caring for Frank's burns. Now you have the complete code to report:

T20.39xA Burn of third degree of multiple sites of head, face, and neck, initial encounter

Excellent!

Extent

The next code you have to report indicates the **extent,** or percentage, of the body involved. The three-character category for reporting the extent of a burn is T31 and the extent of a corrosion is T32. Either of these codes requires a total of five characters to be valid, no matter what the extent of the burn or corrosion.

T31 Burns classified according to extent of body surface involved
T32 Corrosions classified according to extent of body surface involved

Turn to code T31 in the Tabular List. The required fourth character will identify the percentage of the patient's *entire body* that is affected by any and all burns, of all degrees (severity). The code descriptions refer to this as *percentage of body surface,* also known as *total body surface area (TBSA).*

The physician may specify the percentages directly in his or her notes. A statement like "third-degree burns over 10% of the body" or "7% of the body burned" will give you the information you need to find the correct fourth character for code T31 or T32. However, other times, the physician may not use a number, and you will have to calculate the percentage yourself. To calculate, you can use the **rule of nines.**

The rule of nines is used to estimate the total body surface area that has been affected by the burns. The body is divided into sections, each section representing 9% of the human body (see Figure 21-3):

Head and neck 9%

Arm, right 9%

Arm, left 9%

Chest 9%

Abdomen 9%

Upper back 9%

Lower back 9%

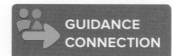

GUIDANCE CONNECTION

Review the ICD-10-CM Coding Guidelines, Section I.C.19, Chapter 19: **Injury, poisoning, and certain other consequences of external causes,** Subsection d(6), **Burns and corrosions classified according to extent of body surface involved,** for more input.

extent
The percentage of the body that has been affected by the burn or corrosion.

rule of nines
A general division of the whole body into sections that each represent 9%; used for estimating the extent of a burn.

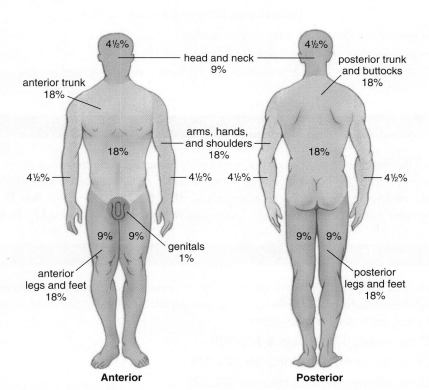

FIGURE 21-3 Using the Rule of Nines to Estimate the Extent of Burns

Leg, right, anterior (front) 9%

Leg, right, posterior (back) 9%

Leg, left, anterior (front) 9%

Leg, left, posterior (back) 9%

Genitalia 1%

As you read through the physician's notes, be aware of the anatomical site, not only for your site code but also for your calculation of the extent of the body involved in the burns.

Next, you must determine the most accurate fifth character for this code. The fifth character identifies the percentage of the patient's body that is *suffering with third-degree burns* only. You can also use the rule of nines to calculate the percentage of area affected by third-degree burns to find the best fifth character.

Of course, these percentages are general—to be used for estimation purposes. As you look at the code descriptions for the fourth and the fifth characters, you will see that the choices for codes T31 and T32 all have descriptors that require you to know the percentage of the body involved only within a 10% range. Therefore, you don't have to worry too much about narrowing down the number.

When you are determining the fourth and fifth characters for code T31 or T32, you may have to add the percentages for several anatomical sites together.

While everyone knows that the rule of nines provides an estimate and is not expected to be precise, it is a professional coder's job to be as specific as possible. Therefore, you want to adjust the percentage as appropriate.

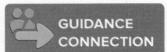

GUIDANCE CONNECTION

Review the ICD-10-CM Coding Guidelines, Section I.C.19, Chapter 19: **Injury, poisoning, and certain other consequences of external causes,** Subsection d(1), **Sequencing of burn and related condition codes,** for more input.

EXAMPLE

Alice suffered third-degree burns on her lower back and the back of her left leg and second-degree burns on her anterior forearm, wrist, and hand:

Lower back (9%) + left leg, back (9%) + anterior forearm (2%) + wrist and hand (1%) = total body surface (21%)

T31.2 Burns involving 20%–29% of body surface

Only her back and leg had third-degree burns:

Lower back (9%) + left leg, back (9%) = 18%

T31.21 Burns involving 20%–29% of body surface with 10–19% third-degree burns

LET'S CODE IT! SCENARIO

Arthur Bucholtz, a 28-year-old male, was trying to start a campfire when the flames flared and burned him on the back of his right hand, right forearm, and right elbow. He was rushed to the emergency room, where Dr. Mathers determined that he had third-degree burns on his hand and forearm and second-degree burns on his elbow.

Let's Code It!

Dr. Mathers diagnosed Arthur with *third-degree burns on his hand and forearm* and *second-degree burns on his elbow*. Go to the Alphabetic Index, and look up *burn, hand*. Find that listing and the others:

Burn, hand, third–degree T23.309

Burn, forearm, third–degree T22.319

Burn, elbow, second–degree T22.229

Does the Tabular List confirm the codes? Let's check each one:

T23 Burn and corrosion of wrist and hand

You can see that a fourth character is required, so read down the column to:

T23.3 Burn of third degree of wrist and hand

The burns on Arthur's hand were documented as third-degree, so that is correct. Now you need to determine the required fifth and sixth characters. Read all of the choices and determine which is the most accurate.

T23.36 Burn of third degree of back of hand

T23.361- Burn of third degree of back of right hand

Don't forget the seventh character. The options are at the beginning of this code category.

T23.361A Burn of third degree of back of right hand, initial encounter

This code tells the whole story about the burn to Arthur's hand. Now look at the other codes suggested by the Alphabetic Index:

Burn, forearm, third degree T22.319

Burn, elbow, second-degree T22.229

Did you notice that both of these burns are reported using the same three-character code category, T22?

T22 Burn and corrosion of shoulder and upper limb, except wrist and hand

You have two codes with the same three-character code category. The guidelines state that you must combine these into one code, T22, but which fourth character should you use? Remember, the guidelines also direct you to use the character that reports the greatest severity (the highest degree) of the burn. Third degree is more severe than second degree, so you will use:

T22.3 Burn of third-degree of shoulder and upper limb, except wrist and hand

Read the fifth-character choices for this code category. Which one code can report the burn to both Arthur's forearm and his elbow?

T22.39 Burn of third-degree of multiple sites of shoulder and upper limb, except wrist and hand

The sixth character will report which forearm and elbow were burned:

T22.391 Burn of third-degree of multiple sites of right shoulder and upper limb, except wrist and hand

And the seventh character will report which encounter this is:

T22.391A Burn of third-degree of multiple sites of right shoulder and upper limb, except wrist and hand, initial encounter

Good! Next, you need a code to report the extent of the burns. Arthur was burned on the following sites:

Hand (part of the arm), 9%

Forearm (part of the same arm), 9%

Elbow (also part of the same arm), 9%

The rule of nines states that one arm represents 9%. Arthur had burns on his hand, forearm and elbow of the same arm. You can see that it would not make sense to add 9% for each of these injuries, as it is still only one arm, so you get a TBSA of 9%. Of this 9%, you must note that only an estimated 4% of his body (his hand and forearm) suffered third-degree burns. Therefore, the next code on Arthur's chart will be:

> **T31.10 Burns involving 10%–19% of body surface with 0%–9% third degree burns**

The codes you have for Arthur's burns are T23.361A, T22.391A, and T31.10 (plus the external cause codes, of course!).

Good work!

Infection in the Burn Site

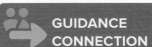

GUIDANCE CONNECTION

Review the ICD-10-CM Coding Guidelines, Section I.C.19, Chapter 19: **Injury, poisoning, and certain other consequences of external causes,** Subsection d(4), **Infected burn,** for more input.

If not treated properly, a burn site can become infected. This can happen because the inner layers of the tissue are exposed, and it might be difficult to keep the wound clean and sterile. If an infection occurs, you should add a code for the specific pathogen. Sequence the infection code after the burn code but before the T31 or T32 code.

Solar and Radiation Burns

When a patient has been burned not by fire or chemicals but by some kind of radiation, the injuries are not reported with codes from the T20–T28 range.

Even with all the ads promoting sunblock lotions and ointments to protect the skin, individuals still manage to get sunburns. These burns are also identified in three degrees to report damage to the skin as a result of overexposure to the natural sun, and each degree has its own code:

> **L55.0 Sunburn (first degree sunburn)**
>
> **L55.1 Sunburn of second degree**
>
> **L55.2 Sunburn of third degree**

Some individuals have a hypersensitivity to the sun, similar to an allergic reaction. Actually, this can be diagnosed as a photoallergic or a phototoxic response to the sun. This type of severe reaction can be determined to be an effect of solar radiation and is reported with one of the following codes:

> **L56.0 Drug phototoxic response**
>
> **L56.1 Drug photoallergic response**
>
> **L56.2 Photocontact dermatitis (berloque dermatitis)**
>
> **L56.3 Solar urticaria**

In addition to physiological sensitivity to the sun, certain medications can cause a patient to develop a sensitivity to the sun. When this is the case, you will need to add an external cause code to report the specific drug that caused this situation.

Sequelae (Late Effects) of Burns and Corrosions

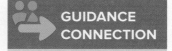

GUIDANCE CONNECTION

Review the ICD-10-CM Coding Guidelines, Section I.C.19, Chapter 19: **Injury, poisoning, and certain other consequences of external causes,** Subsections d(7), **Encounters for treatment of late effects of burns,** and d(8), **Sequelae with a late effect code and current burn,** for more input.

Often, a scar or contracture develops at the site of a healed burn or corrosion. There are times when this lasting condition requires treatment or a procedure. In these cases, you will report the original burn or corrosion code using the seventh character "S," for sequela, to identify that the care and treatment are directed at the late effect of the burn or corrosion.

LO 21.3 Adverse Effects, Poisoning, Underdosing, and Toxic Effects

When an individual comes in contact with a drug or a chemical that has an unhealthy impact, this must be coded. The person might have had an unusual reaction to a medication prescribed by a health care professional or might have been exposed to something noxious. Your first step is to determine whether the patient was **poisoned,** had an **adverse effect** (or reaction), or had a **toxic effect.** Each of these is reported with a code or codes in the range T36–T50.

The type of drug or substance that was responsible for the patient's condition is the first detail identified and will direct you to the correct code category:

> **T36 Poisoning by, adverse effect of, and underdosing of systemic antibiotics**
>
> **T37 . . . of other systemic anti-infectives, and antiparasitics**
>
> **T38 . . . of hormones and their synthetic substitutes and antagonists, not elsewhere classified**
>
> **T39 . . . of nonopioid analgesics, antipyretics and antirheumatics**
>
> **T40 . . . of narcotics and psychodysleptics [hallucinogens]**
>
> **T41 . . . of anesthetics and therapeutic gases**
>
> **T42 . . . of antiepileptic, sedative-hypnotic, and antiparkinsonism drugs**
>
> **T43 . . . of psychotropic drugs, not elsewhere classified**
>
> **T44 . . . of drugs primarily affecting the autonomic nervous system**
>
> **T45 . . . of primarily systemic and hematological agents, not elsewhere classified**
>
> **T46 . . . of agents primarily affecting the cardiovascular system**
>
> **T47 . . . of agents primarily affecting the gastrointestinal system**
>
> **T48 . . . of agents primarily acting on smooth and skeletal muscles and the respiratory system**
>
> **T49 . . . of topical agents primarily affecting skin and mucous membrane and by ophthalmological, otorhinolaryngological, and dental drugs**
>
> **T50 . . . of diuretics and other and unspecified drugs, medicaments, and biological substances**

You can see that these code categories are set up by the classification of drug, rather than generic or brand name of the medication itself. Don't worry. The Table of Drugs and Chemicals will help direct you to the correct code category.

Once you get to the correct code category, you will find that the fourth and fifth characters will enable you to add more specifics about the drug. Then you will need to determine the sixth character that will describe the **intent** of this circumstance—in other words, how the patient came to be affected by this drug or chemical.

Adverse Reaction: Sixth Character 5

Pharmaceuticals (also known as *drugs* or *medications*) are used very often in health care today. They can function as preventive and/or **therapeutic** resources that support positive outcomes for patients. Some drugs are prescribed for patient self-administration (to take at home), while others require the skills of a professional to

---

poisoned
A condition produced by a substance that harms or causes death.

adverse effect
An unexpected bad result; also known as *adverse reaction.*

toxic effect
A health-related reaction caused by a poisonous substance.

intent
The objective or goal of the individual taking the action.

therapeutic
Intended to restore good health or reduce the effect of a disease or negative condition.

be administered. There are circumstances in which a patient may have an unexpected reaction (adverse effect) to a prescribed drug or in which medication may be misused or abused. A patient is diagnosed with an adverse effect, or reaction, when all of the following occur and the patient has an unexpected bad reaction:

- A health care professional correctly prescribes a drug for a patient.
- The correct patient receives the correct drug.
- The correct dosage is given to the patient (or taken by the patient). The correct dosage includes the correct amount in the correct frequency.
- The correct route of administration is used.

Unpredictable reactions can be due to genetic factors, other diseases or allergies, the method of administration of the drug, or other issues. When an adverse reaction has occurred, you will need a minimum of *two codes:*

E = effect: The code or codes will report exactly what reaction or reactions the patient had to the substance, such as a rash, vomiting, or unconsciousness. It might be a confirmed diagnosis of the problem or the signs and/or symptoms experienced by the patient as a result of taking the medicine.

T = type of drug and intent combination code: This code will explain the specific type of drug that the patient took. You can find this code in the Table of Drugs and Chemicals in the column under the heading "Adverse Effect."

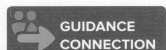

GUIDANCE CONNECTION

Review the ICD-10-CM Coding Guidelines, Section I.C.19, Chapter 19: **Injury, poisoning, and certain other consequences of external causes,** Subsections e, **Adverse effects, poisoning, underdosing, and toxic effects,** and e(5)(a), **Adverse effect,** for more input.

The Five Rights of Drug Administration

This simple list helps remind you of all the components of safely delivering medication to a patient:

1. *Right drug:* the specific pharmaceutical prescribed.
2. *Right dose:* the specific quantity of pharmaceutical prescribed.
3. *Right patient:* the specific individual for whom it was prescribed.
4. *Right time frame (time and frequency):* the specific time schedule (such as every 4 hours or twice a day).
5. *Right route:* the specific route of administration as prescribed.

Administration Routes

When documentation or a codebook refers to the route of administration, it is referring to the delivery method. In other words, how did the professional get the drug into the patient? (See Figure 21-4.)

- *Infusion (INF):* using a mechanism to insert fluid into a vein.
- *Injection (INJ):* using a syringe and needle to insert fluid into the body.
- *Push:* injected into an IV tube that has already been inserted.
- *Buccal (buc):* inside the cheek.
- *Intra-arterial (IA):* into an artery.
- *Intradermal (ID):* into the skin.
- *Intramuscular (IM):* into a muscle.
- *Intranasal (INH):* into the nose.
- *Intrathecal (IT):* into the arachnoid membrane of the brain or spinal cord.
- *Intravenous (IV):* into a vein.
- *Oral (ORAL):* taken by mouth.
- *Percutaneous:* into the skin.

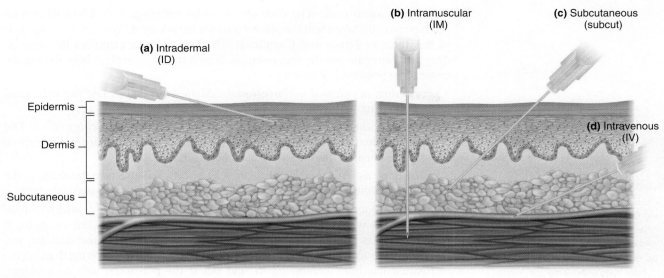

FIGURE 21-4 Injection Routes

Source: Booth et al., MA, 5e. Copyright © 2013 by McGraw-Hill. Figure 53-12, p. 1085

- *Peripherally inserted central venous catheter (PICC):* type of IV catheter that stays in the patient for long-term medication administration.
- *Subcutaneous (SC or sub Q):* into the subcutaneous tissue.
- *Sublingual (SL):* under the tongue.
- *Suppository:* into the rectum (R) or vagina (vag).

Poisoning

Most people think of poisoning as something from a great detective novel or movie. However, poisoning can happen under many different circumstances. In reality, when a person comes in contact with a chemical or drug (not prescribed by a physician or not taken as prescribed) and a health problem results, it is called a *poisoning.* The substance can be ingested, inhaled, absorbed through the skin, injected, or taken by some other method. When a poisoning occurs, you will need a minimum of *two codes:*

E = effect: The code or codes will report exactly what result the poison had on the patient. It might be a confirmed diagnosis of the problem or the signs and/or symptoms experienced by the patient as a result of taking the medicine.

T = type and intent code: The code chosen from the range T36–T50 will explain the type of drug taken and the patient's intent for taking it. You can find the code in the Table of Drugs and Chemicals. The first column identifies the specific drug or chemical, and the five columns across the page explain how the patient came to be poisoned. Was it a:

- *Poisoning, accidental (unintentional)? Sixth character 1.* Did the individual take the drug by mistake? Or possibly take too much by mistake?
- *Poisoning, intentional self-harm (attempted suicide)? Sixth character 2.* Did the individual take the drug, or the wrong amount of the drug, on purpose with the intent of causing himself or herself harm?
- *Poisoning, assault? Sixth character 3.* Did someone else give the drug, or the wrong quantity of the drug, to the patient with the intent of causing harm?
- *Poisoning, undetermined? Sixth character 4.* You may use *undetermined* in cases in which it is impossible to determine the intent. For example, if the patient is brought into the emergency department (ED) unconscious, you might have to wait until the patient regains consciousness or until an investigation has been completed to find out if the poisoning was an accident, assault, or attempted suicide. *Never assume.* Therefore, undetermined would be the correct code.
- *Underdosing? Sixth character 6.* Did the individual take too little of the drug, thereby preventing the desired effect of the drug?

Again, the Table of Drugs and Chemicals will help you find the most accurate external cause code.

The Table of Drugs and Chemicals

Often located directly after the alphabetical listing in Volume 2 is Section 2, the Table of **Drugs** and **Chemicals** (see Figure 21-5). (*Note:* Different published versions of the ICD-10-CM book may place sections in a different order. Therefore, Section 2 of Volume 2 may be in a different location in your book.) The Table of Drugs and Chemicals is used when a drug or chemical caused an adverse reaction, poisoned the patient, or caused a toxic effect. Similar to the Neoplasm Table, the Table of Drugs and Chemicals is organized in columns.

Drug and Chemical Names

The first column of the table lists the names of drugs and chemicals, in alphabetic order. The list includes prescription medications, over-the-counter medications, household and industrial chemicals, and many other items with a chemical basis. Aspirin, indigestion relief medication, drugstore-brand allergy relievers, alcohol (for drinking or sterilization), window cleaner, battery acid, and lots of other similar substances are included, as well as medications prescribed by a physician.

Sometimes, it is easy to find what you're looking for. For example, Giselle had a bad reaction to Nytol. Even though *Nytol* is the brand name of an over-the-counter sleep medication, you will find it easily in the list of substances in the first column of the Table of Drugs and Chemicals.

Other times, it may not be this easy, and the name—whether brand name, generic name, or chemical name—that is documented in the physician's notes may not be in the table. If you don't find it, you may have to do some research. Some of the drugs and chemicals are listed by their brand or common names, such as Metamucil or Nytol. Others are listed by their chemical or generic names, such as barbiturates (sedatives). If you are not certain, consult a ***Physicians' Desk Reference* (PDR),** a group of books that list all the approved drugs, herbal remedies, and over-the-counter medications by brand name, chemical name, generic name, and drug category.

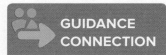

GUIDANCE CONNECTION

Review the ICD-10-CM Coding Guidelines, Section I.C.19, Chapter 19: **Injury, poisoning, and certain other consequences of external causes,** Subsections e, **Adverse effects, poisoning, underdosing, and toxic effects,** and e(5) (b), **Poisoning,** for more input.

drugs
Substances, natural or combined, created to treat or prevent illness or disease. Examples include aspirin, Lipitor, and Prozac.

chemicals
Substances used in, or made by, the process of chemistry. Examples include benzene, turpentine, and bleach.

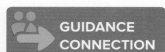

GUIDANCE CONNECTION

Review the ICD-10-CM Coding Guidelines, Section I.C.19, Chapter 19: **Injury, poisoning, and certain other consequences of external causes,** Subsections e, **Adverse effects, poisoning, underdosing, and toxic effects,** and e(1), **Do not code directly from the Table of Drugs,** for more input.

***Physicians' Desk Reference* (PDR)**
A series of reference books identifying all aspects of prescription and over-the-counter medications, as well as herbal remedies.

ICD-10-CM TABLE of DRUGS and CHEMICALS

#|A|B|C|D|E|F|G|H|I|J|K|L|M|N|O|P|Q|R|S|T|U|V|W|X|Y|Z

Substance	Poisoning, Accidental (unintentional)	Poisoning, Intentional self-harm	Poisoning, Assault	Poisoning, Undetermined	Adverse effect	Underdosing
#						
1-propanol	T51.3X1	T51.3X2	T51.3X3	T51.3X4	--	--
2-propanol	T51.2X1	T51.2X2	T51.2X3	T51.2X4	--	--
2,4-D(dichlorophen-oxyacetic acid)	T60.3X1	T60.3X2	T60.3X3	T60.3X4	--	--
2,4-toluene diisocyanate	T65.0X1	T65.0X2	T65.0X3	T65.0X4	--	--
2,4,5-T(trichloro-phenoxyacetic acid)	T60.1X1	T60.1X2	T60.1X3	T60.1X4	--	--
14-hydroxydihydro-morphinone	T40.2X1	T40.2X2	T40.2X3	T40.2X4	T40.2X5	T40.2X6
A						
ABOB	T37.5X1	T37.5X2	T37.5X3	T37.5X4	T37.5X5	T37.5X6
Abrine	T62.2X1	T62.2X2	T62.2X3	T62.2X4	--	--
Abrus(seed)	T62.2X1	T62.2X2	T62.2X3	T62.2X4	--	--
Absinthe	T51.0X1	T51.0X2	T51.0X3	T51.0X4	--	--
- beverage	T51.0X1	T51.0X2	T51.0X3	T51.0X4	--	--
Acaricide	T60.8X1	T60.8X2	T60.8X3	T60.8X4	--	--
Acebutolol	T44.7X1	T44.7X2	T44.7X3	T44.7X4	T44.7X5	T44.7X6
Acecarbromal	T42.6X1	T42.6X2	T42.6X3	T42.6X4	T42.6X5	T42.6X6
Aceclidine	T44.1X1	T44.1X2	T44.1X3	T44.1X4	T44.1X5	T44.1X6
Acedapsone	T37.0X1	T37.0X2	T37.0X3	T37.0X4	T37.0X5	T37.0X6
Acefylline piperazine	T48.6X1	T48.6X2	T48.6X3	T48.6X4	T48.6X5	T48.6X6
Acemorphan	T40.2X1	T40.2X2	T40.2X3	T40.2X4	T40.2X5	T40.2X6
Acenocoumarin	T45.511	T45.512	T45.513	T45.514	T45.515	T45.516
Acenocoumarol	T45.511	T45.512	T45.513	T45.514	T45.515	T45.516
Acepifylline	T48.6X1	T48.6X2	T48.6X3	T48.6X4	T48.6X5	T48.6X6
Acepromazine	T43.3X1	T43.3X2	T43.3X3	T43.3X4	T43.3X5	T43.3X6
Acesulfamethoxypyridazine	T37.0X1	T37.0X2	T37.0X3	T37.0X4	T37.0X5	T37.0X6
Acetal	T52.8X1	T52.8X2	T52.8X3	T52.8X4	--	--
Acetaldehyde(vapor)	T52.8X1	T52.8X2	T52.8X3	T52.8X4	--	--
- liquid	T65.891	T65.892	T65.893	T65.894	--	--
P-Acetamidophenol	T39.1X1	T39.1X2	T39.1X3	T39.1X4	T39.1X5	T39.1X6
Acetaminophen	T39.1X1	T39.1X2	T39.1X3	T39.1X4	T39.1X5	T39.1X6
Acetaminosalol	T39.1X1	T39.1X2	T39.1X3	T39.1X4	T39.1X5	T39.1X6
Acetanilide	T39.1X1	T39.1X2	T39.1X3	T39.1X4	T39.1X5	T39.1X6
Acetarsol	T37.3X1	T37.3X2	T37.3X3	T37.3X4	T37.3X5	T37.3X6
Acetazolamide	T50.2X1	T50.2X2	T50.2X3	T50.2X4	T50.2X5	T50.2X6
Acetiamine	T45.2X1	T45.2X2	T45.2X3	T45.2X4	T45.2X5	T45.2X6
Acetic						
- acid	T54.2X1	T54.2X2	T54.2X3	T54.2X4	--	--
- - with sodium acetate(ointment)	T49.3X1	T49.3X2	T49.3X3	T49.3X4	T49.3X5	T49.3X6
- - ester(solvent)(vapor)	T52.8X1	T52.8X2	T52.8X3	T52.8X4	--	--
- - irrigating solution	T50.3X1	T50.3X2	T50.3X3	T50.3X4	T50.3X5	T50.3X6
- - medicinal(lotion)	T49.2X1	T49.2X2	T49.2X3	T49.2X4	T49.2X5	T49.2X6
- anhydride	T65.891	T65.892	T65.893	T65.894	--	--

FIGURE 21-5 ICD-10-CM Table of Drugs and Chemicals

Vesicare—the brand name.
Solifenacin succinate—the generic or chemical name.
Muscarinic receptor antagonist—the drug category.
Anticholinergic—the general drug category.

In our example, you can see Vesicare is shown as the trade or brand name. The generic or chemical name is solifenacin succinate. If a physician prescribed it for a patient, who then had an adverse reaction or took an overdose, you would most likely see one or the other of those names in the notes. However, you will find neither of them listed in the Table of Drugs and Chemicals. The next piece of information given to you by the PDR is found in the description of the drug: muscarinic receptor antagonist. Unfortunately, there is nothing in the table under *muscarinic* either. Because the patient either had an adverse reaction or had taken an overdose, take a look at the following paragraphs from PDR:

ADVERSE REACTIONS

. . . Expected side effects of antimuscarinic agents . . .

OVERDOSAGE

. . . Overdosage with Vesicare can potentially result in severe *anticholinergic* effects . . .

The two paragraphs provide us with two new descriptors for the drug: antimuscarinic and anticholinergic. Both of them are shown in the Table of Drugs and Chemicals and, interestingly, lead you to the same codes.

LET'S CODE IT! SCENARIO

Jesse Winthrop found an unmarked barrel in the back of the warehouse where he works. He opened the top and leaned over to see what was inside. Vapors from the benzene solvent being stored in that barrel overcame Jesse. He had difficulty breathing. He was taken to the doctor immediately. Dr. Stang diagnosed Jesse with respiratory distress syndrome, a toxic effect from inhaling the benzene, but it was an accident.

Let's Code It!

Jesse had *a toxic effect from inhaling the benzene*. The notes also state that Jesse had *respiratory distress*. You learned that you need at least two codes: toxic effect + external cause code.

The first code identifies the chemical or substance and intent. In Jesse's case, the substance was the vapor from a barrel of benzene solvent. Turn to the Alphabetic Index's Table of Drugs and Chemicals. Look down the first column and find *benzene:*

Benzene

    Homologues (acetyl) (dimethyl) (methyl) (solvent)

You know from the documentation that this was an accidental poisoning, so look across the line to the first column titled "Poisoning, Accidental (Unintentional)":

Benzene   T52.1x1

    Homologues (acetyl) (dimethyl) (methyl) (solvent)   T52.2x1

Hmm. It can be difficult to know what was in that barrel. You can get more information from the Tabular List and see if that helps. Start at the three-character number and be certain to check any notations or directives:

T52 Toxic effect of organic solvents

Be sure to read the *Excludes1* notation. Does it relate to Jesse's diagnosis? No. Good! There are the seventh-character options for later, but first you must determine the rest of the code, so keep reading down the column:

T52.1 Toxic effects of benzene

T52.2 Toxic effects of homologues of benzene

Homologues are not mentioned in the documentation, so review the options for fifth and sixth characters under T52.1:

T52.1x1 Toxic effects of benzene, accidental (unintentional)

Remember, you need to include the seventh character.

T52.1x1A Toxic effects of benzene, accidental (unintentional), initial encounter

Great! You now have the first-listed code for Jesse's encounter.

The next code reports the *effect* that the benzene vapors had on Jesse. The notes state he had respiratory distress. In the main section of the Alphabetic Index, find:

Distress

Respiratory R06.00

Adult J80

Hmm. Again, you have a choice to make. Look up both codes in the Tabular List and compare them:

J80 Acute respiratory distress syndrome

R06.00 Dyspnea, unspecified

Which code description matches Dr. Stang's notes? J80 matches.

Two more codes—remember, you also need external cause codes to report where the accident occurred and Jesse's status (why he was doing this). In the Index to External Causes, turn to "Place of occurrence." The notes state that Jesse was in a warehouse when this accident happened, so read down the list, and you will see:

Place of occurrence

Warehouse Y92.59

Go to the Tabular List, beginning with the code category:

Y92 Place of occurrence of the external cause

Read down the column to review your choices for the required fourth character.

Y92.59 Other trade areas as the place of occurrence of the external cause (warehouse as the place of occurrence of the external cause)

Your last code will report Jesse's status. You know he was at work, so you will use code:

Y99.0 Civilian activity done for income or pay

This completes the report.

T52.1x1A Toxic effects of benzene, accidental (unintentional), initial encounter

J80 Acute respiratory distress syndrome

Y92.59 Other trade areas as the place of occurrence of the external cause (warehouse as the place of occurrence of the external cause)

Y99.0 Civilian activity done for income or pay

You are really becoming a great coder!

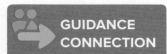

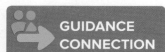

Patient Noncompliance

Sometimes, a patient has an adverse effect because he or she did not take the medication as ordered by the physician or didn't take the drugs at all. When taking too little of the quantity prescribed (known as **underdosing**) is the will of the patient, rather than an error on the part of a health care professional, this is considered noncompliance and is reported with an additional code to explain intent:

Z91.12- Patient's intentional underdosing of medication regimen

Z91.13- Patient's unintentional underdosing of medication regimen

Z91.14- Patient's other noncompliance with medication regimen

Substance Interactions

When the cause of the poisoning or toxic effect is the **interaction** between two substances (e.g., drugs and alcohol), then you will need to report both substances involved. You will need one poisoning code for *each* substance causing the reaction, one or more codes to accurately report the effect of the interaction, and one external cause code to report the intent for *each* substance.

LO 21.4 Abuse, Neglect, and Maltreatment

Some people treat other people terribly. Such treatment may be physical or sexual **abuse,** neglect, or abandonment. Often, people consider unacceptable behavior as being directed toward a child, yet adults also are abused, neglected, and maltreated. As our elder population increases, these adults are also vulnerable and need health care professionals to watch out for them and protect them.

T74 Adult and child abuse, neglect, and other maltreatment, confirmed

T76 Adult and child abuse, neglect, and other maltreatment, suspected

O9A.3 Physical abuse complicating pregnancy, childbirth and the puerperium

O9A.4 Sexual abuse complicating pregnancy, childbirth and the puerperium

O9A.5 Psychological abuse complicating pregnancy, childbirth and the puerperium

Z04.4 Encounter for examination and observation following alleged rape

Z04.7 Encounter for examination and observation following alleged physical abuse

The difference between categories T74 and T76 is important and is determined by the documentation: category T74 reports that the physician knows (confirms) this situation; category T76 records a suspicion. You know that suspected conditions are generally not coded and reported. However, most states require health care professionals to report any instances of abuse or neglect, even if it is just a suspicion at this point.

When applicable, the code from T74 or T76 should be the first-listed or principal diagnosis, followed by the injury code and/or mental health code. For cases in which the circumstances have been confirmed, a code to report the specific cause of the injury should be included, most often from code range X92–Y08. In any case of abuse, neglect, or maltreatment, if the perpetrator is known, an additional code from category Y07 should be included.

CODING TIP

Interactions can occur between two or more drugs, drugs and alcohol or other drinks, drugs and food, or many other combinations. For example, you might notice a warning "Do not take this drug with milk or other dairy products." This is a warning provided to prevent an interaction.

LO 21.5 Complications of Care (T80–T88)

Even though medical procedures and the standards of care are heavily researched and tested, things can go wrong. Complications can occur for any number of reasons. Before a condition can be coded as a "complication of care," the documentation must specifically identify the cause-and-effect relationship between the health care procedure, service, or treatment and the current condition that is noted as a complication.

Pain caused by medical devices and grafts previously implanted is reported with a code from categories T80–T88 (such as T82.847A, Pain from cardiac prosthetic devices, implants and grafts, initial encounter), along with either code G89.18, Other acute postprocedural pain, or G89.28, Other chronic postprocedural pain, as appropriate.

As you might imagine, transplanting an organ from one individual to another is a complex surgical accomplishment and saves thousands of lives. When a complication of the transplantation has been documented, a code from category T86, Complications of transplanted organs and tissue, should be reported, followed by a second code to specify the complication itself.

Not all intraprocedural or postprocedural complications are reported from code categories T80–T88. They may be reported with codes from any chapter of the code set. The Alphabetic Index will guide you.

GUIDANCE CONNECTION

Review the ICD-10-CM Coding Guidelines, Section I.B.16, **Documentation of complications of care,** as well as Section I.C.19, Chapter 19: **Injury, poisoning, and certain other consequences of external causes,** Subsection g, **Complications of care,** for more input.

EXAMPLE

J95.2 Acute pulmonary insufficiency following non-thoracic surgery
K91.840 Postprocedural hemorrhage and hematoma of a digestive system organ or structure following a digestive system procedure

LO 21.6 External Cause Codes

When a patient has been injured traumatically, been poisoned, had an adverse reaction, or been abused or neglected, or harmed in another way as a result of an external cause, you will need to report the details of the event so that you tell the whole story. In addition to the other codes, you will also need to report codes that explain:

- *Cause of the injury,* such as a car accident or a fall off a ladder.
- *Place of the occurrence,* such as the park or the kitchen.
- *Activity during the occurrence,* such as playing basketball or gardening.
- *Patient's status,* such as paid employment, on-duty military, or leisure activity.

Refer to Chapter 16 to remind yourself about reporting external cause codes whenever you are reporting an injury or poisoning.

Chapter Summary

People burn themselves in many different ways under many different circumstances every day. Such patients may go to their family physician's office, the emergency department, a dermatologist, or a plastic surgeon. Burn injuries may be resolved quickly or may cause pain and suffering for the patient for years, resulting in infections, scarring, and other conditions. A professional coding specialist must be able to report burn situations accurately.

Individuals can come into contact with a substance that disagrees with their body chemistry for many reasons. An allergic reaction, the accidental ingestion of too many pills, depression leading to a suicide attempt, environmental factors—any of these and more can cause a person to suffer a health-related incident. Adverse effects, poisonings, and toxic effects can be very serious to the health of an individual. Complex chemical interactions in the human body equate to complex coding processes to accurately report what has happened.

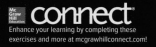

Using Terminology

Match each key term to the appropriate definition.

Part One

_____ **1.** LO 21.1 Injury in which layers of skin are traumatically torn away from the body.

_____ **2.** LO 21.2 Redness of the epidermis (skin).

_____ **3.** LO 21.2 A burn caused by a chemical; chemical destruction of the skin.

_____ **4.** LO 21.3 Substances used in, or made by, the process of chemistry.

_____ **5.** LO 21.2 Destruction of all layers of the skin, with possible involvement of the subcutaneous fat, muscle, and bone.

_____ **6.** LO 21.2 Injury by heat or fire.

_____ **7.** LO 21.2 The level of seriousness.

_____ **8.** LO 21.2 Blisters on the skin; involvement of the epidermis and the dermis layers.

_____ **9.** LO 21.2 A general division of the whole body into sections that each represent 9%; used for estimating the extent of a burn.

_____ **10.** LO 21.1 Damage to the epidermal and dermal layers of the skin made by a sharp object.

_____ **11.** LO 21.2 The location on or in the human body; the anatomical part.

A. Avulsion

B. Burn

C. Chemicals

D. Corrosion

E. First degree

F. Laceration

G. Rule of nines

H. Second degree

I. Severity

J. Site

K. Third degree

Part Two

_____ **1.** LO 21.3 A series of reference books identifying all aspects of prescription and over-the-counter medications, as well as herbal remedies.

_____ **2.** LO 21.2 The percentage of the body that has been affected by the burn or corrosion.

_____ **3.** LO 21.3 An unexpected bad result; also known as *adverse reaction.*

_____ **4.** LO 21.3 A health-related reaction caused by a poisonous substance.

_____ **5.** LO 21.3 Taking too little of the drug, thereby preventing the desired effect.

_____ **6.** LO 21.4 This term is used in different manners: (a) extreme use of a drug or chemical; (b) violent and/or inappropriate treatment of another person.

_____ **7.** LO 21.3 A condition produced by a substance that harms or causes death.

_____ **8.** LO 21.3 The objective or goal of the individual taking the action.

_____ **9.** LO 21.3 Substances, natural or combined, created to treat or prevent illness or disease.

_____ **10.** LO 21.3 Intended to restore good health or reduce the effect of a disease or negative condition.

_____ **11.** LO 21.3 A mixture of two or more substances that changes the effect of any of the individual substances.

A. Abuse

B. Adverse effect

C. Drugs

D. Extent

E. Intent

F. Interaction

G. *Physicians' Desk Reference* (PDR)

H. Poisoned

I. Therapeutic

J. Toxic effect

K. Underdosing

Checking Your Understanding

Choose the most appropriate answer for each of the following questions.

1. LO 21.1 A(n) _____ is damage to the epidermal and dermal layers of the skin made by a sharp object.

   a. contusion.
   b. avulsion.
   c. laceration.
   d. bite.

2. LO 21.1 A bruise or black-and-blue mark is known as a(n)

   a. contusion.
   b. avulsion.
   c. puncture.
   d. bite.

3. LO 21.1 How would you code an avulsion of the scalp?

   a. S01.01XA.
   b. S08.0XXA.
   c. S00.03XA.
   d. S01.03XA.

4. LO 21.2 When you are coding burns, the first-listed code(s) will identify

   a. the percentage of body surface area affected.
   b. the age of the patient.
   c. how the injury occurred.
   d. the site and severity.

5. LO 21.2 Erythema indicates that the epidermis is

   a. necrotic.
   b. blistered.
   c. red.
   d. removed.

6. LO 21.2 An example of a late effect of a burn is

   a. malunion.
   b. scar.
   c. infection.
   d. epidermal loss.

7. LO 21.2 A third-degree burn of the cheek, subsequent encounter, would be coded with which of the following?

   a. T20.36XS.
   b. S01.411A.
   c. S00.83XS.
   d. T20.16XA.

8. LO 21.3 Drugs and chemicals are listed in the Table of Drugs and Chemicals in all of the following manners *except*

   a. the brand name.
   b. the chemical name.
   c. the drug category.
   d. the size of the dose.

9. LO 21.3 The Table of Drugs and Chemicals does not include a specific listing for

    a. lettuce opium.
    b. adhesives.
    c. marsh gas.
    d. vodka.

10. LO 21.3 The columns in the ICD-10-CM Table of Drugs and Chemicals include

    a. Intentional Self-Harm.
    b. malignant.
    c. toxin.
    d. Ca in situ.

Applying Your Knowledge

1. LO 21.1 List four types of traumatic wounds. _____

_____

2. LO 21.2 Explain the difference between a burn and a corrosion to any part of the body. _____

_____

3. LO 21.2 What does the acronym *S/S.E.E.* mean in relation to a burn? What details does it help you remember? _____

_____

4. LO 21.2 How do you identify the severity of burns? Include the description of each stage. _____

_____

5. LO 21.3 Differentiate among adverse effects, poisoning, and toxic effects. _____

_____

6. LO 21.3 What are the five rights of drug administration, and what does each component represent? _____

_____

7. LO 21.3 List six different drug administration routes. _____

_____

8. LO 21.3 Explain patient noncompliance and the different codes that represent noncompliance. _____

_____

9. LO 21.3 What is substance interaction, and how is it coded? _____

_____

Using the techniques described in this chapter, carefully read through the case studies and determine the most accurate ICD-10-CM code(s) and external cause code(s), if appropriate, for each case study.

1. Alfred Rogers, a 15-year-old male, is brought in today by his uncle. Alfred is spending the summer on his uncle's farm. This morning Alfred was milking the cow in the barn, barefoot, and stepped on a nail. Dr. Case thoroughly examines and cleans the site and diagnoses Alfred with a superficial puncture wound to the central part of the plantar aponeurosis, right foot, without foreign body.

   _____

2. Karen Anne Washington, a 6-year-old female, was brought into her pediatrician's office by her mother because Karen is having trouble swallowing. After a thorough examination and the appropriate tests, Dr. Lakemont diagnoses her with a stricture of the esophagus. Karen admitted that her stepfather forced her to drink lye, confirmed by local police.

   _____

3. Steven Harris, a 16-year-old male, is on his school's baseball team. Today at practice, Steven was covering first base and missed catching the ball thrown to him from home plate. The ball hit him in the eye. After a few minutes, Steven began to have trouble opening his eye and the coach brought him to see Dr. Kinlaw. After the examination, Dr. Kinlaw diagnoses Steven with a contusion of the eyelid and periocular area, left eye.

   _____

4. Billy Selas, a 3-year-old male, was brought to the ED by his parents. Billy was found unconscious with an empty bottle of his mother's oral contraceptives next to him. Dr. Daniels, the ED physician, notes Pt is in a coma and has begun to blink his eyes spontaneously.

   _____

5. Kelly Carrison, a 28-year-old female, presents today with a cut on her left hand. Kelly stated that she was preparing lunch in her kitchen at home for her daughter and cut her hand with a knife while slicing a tomato. After the wound is cleaned and no foreign body found, Dr. Garwood diagnoses Kelly with a laceration of the left hand.

   _____

6. Maurice Goodwin, a 5-year-old male, was carried into the ED by his parents due to extreme weakness. Dr. Hearn, the ED on-call pediatrician, examined Maurice and found a chip of paint in his mouth; blood tests show that he was poisoned by

eating the lead paint. Maurice's father admits that the house garage has old lead paint and Maurice likes to play his drums there.

_____

7. Roger Dennis, a 43-year-old male, was found unconscious in his car, which was parked in his house garage. The garage door was closed, and the motor was running. At the emergency room, Dr. Lexington determined that Roger was in a coma due to carbon monoxide poisoning. Paramedics found a suicide note next to Roger on the seat of the car.

_____

8. Bruce Meredith, a 32-year-old male, was landscaping in his home's backyard, and when he finished, he decided to burn the trash. He was almost done when he accidentally stepped on hot coals. Dr. Dillard diagnoses Bruce with a second-degree burn of the left foot.

_____

9. Edward Webber, a 63-year-old male, was at the Benton Medical Center when he suffered a terrible attack of vertigo after being injected with dye for an intravenous pyelogram that his physician had ordered.

_____

10. Jeannette Lyman, a 33-year-old female, comes in today with abdominal pain and nausea. Jeannette stated that she has been taking Motrin over the last few days for general body aches. Dr. Trevani completes a thorough examination and diagnoses her with acute gastritis due to accidental overdose of Motrin.

_____

11. Belle Delong, a 16-year-old female, presents today weak and tired. Belle is trying to lose weight for the prom and admits to taking laxatives; she didn't realize the potential hazards. After an examination and the appropriate tests, she was diagnosed with a vitamin deficiency.

_____

12. Helen Yeager, a 48-year-old female, came home after work today, and when she opened the back door, she said it seemed to smell of hot electricity. A few minutes later her house was on fire and collapsed around her. Helen was taken to the ER, where she was diagnosed with deep third-degree burns on her left forearm. She was taken to the operating room to have her forearm amputated as a result of the burns.

_____

13. Kyle Ketterson, a 15-year-old male, was swimming at the beach and was accidentally stung by a jellyfish. He presents today with a wound on his right thigh. After an examination, Dr. Waters diagnoses Kyle with a jellyfish sting.

_____

14. Gary Monroe, a 16-year-old male, is on his high school volleyball team. At practice today, at the outdoor volleyball court, Gary took his shirt off. Later that afternoon Gary felt like he was having chills, and his torso was red, itchy, and painful to touch. When Gary got home, he was brought to the ER by his mother. The on-call ER physician performed a thorough examination and diagnosed Gary with second-degree sunburn due to overexposure of the sun.

_____

15. Kenneth Caine, a 9-year-old male, is brought in today by his father. Ken burned his forehead while playing with a cigarette lighter in his bedroom at home yesterday. He did not tell his parents when it happened because he was afraid of getting in trouble and just covered the wound with his hair. His hair gel caused the burn to get infected, and it became so painful he had to tell his father. After a thorough examination, Dr. DuBois diagnosed Ken with a second-degree burn to the forehead.

_____

The following exercises provide practice in abstracting physicians' notes and learning to work with SOAP notes from our health care facility, *Taylor, Reader, & Associates.* These case studies (SOAP notes) are modeled on real patient encounters. Using the techniques described in this chapter, carefully read through the case studies and determine the most accurate ICD-10-CM code(s) and external cause code(s), if appropriate, for each case study.

TAYLOR, READER, & ASSOCIATES
A Complete Health Care Facility
975 CENTRAL AVENUE • SOMEWHERE, FL 32811 • 407-555-4321

PATIENT: McCOY, DARLENE
ACCOUNT/EHR #:   MCCODA001
DATE: 09/16/18

Attending Physician: Suzanne R. Taylor, MD

S: This new Pt is a 33-year-old female who works for the landscaping crew of the city parks department. Pyrethrin insecticide was sprayed, after which she spent the last 2 days trimming and working in the flower beds in Central Park. She has since developed blisters and a bleeding rash on her arms and lower legs.

O: Ht 5′5″ Wt. 147 lb. R 16. Pt's skin is blistered and raw, painful to the touch. Rash begins at the shin, directly above the sock line, and on the hands and lower portion of the arms, indicating a contact dermatitis.

A: Blistering rash due to exposure to pyrethrin insecticide

P: 1. Rx oxaprozin
    2. Note to workplace to eliminate outdoor duties for 3 weeks
    3. Return for follow-up in 1 week

Suzanne R. Taylor, MD

SRT/pw   D: 9/16/18 09:50:16   T: 9/18/18 12:55:01

Determine the most accurate ICD-10-CM code(s).

_____

_____

_____

TAYLOR, READER, & ASSOCIATES
A Complete Health Care Facility
975 CENTRAL AVENUE • SOMEWHERE, FL 32811 • 407-555-4321

PATIENT: HINSON, GAYLE
ACCOUNT/EHR #:   HINSGA001
DATE: 09/16/18

Attending Physician: Suzanne R. Taylor, MD

S: This new Pt is a 25-year-old female who presents with splatter burns on the back of her right hand and her right cheek. She stated that she was deep-frying shrimp for a dinner party at her home in the kitchen and the grease splattered up unexpectedly.

O: Ht 5′5″ Wt. 149 lb. R 16. Skin is red and blistered on both sites. There is some epidermal loss. Area was cleansed with antiseptic, and ointment was applied before a clean gauze bandage was put on the hand. The facial area was also cleansed and bandaged.

A: Second-degree burns to back of hand, and face

P: 1. Rx Aspirin for pain, prn
    2. Return in 1 week for dressing change.

_____

Suzanne R. Taylor, MD

SRT/pw   D: 9/16/18 09:50:16   T: 9/18/18 12:55:01

Determine the most accurate ICD-10-CM code(s).

_____

_____

_____

TAYLOR, READER, & ASSOCIATES
A Complete Health Care Facility
975 CENTRAL AVENUE • SOMEWHERE, FL 32811 • 407-555-4321

PATIENT: GONZALES, GRACE
ACCOUNT/EHR #: GONZGR001
DATE: 09/16/18

Attending Physician: Willard B. Reader, MD

S: Pt is a 39-year-old female who has been trying to stop drinking alcohol. She states that she went 3 months without a drink and has been taking Librium as prescribed to assist with the anxiety and other effects of alcohol withdrawal. Last night, she went on a binge and drank vodka. She came in today because she has been experiencing chest pains. Pt states she did not know that drinking while on the Librium would really be a problem.

O: Ht 5'11" Wt. 203 lb. R 20. T 98.6. BP 140/95. EKG indicates a cardiac arrhythmia.

A: Cardiac arrhythmia as a result of alcohol and drug interaction

P: 1. Pt to return PRN
   2. Referral to counseling

Willard B. Reader, MD

WBR/pw   D: 09/16/18 09:50:16   T: 09/18/18 12:55:01

Determine the most accurate ICD-10-CM code(s).

_____

_____

_____

TAYLOR, READER, & ASSOCIATES
A Complete Health Care Facility
975 CENTRAL AVENUE • SOMEWHERE, FL 32811 • 407-555-4321

PATIENT: TRINDLE, TRACY
ACCOUNT/EHR #:   TRINTR001
DATE: 09/16/18

Attending Physician: Willard B. Reader, MD

S: Pt is a 3-year-old female brought in by ambulance with her mother. The mother told me that the child pulled the cord on the iron while it was turned on and sitting on the ironing board in their apartment bedroom. The child was crying violently.

O: Upon examination, we counted 15 triangle-shaped burns, evidently from the front end of the iron, on the child's chest wall, legs, buttocks, and hands. The burn on the buttocks was a third-degree burn, probably the first one inflicted. The rest are second-degree burns.

A: Third-degree burn of the buttocks; second-degree burns of chest wall, anterior lower right leg (multiple sites), and the palm of her right hand.

P: 1. Referral to burn therapy unit
   2. Child abuse hotline is notified

_____

Willard B. Reader, MD

WBR/pw   D: 09/16/18 09:50:16   T: 09/18/18 12:55:01

Determine the most accurate ICD-10-CM code(s).

_____

_____

_____

TAYLOR, READER, & ASSOCIATES
A Complete Health Care Facility
975 CENTRAL AVENUE • SOMEWHERE, FL 32811 • 407-555-4321

PATIENT: DIAZ, PAULA
ACCOUNT/EHR #:   DIAZPA001
DATE: 09/16/18

Attending Physician: Suzanne R. Taylor, MD

S: This new Pt is a 31-year-old female who was seen 2 days ago for a UTI caused by exposure to *E. coli.* Today, she presents with an acute rash all over her body. She states that she has been taking the Gantanol, according to instructions, as prescribed for her infection for the last 2 days. The rash became evident the night before last. She waited, hoping that the rash would go away. She came in today because it got worse, not better.

O: Ht 5′5″ Wt. 147 lb. R 16. Upon examination, it is suspected that the patient is having an allergic reaction to the sulfonamides. Patient is given an injection of antihistamine and given a new prescription. She is told to immediately discontinue the Gantanol.

A: Rash—reaction to sulfonamides

P: Return PRN

_____

Suzanne R. Taylor, MD

SRT/pw   D: 9/16/18 09:50:16   T: 9/18/18 12:55:01

Determine the most accurate ICD-10-CM code(s).

_____

_____

_____

22

FACTORS INFLUENCING HEALTH STATUS AND CONTACT WITH HEALTH SERVICES

Learning Outcomes *After completing this chapter, the student should be able to:*

LO 22.1 Abstract details about preventive services.

LO 22.2 Determine reasons for early detection.

LO 22.3 Demonstrate how to report encounters related to genetic susceptibility.

LO 22.4 Accurately report the reasons for observation services.

LO 22.5 Apply the Official Guidelines for reporting aftercare and follow-up care.

LO 22.6 Interpret documentation for reporting obstetrics and neonatal exams.

LO 22.7 Distinguish indications of antimicrobial drug resistance.

LO 22.8 Employ Z codes accurately.

Key Terms

Abnormal findings

Allogeneic

Autologous

Carrier

Isogeneic

Preventive care

Prosthetic

Screening

Xenogeneic

In Chapter 2, you got an overview of Z codes, which are codes used to report a reason for a visit to a physician for something other than an illness or injury. As you have learned, there must always be a valid, medical reason for a patient's encounter with a health care professional. And there are occasions for patients to seek attention even when they are not currently ill. These codes give you the opportunity to explain.

LO 22.1 Preventive Care

Science and research have provided us with a better understanding of disease and disease progression, as well as etiology (underlying cause of disease). This knowledge has evolved into improved **preventive care** services to stop the onset of illness or injury.

The provision of these services is likely to increase. The enacting of the Affordable Care Act enables more patients to take advantage of more preventive services than ever before. Since September 2010, new health insurance policies must cover preventive services (see Box 22-1), with no copayment, no coinsurance payments, and no requirement for deductible fulfillment.

Reporting the provision of preventive care will require a Z code to explain the specific reason for the encounter, such as a flu shot or measles vaccination (Z23, Encounter for immunization).

The physician or other health care professional may also be able to provide counseling for the patient and/or family members. This type of counseling is not the same as that provided by a psychiatrist or psychologist; instead, the physician would take the time to discuss options for preventing

BOX 22-1 Free Preventive Services under Affordable Care Act

All marketplace plans and many other plans must cover the following list of preventive services without charging you a copayment or coinsurance. This is true even if you haven't met your yearly deductible. This applies only when these services are delivered by a network provider.

1. *Abdominal aortic aneurysm one-time screening* for men of specified ages who have ever smoked.
2. *Alcohol misuse screening and counseling.*
3. *Aspirin use* to prevent cardiovascular disease for men and women of certain ages.
4. *Blood pressure screening* for all adults.
5. *Cholesterol screening* for adults of certain ages or at higher risk.
6. *Colorectal cancer screening* for adults over 50.
7. *Depression screening* for adults.
8. *Diabetes (Type 2) screening* for adults with high blood pressure.
9. *Diet counseling* for adults at higher risk for chronic disease.
10. *HIV screening* for everyone ages 15 to 65, and other ages at increased risk.
11. *Immunization vaccines* for adults—doses, recommended ages, and recommended populations vary:
    - Hepatitis A
    - Hepatitis B
    - Herpes zoster
    - Human papillomavirus
    - Influenza (flu shot)
    - Measles
    - Mumps
    - Rubella
    - Meningococcal
    - Pneumococcal
    - Tetanus
    - Diphtheria
    - Pertussis
    - Varicella
12. *Obesity screening and counseling* for all adults.
13. *Sexually transmitted infection (STI) prevention counseling* for adults at higher risk.
14. *Syphilis screening* for all adults at higher risk.
15. *Tobacco use screening* for all adults and cessation interventions for tobacco users

Source: Preventive care benefits. https://www.healthcare.gov/what-are-my-preventive-care-benefits/

preventive care
Health-related services designed to stop the development of a disease or injury.

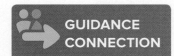

GUIDANCE CONNECTION

Review the ICD-10-CM Coding Guidelines, Section I.C.21, Chapter 21: **Factors influencing health status and contact with health services,** Subsection c(2), **Inoculations and vaccinations,** for more input.

the development of disease or injury. Perhaps this may include dietary counseling and surveillance (Z71.3) to prevent the onset of hypertension, heart disease, obesity, or other nutrition-related condition, or a discussion about the patient's tobacco use (Z72.0) could focus on various methodologies available to quit smoking to prevent the patient from developing lung disease. Couples may come in for genetic counseling (Z31.5) to prevent passing chromosomal abnormalities to their future children; for those who do not want to have children yet, general counseling and advice on contraception (Z30.09) may be provided.

LET'S CODE IT! SCENARIO

Geneva Koti, a 12-year-old female, came into the clinic with her mother. While searching for seashells at the beach, she went up on the boardwalk to get ice cream and she stepped on a nail, puncturing the sole of her left foot. After checking the puncture wound, cleaning it, and dressing it, Dr. Salton gave Geneva a tetanus shot as a precaution.

You are reviewing how to determine Z codes in this chapter, so here's the first code for this encounter: S91.332A Puncture wound without foreign body, left foot, initial encounter. Dr. Salton's notes state that Geneva received a preventive tetanus shot. You have learned that, in medical terminology, this is known as an *immunization*. When you turn to the Alphabetic Index, you see:

Immunization—*see also* Vaccination

Encounter for Z23

When you turn to the Tabular List, you confirm:

Z23 Encounter for immunization

This is great. Are you concerned that this code does not include the specific detail that the immunization was for tetanus? Don't worry. That will be reported with the procedure code explaining what was in the syringe. But you do need an external cause code to explain why Geneva needed this immunization. Turn to the Alphabetic Index to External Causes. Did you find:

Puncture, puncturing—*see also* Contact, with, by type of object or machine

Let's turn to:

Contact

With

Nail W45.0

Now let's find code category W45 in the Tabular List:

W45 Foreign body or object entering through skin

That sounds right. First, read carefully the *Excludes2* notation listing several diagnoses. Take a minute to review them, and determine whether any apply to Geneva's condition. No, none of them do, so you are in the correct location. Notice the seventh-character options here. You will need them for later. First, you need to determine the first six characters, so continue down and review all of the fourth-, fifth-, and sixth-character choices. Which matches Dr. Salton's notes?

W45.0XX Nail entering through skin

Perfect! And the seventh character? The choices are listed at the top of this code category:

W45.0XXA Nail entering through skin, initial encounter

Next, you need the place of occurrence (the beach) and the status code. (Refer to Chapter 16 to remind yourself about reporting external cause codes whenever you are reporting an injury or poisoning.)

Take a look. Did you find:

Y92.832 Beach as the place of occurrence of the external cause

Y99.9 Other external cause status

Fantastic! You have determined all of the codes required for this encounter:

S91.332A Puncture wound without foreign body, left foot, initial encounter

Z23 Encounter for immunization

W45.0XXA Nail entering through skin, initial encounter

Y92.832 Beach as the place of occurrence of the external cause

Y99.9 Other external cause status

You have got this!

LO 22.2 Early Detection

The reason for routine and administrative exams is to ensure continued good health by looking for signs of disease as early as detection may be possible, using a physician's knowledge and technological advancement. Commonly, these health care encounters are known as *annual physicals, well-baby checks,* or *well-woman exams.* These routine encounters, most often prompted by the calendar rather than the way the patient feels, are reported with Z codes, such as code Z00.00, Encounter for general adult medical examination without abnormal findings, or Z00.129, Encounter for routine child health examination without abnormal findings.

Many schools and organizations require that a physician examine a child before the child joins a sports team (Z02.5), companies may require preemployment exams (Z02.1), and virtually all surgeons will order preprocedural exams (Z01.81-) for the patient prior to surgery. These are all considered administrative health encounters because they are determined by a specific circumstance, rather than the calendar or the way the patient feels.

Certain conditions, even after being resolved, may continue to identify the patient as being at risk of a recurrence. The patient had a previous condition; however, prudent health care standards require that the physician keep a watchful eye to catch and treat a recurrent episode. Codes such as Z86.11, Personal history of tuberculosis, and Z87.11, Personal history of peptic ulcer, may provide medical necessity for an extra screening test or encounter.

YOU CODE IT! CASE STUDY

Helen Buckwald, a 53-year-old female, came in to see Dr. Apter to get a colonoscopy. Dr. Apter explained last week that this was an important screening for malignant neoplasms of the colon and was recommended for all adults aged 50 and over. After the screening, Dr. Apter told Helen she was fine and there were no abnormalities.

You Code It!

Go through the steps of coding, and determine the code or codes that should be reported for this encounter between Dr. Apter and Helen Buckwald.

Step 1: Read the case completely.

Step 2: Abstract the notes: Which key words can you identify relating to why Dr. Apter cared for Helen?

_____

Step 3: Query the provider, if necessary.

Step 4: Code the diagnosis or diagnoses.

_____

Step 5: Code the procedure(s): Screening colonoscopy.

Step 6: Link the procedure codes to at least one diagnosis code to confirm medical necessity.

Step 7: Back code to double-check your choices.

Answer:

Did you determine the correct code to be:

Z12.11 Encounter for screening for malignant neoplasm of colon

A **screening** is a test or examination, such as routine lab work or imaging services, administered when there are no current signs, symptoms, or related diagnosis. Report a visit for a screening with a Z code such as code Z13.22, Encounter for screening for metabolic disorder, or Z13.820, Encounter for screening for osteoporosis.

The standards of care have established important examinations and tests to detect illnesses at the earliest possible time. However, these tests are typically recommended for specific population subgroups determined to be at the greatest risk, such as mammograms for women over 40 (see Figure 22-1) or prostate examinations for men over 50. These encounters would be reported with a Z code such as code Z12.5, Encounter for screening for malignant neoplasm of prostate, or Z13.6, Encounter for screening for cardiovascular disorders.

Society, especially in the United States, is designed for interaction between individuals. Shopping malls, concert halls and festival venues, public transport sites, classrooms, playgrounds, and other locations draw friends, families, and strangers together in close proximity to one another. Close physical proximity can put someone in contact with a potential health hazard and facilitate (suspected) exposure to a communicable disease. Think of this: Two children, Jane and Mary, were playing together, and the next day Jane is diagnosed with rubella. This means that Mary was exposed. When Mary's mom takes her to the doctor, this visit will include code Z20.4, Contact with and (suspected) exposure to rubella. Another example: Kenny works for County Animal Control. As he was placing a wild raccoon into his vehicle, the raccoon bit him. Kenny went to the emergency clinic immediately, and code Z20.3, Contact with and (suspected) exposure to rabies, was included on the claim.

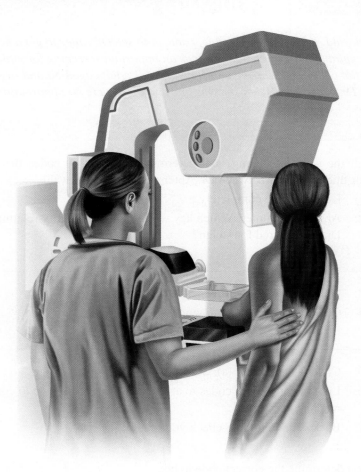

FIGURE 22-1 Mammograms Are Recommended for All Women over 40 Years of Age

With all these tests being done to confirm the patient's good health, there are times when the documentation includes **abnormal findings,** meaning the results indicate something is wrong. This is not the same thing as a confirmed diagnosis, necessarily. It may be a signal that a condition is potential or that more extensive and specific examinations must be done.

EXAMPLE

Z00.01 Encounter for general adult medical examination with abnormal findings
Z01.411 Encounter for gynecological examination (general)(routine) with abnormal findings

YOU CODE IT! CASE STUDY

Raffah Jones, a 53-year-old male, came in to see his regular physician, Dr. Crisppe, for his annual physical. Raffah said he has been feeling great and working out about twice a week. During the digital rectal exam, Dr. Crisppe noted a palpable nodule on the posterior of Raffah's prostate. Dr. Crisppe told Raffah that he appears in good health except for the nodule. They discussed this and scheduled an appointment for a biopsy.

You Code It!

Go through the steps of coding, and determine the code or codes that should be reported for this encounter between Dr. Crisppe and Raffah Jones.

Step 1: Read the case completely.

Step 2: Abstract the notes: Which key words can you identify relating to why Dr. Crisppe cared for Raffah?

_____

Step 3: Query the provider, if necessary.

Step 4: Code the diagnosis or diagnoses.

_____

Step 5: Code the procedure(s): Annual physical exam.

Step 6: Link the procedure codes to at least one diagnosis code to confirm medical necessity.

Step 7: Back code to double-check your choices.

Answer:

Did you determine the correct codes to be:

Z00.01 Encounter for general adult medical examination with abnormal findings

N40.2 Nodular prostate without lower urinary tract symptoms

You did great!

LO 22.3 Genetic Susceptibility

carrier

An individual infected with a disease who is not ill but can still pass it to another person; an individual with an abnormal gene that can be passed to a child, making the child susceptible to disease.

A patient might be a **carrier** or suspected carrier of a disease. He or she needs to know this so the condition is not unintentionally passed on. Or the patient may have an abnormal gene that may increase a patient's chances of developing a disease. This is of particular concern when there is a known family history for conditions that are, or may be, inherited.

In most cases, the documentation will note that the patient has a family history of a condition, such as code Z80.6, Family history of leukemia, or Z83.3, Family history of diabetes mellitus. In these cases, no additional genetic testing may be done. However, the knowledge of family members with a particular condition could support more frequent screenings, such as a patient getting a mammogram every 6 months instead of the standard annual test.

A patient may have reason to believe he or she is the carrier of a disease, such as diphtheria (Z22.2) or viral hepatitis B (Z55.51). A carrier is an individual who has been infected with a pathogen yet has no signs or symptoms of the disease. Carriers, while not ill themselves, are still able to pass the condition to another person.

You may have heard about genetic susceptibility to malignant neoplasm of the breast (Z15.01) and genetic susceptibility to malignant neoplasm of the ovary (Z15.02), identified by the BRCA1 and BRCA2 tests. These tests may be used to confirm, or deny, the presence of an abnormality in a gene that may have been inherited, which can serve as a prediction of the potential for developing a disease—in these cases, cancer. Some patients have opted for prophylactic (preventive) surgery after a positive finding of an abnormal gene. If a patient had this procedure, you would report it with code Z40.01, Encounter for prophylactic removal of breast.

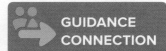

GUIDANCE CONNECTION

Review the ICD-10-CM Coding Guidelines, Section I.C.21, Chapter 21: **Factors influencing health status and contact with health services,** Subsections c(3), **Status,** and c(14), **Miscellaneous Z codes— Prophylactic organ removal,** for more input.

LO 22.4 Observation

There might be a reason that a physician suspects a patient may be ill despite the absence of signs and symptoms. Code categories Z03 and Z04 enable you to report the reason these types of encounters are medically necessary.

Imagine that a mother brings her 2-year-old son into the emergency department because she found him in her bathroom with her allergy pill bottle tipped over and pills strewn about the floor. She does not know whether he ingested any of the pills and, if he did, how many. After an examination showing no signs or symptoms of overdose or poisoning, the doctor decides to keep the boy in the hospital for observation, just in case. The next day, the boy appears to be fine, and his blood tests show no signs of the allergy medication at all. He is discharged with a clean bill of health. You would report this with code Z03.6, Encounter for observation for suspected toxic effect from ingested substance, ruled out.

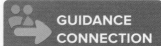

GUIDANCE CONNECTION

Review the ICD-10-CM Coding Guidelines, Section I.C.21, Chapter 21: **Factors influencing health status and contact with health services,** Subsection c(6), **Observation,** for more input.

LO 22.5 Continuing Care and Aftercare

Chronic illness may require long-term use of medication, known as *drug therapy.* When a patient is taking any type of pharmaceutical on an ongoing basis, regular monitoring can identify potential concerns, such as side effects or loss of potency. Some individuals' body chemistry can get used to certain drugs, making them less effective. When coding an encounter for such monitoring, you may begin with Z51.81, Encounter for therapeutic drug level monitoring, along with a code to identify the type of therapeutic drug, such as Z79.01, Long term (current) use of anticoagulants, or Z79.811, Long term (current) use of aromatase inhibitors.

Of course, the physician-patient relationship in treating a specific illness or injury does not end at the end of a surgical procedure or other type of therapeutic service. A healing illness or injury may require aftercare, reported with a code such as Z47.1, Aftercare following joint replacement surgery; Z48.00, Encounter for change or removal of nonsurgical wound dressing (see Figure 22-2); or Z48.45, Encounter for aftercare following lung transplant.

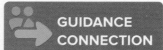

GUIDANCE CONNECTION

Review the ICD-10-CM Coding Guidelines, Section I.C.21, Chapter 21: **Factors influencing health status and contact with health services,** Subsections c(7), **After care,** and c(8), **Follow-up,** for more input.

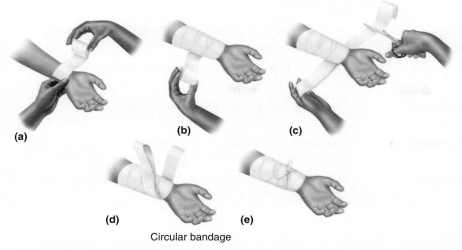

(a)   (b)   (c)

(d)   (e)

Circular bandage

FIGURE 22-2 Nonsurgical Dressing

Patients with implanted medical devices may need more frequent encounters to check the device to ensure it is working properly, as is the case with a patient with a cardiac pacemaker (Z45.01) or a patient with a cochlear implant (Z45.321).

Follow-up examinations may be necessary for a condition that has already been treated or no longer exists. Examples of such follow-ups include an encounter for the removal of sutures (stitches), reported with code Z48.02, or an encounter after the patient has completed treatment for a malignant neoplasm (Z08), once the patient has finished the chemotherapy or radiation treatment plan.

LO 22.6 Obstetrics (Prenatal) and Neonatal Exams

You may remember that in Chapters 19 and 20, you learned about regularly planned obstetrics and neonatal evaluations (see Figure 22-3). Once the baby has arrived, the outcome of delivery, birth status, and health supervision and observations of an infant or child are all reported with a Z code such as Z00.110, Health examination for newborn under 8 days old, or Z37.2, Twins, both liveborn.

Organ Donation

The number of organs and tissues that can be successfully transplanted has dramatically increased over the years, and many can be provided by a living donor. Code category Z52, Donors of organs and tissues, includes various types of blood donors (Z52.0-), skin donors (Z52.1-), and bone donors (Z52.2-). You will notice that all three of these code subcategories require you, as the professional coder, to determine from the documentation whether the donor is **autologous** or is providing another type of graft or donation (see Table 22-1). It is not unusual for a patient to donate his or her own blood prior to having a surgical procedure so that in the event he or she needs a transfusion, his or her own blood will be used. When an injury to the skin is so severe that a graft is needed, there are times when the surgeon will take the graft from another part of the patient's own body and transfer it to the injured site.

A kidney (Z52.4) and cornea (Z52.5), as well as a part of the liver (Z52.6), may come from a living donor. Fertility issues occur, and some women donate their oocytes (eggs) for in vitro fertilization for themselves or someone else (Z52.81-). The donations of any of these organs would almost always be used as an **allogeneic** donation to another individual.

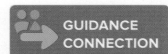

GUIDANCE CONNECTION

Review the ICD-10-CM Coding Guidelines, Section I.C.21, Chapter 21: **Factors influencing health status and contact with health services,** Subsections c(11), **Encounters for obstetrical and reproductive services,** and c(12), **Newborns and infants,** for more input.

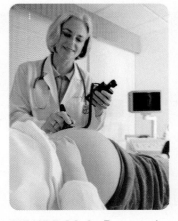

FIGURE 22-3 Prenatal Examination
© Andersen Ross/Getty Images

autologous
The donor tissue is taken from a different site on the same individual's body (also known as an *autograft*).

allogeneic
The donor and recipient are of the same species, e.g., human → human, dog → dog (also known as an *allograft*).

TABLE 22-1 Types of Grafts

Autologous	The donor tissue is taken from a different site on the same individual's body (also known as an *autograft*).
Isogeneic	The donor and recipient individuals are genetically identical (i.e., monozygotic twins).
Allogeneic	The donor and recipient are of the same species, e.g., human → human, dog → dog (also known as an *allograft*).
Xenogeneic	The donor and recipient are of different species, e.g., bovine cartilage → human (also known as a *xenograft* or *heterograft*).
Prosthetic	Lost tissue is replaced with synthetic material such as metal, plastic, or ceramic.

isogeneic
The donor and recipient individuals are genetically identical (i.e., monozygotic twins).

xenogeneic
The donor and recipient are of different species, e.g., bovine cartilage → human (also known as a *xenograft* or *heterograft*).

prosthetic
Lost tissue is replaced with synthetic material such as metal, plastic, or ceramic.

A donation from the recipient's monozygotic twin is called **isogeneic,** while a **xenogeneic** donation involves a donor and recipient who are of different species. Synthetic organ and tissue replacements are referred to as **prosthetic.**

YOU CODE IT! CASE STUDY

Wishanda Robinette, a 27-year-old female, came in to donate her eggs. Her sister, Latisha, had lesions on her ovaries and had to have them removed many years ago. Dr. Post is going to harvest eggs from Wishanda to implant in Latisha so she and her husband, Albert, can have children. Wishanda wanted to help her sister and brother-in-law by donating her eggs.

You Code It!

Go through the steps of coding, and determine the code or codes that should be reported for this encounter between Dr. Post and Wishanda.

Step 1: Read the case completely.

Step 2: Abstract the notes: Which key words can you identify relating to why Dr. Post cared for Wishanda?

_____

Step 3: Query the provider, if necessary.

Step 4: Code the diagnosis or diagnoses.

_____

Step 5: Code the procedure(s): Harvesting donated oocytes.

Step 6: Link the procedure codes to at least one diagnosis code to confirm medical necessity.

Step 7: Back code to double-check your choices.

Answer:

Did you determine the correct code to be:

Z52.811 Egg (oocyte) donor under age 35, designated recipient

Very good!

Of course, prior to the actual procedure to harvest the organ or tissue, an examination will need to be done, reported with code Z00.5, Encounter for examination for potential donor of organ or tissue.

LO 22.7 Resistance to Antimicrobial Drugs

The World Health Organization (WHO) defines *antimicrobial resistance (AMR)* as the "resistance of a micro-organism to an antimicrobial medicine to which it was originally sensitive" ("Antimicrobial Resistance," www.who.int/mediacentre/factsheets/fs194/en/). AMR may be the result of overuse of antibiotics. In the United States, it is estimated that 50% of the time, antibiotics are prescribed for patients who actually do not need them. The CDC's new plan for "antibiotic stewardship" recommends waiting for cultures and lab test results before writing the prescription to ensure that the bacterium or virus proven to cause the patient's infection can be fought off with the most effective drug. These tests will also identify when no prescription is in the patient's best interests.

Less-than-effective infection control and prevention in both inpatient and outpatient facilities is another underlying cause of AMR. The invisibility of microorganisms makes it difficult for some individuals to remember to wash up or at least access antibacterial gel or foam.

Patients with malignancies who are undergoing chemotherapy, those who have recently had complex surgery, those suffering with rheumatoid arthritis (RA), those with end-stage renal disease (ESRD) who are undergoing regular dialysis, and patients who have recently received an organ or bone marrow transplant are all especially susceptible to an AMR infection, and these individuals are seen in every type of health care facility every day.

Take a look at code category Z16, Resistance to antimicrobial drugs. You can see that ICD-10-CM provides a note with some direction about the proper use of these Z codes:

> *Note:* The codes in this category are provided for use as additional codes to identify the resistance and non-responsiveness of a condition to antimicrobial drugs.

And you can see the *code first the infection* notation that provides sequencing direction.

Z16.10 Resistance to unspecified beta lactam antibiotics

Z16.11 Resistance to penicillins (amoxicillin)(ampicillin)

Z16.12 Extended spectrum beta lactamase (ESBL) resistance

Z16.19 Resistance to other specified beta lactam antibiotics (cephalosporins)

Z16.20 Resistance to unspecified antibiotic (antibiotics NOS)

Z16.21 Resistance to vancomycin

Z16.22 Resistance to vancomycin related antibiotics

Z16.23 Resistance to quinolones and fluoroquinolones

Z16.24 Resistance to multiple antibiotics

Z16.29 Resistance to other single specified antibiotic (aminoglycosides)(macrolides) (sulfonamides)(tetracylines)

Z16.342 Resistance to multiple antimycobacterial drugs

Z16.35 Resistance to multiple antimicrobial drugs

[Excludes1 resistance to multiple antibiotics only (Z16.24)]

Reporting these conditions is not exclusive to the Z code chapter. When a patient is confirmed to have an infection that is resistant, you might report one of these codes instead:

A41.02 Sepsis due to methicillin resistant *Staphylococcus aureus*

B95.62 Methicillin resistant *Staphylococcus aureus* infection as the cause of diseases classified elsewhere

A49.02 Methicillin resistant *Staphylococcus aureus* infection, unspecified site

J15.212 Pneumonia due to methicillin resistant *Staphylococcus aureus*

LO 22.8 Z Codes As First-Listed/Principal Diagnosis

During most encounters, a Z code may be the only code you report, or it may be reported along with others, determined by the specific circumstances. Except for 20 of the Z codes, sequencing is determined by the facts of the encounter and the Official Guidelines, as explained in Sections II and III. The other 20 Z codes are permitted to be *only* first-listed or principal diagnosis codes:

Z00 Encounter for general examination without complaint, suspected or reported diagnosis

Z01 Encounter for other special examination without complaint, suspected or reported diagnosis

Z02 Encounter for administrative examination

Z03 Encounter for medical observation for suspected diseases and conditions ruled out

Z04 Encounter for examination and observation for other reasons

Z33.2 Encounter for elective termination of pregnancy

Z31.81 Encounter for male factor infertility in female patient

Z31.82 Encounter for Rh incompatibility status

Z31.83 Encounter for assisted reproductive fertility procedure cycle

Z31.84 Encounter for fertility preservation procedure

Z34 Encounter for supervision of normal pregnancy

Z39 Encounter for maternal postpartum care and examination

Z38 Liveborn infants according to place of birth and type of delivery

Z42 Encounter for plastic and reconstructive surgery following medical procedure or healed injury

Z51.0 Encounter for antineoplastic radiation therapy

Z51.1- Encounter for antineoplastic chemotherapy and immunotherapy

Z52 Donors of organs and tissues

    Except: Z52.9, Donor of unspecified organ or tissue

Z76.1 Encounter for health supervision and care of foundling

Z76.2 Encounter for health supervision and care of other healthy infant and child

Z99.12 Encounter for respirator [ventilator] dependence during power failure

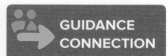

GUIDANCE CONNECTION

Review the ICD-10-CM Coding Guidelines, Section I.C.21, Chapter 21: **Factors influencing health status and contact with health services,** Subsection c(16), **Z codes that may only be principal/first-listed diagnosis,** for more input.

Chapter Summary

As a professional coder, you are responsible to ensure that every physician-patient encounter is supported as medically necessary. You probably know from your own personal experience that there are legitimate reasons for a healthy person to seek the attention of a physician or other health care professional. In ICD-10-CM, virtually all of the codes used to explain these valid reasons are found in the Z code chapter. Here, you will find codes to report the medical necessity for providing preventive care services, performing a screening, observing a patient, and checking for the viability of a potential organ donor.

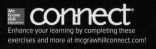

Using Terminology

Match each key term to the appropriate definition.

_____ **1.** LO 22.6 The donor and recipient individuals are genetically identical.

_____ **2.** LO 22.3 An individual infected with a disease who is not ill but can still pass it to another person; an individual with an abnormal gene that can be passed to a child, making the child susceptible to disease.

_____ **3.** LO 22.2 Test results that indicate a disease or condition may be present.

_____ **4.** LO 22.6 The donor and recipient are of different species.

_____ **5.** LO 22.2 An examination or test of a patient who has no signs or symptoms that is conducted with the intention of finding any evidence of disease as soon as possible, thus enabling better patient outcomes.

_____ **6.** LO 22.6 Lost tissue is replaced with synthetic materials such as metal, plastic, or ceramic.

_____ **7.** LO 22.6 The donor tissue is taken from a different site on the same individual's body.

_____ **8.** LO 22.1 Health-related services designed to stop the development of a disease or injury.

_____ **9.** LO 22.6 The donor and recipient are of the same species.

A. Abnormal findings
B. Allogeneic
C. Autologous
D. Carrier
E. Isogeneic
F. Preventive care
G. Prosthetic
H. Screening
I. Xenogeneic

Checking Your Understanding

Choose the most appropriate answer for each of the following questions.

1. LO 22.1 Health care–related services designed to stop the development of a disease or injury are known as

  a. abnormal findings.
  b. autologous.
  c. aftercare.
  d. preventive care.

2. LO 22.2 Abnormal findings are

  a. test results that indicate a disease or condition may be present.
  b. test results that are negative.
  c. test results showing that the donor and recipient are of the same species.
  d. test results that are inconclusive.

3. LO 22.6 If the donor and recipient are of different species, the graft is

  a. isogeneic.
  b. allogeneic.
  c. xenogeneic.
  d. autologous.

4. LO 22.1 When the patient has a preventive care encounter, you will use a _____ code.

   a. W.
   b. Z.
   c. X.
   d. Y.

5. LO 22.2 The patient, a 38-year-old adult, presents for an annual physical examination, without abnormal findings. You would use code

   a. Z00.00.
   b. Z01.00.
   c. Z00.2.
   d. Z00.70.

6. LO 22.2 A physical examination may be required before all of the following *except*

   a. joining a sports team.
   b. starting a new job.
   c. having a medical procedure.
   d. kayaking.

7. LO 22.3 An individual with an abnormal gene that can be passed to a child, making the child susceptible to disease, is known as a(n)

   a. screen.
   b. abnormal finding.
   c. carrier.
   d. observation.

8. LO 22.4 If a patient is without signs or symptoms and is being watched for a suspected illness, then the patient is under

   a. preventive care.
   b. observation.
   c. continuous care.
   d. aftercare.

9. LO 22.5 The patient presents today to have his surgical wound dressing changed. You would use code

   a. Z48.00.
   b. Z48.01.
   c. Z48.02.
   d. Z48.03.

10. LO 22.8 A professional coder's responsibility is to ensure that every patient encounter is supported by

   a. medical antimicrobial drugs.
   b. medical observation.
   c. medical necessity.
   d. medical prophylactic action.

Applying Your Knowledge

1. LO 22.1 Explain preventive care. _____

   _____

2. LO 22.1 List six free preventive services under the Affordable Care Act. _____

   _____

3. LO 22.2 Why is early detection important? Include examples of early detection encounters. _____

   _____

4. LO 22.2 What is a screening, and why is it important? _____

   _____

5. LO 22.3 Why is it important for a patient to know if he or she has a genetic susceptibility? _____

   _____

6. LO 22.5 Why would a patient need continuing care or aftercare? _____

   _____

7. LO 22.6 Explain the difference between *autologous, allogeneic,* and *xenogeneic.* _____

   _____

8. LO 22.8 List 10 of the Z codes, including descriptions, that are permitted to be only first-listed or principal codes. _____

   _____

Using the techniques described in this chapter, carefully read through the case studies and determine the most accurate ICD-10-CM code(s) and external cause code(s), if appropriate, for each case study.

1. Deborah Bartley, a 23-year-old female, gave birth to a beautiful baby girl 1 month ago. Deborah comes in today for a routine follow-up maternal postpartum care and examination. Dr. McClure tells Deborah she is doing fine.

   _____

2. Victor Casada, an 18-year-old male, wants to join the U.S. Navy when he graduates from high school in a few weeks. The U.S. Navy recruiting officer tells Victor that a physical examination is required before he can join. Victor comes in today to see Dr. Cashwell for a prerecruitment examination. Dr. Cashwell completes the exam with no noted abnormalities and signs Victor's recruitment papers.

   _____

3. Elena Cavallas, a 34-year-old female, presents today for her annual gynecologic examination. Dr. Freeman completes the exam and informs Elena there are no abnormal findings.

   _____

4. Billy Williams, a 6-month-old male, is brought in by his mother and Dante Kibler to determine whether Dante is the biological father. Billy's mother is applying for child support and social welfare benefits and needs proof of the biological father before she can proceed. Dr. Paterson completes a paternity test, and the results show 99.99% that Dante is the biological father.

   _____

5. Janie Davis, a 42-year-old female, was plugging in a light fixture at work when it shocked her badly. She was taken to the ER by the office manager. After the appropriate tests were completed, Dr. Anderson, the ER physician, put Janie under observation.

   _____

6. Charles Fredrick, a 65-year-old male, comes in today with the complaint that it is getting difficult to hear low conversations, and he is concerned about his ability to hear. Dr. Pennington performs a hearing test using an audiometer; results are within normal at 18 dB SPL.

   _____

7. Chiquita Goodnough, an 18-year-old female, presents today with the complaint that she has missed her last two periods, and she thinks that she might be pregnant. Dr. Lindsey performs a pregnancy test with a positive result.

   _____

8. Roberta Kelly, a 36-year-old female, comes in today with the complaint of painful and burning urination. Dr. Keyton completes the appropriate tests and diagnoses Roberta with a UTI due to *Staphylococcus aureus;* the culture shows that the UTI is resistant to vancomycin.

   _____

9. Elizabeth McCormac, a 53-year-old female, presents today for a screening for malignant neoplasm of the ovaries. Elizabeth's mother died at age 58 of ovarian cancer. Dr. Noles performs the screening; results were negative.

   _____

10. Paul Platter, a 34-year-old male, presents today for the removal of his tube drain, which was inserted during his hand surgery 5 weeks ago. Dr. Pitts removes the drain without complications.

    _____

11. Ifad Rahman, a 45-day-old male, is brought in by his parents for a well-baby check. Dr. Scott notes that Ifad's heelprick is slow to coagulate and stop bleeding. After the appropriate tests, Dr. Scott diagnoses Ifad with hemophilia A, symptomatic carrier.

    _____

12. Andy Suber, a 19-year-old male, presents today to see Dr. Gates with the complaint of generalized pain and headaches. Andy's last visit here, for a sports participation exam 9 months ago, revealed a healthy young man without any significant medical history. Andy graduated from high school 3 months ago and does not plan to go to college; he's *happily* unemployed, living at his parents' home. Andy states that his father wants him to join the family landscaping business, but he hates the idea of working. Dr. Gates completes a thorough examination and appropriate tests, and all of Andy's test results are within the normal range. Dr. Gates diagnoses Andy as a malingerer.

    _____

13. Christopher Gerringer, a 7-year-old male, is brought in today by his mother. One of Chris's classmates has been diagnosed with varicella, and she wants to have Chris checked for the disease.

    _____

14. James Norris, a 46-year-old male, presents today to donate bone marrow for his brother, who has been diagnosed with multiple myeloma.

_____

15. Barbara Outen, a 37-year-old female, presents today for her annual eye examination. Dr. Walters completes the eye examination without complications or abnormalities.

_____

The following exercises provide practice in abstracting physicians' notes and learning to work with SOAP notes from our health care facility, *Taylor, Reader, & Associates.* These case studies (SOAP notes) are modeled on real patient encounters. Using the techniques described in this chapter, carefully read through the case studies and determine the most accurate ICD-10-CM code(s) and external cause code(s), if appropriate, for each case study.

TAYLOR, READER, & ASSOCIATES
A Complete Health Care Facility
975 CENTRAL AVENUE • SOMEWHERE, FL 32811 • 407-555-4321

PATIENT: CANIN, ROXIE
ACCOUNT/EHR #:   CANIRO001
DATE: 10/16/18

Attending Physician: Suzanne R. Taylor, MD

S: Roxie Canin, a 27-year-old female, came in to see Dr. Taylor for a physical. Roxie is an established patient of Dr. Taylor's. She is starting a new job on the first of next month and is required by her employment contract to get a complete physical including blood pressure check, cholesterol screening, blood glucose levels, tetanus-diphtheria and acellular pertussis (TdAP) (or documentation of this immunization within the last 10 years), and flu vaccine within the last 12 months.

O: Dr. Taylor's notes include all vital signs, height, weight, and BMI. Finger stick glucose test was normal, showing there were no indications of Roxie being prediabetic. Cholesterol screening shows Roxie is within normal limits. Dr. Taylor also notes the TdAP immunization was administered on 5/24/2010. The flu vaccine was administered on 09/28/2016.

A: Preemployment examination.

P: Dr. Taylor completed the form, and attached the documentation showing the TdAP and flu administration dates, for Roxie's job and signed it.

Suzanne R. Taylor, MD

SRT/pw   D: 10/16/18 09:50:16   T: 10/18/18 12:55:01

Determine the most accurate ICD-10-CM code(s).

_____

_____

_____

TAYLOR, READER, & ASSOCIATES
A Complete Health Care Facility
975 CENTRAL AVENUE • SOMEWHERE, FL 32811 • 407-555-4321

PATIENT: LONGMIRE, JACE
ACCOUNT/EHR #:   LONGJA01
DATE: 10/16/18

Attending Physician: Willard B. Reader, MD

S: Jace Matthew Longmire was born 12 hours ago via spontaneous vaginal delivery, full-term.

O: Newborn screening exam performed in the well-baby nursery included pulse oximetry showing normal percentage of hemoglobin in his blood that is saturated with oxygen. However, the test for hypothyroidism was found to be a concern. Prior to discharge, Dr. Reader met with Jace's parents and explained this condition and discussed thyroxine, the medication required so Jace can avoid problems such as slowed growth and brain damage, seen in newborns with untreated hypothyroidism.

A: Congenital hypothyroidism without goiter

P: Rx: Thyroxine
    Follow-up in office in 2 days

Willard B. Reader, MD

WBR/pw   D: 10/16/18 09:50:16   T: 10/18/18 12:55:01

Determine the most accurate ICD-10-CM code(s).

_____

_____

_____

TAYLOR, READER, & ASSOCIATES
A Complete Health Care Facility
975 CENTRAL AVENUE • SOMEWHERE, FL 32811 • 407-555-4321

PATIENT: MCCARTHY, FELICIA
ACCOUNT/EHR #:   MCCAFE001
DATE: 10/17/18

Attending Physician: John S. Warwick, MD

Ronan and Felicia McCarthy are thinking about starting a family, so they came in to see Dr. Warwick to learn about genetic screenings. They wanted to get all the information possible before Felicia gets pregnant so preparations can be employed to have a healthy child. Dr. Warwick counseled them and discussed many options. Both Ronan and Felicia decided to complete a preconception genetic test, and family histories were reviewed.

_____

John S. Warwick, MD

JSW/pw   D: 10/16/18 09:50:16   T: 10/18/18 12:55:01

Determine the most accurate ICD-10-CM code(s).

_____

_____

_____

TAYLOR, READER, & ASSOCIATES
A Complete Health Care Facility
975 CENTRAL AVENUE • SOMEWHERE, FL 32811 • 407-555-4321

PATIENT: GOODING, MASON
ACCOUNT/EHR #: GOODMA001
DATE: 10/17/18

Attending Physician: Suzanne R. Taylor, MD

S: Mason Gooding, a 15-year-old male, presents to Dr. Taylor complaining of a cough and a sore throat, lasting about 1 week. He and his mother deny fever, nasal congestion, or runny nose. He says he feels more tired than usual, and his mom states that he hasn't been getting out of bed to go to school. Mom seems most worried that he is much less active than he usually is and that he has been truant from school over the last 3–4 weeks. Patient states that his "mom won't get off my back." He admits that his grades have been dropping and he quit the baseball team. Mom leaves the room, and patient admits to smoking pot every day, sometimes several times a day, for the last month or so. He denies any other drug use and states smoking pot is "no big deal." His last visit here, for his back-to-school annual exam 3 months ago, revealed a healthy young man without any significant medical history.

O: Physical examination is remarkable only for a mildly erythematous throat without petechiae. Lungs are clear, and the rest of his exam is normal. Vital signs are also unremarkable.

COUNSELING: Discussion with patient about side effects and risks of abusing pot. He states he has tried to quit but can't make it through an entire day without smoking. It is pointed out to him that his pot use is already having a negative impact on his life (his absence from and lack of interest in school). He understands that his parents need to know about this, but that he must tell them himself. He is assured that doctor-patient confidentiality is secure. We discussed options and methodologies for his quitting with reduced effects. He agrees to regular surveillance.

A: Marijuana abuse counseling

P: Refer to drug counselor

_____

Suzanne R. Taylor, MD

SRT/pw   D: 10/17/18 09:50:16   T: 10/18/18 12:55:01

Determine the most accurate ICD-10-CM code(s).

_____

_____

_____

TAYLOR, READER, & ASSOCIATES
A Complete Health Care Facility
975 CENTRAL AVENUE • SOMEWHERE, FL 32811 • 407-555-4321

PATIENT: BOWEN, CLIVE
ACCOUNT/EHR #:   BOWECL001
DATE: 10/17/18

Attending Physician: Willard B. Reader, MD

S: Clive Bowen, a 37-year-old male, came to see Dr. Reader for his annual physical exam. Dr. Reader has a lab on the premises, so blood was taken and processed while the rest of the exam was completed. The results of his blood work revealed a random elevated transferrin saturation of 82%.

O: Past Medical History: No relevant past medical history; denies routine blood donation.

     Family History: No relevant family history.

     Social History: Active, states he works out in the gym 2–3 times a week; apparently healthy; married for 3 years to Denise, no children. He states that his wife gives him a multivitamin daily, but he is not certain which one or its exact contents. His diet includes raw oysters on the half shell and sushi about once a week; denies eating red meat or organ meat; drinks coffee, about 3 cups a day, but denies drinking teas or caffeinated beverages.

     Physical Exam: Unremarkable; Height: 5'11"; Weight: 205 lb.; Vital signs: within normal limits.

A: Hemochromatosis

P: Quantitative phlebotomy of 500 mL of whole blood per week for an estimated 5 months.
     Regular monitoring via blood tests every month: serum ferritin, hemoglobin, and hematocrit over the course of the phlebotomy treatments
     Dietary modifications, including elimination of all iron supplements and multivitamins containing iron, as well as no more consumption of raw shellfish.

Willard B. Reader, MD

WBR/pw   D: 10/17/18 09:50:16   T: 10/19/18 12:55:01

Determine the most accurate ICD-10-CM code(s).

_____

_____

_____

Learning Outcomes *After completing this chapter, the student should be able to:*

LO 23.1 Evaluate concurrent and discharge coding methodologies.

LO 23.2 Understand the Official Guidelines specific for inpatient reporting.

LO 23.3 Apply the proper application of present on admission (POA) indicators.

LO 23.4 Determine the impact of diagnosis-related groups on the coding process.

LO 23.5 Identify complications and co-morbidities.

LO 23.6 Recognize the importance of the Uniform Hospital Discharge Data Set (UHDDS).

For the most part, coding hospital encounters and coding outpatient encounters use the same guidelines and the same coding process. However, emergency room and outpatient surgery departments, even though they may be under the same roof as the inpatient acute care facility, will typically be coded as outpatient encounters.

This chapter reviews the few aspects of coding inpatient cases that differ somewhat from what you have learned throughout this book.

LO 23.1 Concurrent and Discharge Coding

Some acute care facilities have patients who may spend weeks or months in the hospital. In these cases, professional coding specialists may do what is called **concurrent coding.** This means that coders actually go up to the nurse's station on the floor of the hospital and code from the patient's chart while the patient is still in the hospital. Concurrent coding enables the hospital to gain reimbursement to date without having to wait until the patient is discharged, improving cash flow for the facility. Figure 23-1 shows you an example of progress notes that might be found in a patient's chart. A coder performing concurrent coding would read these, as well as other documentation, to determine what diagnoses to report.

Once a patient is discharged, you will go through the complete patient record. The most important documentation to look for includes:

- *Discharge summary or discharge progress notes,* signed by the attending physician.
- *Hospital course,* which is a summary of the patient's hospital stay.
- *Discharge instructions,* a copy of which is given to the patient.
- *Discharge disposition,* which contains orders for the patient to be transferred home with special services, transferred to another facility, etc.
- *The death/discharge summary,* which is used if the patient expired prior to discharge.

Key Terms

Comorbidity

Complication

Concurrent coding

Diagnosis-related groups (DRG)

Hospital-acquired conditions (HAC)

Major complications and co-morbidities (MCC)

Present on admission (POA)

Uniform Hospital Discharge Data Set (UHDDS)

concurrent coding
System in which coding processes are performed while a patient is still in the hospital receiving care.

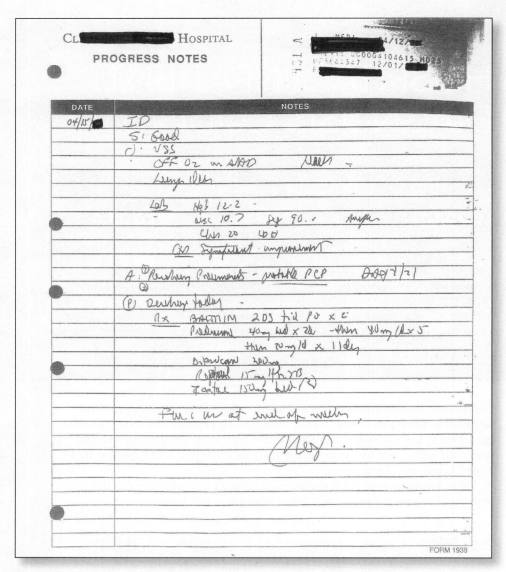

FIGURE 23-1 Progress Notes

All of these documents should be reviewed to provide you with a complete picture of what procedures, services, and treatments were provided to the patient, along with signs, symptoms, and diagnoses to support medical necessity.

LET'S CODE IT! SCENARIO

The attending physician, Milo Sternan, MD, included this in the discharge summary:

> *Admission Diagnosis: Abdominal pain, status post appendectomy*
>
> *Final Diagnosis: Abdominal pain, unknown etiology, status post appendectomy*
>
> *Brief History: Patient underwent an appendectomy for perforated appendicitis 6 weeks ago. . . . Three days prior to admission, she had a recurrent bout of diffuse, dull abdominal pain in the right upper quadrant with associated nausea and anorexia. She was admitted to the hospital at the time for workup of this pain.*
>
> *At this time, the patient has just had a regular meal without difficulty and feels like returning home. She will be discharged home at this time and can follow up with her primary MD. We will see her on an as-needed basis.*

This discharge documentation provides you the information you need to code the diagnosis supporting this patient's stay in the hospital. (To code the procedures, you would have to review the complete record.)

You have the admitting diagnosis and the final diagnosis. Remember, the Official Guidelines state that the principal diagnosis is "that condition established after study." This tells you that the final diagnosis would be used. You have two conditions to report: *abdominal pain, unknown etiology,* and *status post appendectomy.*

As always, begin in the Alphabetic Index, and find:

Pain
    Abdominal R10.9

Turn to the Tabular List to review the complete code description:

R10 Abdomen and pelvis pain

The *Excludes1* and *Excludes2* notes do not appear to include any diagnosis documented in these notes, so continue reading down the column to determine the most accurate fourth character:

R10.1 Pain localized to upper abdomen

Virtually all of the choices you have for the fifth character are specific to the location of the pain in the abdomen. Dr. Sternan did state that when the patient was admitted, she had "abdominal pain in the right upper quadrant," leading you to the fifth character 1. So this diagnosis code will be reported as:

R10.11 Right upper quadrant pain

Are you done? Do you need to report that the patient was status post appendectomy? Yes, you do. It is not known if the pain is related to the surgical procedure or the condition for which it was performed. So let's turn back to the Alphabetic Index and look up:

Status (post)

Appendectomy is not listed. What can you look up? Think about the patient status post: What exactly is an appendectomy? Surgery. No, *surgery* is not listed in this index either. Hmmmm. Try looking at *postsurgical.* Aha!

Status (post)
    Postsurgical NEC Z98.89

(Postoperative NEC is also shown, leading to the same code.)

Let's turn to the Z code section and check this code out:

Z98 Other postprocedural states

The *Excludes2* notes don't relate to this discharge summary, so continue reading down the column to find the correct fourth character. No other fourth character is accurate to report postappendectomy, so let's take a look at what the Alphabetic Index suggested:

Z98.8 Other specified postprocedural status
Z98.89 Other specified postprocedural states

When you review the other procedures included in this classification, none seem to relate to an appendectomy. This code description is the most accurate of those available. So the diagnosis codes you will report for this case are:

R10.11 Right upper quadrant pain
Z98.89 Other specified postprocedural states

Good job!

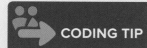

CODING TIP

What about the part of the diagnosis where Dr. Sternan wrote "Abdominal pain, *unknown etiology*"? How is that reported? Notice that the code R10.11 for the abdominal pain is located in the "Symptoms, signs, and ill-defined conditions" chapter. This is the part that reports the physician could not determine the cause (etiology) of the pain. Had the cause of the pain been identified, you would be reporting that with a different code.

LO 23.2 Official Coding Guidelines

The Official Coding Guidelines located in your ICD-10-CM book will still provide you guidance. However, there are two instances in which the guidelines direct inpatient coders differently than outpatient.

Uncertain Diagnosis

Remember, you learned for outpatient coding that you are *not permitted* to ever code something identified by the physician in his or her documentation as "rule out," "probable," "possible," "suspected," or other similar terms of an unconfirmed nature. This guidance (as shown in Section IV, Subsection I, Uncertain diagnosis) is different from that provided to inpatient coders.

The guidance for inpatient coders is that you *are permitted* to "code the condition as if it existed or was established." This is done so that medical necessity can be reported for tests, observation, or other services and resources used to care for the patient whether or not these efforts resulted in a confirmed diagnosis.

Patient Receiving Diagnostic Services Only

In the outpatient world, the guidelines instruct you to wait until the test results have been determined and interpreted by the physician as documented in the final report before coding. At that time, confirmed diagnoses, or the signs and symptoms that were documented as the reason for ordering the test, are reported.

When you are coding for inpatient services, abnormal test results are not reported unless the physician has documented the clinical significance of those results. Interestingly, in this section of the guidelines, it is reiterated that if the coding professional notices abnormal test results and documentation is unclear from the physician, it is "appropriate to ask the provider whether the abnormal finding should be added."

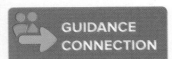

GUIDANCE CONNECTION

Review the ICD-10-CM Coding Guidelines, Section II, **Selection of Principal Diagnosis,** Subsection H, **Uncertain diagnosis,** for more input.

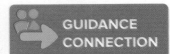

GUIDANCE CONNECTION

Review the ICD-10-CM Coding Guidelines, Section III, **Reporting Additional Diagnoses,** Subsection B, **Abnormal findings,** for more input.

YOU CODE IT! CASE STUDY

The attending physician, Oscar Medina, MD, included this in the discharge summary:

Admission Diagnosis: Acute cervical pain admitted through ED after MVA

Final Diagnosis: Acute cervical pain and radiculitis secondary to degenerative disc disease with posttraumatic activation of pain

Brief History: Patient is a 37-year-old male who was involved in a motor vehicle accident, admitted after being brought to the ED by the ambulance that responded to the accident scene. Patient showed signs of neck and arm pain associated with cervical radiculopathy, radiating into the shoulders along with constant headaches. He has numbness and tingling into the hands and fingers.

Radiology: X-rays AP and lateral cervical spinal x-rays demonstrate evidence of significant degenerative disc disease at C5–6 and C6–7 levels. MRI of cervical spine demonstrates evidence of significant degenerative disc disease at the C5–6 and C6–7 levels with osteophyte formation and canal compromise with the spinal canal diameter reduced to approximately 9 mm. Lumbar spine MRI demonstrates mild degenerative disc disease; otherwise normal.

Recommendation to patient is to undergo an anterior cervical diskectomy and fusion utilizing an autologous iliac bone grafting and placement of anterior titanium plate. After reviewing with patient regarding risks and benefits of surgery, the patient refused and requested to be discharged immediately.

You Code It!

In this case, the patient received only diagnostic services. Determine the most accurate diagnosis codes for this inpatient encounter.

Answer:

Did you determine the accurate codes?

M50.12 Cervical disc disorder with radiculopathy, mid-cervical region

G89.11 Acute pain due to trauma

V43.92xA Unspecified car occupant injured in collision with other type car in traffic accident

Good job!

LO 23.3 Present on Admission Indicators

Present on admission (POA) indicators are required for each diagnosis code reported on UB-04 and 837 institutional claim forms. They are used to report additional detail about the patient's condition.

Centers for Medicare and Medicaid Services (CMS), in CR5499, requires a POA indicator for every diagnosis appearing on a claim from an acute care facility. Claims are returned stamped "unpaid" to the facility if POA indicators are not included. Hospitals are permitted to enter the POA indicators and refile the claim; however, think about all the time and work wasted by having to do this.

General Reporting Guidelines

According to CMS Publication 100-04, "Present on admission is defined as present at the time the order for inpatient admission occurs—conditions that develop during an outpatient encounter, including emergency department, observation, or outpatient surgery, are considered as present on admission."

What does this mean? This means professional coders must carefully review the admitting physician's history and physical (H&P)—the documentation that supports the order to admit the patient into the hospital (see Figure 23-2 for an example)—to determine whether or not the condition was identified at that time. Then you will assign the POA indicator to report this fact: Yes—this diagnosis was present when the patient was admitted; No—it was not present; and so on.

One reason for the importance of gathering POA data is to identify **hospital-acquired conditions (HACs).** A hospital-acquired condition is exactly what it sounds like: an illness or injury that the patient contracted solely due to the fact that he or she was in the hospital at the time. HAC data are used for many different purposes, including evaluating patient safety directives and limiting payment to a facility for errors it may have made that caused the problem.

POA Indicators

The POA indicators are used to clearly identify whether or not the signs, symptoms, and diagnoses reported on the claim form were documented by the admitting physician at the time the patient was admitted into the hospital.

present on admission (POA)
A one-character indicator reporting the status of the diagnosis at the time the patient was admitted to the acute care facility.

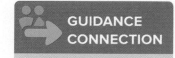

GUIDANCE CONNECTION

Review the ICD-10-CM Coding Guidelines, Appendix I, **Present on Admission Reporting Guidelines,** for more input.

hospital-acquired condition (HAC)
A condition, illness, or injury contracted by the patient during his or her stay in an acute care facility; also known as *nosocomial condition.*

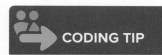

CODING TIP

POA indicators are not required for external cause codes unless the code is being reported as an "other diagnosis."

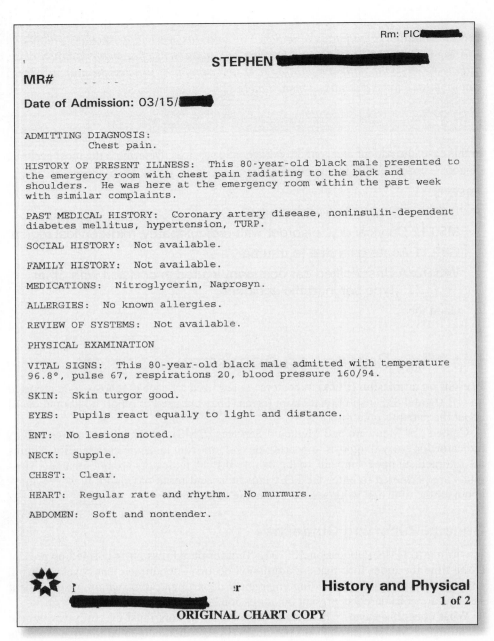

Rm: PIC

STEPHEN

MR#

Date of Admission: 03/15/

ADMITTING DIAGNOSIS:
     Chest pain.

HISTORY OF PRESENT ILLNESS: This 80-year-old black male presented to
the emergency room with chest pain radiating to the back and
shoulders. He was here at the emergency room within the past week
with similar complaints.

PAST MEDICAL HISTORY: Coronary artery disease, noninsulin-dependent
diabetes mellitus, hypertension, TURP.

SOCIAL HISTORY: Not available.

FAMILY HISTORY: Not available.

MEDICATIONS: Nitroglycerin, Naprosyn.

ALLERGIES: No known allergies.

REVIEW OF SYSTEMS: Not available.

PHYSICAL EXAMINATION

VITAL SIGNS: This 80-year-old black male admitted with temperature
96.8°, pulse 67, respirations 20, blood pressure 160/94.

SKIN: Skin turgor good.

EYES: Pupils react equally to light and distance.

ENT: No lesions noted.

NECK: Supple.

CHEST: Clear.

HEART: Regular rate and rhythm. No murmurs.

ABDOMEN: Soft and nontender.

History and Physical
1 of 2

ORIGINAL CHART COPY

FIGURE 23-2 Admitting History and Physical (H&P)

The indicators are:

- Y   Yes   This condition was documented by the admitting physician as present at
the time of inpatient admission.

EXAMPLE of POA—"Y" Indicator

Serena was admitted to the hospital from the emergency department with severe angina (chest pains), dyspnea (shortness of breath), and paresthesia (tingling) in her left arm. After all the tests were run, Dr. Abaddi diagnosed her with an acute myocardial infarction (AMI) of the anterior wall, discussed diet, exercise, medications, and discharged her. Reported with I21.02, ST elevation (STEMI) myocardial infarction involving other coronary artery of anterior wall, would be POA indicator

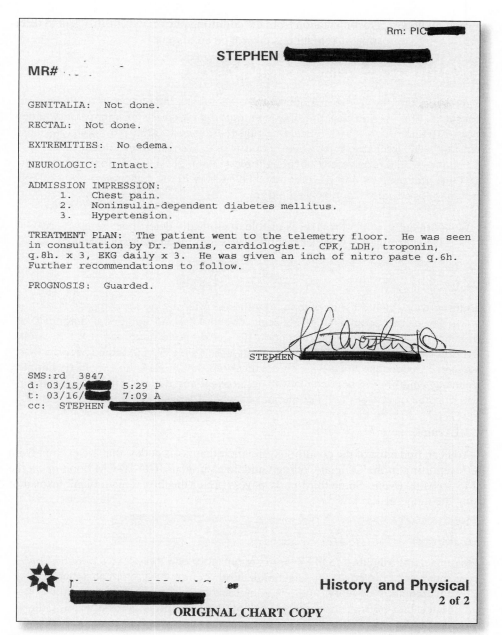

GENITALIA: Not done.

RECTAL: Not done.

EXTREMITIES: No edema.

NEUROLOGIC: Intact.

ADMISSION IMPRESSION:
1. Chest pain.
2. Noninsulin-dependent diabetes mellitus.
3. Hypertension.

TREATMENT PLAN: The patient went to the telemetry floor. He was seen in consultation by Dr. Dennis, cardiologist. CPK, LDH, troponin, q.8h. x 3, EKG daily x 3. He was given an inch of nitro paste q.6h. Further recommendations to follow.

PROGNOSIS: Guarded.

STEPHEN ████████████.

SMS:rd 3847
d: 03/15/█████   5:29 P
t: 03/16/█████   7:09 A
cc: STEPHEN ████████████

History and Physical
2 of 2

ORIGINAL CHART COPY

FIGURE 23-2 (*Continued*)

Y because the signs and symptoms that caused her admission to the hospital were those of an AMI. Her heart attack was present on admission.

- N   No   This condition was *not* present at the time of inpatient admission.

EXAMPLE of POA—"N" Indicator

Elijah was admitted with an esophageal ulcer that did not begin bleeding until after admission. Reported with code K22.11, Ulcer of esophagus with bleeding, is POA indicator N because the entire description of this code was not present at admission.

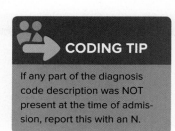

CODING TIP

If any part of the diagnosis code description was NOT present at the time of admission, report this with an N.

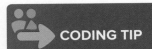
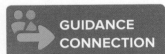
- U Unknown Documentation from the admitting physician is insufficient to determine if condition is present on admission.

EXAMPLE of POA—"U" Indicator

Zach was admitted to the hospital to have his tonsils removed due to his chronic tonsillitis. The second day, the physician noted a diagnosis of urinary tract infection (UTI) and ordered antibiotics. Upon discharge, code J35.01, Chronic tonsillitis, will get POA indicator Y; however, code N39.0, Urinary tract infection, site not specified, would receive a U because the documentation is not clear whether the UTI was not present and developed while he was in the hospital or present and not diagnosed when Zach was admitted.

- W Clinically Provider is unable to clinically determine
     Undetermined whether condition was present on admission or not.

EXAMPLE of POA—"W" Indicator

Clarissa was admitted with diabetic gangrene. After a blood workup early on her third day in the hospital, the physician documented an additional diagnosis of septicemia. Upon discharge, the code for the diabetic gangrene (E11.52) would be reported with a POA of Y; however, the septicemia (A41.9) would receive POA indicator W because the physician documented that there is no way to be certain clinically whether the septicemia was not present and developed while she was in the hospital or present and not diagnosed when Clarissa was admitted.

- 1 Exempt

You can find a list of the conditions, and their diagnosis codes, that are exempt from POA reporting in the Official Coding Guidelines in your ICD-10-CM book or on the CMS website. (*Note:* Some third-party payers prefer this box remain blank instead of using the numeral 1.)

EXAMPLE of POA—"Exempt" Diagnoses

Makenzie was admitted to the hospital in full labor and delivered a beautiful baby boy the next morning. Upon discharge, both codes O80, Normal delivery, and Z37.0 Outcome of delivery, single liveborn, are reported with POA indicator 1. You will notice that both of these codes are on the Exempt list shown in the Official Coding Guidelines in ICD-10-CM.

LET'S CODE IT! SCENARIO

Roberta was admitted into the hospital because she was suffering acute exacerbation of her obstructive chronic bronchitis. After 2 days of treatment, while still in the hospital, she tried to get out of bed without help, fell, and broke her left wrist.

Let's Code It!

The reason Roberta was admitted into the hospital was because she was having exacerbation of her bronchitis. Therefore, the documentation (the physician's H&P) identifies this as being present when she was admitted:

J44.1 Chronic obstructive pulmonary disease with (acute) exacerbation POA: Y

When she was discharged, Roberta also had her wrist in a cast, due to the break suffered from her fall. This is very clearly a condition she did not have when she was admitted:

S62.102A Fracture of unspecified carpal bone, left wrist, initial encounter POA: N

LO 23.4 Diagnosis-Related Groups

In addition to dealing with diagnosis and procedure codes, hospitals must work with **diagnosis-related groups (DRGs)** for Medicare reimbursement, under Medicare Part A—Hospital Insurance. To determine how much an acute care facility will be paid, the Inpatient Prospective Payment System (IPPS) was developed. Within IPPS, each and every patient case is sorted into a DRG.

Each DRG has a payment weight assigned to it determined by the typical resources used to care for the patient in that case. This calculation includes the labor costs, such as nurses and technicians, as well as nonlabor costs, such as maintenance for equipment and supplies.

Typically, professional coding specialists do not have to worry about assigning the DRG for a patient's case. This is determined, most often, by a special software program known as a "DRG grouper."

diagnosis-related group (DRG)
An episodic-care payment system basing reimbursement to hospitals for inpatient services upon standards of care for specific diagnoses grouped by their similar usage of resources for procedures, services, and treatments.

Principal Diagnosis

So why do you need to know all this? The *principal* diagnosis assigned is one of the factors used to determine which DRG is most accurate. Particularly when it comes to coding for reporting inpatient services to a Medicare beneficiary, the sequence in which you place the diagnosis codes can make a big difference in how accurately the hospital will be reimbursed.

Remember that the principal, or first-listed, diagnosis as defined by the guidelines is "that condition established after study to be chiefly responsible for occasioning the admission of the patient to the hospital for care." This is the diagnosis that explains the most serious reason for the patient to be in the hospital. This might be the reason for admission, it might be the most serious condition, or it might be the condition that required the greatest number of services, treatments, or procedures during the patient's stay in the hospital.

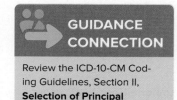

GUIDANCE CONNECTION

Review the ICD-10-CM Coding Guidelines, Section II, **Selection of Principal Diagnosis,** for more input.

LO 23.5 Complications and Co-morbidities

As each diagnosis is evaluated for its standard of care, CMS understands that a patient in a hospital may have multiple conditions or concerns (signs, symptoms, diagnoses) that are interrelated and create a more complex need for care. These may be *complications and/or co-morbidities (CCs).*

In some cases, regardless of the precautions that may be taken, **complications** of a procedure or treatment may arise during the patient's stay. Such a condition must be coded and reported to support the medical necessity for the treatment provided to resolve the concern.

complication
An unexpected illness or other condition that develops as a result of a procedure, service, or treatment provided during the patient's hospital stay.

EXAMPLE

Curtis had surgery this morning and is now having a bronchospasm, a reaction to the general anesthesia. This bronchospasm is a complication of the administration of general anesthesia and must be coded and reported to identify the medical necessity for the treatments to help alleviate this condition.

You have learned that a patient may have, or end up with, several different conditions treated during a stay in the hospital. The individual may also have preexisting conditions that have nothing to do with the reason for admission but still need attention by hospital personnel.

co-morbidity
A separate condition or illness present in the same patient at the same time as another, unrelated condition or illness.

major complication and co-morbidity (MCC)
A complication or co-morbidity that has an impact on the treatment of the patient and makes care for that patient more complex.

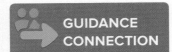

GUIDANCE CONNECTION

Review the ICD-10-CM Coding Guidelines, Section III, **Reporting Additional Diagnoses,** for more input.

Uniform Hospital Discharge Data Set (UHDDS)
A compilation of data collected by acute care facilities and other designated health care facilities.

Major Complications and Co-morbidities

Conditions, illnesses, injuries come in all shapes and sizes, as well as severities, and so do complications and co-morbidities. Typically, a **major complication and co-morbidity (MCC)** is a condition that is systemic, making treatment for the principal diagnosis more complex and/or making the health concern life-threatening.

LO 23.6 Uniform Hospital Discharge Data Set

The **Uniform Hospital Discharge Data Set (UHDDS)** is a collection of specific data gathered about hospital patients at discharge. No, this is not an invasion of privacy, nor is it a collection of personal data. The information pulled from hospital claim forms is related to demographic and clinical details.

Demographic data include:

- *Gender.*
- *Age.*
- *Race and ethnicity.*
- *Geographic location.*
- *Provider information,* such as the hospital facility National Provider Identifier (NPI) as well as attending and operating physician(s).
- *Expected sources of payment,* including primary and other sources of payment for this care.
- *Length of stay (LOS),* determined by date of admission and date of discharge.
- *Total charges billed by the hospital* for this admission (this will not include physician and other professional services billed).

Clinical data collected evaluate:

- *Type of admission,* described as *scheduled* (planned in advance with preregistration at least 24 hours prior) or *unscheduled.*
- *Diagnoses,* including principal and additional diagnoses.
- *Procedures, services, and treatments provided* during this admission period.
- *External causes of injury,* determined by the reporting of external cause codes.

Definitions of these, and other, categories as determined by the UHDDS are used by ICD-10-CM in the official coding guidelines. Over the years that the UHDDS has been in place, these definitions have been used to assist the reporting of patient data not only in acute care facilities (hospitals) but also for inpatient short-term care, long-term care, and psychiatric hospitals. Outpatient providers including home health agencies, nursing homes, and rehabilitation facilities also use these definitions for their data.

Chapter Summary

The coding process remains the same for inpatient and outpatient services for which coders are determining and reporting accurate diagnosis codes. The same code set, ICD-10-CM, is used; the same guidelines are used (with the exception of the two specific guidelines). Therefore, with the additional knowledge provided in this chapter, a professional coder can be successful in any type of facility.

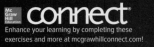

Using Terminology

Match each key term to the appropriate definition.

_____ **1.** LO 23.5 A complication or co-morbidity that has an impact on the treatment of the patient and makes care for that patient more complex.

_____ **2.** LO 23.5 A separate condition or illness present in the same patient at the same time as another, unrelated condition or illness.

_____ **3.** LO 23.6 A compilation of data collected by acute care facilities and other designated health care facilities.

_____ **4.** LO 23.1 System in which coding processes are performed while a patient is still in the hospital receiving care.

_____ **5.** LO 23.3 A condition, illness, or injury contracted by the patient during his or her stay in an acute care facility; also known as *nosocomial condition.*

_____ **6.** LO 23.5 An unexpected illness or other condition that develops as a result of a procedure, service, or treatment provided during the patient's hospital stay.

_____ **7.** LO 23.4 An episodic-care payment system basing reimbursement to hospitals for inpatient services upon standards of care for specific diagnoses grouped by their similar usage of resources for procedures, services, and treatments.

_____ **8.** LO 23.3 A one-character indicator reporting the status of the diagnosis at the time the patient was admitted to the acute care facility.

A. Co-morbidity

B. Complication

C. Concurrent coding

D. Diagnosis-related group (DRG)

E. Hospital-acquired condition (HAC)

F. Major complication and co-morbidity (MCC)

G. Present on admission (POA)

H. Uniform Hospital Discharge Data Set (UHDDS)

Checking Your Understanding

Choose the most appropriate answer for each of the following questions.

1. LO 23.4 The acronym DRG stands for

   a. diagnostic and radiologic guidelines.
   b. discharge restrictive guidance.
   c. diagnosis-related group.
   d. detailed radiologic groups.

2. LO 23.3 All of the following are POA indicators *except*

   a. W.
   b. X.
   c. Y.
   d. 1.

3. LO 23.1 The term *concurrent coding* means coding
   a. the case while the patient is still in the hospital.
   b. diagnosis and procedure codes at the same time.
   c. signs and symptoms along with confirmed diagnoses.
   d. all of these.

4. LO 23.2 Inpatient coders are not permitted to ever code something identified in the physician's notes as "suspected" or "probable."
   True.
   False.

5. LO 23.6 The UHDDS is a new code set that will replace ICD-10-CM in 2020.
   True.
   False.

6. LO 23.3 Felicia was admitted into the hospital with a compound fracture of the left femur head. Three days later, during her stay, she developed pneumonia. The POA indicator for the pneumonia is
   a. Y.
   b. N.
   c. W.
   d. 1.

7. LO 23.6 The UHDDS collects all of these data elements *except*
   a. gender.
   b. principal diagnosis.
   c. payment sources.
   d. credit card numbers.

8. LO 23.5 An example of a complication is
   a. postoperative wound infection.
   b. known allergy to penicillin.
   c. family history of breast cancer.
   d. high-risk pregnancy.

9. LO 23.4 DRGs are used for reimbursement from Medicare to
   a. physician offices.
   b. ambulatory surgical centers.
   c. acute care facilities.
   d. walk-in clinics.

10. LO 23.3 POA indicators are appended to the data element related to the admitting procedure code.
    True.
    False.

Applying Your Knowledge

1. LO 23.1 Explain concurrent coding. _____

_____

2. LO 23.3 Define *Present on admission,* according to CMS Publication 100-04. _____

_____

3. LO 23.3 What are POA indicators? Who requires their use, and what type of facility must use them? _____

_____

4. LO 23.3 List all of the POA indicators, and give their definitions. _____

_____

5. LO 23.4 Define and explain *DRG.* _____

_____

6. LO 23.4 What is a principal diagnosis? Why is it important? _____

_____

7. LO 23.5 Differentiate between a co-morbidity and a complication. _____

_____

8. LO 23.6 What does UHDDS stand for, and what is its function? _____

_____

9. LO 23.6 Discuss the types of data UHDDS collects. _____

_____

The following exercises provide practice in abstracting physicians' notes and learning to work with SOAP notes from our health care facility, Hillside Hospital. These case studies (SOAP notes) are modeled on real patient encounters. Using the techniques described in this chapter, carefully read through the case studies and determine the most accurate ICD-10-CM code(s) and external cause code(s), if appropriate, for each case study.

HILLSIDE HOSPITAL
359 Mountain Pass Road
Langston, FL 33993

DISCHARGE SUMMARY

PATIENT:	MASCONNI, ANGELO
DATE OF ADMISSION:	05/30/18
DATE OF SURGERY:	05/31/18
DATE OF DISCHARGE:	06/01/18
ADMITTING DIAGNOSIS:	Right breast mass
DISCHARGE DIAGNOSIS:	Malignant neoplasm of areola, right breast, estrogen receptor status negative; postsurgical respiratory congestion

This 39-year-old African-American male was admitted to the hospital with a palpable 2-cm nodule in the right breast in the superficial aspect of the right breast in the 5 o'clock axis near the periphery.

Excision of the right breast mass with an intermediate wound closure of 3 cm was accomplished. Patient tolerated the procedure well; however, some respiratory complications were realized as a result of the general anesthesia so the patient was kept in the facility for an extra day.

Patient is discharged home with his wife. Discharge orders instruct him to make a follow-up appointment with Dr. Facci, the oncologist, to discuss treatment.

Suzanne R. Taylor, MD—2222

556839/mt98328: 06/01/18 09:50:16   T: 06/01/18 12:55:01

Determine the most accurate ICD-10-CM code(s).

_____

_____

_____

HILLSIDE HOSPITAL
359 Mountain Pass Road
Langston, FL 33993

DISCHARGE SUMMARY

PATIENT: COLLIER, ROBIN
DATE OF ADMISSION: 07/15/18
DATE OF SURGERY: 07/29/18
DATE OF DISCHARGE: 08/01/18

ADMITTING DIAGNOSIS: Schizoaffective disorder
DISCHARGE DIAGNOSIS: Schizoaffective disorder; hypothyroidism; hypercholesterolemia;
                                                 borderline hypertension

The patient is a 57-year-old white female with a long history of schizoaffective disorder with numerous hospitalizations, brought in by ambulance for increasing paranoia; increasing arguments with other people; and, in general, an exacerbation of her psychotic symptoms, which had been worsening over the previous 2 weeks.

She is now discharged to return to her home at the YMCA and also to return to her weekly psychiatric appointments with Dr. Yahia. The patient also is advised to follow up with her medical doctor for her hypertension.

The patient was advised during this admission to start on hydrochlorothiazide 12.5 mg daily, but she refused.

She has been compliant with her medication until the recently refused hydrochlorothiazide. She is irritable at times, but overall she is redirectable and is considered to be at or close to her best baseline. She is considered in no imminent danger to herself or to others at this time.

Willard B. Reader, MD—4444

556848/mt98328: 08/01/18 09:50:16   T: 08/01/18 12:55:01

Determine the most accurate ICD-10-CM code(s).

_____

_____

_____

HILLSIDE HOSPITAL
359 Mountain Pass Road
Langston, FL 33993

DISCHARGE SUMMARY

PATIENT: DRONICA, BRUCE
DATE OF ADMISSION: 03/05/18
DATE OF DISCHARGE: 03/17/18

ADMITTING DIAGNOSIS: Major depressive disorder
DISCHARGE DIAGNOSIS: Alcohol dependence; cocaine dependence; major depressive
                                disorder, recurrent; HIV positive; hepatitis C; and history of
                                asthma

This 23-year-old single male was referred for this admission, his second lifetime rehabilitation.
The patient has a history of alcohol and cocaine dependence since age 17.

During the course of admission, the patient was placed on hydrochlorothiazide 25 milligrams for
hypertension, to which he responded well. He participated in this rehabilitation program and worked
rigorously throughout.

On discharge, the patient is alert and oriented ×3. Mood is euthymic. Affect is full range. The patient
denies SI, HI, denies AH, VH. Thought process is organized. Thought content—no delusions elicited.
There is no evidence of psychosis. There is no imminent risk of suicide or homicide.

John S. Warwick, MD—8888

556845/mt98328: 03/17/18 09:50:16   T: 03/17/18 12:55:01

Determine the most accurate ICD-10-CM code(s).

_____

_____

_____

HILLSIDE HOSPITAL
359 Mountain Pass Road
Langston, FL 33993

DISCHARGE SUMMARY

PATIENT: PREGGER, LOUIS
DATE OF ADMISSION: 01/15/18
DATE OF DISCHARGE: 01/17/18

ADMITTING DIAGNOSIS: Mass in bladder
DISCHARGE DIAGNOSIS: High-grade transitional cell carcinoma of the left bladder wall;
                                  low-grade transitional cell carcinoma in situ, bladder; underlying
                                  mild chronic inflammation, bladder

This 63-year-old male was admitted with a suspicious mass identified in the lateral bladder wall. Biopsy was performed, and upon pathology report of malignancy, a transurethral resection of the bladder tumors was performed. Patient was kept overnight. Foley catheter removed second day, and discharged with orders to make appointment to be seen in the office in about 2 weeks to start weekly BCG bladder installation treatments for recurrent bladder tumors.

Suzanne R. Taylor, MD—2222

556839/mt98328: 01/17/18 09:50:16   T: 01/17/18 12:55:01

Determine the most accurate ICD-10-CM code(s).

_____

_____

_____

HILLSIDE HOSPITAL
359 Mountain Pass Road
Langston, FL 33993

DISCHARGE SUMMARY

PATIENT: WOLSZCZAK, LEE
DATE OF ADMISSION: 10/07/18
DATE OF DISCHARGE: 10/09/18

ADMITTING DIAGNOSIS: Hematuria
DISCHARGE DIAGNOSIS: Benign prostatic hypertrophy; hematuria

This 45-year-old male had a transurethral resection of prostate 10 years ago, complicated by a postoperative bleed as well as evaluation with an attempted ureteroscopy. This hematuria is secondary to prostatic varices.

Flexible cystoscopy demonstrated a normal urethra and obstructed bladder outlet secondary to a very large nodular regrowth of the prostate at the medium lobe.

A transurethral resection of prostate was performed with success.

John S. Warwick, MD—8888

556845/mt98328: 10/09/18 09:50:16   T: 10/09/18 12:55:01

Determine the most accurate ICD-10-CM code(s).

_____

_____

_____

HILLSIDE HOSPITAL
359 Mountain Pass Road
Langston, FL 33993

DISCHARGE CLINICAL RESUME

PATIENT: BOLIVAR, STEPHEN
DATE OF ADMISSION: 05/09/18
DATE OF DISCHARGE: 05/14/18

ADMITTING DIAGNOSES:
1. Dyspnea
2. Congestive heart failure (CHR) exacerbation
3. Hypertension
4. Heart murmur
5. Inferior vena cava filter placed July 2010 secondary to lower extremity deep venous thrombosis (DVT)
6. Hypothyroidism with TSH 9.1
7. Peripheral vascular disease—peripheral arterial disease

DISCHARGE DIAGNOSES:
1. Dyspnea, resolved
2. Diastolic CHR, ejection fraction 70%
3. Hypertension, controlled
4. Aortic stenosis with insufficiency
5. Catheter placed secondary to deep venous thrombosis, on Coumadin, INR in 2 on discharge
6. Hypothyroidism
7. Peripheral vascular disease
8. Renal ultrasound with medical disease

HISTORY: An 88-year-old male who was admitted with dyspnea. He was found with diastolic CHF exacerbation. The patient was seen by Dr. Patel, vascular surgeon, who believed that he had some mild arterial insufficiency and continued anticoagulation. He wants to see him in his office as an outpatient. During admission, on and off he was having numbness in bilateral feet and hands and cyanosis that resolved by themselves with no problems. Probably Raynaud phenomenon. During the admission also was seen by cardiologist, who diuresed the patient with no complications. He believes that the patient needs to be started on 1 mg po Bumex. Weigh every day. If the weight gain is more than 3 pounds, Bumex is to be increased by 1 mg po. The patient also was seen by Dr. Bommineni, who believed that the patient can go home and continue follow-up as an outpatient. Pulmonology saw the patient as well and believed the same thing. The patient has been stable. Vital signs stable, afebrile, 98% 02 stat on room air. He was complaining of some biting itching. The daughter had taken him to the dermatologist and wants to continue follow-up with the dermatologist as an outpatient.

RECOMMENDATIONS: Discharge patient home. Follow up with Dr. Yablakoff in the nursing home.

(Continued)

DISCHARGE MEDICATIONS

1. The patient is going with alendronate 70 mg every week, bumetanide 1 mg twice a day if the weight gain is more than 3 pounds
2. Diovan 80 mg once a day
3. Levothyroxine was increased to 200 mcg every day, and check TSH in 4 weeks with Dr. Yablakoff
4. Metolazone 2.5 mg once a day
5. Potassium 20 prn every day
6. Warfarin 5 mg every day. Check INR every day and let Dr. Yablakoff know if the INR is more than 2.5
7. Medrol Dosepak as directed

The outpatient care plan was discussed with the patient and his daughter. They understood, had no questions, agreed with the plan.

_____

Roger Casey, MD—9999

556842/mt98328 05/14/18 12:13:56 05/14/18 17:51:58
cc. Carole Yablakoff, MD

Determine the most accurate ICD-10-CM code(s).

_____

_____

_____

HILLSIDE HOSPITAL
359 Mountain Pass Road
Langston, FL 33993

DISCHARGE CLINICAL RESUME

PATIENT:	NATUZZI, BARRY
DATE OF ADMISSION:	06/03/18
DATE OF DISCHARGE:	06/06/18

ADMITTING DIAGNOSIS: Ischemia transient ischemic attack, rule out myocardial infarction, arrythmia

DISCHARGE DIAGNOSES: Transient ischemic attack (TIA)
Hyperlipidemia
Coronary artery disease, status post coronary artery bypass graft and cardioversion
Urinary tract infection

CONSULTATIONS: Dr. Falkner for neurology and Dr. Mathias for cardiology

PROCEDURES: Echocardiogram, TEE, Thallium stress test

COMPLICATIONS: None

INFECTIOUS: None

HISTORY: Seventy-one-year old white male with significant history of coronary artery disease, status post coronary artery bypass graft 3 years ago and cardioversion in February 2016, who presented with difficulty speaking. He stated that he had difficulty obtaining the right words when he spoke. This lasted about 15 minutes; however, when the patient came to the emergency room he was completely okay. He did not have any deficits. The patient was admitted and consultants were called in to provide evaluation of possible TIA with rule out cardiac source. Carotid Doppler was done. Echocardiogram was done. This showed dilated left ventricle, severe global left ventricular dysfunction, estimated ejection fraction 20% and left atrial enlargement, mitral annular calcification with severe mitral regurgitation, aortic sclerosis with moderate aortic insufficiency and severe tricuspid regurgitation with estimated pulmonary study pressure of 70 mm. Thallium stress test was uneventful. Persantine infusion protocol and no clinical EKG changes of ischemia and radionuclide showed fixed defect anteroseptal, anteroapical, and adjacent inferior wall with hypokinesis; no ischemia seen. The ejection fraction was calculated 40%. CT of the brain showed white matter ischemic changes and atrophy, no acute intracranial abnormalities. MRI showed extensive periventricular white matter ischemia changes. MRA was normal. EKG was within normal limits, showing sinus bradycardia with average of 50 to 56.

The patient went to TEE to rule out cardiac source. The TEE was not conclusive and there was no hypokinesis, as described in the previous echocardiogram, and it was considered the patient needs to have lifetime Coumadin because of previous events.

(Continued)

The hospital course was uneventful. He never presented with any other new deficit or any new symptoms.

Today, the patient is asymptomatic; vital signs are stable. Monitor shows sinus rhythm, and he is discharged in stable condition to be followed by Dr. Roman in 1 week; by Dr. Falkner in 2 weeks, and by Dr. Mathias in 2 weeks. He will have home health nurse to inject him Lovenox until PT and INR reach therapeutic levels of 2/3. He will be on Coumadin 5 mg po qd, and home health nurse will draw PT and INR daily until Dr. Roman thoroughly assesses the patient. He will receive the last dose of Bactrim today for urine; however, urine culture has been negative.

Roger Casey, MD—9999

556842/mt98328 06/06/18 1:23:36 06/06/18 10:11:59
cc. Kevin Roman, MD

Determine the most accurate ICD-10-CM code(s).

_____

_____

_____

HILLSIDE HOSPITAL
359 Mountain Pass Road
Langston, FL 33993

DISCHARGE DOCUMENT SUMMARY

PATIENT: BRINKLEY, CAROLE
DATE OF ADMISSION: 02/09/18
DATE OF DISCHARGE: 02/10/18

ADMISSION DIAGNOSIS: Abdominal pain, status postappendectomy

DISCHARGE DIAGNOSIS: Abdominal pain, unknown etiology, status postappendectomy

BRIEF HISTORY: The patient is an 18-year-old female who, 6 weeks ago, underwent an appendectomy for perforated appendicitis. About 3 weeks following that, she had episodes of nausea and vomiting and diffuse abdominal pain. This was worked up at McGraw Medical Center, including CT scan, Meckel scan, and laboratory, which were unremarkable. It resolved spontaneously over a 3-day period. Three days prior to admission, she had a recurrent bout of diffuse, dull, abdominal pain with associated nausea and anorexia. She was admitted to the hospital at the time for workup of this pain.

CLINICAL COURSE: On examination, the patient was found to have a diffuse, mild tenderness without any rebound or peritoneal signs. Plain radiographs of the abdomen were obtained, which were within normal limits. A CT scan of the abdomen and pelvis was also obtained, which was unremarkable. She was without leukocytosis. Dr. Andrews of GI saw the patient in consultation, and an upper GI with small bowel follow-through was obtained. This was performed today and was found to be normal.

At this time, the patient has just had a regular meal without difficulty and feels like returning home. She will be discharged home at this time and can follow up with her primary MD. We will see her on an as-needed basis.

_____

Gail Robbins, MD—7777

6582411/mt98328 02/10/18 12:13:56 02/10/18 17:51:58

Determine the most accurate ICD-10-CM code(s).

_____

_____

_____

HILLSIDE HOSPITAL
359 Mountain Pass Road
Langston, FL 33993

DISCHARGE DOCUMENT SUMMARY

PATIENT: LOWENSON, MARC

DATE OF ADMISSION: 08/01/18

DATE OF DISCHARGE: 08/22/18

FINAL DIAGNOSES:

1. Alcohol dependence, methamphetamine dependence
2. Major depressive disorder, recurrent, current episode severe
3. HIV
4. Tuberculosis of the lung, primary
5. Hepatitis C, chronic

DISCHARGE MEDICATIONS:

1. Zoloft 100 mg, po, qam
2. Seroquel 50 mg po qhs
3. Truvade 1 tab qam
4. Regataz 300 mg po qam
5. Norvir 100 mg po qam with breakfast
6. Dapsone 100 mg po qam
7. Hydrochlorothiazide 25 mg po qam

DISPOSITION: The patient will return to his residence at the Midtown Hotel. He will attend the hospital continuing day treatment program.

PROGNOSIS: Guarded

HISTORY: He is noted to have significant immunosuppression related to his HIV. Currently there is no stigmata of opportunistic infection.

During the course of admission, the patient was placed on hydrochlorothiazide 25 mg for hypertension, which he responded well to.

CONDITION ON DISCHARGE: The patient is a 54-year-old single black male referred for his first BRU admission, his second lifetime rehabilitation. The patient has a history of alcohol and methamphetamine dependence since age 21. Prior to this admission, he had attained no significant period of sobriety other than time spent incarcerated.

The patient participated in a 21-day MICA rehabilitation program. He worked rigorously throughout the entire program. He had perfect attendance and participated well as a peer support provider. The patient attended eight groups daily. He worked well in individual therapy with his nurse practitioner and social worker.

(Continued)

On discharge, the patient is alert and oriented ×3. Mood is euthymic. Affect is full range. The patient denies SI, HI, denies AH, VH. Thought process is organized. Thought content—no delusions elicited. There is no evidence of psychosis. There is no imminent risk of suicide or homicide.

Keith Masters, MD—5555

517895221/mt98328 08/22/18 12:13:56 08/22/18 17:51:58

Determine the most accurate ICD-10-CM code(s).

_____

_____

_____

HILLSIDE HOSPITAL
359 Mountain Pass Road
Langston, FL 33993

DISCHARGE CLINICAL RESUME

PATIENT: WYLER, WENDY
DATE OF ADMISSION: 11/05/18
DATE OF DISCHARGE: 11/18/18

This is a 36–37-week female delivered to a 22-year-old, gravida 2, para 1, who was a known breech presentation. Mother presented with complaint of vaginal bleeding, rupture of membranes, and abdominal pain and cramping. On exam found to be complete with large fecal impaction. Fetal heart rate 120 by monitor. To c-section room for disimpaction and cesarean section for breech. Delivered precipitously immediately after impaction was removed, breech presentation. OB moved baby to warmer. She was pale with no respiratory effort or heart rate. Ambu bagged with mask for 30 seconds. Intubation attempted. Code called. UAC was placed. ENT in place and bagged. No heart rate, no breath sounds, pale, cyanotic. Reintubated with chest rise, heart rate about 60. Chest compression stopped when heart rate above 120, color improved. Apgar 0 at 1 minute, 1 at 5 minutes, and 4 at 10 minutes. No spontaneous respiratory effort. Received sodium bicarbonate, epinephrine, and calcium. No grimace, no spontaneous movements. Pupils midpoint, nonreactive to light. NG placed for distended abdomen. Cord pH 7.33. Mother noted to have 50% abruptio placenta. Transferred to Neo. UAC was removed and replaced. UVC also placed.

Physical exam: weight 2,620 grams, pink, fontanelle soft, significant clonus of extremities, tone decreased. Pupils 2 cm and round, nonreactive to light. No movement, no grimace, no suck, good chest rise. Equal breath sounds, no murmur. Pulses 2+. Perfusion good. Abdomen soft and full. No masses. Normal female genitalia externally. Anus patent. Extremities no edema. Skin—Mongolian spot sacrum and both arms, single café-au-lait spot left flank 1.5 cm × 0.5 cm. Palate intact.

IMPRESSION:
1. 36–37 week AGA female
2. Status postcardiopulmonary arrest
3. Rule out sepsis
4. At risk for hypoxic ischemic encephalopathy

PHYSICAL EXAM: 43 days of age, weight 2,520 grams, head circumference 35, pink. Anterior fontanelle soft. Heart—II/VI murmur radiating to the axilla. Chest clear. Abdomen soft, positive bowel sounds, gastrostomy tube intact, wound is okay. Neuro—irritable. The infant has an anal fissure at 12 o'clock which has caused some blood streaks in the stool.

(Continued)

FINAL DIAGNOSES:
1. 36–37 week appropriate for gestational age female
2. History post cardiac arrest
3. Respiratory arrest
4. Rule out sepsis
5. Hypoxic ischemic encephalopathy, mild
6. Seizures
7. Gastroesophageal reflux and feeding problems
8. Postoperative cesarean wound disruption

Gary Benjamin, MD—3333

2564821/mt98328 11/18/18 12:13:56 11/18/18 17:51:58

Determine the most accurate ICD-10-CM code(s).

_____

_____

_____

YOU CODE IT! PRACTICE AND APPLICATION
Complete Diagnostic Coding Review

Learning Outcomes *After completing this chapter, the student should be able to:*

LO 24.1 Abstract physician's notes accurately to determine the appropriate key words.

LO 24.2 Assess the reasons the patient came to see the health care professional.

LO 24.3 Correctly apply the guidelines to find the most accurate diagnosis code or codes.

LO 24.4 Identify the circumstances that require an external cause code or codes.

LO 24.5 Apply the rules and policies in determining if additional codes are needed.

LO 24.6 Determine the correct sequencing when multiple codes are required.

The following exercises provide practice in abstracting physicians' notes from our health care facility, *Taylor, Reader, & Associates.* These case studies are modeled on real patient encounters. Using the techniques described in this textbook, carefully read through the case studies and determine the most accurate ICD-10-CM code(s), including external cause code(s) when appropriate, for each case study.

Using the techniques described in this textbook, carefully read through the case studies and determine the most accurate ICD-10-CM code(s), and external cause code(s) when appropriate, for each case study or scenario.

1. Isaac Thomas, a 73-year-old male, is admitted to the observation unit today after collapsing at church during services. He continues to have an irregular heartbeat.

_____

2. Johanna Arthur, a 7-year-old female, is brought into the ER by her parents due to a painful rash on her legs. The ER physician admits Johanna to the hospital with the diagnosis of severe poison ivy. Johanna's mother admitted Johanna was walking their dog at the local park this morning and must have come in contact with the poison ivy there.

_____

3. Dr. Maxwell calls in Dr. Frizzola for a consultation on 8-year-old David Harrison to determine if a tonsillectomy should be performed. David is currently in the hospital for treatment of his previously diagnosed acute lymphoblastic leukemia. Dr. Frizzola gathers a comprehensive history, performs a comprehensive examination in the hospital room, and spends time reviewing all prior test results. He then confirms the diagnosis of tonsillitis and schedules the procedure. Select the correct code(s).

   a. C91.00, J03.10
   b. J03
   c. J03.01, C91.00
   d. C91.00

_____

4. Jamie Farmer, a 19-year-old male, came into the hospital for initial observation for lower right quadrant pain, accompanied by nausea, vomiting, and a low-grade fever. Dr. Wadhwa was brought in for a surgical consultation, and he recommended that Jamie stay in the hospital overnight to rule out the possibility of a ruptured appendix.

_____

5. Randy Taylor, a 2-year-old male, is admitted into the hospital with bacterial pneumonia after 5 days of antibiotic therapy. At admittance, his vitals show a temperature of 38.3°C (101°F) with a mild rash on his torso. Select the correct code(s).

   a. R21, J15.8
   b. J15.211
   c. J15.9, R21
   d. R20.1, J15.211

_____

6. Loretta Gerbil, a 47-year-old female, was sent to Dr. Harrington, an OB/GYN, for an office consultation. She had been suffering with moderate pelvic pain, a heavy sensation in her lower pelvis, and marked discomfort during sexual intercourse. In a detailed history, Dr. Harrington noted the location, severity, and duration of her pelvic pain and related symptoms. In the review of systems, Loretta had positive findings related to her genitourinary system. Dr. Harrington noted that her past medical history was noncontributory to the present problem. The detailed physical examination centered on her genitourinary system with a complete pelvic exam. Dr. Harrington ordered lab tests and a pelvic ultrasound in order to consider uterine fibroids, endometritis, or other internal gynecologic pathology.

_____

7. Martin Mazzenthorp, a 52-year-old male, presents today to Dr. Appleton's office for a confirmatory consultation regarding his own physician's recommendation for surgical repair of a hiatal hernia. After a brief problem-focused exam of the affected body area and organ system, Dr. Appleton concurs with the diagnosis of a hiatal hernia and supports the original recommendation for surgery. Select the correct code(s).

a. K40.41
b. K44.9
c. K44.1
d. K44.0

_____

8. Carolina Tanner, an 18-year-old female, came into the emergency department with a wrist sprain where a ball had hit her. She is on her school baseball team and was at a practice game being played on the school baseball field when she got hit by the ball. She was in obvious pain, and the wrist was swollen and too painful upon attempts to flex. After Dr. Ramada reviewed the x-ray, Carolina was diagnosed with a Salter-Harris type II fracture of the distal radius, left.

_____

9. Bernard Kristenson, an 82-year-old male, was diagnosed with advanced Alzheimer's disease about 1 year ago. Today he is being seen by the nursing facility's physician, Dr. Mintz, over concern of the development of urinary and fecal incontinence. Dr. Mintz performs a comprehensive physical exam to assess all body systems. Bernard is diagnosed with Alzheimer's disease with dementia, and with fecal and urinary incontinence due to his severe physical immobility.

_____

10. Karyn Cassey, a 3-year-old female, is brought in by her mother to see Dr. Fahey, her pediatrician. Karyn has itchy spots all over her body. After a detailed examination, Dr. Fahey diagnoses her with chickenpox. Select the correct code.

a. B01
b. B01.89
c. B01.9
d. B01.12

_____

11. Verniece Dantini, a 61-year-old female, comes to see Dr. Smallerman for her regular annual physical examination. She has insulin-dependent diabetes mellitus with retinal edema and chronic kidney disease, stage 1. In addition, she suffers from hypertensive heart disease with episodes of congestive heart failure. After the exam, Dr. Smallerman spends some time talking with Verniece about her day-to-day activities, her diet and overall eating habits, whether or not she is engaging in regular exercise, and her overall mental attitudes as well as physical well-being. The patient states it can be difficult to get around by herself due to the problems with her eyes, and she is finding it more and more difficult to give herself the insulin injections. Dr. Smallerman provides her with some information about an insulin pump, and she states she will go over it and discuss it with her son.

12. Kimberly Huggins, an 18-year-old female, was deep-frying fish and the kettle fell over and burned her right thigh. Kimberly was rushed to the ER by her parents, where the ER physician, Dr. Humes, diagnosed her with a second-degree burn on her right thigh. Dr. Humes dressed the wounds and sent her to the burn unit. Select the correct code(s).

    a. T24.212A, T31.11, X15.3XXA, Y93.E5
    b. T24.211A, T31.0, X10.2XXA, Y93.G3
    c. T24.219D, T31.10, X12.XXA, Y93.41
    d. T31.0, T24.212A, X19.XXXA, Y93.A4

13. Karina Wilmington, a 33-year-old female, came to the office to see Dr. Grace because of a cough, fever, excessive sputum production, and shortness of breath. She had been reasonably well until now. Dr. Grace did a detailed exam of the respiratory system, as well as a review of the patient's cardiovascular system. Dr. Grace ordered a chest x-ray to rule out pneumonia and told Karina to come back in a week to discuss the test results.

14. Zena Johnson, a 37-year-old female, presents today with a painful and swollen leg just below the right knee. Zena states that the pain is worse at night and the pain comes and goes. Dr. Anthony does a thorough examination and the appropriate tests. Zena is diagnosed with parosteal osteogenic sarcoma. Select the correct code.

    a. C41.9
    b. C79.51
    c. D16.9
    d. D48.0

15. George Carter, a 17-month-old male, is brought in by his mother to see his pediatrician, Dr. Mitchell. George has a cough and fever and is breathing fast. After Dr. Mitchell completes a thorough examination and reviews the chest x-ray, he admits George to the hospital with pneumonia.

16. Tricia Thornwell, a 68-year-old female, was going walking when she fell down the icy front steps of her house; now she can't bear weight on her right leg. She was brought into the ER by ambulance. After the ER physician completed a thorough exam and reviewed the x-ray, Tricia was diagnosed with a femoral neck base fracture, nondisplaced.

17. Ellen Onoton, a 45-year-old female, recently diagnosed with asthma, comes to see Dr. Pashma with the complaint of headache, facial pain, and trouble sleeping due to shortness of breath. After the appropriate tests and a thorough examination, Dr. Pashma diagnoses Ellen with persistent moderate asthma, exacerbation.

18. Marie Neal, a 3-year-old female, is brought in today to see her pediatrician, Dr. Conyers, by her mother. Marie was playing in her mother's dresser and found a penny, and before her mother could get it from Marie, she put the penny in her mouth and swallowed it. Dr. Conyers notes Marie is breathing normally and orders x-rays. The x-rays confirmed the penny is in Marie's stomach. Dr. Conyers admits Marie in order to retrieve the penny. Select the correct code.

    a. T18.0XXA
    b. T18.100D
    c. T18.198A
    d. T18.2XXA

19. Frank Childers, a 72-year-old male in good health, came to see his regular family physician, Dr. Rappoport, for his yearly physical exam. No problems were found during the examination.

20. Raymond Catertell, a 20-year-old male, was admitted into the hospital 2 days ago for bronchitis. Raymond requested that his family physician, Dr. Kaminsky, perform a circumcision, so Dr. Kaminsky called in Dr. Longwell, a urologist, for a consultation. Dr. Longwell performed a problem-focused history and problem-focused physical exam and made the straightforward decision to recommend that Raymond have the surgical procedure done as an outpatient at a later date. Code for Dr. Longwell's consultation.

21. Maribelle Johannsen, a 23-year-old female, presents today with the complaints of loss of appetite, diarrhea, stomach cramps, and some vomiting and excessive gas. Dr. Benton asks Maribelle if she had been traveling recently. Maribelle states she went hiking with friends in the mountains last week. After the appropriate tests and examination, Dr. Benton diagnoses Maribelle with beaver fever (giardiasis).

22. Wilson McGraw, a 48-year-old male, comes in today to see Dr. Avenavour because he doesn't feel like eating and, when he does eat, he becomes nauseated and sometimes vomits. He also states he aches all over. Dr. Avenavour notes a low-grade fever (100.2°F), and eyes and skin are jaundiced. After a comprehensive examination and appropriate tests, Wilson is diagnosed with acute hepatitis B with delta-agent.

_____

23. Janet Windham, a 1-month-old female, is brought in today by her mother, who is concerned about the size of Janet's lips—they seem out of proportion to the rest of Janet's features. Dr. Young, her pediatrician, notes microcheilia, congenital. Select the correct code.

a. Q18.6
b. Q18.7
c. Q18.8
d. Q18.9

_____

24. Clifford Mickens, a 49-year-old male, comes in today to see Dr. Marasco because he has a hoarse-sounding voice for no reason that he is aware of, and it has lasted for over 7 weeks. Dr. Marasco performs a comprehensive examination and appropriate tests, and diagnoses Clifford with a benign neoplasm of the hypopharynx.

_____

25. Oscar Unger, a 40-year-old male, goes to his family physician, Dr. Carter, because he is experiencing jerky and uncontrolled movements. Dr. Carter notes lack of coordination, motor abnormalities, and some cognition issues. After the appropriate tests are completed and a comprehensive examination is completed, Dr. Carter diagnoses Oscar with Huntington's chorea with dementia.

_____

26. George Hackworth, a 64-year-old male, presents today with a painful groin area. Dr. Graham notes the area is filled with dead tissue, fluid, and pus. After an examination, Dr. Graham diagnoses George with a groin carbuncle. Select the correct code.

a. L02.214
b. L02.231
c. L02.224
d. L02.234

_____

27. Dr. Pittman goes to see his patient, Matilda Grinowski, a 78-year-old female, who has been homebound since having a stroke 1 year ago. Matilda has essential benign hypertension and peripheral vascular disease and is post-CVA hemiplegic on her dominant side. Dr. Pittman does an expanded problem-focused interval history and a problem-focused examination. Due to his familiarity with Matilda and her concerns, his medical decision making is straightforward. He renews her prescriptions.

_____

28. Ronald Walden, a 53-year-old male, presents today with the complaint of pain, swelling, and redness of the throat. After Dr. Limb completes an examination, he diagnoses Ronald with acute sialoadenitis.

_____

29. A 15-year-old female, Lakeesha Jones, sprained her left ankle and was brought to the emergency department by her mother. Lakeesha had been rollerblading and tripped, falling on the sidewalk. Lakeesha was in pain and unable to flex her ankle, which had already begun to swell. Dr. Carole talked with the girl about her ankle and gathered a brief history of the incident that caused the sprain, as well as any history relating to her legs and feet. He then performed a limited examination of her left leg, ankle, and foot. The imaging confirmed a sprained calcaneofibular ligament and a sprained anterior tibiofibular ligament.

_____

30. Michael Wright, a 69-year-old male, presents today with the complaint of frequent nighttime urination. Dr. Wells completes a comprehensive examination and diagnoses Michael with nocturia due to enlarged prostate. Select the correct codes.

a. R35.1, N40.0
b. R35.8, N40.1
c. N40.1, R35.1
d. N40.0, R35.0

_____

31. Elnora McWarren, a 28-year-old female at 41 weeks gestation, comes to see Dr. Farmer. Dr. Farmer diagnoses Elnora with postmature pregnancy and admits her to the hospital.

_____

YOU CODE IT! Application

The following exercises provide practice in abstracting physicians' notes and learning to work with SOAP notes from our health care facility, *Taylor, Reader, & Associates*. These case studies (SOAP notes) are modeled on real patient encounters. Using the techniques you have learned in this textbook, carefully read through the case studies and determine the most accurate ICD-10-CM code(s) and external cause code(s), if appropriate, for each case study.

TAYLOR, READER, & ASSOCIATES
A Complete Health Care Facility
975 CENTRAL AVENUE • SOMEWHERE, FL 32811 • 407-555-4321

PATIENT: GONZALEZ, RENITA
ACCOUNT/EHR #:   GONZRE001
DATE: 09/16/18

Attending Physician: Suzanne R. Taylor, MD

S: This new Pt is a 72-year-old female brought in by her daughter. She has been anxious, hyperventilating, labored breath, short of breath—worse since taking medication for anxiety. She is allergic to PCN, Biaxin, and ASA.

Patient has a history of asthma and kidney stones. She is retired. Patient is extremely anxious. She states her husband died 2 years ago, and she has been having trouble. She started seeing a psychiatrist 1 week ago, and he prescribed Zoloft 50 mg bid. She is also taking Liseropril 1 tab qd, potassium 20 mg qd. She denies pain but has trouble breathing at times when she is anxious.

O: Wt. 160 lb. Ht 5′6″. T 97.5. P 95. R 26. BP 155/83. Lungs clear. Pt calmed down with reassurance and emotional support. EKG abnormal, cardiac enzyme in normal range. Automated differential, PT, PTT, EKG show normal sinus rhythm. Left ventricular hypertrophy with repolarization abnormality, Chest x-rays (PA and Lat) show no acute intrathoracic abnormality. CBC: Glucose is elevated; sodium, potassium, and chloride are low. All other labs are unremarkable.

A: Anxiety

P: 1. Rx Xanax 1 mg po tid
     2. Follow-up with psychiatrist

_____

Suzanne R. Taylor, MD

SRT/pw   D: 09/16/18 09:50:16   T: 09/18/18 12:55:01

Determine the most accurate ICD-10-CM code(s).

_____

_____

_____

TAYLOR, READER, & ASSOCIATES
A Complete Health Care Facility
975 CENTRAL AVENUE • SOMEWHERE, FL 32811 • 407-555-4321

PATIENT: DEPARI, WILLARD
ACCOUNT/EHR #:   DEPAWI001
DATE: 08/11/18
Physical Therapist: Donata R. Chen, MPT

Attending Physician: Willard B. Reader, MD

DX. Derangement of anterior horn medial meniscus due to old tear, right knee

Order for physical therapy:
    Moist heat, cryotherapy, muscle stimulation, whirlpool, massage
    ROM: active, active assistive, passive
    Exercise: isometric, isotonic ambulation training, as tolerated

3 a week for 6 weeks

Session # 3/6:   Pain Level: 4/10
Pt states pain shooting down right medial lower leg and numbness in toes.
                  Total time: 35 minutes
                  10 minutes. Cold pack/right knee
                  25 minutes. Therapeutic exercise . . . to increase strength and ROM

Symptoms began to return in right lower leg toward the end of the exercise. No new exercises added.

_____

Donata R. Chen, MPT

DRC/pw   D: 08/11/18 09:50:16   T: 08/13/18 12:55:01

Determine the most accurate ICD-10-CM code(s).

_____

_____

_____

TAYLOR, READER, & ASSOCIATES
A Complete Health Care Facility
975 CENTRAL AVENUE • SOMEWHERE, FL 32811 • 407-555-4321

PATIENT: BENJAMIN, DAVIDA
ACCOUNT/EHR #:   BENJDA001
DATE: 09/16/18

Attending Physician: Suzanne R. Taylor, MD

S: Pt is a 49-year-old female complaining of abdominal pain. She states that the pain has been consistent since noon and vomiting since 2 p.m. She has been experiencing chills and weakness, as well. No diarrhea. Last BM was a small one at 7 a.m. and again at 2 p.m. She was in good health prior to the symptoms at noon. She also has GERD.

O: Wt. 140 lb. Ht 5′2″. T 99. P 90. R 18. BP 128/73. Abdomen distended, tympanic, tender. CT Scan abd/pelvis: Dilated small bowel loop appears to contain semisolid material in RLQ, compatible with early small bowel obstruction. EKG: Sinus tachycardia, otherwise normal EKG. Bowel sounds are normal and hypoactive. Breathing pattern is nonlabored; breath sounds clear. Heart rhythm: regular. Neck veins: nondistended. Skin: warm, dry, intact. Peripheral pulses: Normal.

CBC w/differential: WBC, RBC, HGB, and HCT are high; MCHC is low; all other results unremarkable. Glucose and BUN/Creat are high; anion gap is low; all other chemistry unremarkable. UA: UR is cloudy, glucose high.

A: Small bowel obstruction; pure hypercholesterolemia; diaphragmatic hernia; esophageal reflux with esophagitis

P: Admit to hospital for surgery

Suzanne R. Taylor, MD

SRT/pw   D: 09/16/18 09:50:16   T: 09/18/18 12:55:01

Determine the most accurate ICD-10-CM code(s).

_____

_____

_____

TAYLOR, READER, & ASSOCIATES
A Complete Health Care Facility
975 CENTRAL AVENUE • SOMEWHERE, FL 32811 • 407-555-4321

PATIENT: BLACK, YVONDA
ACCOUNT/EHR #: BLACYV001
DATE: 08/11/18

Attending Physician: Willard B. Reader, MD

S: Pt is a 6-year-old female seen in our emergency facility. She was brought in by ambulance, accompanied by her mother. Mother states that they were baking cookies when the phone rang. She turned to answer it, and when she returned, the child was unconscious on the kitchen (apartment) floor. A bottle of wintergreen oil was found empty next to the patient.

O: Pt is listless and unresponsive. Respiration labored, BP 80/65, P slow and erratic. Skin is pale and moist. Stomach pumped. Pt responding to treatment.

A: Poisoning by overdose of wintergreen oil, accidental

P: Admit to observation unit

_____

Willard B. Reader, MD

WBR/pw   D: 08/11/18 09:50:16   T: 08/13/18 12:55:01

Determine the most accurate ICD-10-CM code(s).

_____

_____

_____

TAYLOR, READER, & ASSOCIATES
A Complete Health Care Facility
975 CENTRAL AVENUE • SOMEWHERE, FL 32811 • 407-555-4321

PATIENT: WEBSTER, LEOPOLD
ACCOUNT/EHR #:   WEBSLE001
DATE: 09/16/18

Attending Physician: Suzanne R. Taylor, MD

S: Pt is a 47-year-old male brought in by ambulance and accompanied by his wife. Wife states he has been confused, dizzy, and vomiting all morning.

O: Ht 5'11". Wt. 187 lb. R 16. During the physical examination the patient has a dramatic drop in vital sign measurements and suffers cardiac arrest. The crash team takes over and patient is successfully resuscitated. Blood work reveals overdose of digoxin. After Pt is stabilized, he states he was in a rush to get to work this morning and couldn't remember if he had taken his medication, so he took it again.

A: Cardiac arrest due to overdose of digoxin, accidental

P: Admit for stabilization
 Oxygenation
 Hydration IV fluids
 Monitor electrolyte balance

Suzanne R. Taylor, MD

SRT/pw D: 09/16/18 09:50:16 T: 09/18/18 12:55:01

Determine the most accurate ICD-10-CM code(s).

_____

_____

_____

TAYLOR, READER, & ASSOCIATES
A Complete Health Care Facility
975 CENTRAL AVENUE • SOMEWHERE, FL 32811 • 407-555-4321

PATIENT: STARKER, SHARON
ACCOUNT/EHR #:   STARSH001
DATE: 08/11/18

Attending Physician: Willard B. Reader, MD

S: Patient is a 41-year-old female, who comes in with a complaint of severe neck pain and difficulty turning her head. She states she was in a car accident 2 days ago, her car struck from behind when she was driving home from work on the freeway near her home.

O: PE reveals tightness upon palpation of ligaments in neck and shoulders, most pronounced C3 to C5. X-rays are taken of head and neck, including the cervical vertebrae. Radiologic review denies any fracture.

A: Anterior longitudinal cervical sprain

P: 1. Applied cervical collar to be worn during all waking hours
    2. Rx Vicodin (hydrocodone) 500 mg po prn
    3. 1,000 mg aspirin qid
    4. Pt to return in 2 weeks for follow-up

Willard B. Reader, MD

WBR/pw   D: 08/11/18 09:50:16   T: 08/13/18 12:55:01

Determine the most accurate ICD-10-CM code(s).

_____

_____

_____

TAYLOR, READER, & ASSOCIATES
A Complete Health Care Facility
975 CENTRAL AVENUE • SOMEWHERE, FL 32811 • 407-555-4321

PATIENT: WESTERBY, ELMO
ACCOUNT/EHR #:   WESTEL001
DATE: 09/16/18

Attending Physician: Suzanne R. Taylor, MD

Preoperative DX: Eyelid edema, OD

Postoperative DX: Blepharochalasis, OD

Procedure: Repair, right superior orbit

Surgeon: Raul Sanchez, MD

Anesthesia: Local

PROCEDURE: After proparacaine was instilled in the eye, it was prepped and draped in the usual sterile manner, and 2% lidocaine with 1:200,000 epinephrine was injected into the superior aspect of the right orbit. A corneal protective shield was placed in the eye. The eye was placed in down-gaze.

The upper right lid was everted and examined.

The damage to the levator palpebrae superioris muscle was repaired using running suture of 6-0 plain gut. Bacitracin ointment was applied to the eye followed by an eye pad. The patient tolerated the procedure well and left the operating room in good condition.

Suzanne R. Taylor, MD

SRT/pw   D: 09/16/18 09:50:16   T: 09/18/18 12:55:01

Determine the most accurate ICD-10-CM code(s).

_____

_____

_____

TAYLOR, READER, & ASSOCIATES
A Complete Health Care Facility
975 CENTRAL AVENUE • SOMEWHERE, FL 32811 • 407-555-4321

PATIENT: CAPOZZI, VINCENT
ACCOUNT/EHR #:   CAPOVI001
DATE: 08/11/18

Attending Physician: Willard B. Reader, MD

S: Patient is a 62-year-old male previously seen by Dr. David Bush 18 months ago. The patient has a history of coronary artery disease and hyperlipidemia. He underwent coronary bypass surgery in 1973, by Dr. Howard, that involved a left internal mammary artery to left anterior descending. In 1989, he underwent a redo operation consisting of a right internal mammary artery to left anterior descending, saphenous vein graft to circumflex, and saphenous vein graft to right coronary artery.

He did well until yesterday afternoon when he developed an episode of moderate retrosternal chest pressure radiating to the right shoulder, which was prolonged and lasted until 3:00 a.m., at which time he presented to the ED. He apparently was given one nitroglycerin sublingual, with resolution of symptoms. The patient is currently asymptomatic on examination, and his review of systems is noncontributory.

O: He is alert, oriented times three, in no acute distress. HEENT: unremarkable. Lungs: clear. Cardiovascular: Regular rate and rhythm. No murmurs and no gallops. Abdomen: benign. Extremities: no edema. EKG: normal sinus rhythm with myocardial changes. Lipid Panel: all unremarkable except for a cholesterol of 255. CBC: within normal limits. PT and PTT within normal limits. Cardiac enzymes times one: negative. Chest x-ray: unremarkable.

Admitting DX: Prolonged chest pain with negative electrocardiogram and negative enzymes times one. Admit for observation to telemetry. In view of the atypical nature of prolonged chest pain, we will proceed with a screening Cardiolite stress test later today. Nitroglycerin paste was applied on admission; however, it will be held until the stress test is completed. One aspirin a day was started. Further recommendation and interventions will depend on the results from the stress test.

Discharge DX: Coronary atherosclerosis of native coronary artery

Willard B. Reader, MD

WBR/pw   D: 08/11/18 09:50:16   T: 08/13/18 12:55:01

Determine the most accurate ICD-10-CM code(s).

_____

_____

_____

TAYLOR, READER, & ASSOCIATES
A Complete Health Care Facility
975 CENTRAL AVENUE • SOMEWHERE, FL 32811 • 407-555-4321

PATIENT: GAYLORD, NITA
ACCOUNT/EHR #: GAYLNI001
DATE: 09/16/18

Attending Physician: Suzanne R. Taylor, MD

S: The patient is a 35-year-old female who comes in with severe lower-right-quadrant pain and vomiting. Nita states she has been nauseated for the last few days.

O: Ht 5′4″. Wt. 135 lb. P 103. R 21. T 101.4. BP 135/85. Abdomen is positive for rebound tenderness upon manual examination. Comprehensive metabolic blood test, general health panel blood workup, and an MRA, abdomen, angiography are taken. Results of all tests confirm a diagnosis of appendicitis.

A: Acute appendicitis with generalized peritonitis

P: Admit patient to hospital immediately for appendectomy.

Suzanne R. Taylor, MD

SRT/pw   D: 09/16/18 09:50:16   T: 09/18/18 12:55:01

Determine the most accurate ICD-10-CM code(s).

_____

_____

_____

TAYLOR, READER, & ASSOCIATES
A Complete Health Care Facility
975 CENTRAL AVENUE • SOMEWHERE, FL 32811 • 407-555-4321

PATIENT: KELLO, JOAN
ACCOUNT/EHR #:   KELLJO001
DATE: 09/16/18

Attending Physician: Suzanne R. Taylor, MD

S: The patient is a 25-year-old female with a history of recurrent sinus infections and was well until 5 days ago. She presents with fever, severe frontal headache, facial pain, and runny nose. Patient states she has been having difficulty concentrating.

O: T 101.5°. HEENT: Tenderness over frontal and left maxillary sinuses. Nasal congestion visible.
   CT scan reveals opacification of both frontal and left maxillary, sphenoid sinuses, and a possible large nonenhanced lesion in the brain.
   Parasagittal MRI and axial MRI show a large (7-cm) well-circumscribed epidural collection compressing the left frontal lobe.

A: Epidural abscess with frontal lobe lesions caused by significant compression on frontal lobe. Recommendation for surgery to evacuate the abscess.

P: Rx antibiotics and pseudoephedrine.

_____

Suzanne R. Taylor, MD

SRT/pw   D: 09/16/18 09:50:16   T: 09/18/18 12:55:01

Determine the most accurate ICD-10-CM code(s).

_____

_____

_____

TAYLOR, READER, & ASSOCIATES
A Complete Health Care Facility
975 CENTRAL AVENUE • SOMEWHERE, FL 32811 • 407-555-4321

PATIENT: RUBEN, BETTY
ACCOUNT/EHR #: RUBEBE01
DATE: 09/23/18

Attending Physician: James Healer, MD

Preoperative Diagnosis: C5 Traumatic spondylolisthesis, type III, initial encounter

Postoperative Diagnosis: same

Procedure: C5 corpectomy and fusion fixation with fibular strut graft and Atlantis plate

Anesthesia: General endotracheal

This is a 25-year-old female status post assault. The Pt sustained a C5 traumatic spondylolisthesis, type III. MRI scan showed evidence of posterior ligamentous injury. The patient was subsequently set up for the surgical procedure. The procedure was described in detail including the risks. The risks included but were not limited to bleeding, infection, stroke, paralysis, death, cerebrospinal fluid (CSF) leak, loss of bladder and bowel control, hoarse voice, paralyzed vocal cord, death and damage to adjacent nerves and tissues. The Pt understood the risks. The Pt also understood that back bone instrumentation would be used and that the back bone could collapse and the instrumentation could fail, break, or the screws could pull out. The Pt provided consent.

The Pt was taken to the OR. Endotracheal tube was placed. A Foley was placed. The Pt was given preoperative antibiotics. The Pt was placed in slight extension. The right neck was prepped and draped in the usual manner. A linear incision was made over the C5 vertebral body. The platysma was divided. Dissection was continued medial to the sternocleidomastoid to the prevertebral fascia. This was cauterized and divided.

The longus colli was cauterized and elevated. A spinal needle was used to verify the location using fluoroscopy. The C5 vertebral body was drilled out. The bone was saved. The disks above and below were removed. The posterior longitudinal ligament was removed. The bone was quite collapsed and fragmented. Distraction pins were then packed with bone removed from the C5 vertebral body prior to implantation. A plate was then placed with screws in the C4 and C6 vertebral bodies. The locking screws were tightened. The wound was irrigated. Bleeding was helped with the bipolar. The retractors were removed. The incision was approximated with simple interrupted Vicryl. The subcutaneous tissue was approximated and skin edges approximated subcuticularly. Steri-Strips were applied. A dressing was applied. The Pt was placed back in an Aspen collar. The Pt was extubated and transferred to recovery.

James Healer, MD

JH/mgr   D: 09/23/18 12:33:08 PM   T: 09/25/18 3:22:54 PM

Determine the most accurate ICD-10-CM code(s).

_____

_____

_____

TAYLOR, READER, & ASSOCIATES
A Complete Health Care Facility
975 CENTRAL AVENUE • SOMEWHERE, FL 32811 • 407-555-4321

PATIENT: KLOTSKY, STACY
ACCOUNT/EHR #:   KLOTST01
Admission Date: 10/05/18
Discharge Date: 10/05/18
DATE: 10/05/18

Preoperative DX: Rule out bladder tumor
Postoperative DX: Chronic cystitis with squamous cell metaplasia
Procedure: Cystoscopy, biopsy, and fulguration of bladder

Surgeon: Leonard Dupont, MD

Assistant: None
Anesthesia: Spinal

Indications: The Pt is a 73-year-old female with a history of grade II superficial transitional cell carcinoma of the bladder. Cystoscopy showed a suspicious erythematous area on the right trigone. She presented today for cystoscopy, biopsy, and fulguration. Findings—the urethra was normal, the bladder was 1+ trabeculated, the mid and right trigone areas were slightly erythematous and hypervascular. No papillary tumors were noted; no mucosal abnormalities were noted.

Procedure: The Pt was placed on the table in supine position. Satisfactory spinal anesthesia was obtained. She was placed in dorsolithotomy position. She was prepped sterilely with Hibiclens and draped in the usual manner. A #22 French cystoscopy sheath was passed per urethra in atraumatic fashion. The bladder was resected with the 70-degree lens with findings as noted above. Cup biopsy forceps were placed, and three biopsies were taken of the suspicious areas of the trigone. These areas were fulgurated with the Bugby electrode; no active bleeding was seen. The scope was removed; the Pt was returned to recovery having tolerated the procedure well. Estimated blood loss was minimal.

Pathology report: Chronic cystitis with squamous cell metaplasia.

Leonard Dupont, MD

LD/pw   D: 10/05/18 09:50:16   T: 10/05/18 12:55:01

Determine the most accurate ICD-10-CM code(s).

_____

_____

_____

TAYLOR, READER, & ASSOCIATES
A Complete Health Care Facility
975 CENTRAL AVENUE • SOMEWHERE, FL 32811 • 407-555-4321

PATIENT: VALLARDI, CARMINE
ACCOUNT/EHR #: VALLCA001
DATE: 09/16/18

Attending Physician: Suzanne R. Taylor, MD

Pt is an 18-month-old male, brought to the emergency department by his mother. The mother found the child in the bathroom at home chewing on children's Tylenol tablets. She stated that she had just purchased the bottle the day before and had only used one tablet. When she found the boy, the bottle was nearly empty. She also states that he has been going in and out of consciousness.

Child was taken immediately into the procedure room, and we pumped his stomach. It appeared that many tablets had not yet dissolved. Transient alteration of awareness appears to be lessening. We will continue to monitor the child for the next 12 to 24 hours. Blood tests show a low but toxic level of acetaminophen.

Suzanne R. Taylor, MD

SRT/pw   D: 9/16/18 09:50:16   T: 9/18/18 12:55:01

Determine the most accurate ICD-10-CM code(s).

_____

_____

_____

TAYLOR, READER, & ASSOCIATES
A Complete Health Care Facility
975 CENTRAL AVENUE • SOMEWHERE, FL 32811 • 407-555-4321

PATIENT: JABELONE, JAMAL
ACCOUNT/EHR #: JABEJA01
Admission Date: 10/09/18
Discharge Date: 10/09/18
DATE: 10/09/18

Preoperative DX: Lacerations of arm, hand, and leg
Postoperative DX: same
Procedure: Layered repair of leg laceration; simple repair of arm and hand lacerations

Surgeon: Geoff Conner, MD

Assistant: None
Anesthesia: General

Indications: The patient is a 4-year-old male brought to the emergency room by his father. He was helping his father install a new dining room window at home when the window fell and shattered. The boy suffered lacerations on his left hand, left arm, and left leg.

Procedure: The patient was placed on the table in supine position. Satisfactory anesthesia was obtained. The area was prepped, and attention to the deeper laceration of the left thigh, right above the patella, was first. A layered repair was performed and the 5.1-cm laceration was closed successfully with sutures. The lacerations on the upper extremity, 2-cm laceration on the left hand at the base of the fifth metacarpal, and the 3-cm laceration on the left arm, just below the joint capsule in the posterior position, were successfully closed with 4-0 Vicryl as well. The patient tolerated the procedures well, and was transported to the recovery room.

Geoff Conner, MD

GC/pw   D: 10/09/18 09:50:16   T: 10/09/18 12:55:01

Determine the most accurate ICD-10-CM code(s).

_____

_____

_____

TAYLOR, READER, & ASSOCIATES
A Complete Health Care Facility
975 CENTRAL AVENUE • SOMEWHERE, FL 32811 • 407-555-4321

PATIENT: BACHELDER, JEFFREY
ACCOUNT/EHR #:   BACHJE01
Admission Date: 10/13/18
Discharge Date: 10/13/18
DATE: 10/13/18

Preoperative DX: Malignant neoplasm, scrotum, CA in situ
Postoperative DX: same
Procedure: Resection of scrotum, needle biopsy of testis, laparoscopy with a
                           ligation of spermatic veins

Surgeon: Daniel Macintosh, MD

Assistant: None
Anesthesia: General

Indications: The Pt is a 59-year-old male with a recent diagnosis of malignancy of the scrotum.

Procedure: The Pt was placed on the table in supine position. Dr. Cattan administered general anesthesia. The Pt was placed in proper position. A needle biopsy was taken of the testis, and then a surgical resection of the scrotum was performed. Before closing, a surgical laparoscopy with a ligation of the spermatic veins was performed as well.

_____

Daniel Macintosh, MD

DM/pw   D: 10/13/18 09:50:16   T: 10/13/18 12:55:01

Determine the most accurate ICD-10-CM code(s).

_____

_____

_____

TAYLOR, READER, & ASSOCIATES
A Complete Health Care Facility
975 CENTRAL AVENUE • SOMEWHERE, FL 32811 • 407-555-4321

PATIENT: DENNISON, DANIEL

ACCOUNT/EHR #:   DENNDA01

DATE: 11/23/18

Procedure Performed: Vasectomy

Physician: Sunil Kaladuwa, MD

Indications: Elective sterilization

Procedure: The Pt was given Versed for anxiety, and local anesthesia was administered. Removal of a segment of the deferent duct was accomplished bilaterally. Pt tolerated the procedure well.

Impression: Successful outcome.

Plan: Postoperative semen examination is scheduled for 1 week.

_____

Sunil Kaladuwa, MD

MA/mg   D: 11/23/18 09:50:16   T: 11/25/18 12:55:01

Determine the most accurate ICD-10-CM code(s).

_____

_____

_____

TAYLOR, READER, & ASSOCIATES
A Complete Health Care Facility
975 CENTRAL AVENUE • SOMEWHERE, FL 32811 • 407-555-4321

PATIENT: KLACKSON, KEVIN
ACCOUNT/EHR #:   KLACKE01
DATE: 09/15/18

Diagnosis: Constrictive cardiomyopathy with chest pain
Procedure: Arterial catheterization

Physician: Frank Vincent, MD

Anesthesia: Local

Procedure: The Pt was placed on the table in supine position. Local anesthesia was administered. Once we were assured that the Pt had achieved no nervous stimuli, the incision was made and the catheter was introduced percutaneously. The incision was sutured with a simple repair. The Pt tolerated the procedure well and was transferred to the recovery room.

Frank Vincent, MD

FV/mg D: 09/15/18 09:50:16 T: 09/15/18 12:55:01

Determine the most accurate ICD-10-CM code(s).

_____

_____

_____

TAYLOR, READER, & ASSOCIATES
A Complete Health Care Facility
975 CENTRAL AVENUE • SOMEWHERE, FL 32811 • 407-555-4321

PATIENT: UNDERWOOD, PRICILLA
ACCOUNT/EHR #: UNDEPR01
DATE: 09/25/18

Diagnosis: Medulloblastoma at the temporal lobe

Procedure: Central venous access device (CVAD) insertion

Physician: Frank Vincent, MD

Anesthesia: Conscious sedation

Procedure: Pt is a 4-year-old female, with a recent diagnosis of malignancy. Due to an upcoming course of chemotherapy, the CVAD is being inserted to ease administration of the drugs. The Pt was placed on the table in supine position. The Pt was given Versed to achieve conscious sedation. The incision was made to insert a central venous catheter, centrally. During the placement of the catheter, a short tract (non-tunneled) is made as the catheter is advanced from the skin entry site to the point of venous cannulation. The catheter tip is set to reside in the subclavian vein. The Pt was gently aroused from the sedation and was awake when transported to the recovery room.

Frank Vincent, MD

FV/mg   D: 09/25/18 09:50:16   T: 09/25/18 12:55:01

Determine the most accurate ICD-10-CM code(s).

_____

_____

_____

TAYLOR, READER, & ASSOCIATES
A Complete Health Care Facility
975 CENTRAL AVENUE • SOMEWHERE, FL 32811 • 407-555-4321

PATIENT: WALLACE, MARSHAL
ACCOUNT/EHR #: WALLMA001
DATE: 09/25/18

Attending Physician: Willard B. Reader, MD

S: Pt is a 29-year-old male who was caught in a house fire 6 months ago. He suffered deep third-degree burns on his chest wall and right leg. Pt is concerned about the scars on his body. He states he is self-conscious of the scars and will not go outside in shorts and will not go to the beach with his friends, something he used to do often.

O: Ht 6'0". Wt. 199 lb. R 18. T 98.6. BP 120/95. Examination shows disfiguring scars across the chest wall and covering almost all of the patient's right leg.

A: Severe scarring and disfigurement of chest wall and right leg

P: Referral to plastic surgeon

Willard B. Reader, MD

WBR/pw   D: 09/25/18 09:50:16   T: 09/27/18 12:55:01

Determine the most accurate ICD-10-CM code(s).

_____

_____

_____

TAYLOR, READER, & ASSOCIATES
A Complete Health Care Facility
975 CENTRAL AVENUE • SOMEWHERE, FL 32811 • 407-555-4321

PATIENT: BRADLEY, MICHAEL
ACCOUNT/EHR #: BRADMI001
DATE: 09/25/18

Attending Physician: Willard Reader, MD

S: Pt is a 37-year-old male who was involved in a fistfight at a local bar the previous evening. He complained of an ache in the area of his right eye as well as severe pain around his left ear.

O: Ht 5′10.5″. Wt. 209 lb. R 19. Surface hematoma evident in the area surrounding the left eye socket reaching to the upper cheek. Head x-ray of the right side confirmed a closed fracture of the right mandible.

A: Black eye, right; fracture of the right mandible, angle

P: 1. Wire right jaw
   2. NPO except liquids for 3 weeks
   3. Cold wet compresses on eye prn. Return for follow-up in 3 weeks

_____

Willard Reader, MD

WR/mg   D: 09/25/18 09:50:16   T: 09/27/18 12:55:01

Determine the most accurate ICD-10-CM code(s).

_____

_____

_____

GLOSSARY

A

Abnormal findings Test results that indicate a disease or condition may be present.

Abortion The end of a pregnancy prior to or subsequent to the death of a fetus.

Abuse (a) Ongoing, regular consumption of a substance with resulting clinical manifestations or wrong action or handling of a drug; (b) violent and/or inappropriate treatment of another person (child, adult, elder).

Accessory organs Organs that assist the digestive process and are adjacent to the alimentary canal: the gallbladder, liver, and pancreas.

Accommodation Adaptation of the eye's lens to adjust for varying focal distances.

Activities of daily living (ADLs) Daily tasks involved in normal function: bathing, dressing, eating, mobility, and personal hygiene.

Acute Severe; serious.

Adrenal glands Glands situated on the superior aspect of each kidney that secrete critical hormones, including epinephrine; also known as *suprarenal glands.*

Adverse effect An unexpected bad reaction to a drug or other treatment; also known as *adverse reaction.*

Aftercare Follow-up monitoring of the patient's condition after the primary treatment has been completed.

Agglutination The process of red blood cells combining together in a mass or lump.

Alimentary canal The digestive pathway from the oral cavity to the anus.

Allogeneic The donor and recipient are of the same species.

Alveolar sac A tiny bubble, grouped in clusters at the end of each bronchiole, that holds air.

Anatomical cavity A space or area that is hollow and often houses organs and vessels.

Anatomical direction Medical terminology used to provide the location of a health problem or an approach for a surgical procedure.

Anatomical position Medical terminology that describes the patient's position (on the surgical or examination table).

Anatomical site A specific location within the anatomy (body).

Anatomy The structure of the human body.

Anemic Any of various conditions marked by deficiency in red blood cells or hemoglobin.

Angina pectoris Chest pain.

Anomaly An abnormal, or unexpected, condition.

Antepartum Before the onset of labor.

Antigen A substance that promotes the production of antibodies.

Anus The portion of the large intestine that leads outside the body.

Anxiety The feelings of apprehension and fear, sometimes manifested with physical manifestations such as sweating and palpitations.

Apgar Assessment of a neonate's condition on the basis of five factors: muscle tone, heart rate, reflex response, skin color, and breathing.

Appendicular skeleton The bones that construct the upper and lower extremities.

Articulation A joint.

Ascending colon The portion of the large intestine that connects the cecum to the hepatic flexure.

Asymptomatic No symptoms or manifestations.

Atherosclerosis A condition resulting from plaque buildup on the interior walls of the arteries, causing reduced blood flow; also known as *arteriosclerosis.*

Atrium An upper chamber of the heart that receives blood returning to the heart.

Autologous The donor tissue is taken from a different site on the same individual's body.

Autonomic nervous system The nerve fiber bundles that initiate automatic body functions, such as heart contraction.

Avulsion Injury in which layers of skin are traumatically torn away from the body.

Axial skeleton The bones that construct the central segment of the body.

B

Bacteria A single-celled microorganism that causes disease.

Basal ganglia Groups of nerve cell bodies involved with musculoskeletal movement; the control mechanism for coordination and stability.

Behavioral disturbance A type of common behavior that includes mood disorders, sleep disorders, psychotic symptoms, and agitation.

Benign Nonmalignant characteristic of a neoplasm; not infectious or spreading.

Benign hypertension Hypertension kept under control with diet and medication.

Benign prostatic hyperplasia (BPH) Enlarged prostate that results in depressing the urethra.

Bladder cancer Malignancy of the urinary bladder.

Blepharitis Inflammation of the eyelid.

Blister A bubble or sac formed on the surface of the skin, typically filled with a watery fluid or serum.

Blood Fluid pumped throughout the body, carrying oxygen and nutrients to the cells and wastes away from the cells.

Blood type A system of classifying blood based on the antigens present on the surface of the individual's red blood cells.

Body area A region of the human structure.

Bony thorax The rib cage.

Brain An organ within the skull that controls body functions and external interactions; part of the central nervous system.

Breasts Two mammary glands that extend from the chest in women after puberty.

Bronchi Bilateral air passageways that connect the trachea to the lungs.

Bronchioles Bilateral tubes, small branches of the bronchi, leading to the air sacs.

Bulbar conjunctiva A mucous membrane on the surface of the eyeball.

Bulla A large vesicle that is filled with fluid.

Burn Injury by heat or fire.

Bursa A synovial-membrane-lined sac filled with fluid and located adjacent to an articulation.

C

Cancellous Latticelike shaped bone; also known as *spongy bone*.

Carbuncle A painful, pus-filled boil due to infection of the epidermis and underlying tissues, often caused by staphylococcus.

Carcinoma A malignant neoplasm or cancerous tumor.

Cardio Heart.

Carrier An individual infected with a disease who is not ill but can still pass it to another person; an individual with an abnormal gene that can be passed to a child, making the child susceptible to disease.

Cartilage Connective tissue.

Cataract Clouding of the lens or lens capsule of the eye.

Cecum A pouchlike organ that connects the ileum with the large intestine; the point of connection for the vermiform appendix.

Central nervous system (CNS) The brain and spinal cord.

Cerebellum The posterior portion of the brain responsible for coordinating motor activities with sensory impulses and maintaining balance and muscle tone.

Cerebral hemispheres The two halves of the cerebrum of the brain.

Cerebral infarction An area of dead tissue (necrosis) in the brain caused by a blocked or ruptured blood vessel.

Cerebral meninges Three protective layers of membrane that insulate the brain.

Cerebrovascular accident (CVA) Rupture of a blood vessel causing hemorrhaging in the brain or an embolus in a blood vessel in the brain causing a loss of blood flow; also known as *stroke*.

Cerumen A yellow waxy substance secreted into the ear canal.

Cervix A necklike structure connecting from the lower part of the uterus to the vagina.

Cheeks The walls of the oral cavity that form both sides of the face; the buccal area.

Chemicals Substances used in, or made by, the process of chemistry.

Cholelithiasis Gallstones.

Choroid The vascular layer of the eye that lies between the retina and sclera.

Chronic Long duration; continuing over a long period of time.

Chronic kidney disease (CKD) Ongoing malfunction of one or both kidneys.

Chronic obstructive pulmonary disease (COPD) An ongoing obstruction of the airway.

Ciliary body The vascular layer of the eye that lies between the sclera and the crystalline lens.

Clinically significant Signs, symptoms, and/or conditions present at birth that may impact the child's future health status.

Clitoris An erectile mass of tissue, the primary site of female sexual arousal, at the superior, anterior aspect of the vulva.

Closed fracture A fracture in which the broken bone has not protruded through the skin.

Coagulation Clotting; the change from a liquid into a thickened substance.

Coding for coverage Choosing a code on the basis of what the insurance company will cover (pay for) rather than accurately reflecting the truth.

Common bile duct The juncture of the cystic duct of the gallbladder and the hepatic duct from the liver.

Co-morbidity A separate condition or illness present in the same patient at the same time as another, unrelated condition or illness.

Complication An unexpected illness or other condition that develops as a result of a procedure, service, or treatment provided during the patient's hospital stay.

Concurrent coding System in which coding processes are performed while a patient is still in the hospital receiving care.

Condition A health-related situation.

Conductive hearing loss A problem in the outer or middle ear that interferes with the passage of sound waves.

Cone A receptor in the retina that is responsible for light and color.

Confirmed Found to be true or definite.

Congenital A condition existing at the time of birth.

Conjunctivitis Inflammation of the conjunctiva.

Contracture An abnormal tightening or shortening, often resulting in a deformity.

Controlled hypertension Hypertension that is successfully being treated.

Contusion The result of a minor trauma to a muscle, causing a bruise.

Cornea Transparent tissue covering the eyeball; responsible for focusing light into the eye and transmitting light.

Corneal dystrophy Growth of abnormal tissue on the cornea, often related to a nutritional deficiency.

Corrosion A burn caused by a chemical; chemical destruction of the skin.

Cranial nerves Twelve pairs of nerves, each having specific responsibilities, that extend from the brain and brainstem throughout the body.

Cranium Bones that comprise the skull segments that cover the brain.

Cushing's syndrome A condition resulting from the hyperproduction of corticosteroids, most often caused by an adrenal cortex tumor or a tumor of the pituitary gland.

Cyst A fluid-filled or gas-filled bubble in the skin.

D

Dacryocystitis Lacrimal gland inflammation.

Decibel (dB) Unit of measurement used to determine the intensity, or loudness, of sound.

Decubitus ulcer A skin lesion caused by continuous pressure on one spot, particularly on a bony prominence.

Deformity A size or shape (structural design) that deviates from that which is considered normal.

Dependence Ongoing, regular consumption of a substance with resulting significant clinical manifestations and a dramatic decrease in the effect of the substance with continued use, therefore requiring an increased quantity of the substance to achieve intoxication.

Depressive An emotional state that includes sadness, hopelessness, and gloom.

Dermis The internal layer of the skin; the location of blood vessels, lymph vessels, hair follicles, sweat glands, and sebum.

Descending colon The segment of the large intestine that connects the splenic flexure to the sigmoid colon.

Diabetes mellitus (DM) A chronic systemic disease that results from insulin deficiency or resistance and causes the body to improperly metabolize carbohydrates, proteins, and fats.

Diagnosis A physician's determination of a patient's condition, illness, or injury.

Diagnosis-related group (DRG) An episodic-care payment system basing reimbursement to hospitals for inpatient services upon standards of care for specific diagnoses grouped by their similar usage of resources for procedures, services, and treatments.

Diaphragm A transverse muscle that divides the torso between the chest and the abdomen; its motion aids respiration.

Diaphysis Shaft of a long bone.

Dislocation The displacement of a limb, bone, or organ from its customary position.

Double billing Sending a claim for the second time to the same insurance company for the same procedure or service, provided to the same patient on the same date of service.

Drugs Substances, natural or combined, created to treat or prevent illness or disease.

Duodenum The first segment of the small intestine, connecting the stomach to the jejunum.

Dyslipidemia Abnormal lipoprotein metabolism.

E

Edema An overaccumulation of fluid in the cells of the tissues.

Edentulism Absence of teeth.

Elevated blood pressure An occurrence of high blood pressure; an isolated or infrequent reading of a systolic blood pressure above 140 mmHg and/or a diastolic blood pressure above 90 mmHg.

Embolus A thrombus that has broken free from the vessel wall and is traveling freely within the vascular system.

Endemic The spread of the pathogen is contained within a small area.

Endocrine system All the organs and tissues responsible for creating and secreting hormones and controlling metabolic activity; consists of the hypothalamus, pituitary gland, pineal gland, thyroid gland, parathyroid glands, thymus gland, adrenal glands, and pancreas, as well as the testes in men and the ovaries in women.

Endometrium The mucosal lining of the uterus.

Epidemic The pathogen spreads quickly and easily.

Epidermis The external layer of the skin, the majority of which is squamous cells.

Epiglottis A flap made of cartilage that covers the superior end of the larynx.

Epiphysis The end of a long bone, either the distal or proximal end.

Eponym A condition named after a person.

Esophagus The tubular organ that connects the pharynx to the stomach for the passage of nourishment.

Etiology The study of the causes of disease.

Exacerbation An increase in the severity of a disease or its symptoms.

Expiration The physical process of expulsing carbon dioxide.

Extent The percentage of the body that has been affected by the burn or corrosion.

External cause An event, outside the body, that causes injury, poisoning, or an adverse reaction.

External cause codes Codes that report *how* and/or *where* an injury or poisoning happened.

External ear The portion of the auditory system that includes the pinna (helix), earlobe, and external auditory canal.

Extraocular muscles The muscles that control the eye.

F

Fallopian tubes A pair of tubular structures that reach from the ovaries to the uterus.

First degree Redness of the epidermis (skin).

Fracture Broken cartilage or bone.

Functional activity Glandular secretion in abnormal quantity.

Fundus The section of an organ farthest from its opening.

Fungi Group of organisms, including mold, yeast, and mildew, that cause infection.

Furuncle A staphylococcal infection in the subcutaneous tissue; commonly known as a *boil.*

G

Gallbladder A pear-shaped organ that stores bile until it is required to aid the digestive process.

Gangrene Necrotic tissue resulting from a loss of blood supply; death and decay of tissue due to inadequate blood supply.

Genetic abnormality An error in a gene (chromosome) that affects development during gestation; also known as a *chromosomal abnormality.*

Gestation The length of time for the complete development of a baby from conception to birth; on average, 40 weeks.

Gestational diabetes mellitus (GDM) A temporary diabetes mellitus occurring during pregnancy.

Gestational hypertension Hypertension that develops during pregnancy and typically goes away once the pregnancy has ended.

Glands of Zeis Altered sebaceous glands that are connected to the eyelash follicles.

Glaucoma The condition that results when poor draining of fluid causes an abnormal increase in pressure within the eye, damaging the optic nerve.

Glomerular filtration rate (GFR) The measurement of kidney function; used to determine the stage of kidney disease.

Gravida An alphanumeric (G1, G2, G3, etc.) that indicates how many times a woman has been pregnant in her life.

Gross Inspection of the specimen by the naked eye.

Gynecologist A physician specializing in the care of the female genital tract.

H

Hair A pigmented, cylindrical filament that grows out from the hair follicle within the epidermis.

Hair follicle A saclike bulb containing the hair root.

Hematopoiesis The formation of blood.

Hemoglobin (hgb or Hgb) The part of the red blood cell that carries oxygen.

Hemolysis The destruction of red blood cells, resulting in the release of hemoglobin into the bloodstream.

Hemorrhage Excessive or severe bleeding.

Hemostasis The interruption of bleeding.

Hernia A condition in which one anatomical structure pushes through a perforation in the wall of the anatomical site that normally contains that structure.

Histology The study of the microscopic composition of tissues.

Hospital-acquired condition (HAC) A condition, illness, or injury contracted by the patient during his or her stay in an acute care facility; also known as *nosocomial condition.*

Human immunodeficiency virus (HIV) A condition affecting the immune system.

Hyperglycemia Abnormally high levels of glucose.

Hypertension High blood pressure, usually a chronic condition; often identified by a systolic blood pressure above 140 mmHg and/or a diastolic blood pressure above 90 mmHg.

Hypoglycemia Abnormally low glucose levels.

Hypotension Low blood pressure; systolic blood pressure below 90 mmHg and/or a diastolic measurement of lower than 60 mmHg.

Hypothalamus The part of the brain responsible for autonomic responses such as body temperature control, appetite, blood pressure, respiration, stress reactions, and sleeping patterns; located within the third ventricle of the brain.

Hypothyroidism A condition in which the thyroid converts energy more slowly than normal, resulting in an otherwise unexplained weight gain and fatigue.

I

ICD-9-CM The acronym for International Classification of Diseases, Ninth Revision, Clinical Modification.

ICD-10-CM The acronym for International Classification of Diseases, Tenth Revision, Clinical Modification.

Ileum The last segment of the small intestine.

Incus The small bone within the middle ear that is shaped like an anvil and transfers sound waves from the malleus to the stapes.

Infarction Tissue or muscle that has deteriorated or died (necrotic).

Infection The invasion of pathogens into tissue cells.

Infectious A condition that can be transmitted from one person to another.

Inflammation The reaction of tissues to infection or injury; characterized by pain, swelling, and erythema.

Influenza An acute infection of the respiratory tract caused by the influenza virus.

Inner ear The innermost and most complex segment of the auditory system; contains the semicircular canals, vestibule, and cochlea and is responsible for transmitting sound to the auditory nerve and maintaining equilibrium.

Inpatient facility An establishment that provides health care services to individuals who stay overnight on the premises.

Inspiration The physical process of acquiring oxygen.

Intent The objective or goal of the individual taking the action.

Interaction A mixture of two or more substances that changes the effect of any of the individual substances.

Intervertebral disc A fibrocartilage segment that lies between vertebrae of the spinal column and provides cushioning and support.

Involuntary Automatically; a systemic response.

Iris The round, pigmented muscular curtain in the eye.

Isogeneic The donor and recipient individuals are genetically identical.

J

Jejunum The segment of the small intestine that connects the duodenum to the ileum.

K

Keratitis An inflammation of the cornea, typically accompanied by an ulceration.

Kidney A bean-shaped organ that filters blood and excretes urine.

L

Labium majus One of a pair of liplike folds of skin surrounding the opening of the vagina.

Labium minus One of a set of two thin, liplike folds of skin on either side of the vaginal opening to the outside; located inside the labium majus.

Labyrinth A sequence of canals located within the inner ear that is responsible for maintaining equilibrium.

Laceration Damage to the epidermal and dermal layers of the skin made by a sharp object.

Lacrimal apparatus A system in the eye that consists of the lacrimal glands, the upper canaliculi, the lower canaliculi, the lacrimal sac, and the nasolacrimal duct.

Larynx A tubular organ that connects from the pharynx to the trachea; commonly known as the voice box.

Late effect Cause-and-effect relationship between an original condition, illness, or injury and an additional problem caused by the existence of that original condition; also called *sequela*.

Laterality The right or left side of anatomical sites that have locations on both sides of the body.

Lens A transparent, crystalline segment of the eye, situated directly behind the pupil, that is responsible for focusing light rays as they enter the eye and travel back to the retina.

Ligament A band of connective tissues that bind the components of a joint and facilitate movement.

Lingual tonsils Lymphoid tissue located at the root of the tongue, bilaterally.

Lips A muscular structure around the external area of the oral cavity.

Liver The organ, located in the upper right area of the abdominal cavity, that is responsible for regulating blood sugar levels; secreting bile for the gallbladder; metabolizing fats, proteins, and carbohydrates; manufacturing some blood proteins; and removing toxins from the blood.

Low birth weight (LBW) A baby born weighing less than 5 pounds 8 ounces, or 2,500 grams.

Lungs Bilateral lobed organs that function like balloons, expanding on inspiration and deflating on expiration.

M

Macule A flat lesion with a different pigmentation (color) when compared with the surrounding skin. An ephelidis (freckle) is a small macule.

Major complication and co-morbidity (MCC) A complication or co-morbidity that has an impact on the treatment of the patient and makes care for that patient more complex.

Malformation An irregular structural development.

Malignant Invasive and destructive characteristic of a neoplasm; possibly causing damage or death.

Malignant hypertension Hypertension accompanied by optic nerve swelling and other serious manifestations.

Malleous The small bone within the middle ear that resembles a hammer and transfers sound waves from the eardrum to the incus.

Malunion A fractured bone that did not heal correctly; healing of bone that was not in proper position or alignment.

Manic An emotional state that includes elation, excitement, and exuberance.

Manifestation A condition caused or developed from the existence of another condition.

Mass Abnormal collection of tissue.

Medical necessity The determination that the health care professional was acting according to standard practices in providing a particular procedure for an individual with a particular diagnosis.

Medulla oblongata The bottom portion of the brainstem, at the junction of the spinal cord; consists of nerves responsible for respiration, circulation, and other functions.

Meibomian glands Sebaceous glands that secrete a tear film component that prevents tears from evaporating so that the area stays moist.

Mesentary A fold of a membrane that carries blood to the small intestine and connects it to the posterior wall of the abdominal cavity.

Metastasize To proliferate, reproduce, or spread.

Microscopic Inspection of the specimen using a microscope.

Middle ear A membrane-lined cavity that transmits sound waves from the eardrum to the inner ear.

Moll's glands Ordinary sweat glands.

Mons pubis A plot of adipose (fatty) tissue that lies over the juncture of the two pubic bones in women.

Morbidity Unhealthy.

Morphology The study of the configuration or structure of living organisms.

Mortality Death.

Motor (efferent) fibers Nerve fibers that convey stimuli from the CNS to muscles and glands.

Muscle Tissue that contracts, causing an organ and/or other component of the body to move.

Myalgia Pain in a muscle.

Myocardial infarction (MI) Malfunction of the heart due to necrosis or deterioration of a portion of the heart muscle; also known as a *heart attack*.

N

Nasal septum A ridge of bone and cartilage that forms a barrier between the left and right nares.

Necrosis The death of tissue.

Neonate An infant from birth to 1 month of age.

Neoplasm Abnormal tissue growth; tumor.

Neurologic function assessments Diagnostic examinations, observations, and questions/answers designed to evaluate the patient's neurologic function.

Nevus An abnormally pigmented area of skin. A birthmark is an example.

Nodule A papule larger than 5 mm.

Nonessential modifiers Descriptors whose inclusion in the physician's notes is not absolutely necessary and that are provided simply to further clarify a code description; optional terms.

Nonunion A fractured bone that did not heal back together; no mending or joining together of the broken segments.

Nosocomial A hospital-acquired condition.

Not elsewhere classifiable (NEC) Specifics that are not described in any other code in the ICD-10-CM book; also known as *not elsewhere classified*.

Not otherwise specified (NOS) The absence of additional details documented in the notes.

NSTEMI A heart event during which the coronary artery is partially occluded (blocked).

O

Obstetrics A health care specialty focusing on the care of women during pregnancy, and the puerperium.

Obstruction A blockage or closing.

Open fracture A fracture in which the broken bone has protruded through the skin; fracture with a wound.

Oral cavity The opening in the face that begins the alimentary canal and is used for the input of nutrition; also known as the *mouth*.

Orbit The bony cavity in the skull that houses the eye and its ancillary parts (muscles, nerves, blood vessels).

Organ system A group of anatomical sites working together to perform a specific bodily function.

Osseous Bonylike substance.

Ossicles The three small bones within the middle ear: the incus, the malleus, and the stapes.

Other specified Additional information the physician specified that isn't included in any other code description.

Outpatient services Health care services provided to individuals without an overnight stay in the facility.

Ovaries Two small oval organs, located laterally and above the uterus, within the pelvic cavity that produce female hormones and produce and store eggs (oocytes).

Overlapping boundaries Multiple sites of carcinoma without identifiable borders.

P

Palatine tonsils Lymphoid tissue situated at the entrance to the throat, bilaterally.

Palpebrae The eyelids.

Palpebral conjunctiva A mucous membrane that lines the palpebrae.

Pancreas A gland that secretes insulin and other hormones from the islet cells into the bloodstream and manufactures digestive enzymes that are secreted into the duodenum; functions in the processing of nourishment to the body as a part of the digestive system.

Pancreatic islets Cells within the pancreas that secrete insulin and other hormones into the bloodstream.

Pandemic The pathogen has infected a large geographic area.

Papule A raised lesion with a diameter of less than 5 mm.

Para An alphanumeric that identifies the number of times a woman has given birth, designated on the chart as P1, P2, etc., or had a fetus reach viability.

Paranasal sinuses Bilateral facial sinuses.

Parasites Tiny living things that can invade and feed off other living things.

Parathyroid glands Four small glands situated on the back of the thyroid gland that secrete parathyroid hormone.

Patch a flat, small area of differently colored or textured skin; a large macule.

Pathogen Any agent that causes disease; a microorganism such as a bacterium or virus.

Pathologic Related to, or caused by, disease.

Pathology The study of disease.

Pathophysiology The study of physiological processes of disease.

Perforation An atypical hole in the wall of an organ or anatomical site.

Perinatal The time period from before birth to the 28th day after birth.

Peripheral nervous system (PNS) Components of the nervous system other than the brain and spinal cord; includes ganglia and neurons.

Phalanges Fingers and toes.

Pharmaceuticals Medication (drugs).

Pharyngeal tonsils Lymphoid nodules located on the wall of the pharynx, bilaterally.

Pharynx The section of the tubular organ that leads from the oral cavity to the esophagus.

Phobia Irrational and excessive fear of an object, activity, or situation.

***Physicians' Desk Reference* (PDR)** A series of reference books identifying all aspects of prescription and over-the-counter medications, as well as herbal remedies.

Pineal gland A gland situated within the brain and responsible for the release of melatonin.

Pituitary gland A two-lobed gland that creates and secretes hormones; consists of the adenohypophysis, the larger lobe sitting anteriorly, and the neurohypophysis, which is smaller and toward the posterior.

Plasma The fluid part of the blood.

Platelets (Plats) Large cell fragments in the bone marrow that function in clotting; also called *thrombocytes*.

Pleura A double-layered membrane that envelops the lungs and lines the chest wall.

Pneumonia An inflammation of the lungs.

Pneumothorax A condition in which air or gas is present within the chest cavity but outside the lungs.

Point of insertion The flexible or movable end of the muscle.

Point of origin The secure side of the muscle.

Poisoned A condition produced by a substance that harms or causes death.

Polydipsia Excessive thirst.

Polyuria Excessive urination.

Pons The part of the posterior of the brain, superior to the medulla, that participates in brainstem functions.

Postpartum The first 6 weeks after childbirth.

Posttraumatic stress disorder (PTSD) An ongoing sense of fear after the danger has gone.

Prematurity Birth occurring prior to the completion of 37 weeks gestation.

Prenatal Prior to birth; also referred to as *antenatal.*

Present on admission (POA) A one-character indicator reporting the status of the diagnosis at the time the patient was admitted to the acute care facility.

Preventive care Health-related services designed to stop the development of a disease or injury.

Principal diagnosis The condition that is the primary, or main, reason for the encounter.

Proptosis Bulging out of the eye; also known as *exophthalmos.*

Prostatitis Inflammation of the prostate.

Prosthetic Lost tissue is replaced with synthetic materials such as metal, plastic, or ceramic.

Pterygium A flap of thick-tissue, often triangularly shaped, abnormal growth on the conjunctiva.

Puerperium The time period from the end of labor until the uterus returns to normal size, typically 3 to 6 weeks.

Pupil The opening in the center of the iris that permits light to enter and continue on to the lens and retina.

Pustule A swollen area of skin; a vesicle filled with pus.

R

Rectum The last segment of the large intestine, connecting the sigmoid colon to the anus.

Red blood cells (RBCs) Cells within the blood that contain hemoglobin responsible for carrying oxygen to tissues; also called *erythrocytes.*

Respiration The physical process of acquiring oxygen and releasing carbon dioxide.

Respiratory disorder A malfunction of the organ system relating to respiration.

Retina A membrane in the back of the eye that is sensitive to light and functions as the sensory end of the optic nerve.

Retinal detachment A break in the connection between the retinal pigment epithelium layer and the neural retina.

Retinopathy Degenerative condition of the retina.

Rh (Rhesus) factor An antigen located on the red blood cell that produces immunogenic responses in those individuals without it.

Risk factor A characteristic that increases a person's susceptibility to a disease or injury.

Rod An elongated, cylindrical cell within the retina that is photosensitive in low light.

Rule of nines A general division of the whole body into sections that each represent 9%; used for estimating the extent of a burn.

Rupture A tear in an organ or tissue.

S

Salivary glands Three sets of bilateral exocrine glands that secrete saliva: parotid glands, submaxillary glands, and sublingual glands.

Scale Flaky exfoliated epidermis; a flake of skin.

Schizophrenia A psychotic disorder with no known cause.

Sclera The membranous tissue that covers the entire eyeball (except the cornea); also known as *the white of the eye.*

Screening An examination or test of a patient who has no signs or symptoms that is conducted with the intention of finding any evidence of disease as soon as possible, thus enabling better patient outcomes.

Second degree Blisters on the skin; involvement of the epidermis and the dermis layers.

Secondary diabetes mellitus Diabetes caused by medication or another condition or disease.

Secondary hypertension The condition of hypertension caused by another condition or illness.

Sensorineural hearing loss Damage to the nerves that detect sound in the ear; damage may occur by trauma, pathogen, or congenital anomaly.

Sensory (afferent) fibers Nerve fibers that convey stimuli to the brain or spinal cord.

Sepsis Condition typified by two or more systemic responses to infection; a specified pathogen.

Septic shock Severe sepsis with hypotension; unresponsive to fluid resuscitation.

Septicemia Generalized infection spread through the body via the bloodstream; blood infection.

Sequela Cause-and-effect relationship between an original condition, illness, or injury and an additional problem caused by the existence of that original condition; also called *late effect.*

Severe sepsis Sepsis with signs of acute organ dysfunction.

Severity The level of seriousness.

Sigmoid colon The dual-curved segment of the colon that connects the descending colon to the rectum; also referred to as the *sigmoid flexure.*

Sign Objective evidence of a disease or condition.

Site The specific anatomical location of the disease or injury; the location on or in the human body.

Skin The external membranous covering of the body.

Skull The bones that protect the head and create the face.

Somatoform disorder The sincere belief that one is suffering an illness that is not present.

Sphincter A circular muscle that contracts to prevent passage of liquids or solids.

Spinal cord Nerve tissue that runs through the vertebral bodies along the dorsal (posterior) surface of the torso and from which peripheral nerves extend; part of the CNS.

Spinal nerves Nerves that extend from the spinal cord to the peripheral aspects of the body.

Sprain A partially torn, or overstretched, ligament.

Stapes The small bone within the middle ear that is shaped like a stirrup and transmits sound waves from the incus to the inner ear.

Status asthmaticus The condition of asthma that is life-threatening and does not respond to therapeutic treatments.

STEMI An ST elevation myocardial infarction—a heart event during which the coronary artery is completely blocked by a thrombus or embolus.

Stomach A saclike organ within the alimentary canal designed to contain nourishment during the initial phase of the digestive process.

Strain A tearing of the fibers of the muscle involved, most often the result of overstretching the muscle during movement.

Subcutaneous The layer beneath the dermis; also known as the *hypodermis.*

Subluxation A partial dislocation.

Supporting documentation The paperwork in the patient's file that corroborates the codes presented on the claim form for a particular encounter.

Sutures The junctures of the parts of the cranium and skull.

Symptom A subjective sensation or departure from the norm as related by the patient.

Systemic Spread throughout the entire body.

Systemic inflammatory response syndrome (SIRS) A definite physical reaction, such as fever or chills, to an unspecified pathogen.

T

Tear (muscle tear) A separation within the muscle fibers. A bowstring tear, also known as a *bucket-handle tear,* occurs longitudinally in the meniscus.

Tendon An anatomical structure that connects a muscle to a bone.

Testes Two male reproductive glands located within the scrotum; singular *testis.*

Thalamus The part of the brain responsible for transmitting impulses to the specific, appropriate part of the cerebellum, similar to a dispatcher.

Therapeutic Intended to restore good health or reduce the effect of a disease or negative condition.

Third degree Destruction of all layers of the skin, with possible involvement of the subcutaneous fat, muscle, and bone.

Thrombosis The formation of a blood clot in a blood vessel.

Thrombus A blood clot in a blood vessel; plural *thrombi.*

Thymus gland A gland that assists in the development of the immune system prior to puberty; produces several hormones that encourage T-lymphocyte production.

Thyroid gland A two-lobed gland that produces hormones used for metabolic function; the lobes, located in the neck, reach around the trachea laterally and connect anteriorly by an isthmus.

Tongue Sensory organ attached to the bottom of the mouth; enables speech, eating, and tasting.

Toxic effect A health-related reaction caused by a poisonous substance.

Trachea Tubular membrane that connects the larynx to the bronchi; commonly known as the *windpipe.*

Transfusion The provision of one person's blood or plasma to another individual.

Transverse colon The portion of the large intestine that connects the hepatic flexure to the splenic flexure.

Tuberculosis An infectious condition that causes small, rounded swellings on mucous membranes throughout the body.

Tuberosity A rounded nodule at the end of a bone where a muscle or ligament attaches.

Type 1 diabetes mellitus A sudden onset of insulin deficiency that may occur at any age but most often arises in childhood and adolescence; also known as *insulin-dependent diabetes mellitus (IDDM), juvenile diabetes,* or *type I.*

Type 2 diabetes mellitus A form of diabetes mellitus with a gradual onset that may develop at any age but most often occurs in adults over the age of 40; also known as *non-insulin-dependent diabetes mellitus (NIDDM)* or *type II.*

U

Ulcer An open wound or sore caused by pressure, infection, or inflammation; an erosion or loss of the full thickness of the epidermis.

Unbundling Coding the individual parts of a specific diagnosis or procedure rather than one combination or bundle that includes all of those components.

Uncontrolled Diabetes for which current therapies and/or treatments are not maintaining a proper blood sugar level in the patient.

Underdosing Taking too little of the drug, thereby preventing the desired effect.

Underlying condition One disease that affects or encourages another condition.

Uniform Hospital Discharge Data Set (UHDDS) A compilation of data collected by acute care facilities and other designated health care facilities.

Unspecified The absence of additional specifics in the physician's documentation.

Upcoding Using a code on a claim form that indicates a higher level of service, or a more severe aspect of disease or injury, than that which was actual and true.

Urea A compound that results from the breakdown of proteins and is excreted in urine.

Ureter A long tubular passageway for urine traveling from the kidney to the urinary bladder.

Urethra A tubular structure that carries urine from the urinary bladder to the outside of the body.

Urinary bladder A hollow organ that collects and temporarily stores urine.

Urinary system The organ system responsible for removing waste products that are left behind by protein, excessive water, disproportionate amounts of electrolytes, and other nitrogenous compounds from the blood and the body.

Urinary tract infection (UTI) Inflammation of any part of the urinary tract: kidney, ureter, bladder, or urethra.

Use Consumption of a substance without significant clinical manifestations.

Uterus A hollow, pear-shaped organ in the lower abdominal cavity of the female body; responsible for menstruation and for the housing of a fetus during pregnancy.

Uveal tract The middle layer of the eye, consisting of the iris, ciliary body, and choroid.

Uvula Hanging, fleshy tissue suspended from the soft palate at the opening of the throat.

Vagina A passageway extending from the cervix of the uterus to the vulva and the outside of the body.

Vascular Veins and arteries.

Ventricle A lower chamber of the heart that pushes blood away from the heart.

Vermiform appendix A long, narrow mass of tissue attached to the cecum; also called *appendix*.

Vertebra A bone that is a part of the construction of the spinal column.

Virus A microscopic particle that initiates disease, mimicking the characteristics of a particular cell, and can reproduce only within the body of the cell which it has invaded.

Vitreous chamber The interior segment of the eye that contains the vitreous body.

Voluntary With conscious purpose.

Vulva The external genital organs of a woman.

White blood cells (WBCs) Cells within the blood that help to protect the body from pathogens; also called *leukocytes*.

Xenogeneic The donor and recipient are of different species.

Note: Page numbers followed by *f* designate figures; *b*, boxes; and *t*, tables. A page number in **boldface** indicates the definition of the term on that page.

B

Bacilli, 98, 99f
Background retinopathy, 188
Bacteria, **98**–99
Bacterial infections, 115–116
Bacterial pneumonia, 362
Bacterial vaginosis (BV), 539
Bartholin glands, 526
Basal cell carcinoma, 134f
Basal ganglia, **241**
Beau's lines, 424
Bedsore. *See* Pressure ulcers
Behavioral disorders, 216–218
    due to physiological condition, 215
Benign neoplasm, **134,** 137
Benign prostatic hyperplasia
    (BPH), **510**
Bicarbonate test, 163
Bipolar disorders, 222
Birth defect, 559
Bladder cancer, **510**
Blepharitis, **276**
Blister, 417
Blood, **158, 159**
    culture test, 163
    differential (Diff) test, 163
    formation of, 158–159
    loss anemia, 165
    oxygen and carbon dioxide
        exchanging, 162f
    role of, 161
    tests, 163, 164f, 165
    transfusions, 160
    type, **159**
Blood disorders
    anemia, 165
    clotting disorders, 166–168
Blood pressure cuff, 4
Blood urea nitrogen (BUN) test, 163
Body areas, **13–14**
Body mass index (BMI), 196–197
Body planes, 16, 16f
    frontal, 16f, 17
    sagittal, 16f, 17
    transverse, 16, 16f
Bone marrow, 159f
Bony thorax, **465,** 470, 471f
Bowman's membrane, 269
Bradycardia, 322
Brain, **240,** 240f, **241**
    MRI image of, 247f
Brain cancer (C71), **6**
Brain neurons, 212–213
    anxiety disorders, 225–227
    behavioral disorders, 216–218
    delusional disorders, 220–221
    dissociative disorders, 225–227
    mental disorders, 213–215
    mood (affective) disorders, 222–223

    nonmood psychotic disorders,
        220–221
    nonpsychotic mental disorders,
        225–227
    schizophrenia disorders, 220–221
    schizotypal disorders, 221
    somatoform, 225
    stress-related disorders, 225–227
Brainstem, **241**
Breastbone, 470
Bronchi, **353**
Bronchioles, 353, **354**
Buckle fracture. *See* Torus fracture
Bulbar conjunctiva, **274**
Bulla, **420**
Bundle of His, 321
Burns, **578**
    extent, 583–586
    infection, 586
    multiple sites fall, 581
    sequelae (late effects) of, 586
    severity, **579,** 579f
    site, **579**
    solar and radiation, 586
    specific site, 580
Bursae, **438**
Bursitis, 446
Burst fractures, 479

C

Campylobacter, 115
Cancellous bone, **464, 465**
Cancer, in alphabetic index, 41
Candida albicans, 276
Carbuncles, **421**
Carcinoma, **134**
Cardiac arrest, 322
Cardiovascular disease
    atherosclerotic coronary artery
        disease, 337–338
    atrial fibrillation, 340
    cerebrovascular accident, 333–334
    deep vein thrombosis, 337
    heart failure, 334–335
    hypercholesterolemia, 340
    hypertension, 323–332
    hypotension, 322
    mitral valve prolapse, 340
    myocardial infarction, 335–336
    sequelae of, 338–339
    signs and symptoms, 321–322
Cardiovascular system, 13, 317f
    conduction mechanisms,
        320–321, 320f
    heart, 318, 319f, 320
Carrier, **614**
Cataract, **280**
Catatonia, 220
Catatonic schizophrenia, 220
Catecholamines, 186

Category notes, 74
Cauda equina, 244
Cecum, **389**
Central nervous system (CNS), **239**
    brain, 240–241, 240f
    hereditary and degenerative diseases,
        249
    inflammatory conditions of, 248
    spinal cord, 242
Central pain syndrome, 255
Cerebellum, **241**
Cerebral aneurysm, 252
Cerebral cortex, 241
Cerebral hemispheres, **241**
Cerebral infarction, **334**
Cerebral meninges, **241**
Cerebrovascular accident (CVA), 252,
    333, 334
Cerebrum, 240–241
Cerumen, 296, **298**
Cervical enlargement, 242
Cervical nerves, 244
Cervical vertebrae, 469
Cervicocranial syndrome, M53.0, 17
Cervix, **524**
Cheeks, **383**
Chemical, **590**
Chemotherapy and radiation therapy,
    145–146
Chickenpox, 118
Childbirth, code, 553–554
Chlamydia, 539
Cholecystitis, **399**
Cholelithiasis, 399
Chorionic villus sampling, 560
Choroid, **271**
    disorders of, 281
Choroid plexi, 241
Chromosomal abnormalities, 560–561
    Down syndrome (trisomy 21),
        560–561, 561f
    Klinefelter's syndrome, 561
Chronic conditions, 82, 101
Chronic kidney disease (CKD), **503**
    acute renal failure, 507
    anemia, 506
    diabetes with renal manifestations,
        504–505
    dialysis, 506
    glomerular filtration rate, 503
    hypertensive, 504
Chronic obstructive pulmonary disease
    (COPD), 364–366
Chronic pain syndrome, **253**
Ciliary body, **271**
    disorders of, 278–279
Circulatory manifestations, 189
Circulatory system. *See* Cardiovascular
    system
Cirrhosis, 398
Clavicle, 471

Muscles, **437, 438**
  diseases of, 447
  face, 439t–440t
  facts about, 452t
  foot, 443t
  head, 439t–440t, 440f
  infection and inflammation, 445–447
  joint-related components, 439–445
  leg, 443t
  neck, 439t–440t, 440f
  optical system, 441f, 441t
  reporting external causes, 448–452
  throat, 439t–440t
  throughout body, 439, 439t–444t
  traumatic injury to, 445
  trunk, 443t, 444f
  types, muscle actions, 437–439
Musculoskeletal system, 13
Musculoskeletal system and connective
    tissue diseases, 69
Myalgia, **445**
Myasthenia gravis, 447
Myocardial infarction, 335–336
Myocardial infarction (MI), **335**
Myocardium, 320
Myositis, 446
Myotonic muscular dystrophy, G71.11, 17

N

Nail disorders, 424
Nail plate, 414
Nails, 414–415, 414f
Nasal bones, 466
Nasal cavity, 19
Nasal septum, 351, **352**
Nasolacrimal duct. *See* Lacrimal apparatus
Nasopharynx, 386
National Pressure Ulcer Advisory Panel
    (NPUAP), 417
Nausea, 11
Nausea with vomiting, R11.2, 11
Neck, muscles of, 439t–440t, 440f
Neonatal sepsis, 112
Neonate, **553**
Neoplasm, **131**
  admissions for treatment, 146
  chemotherapy and radiation therapy,
    145–146
  coding sequences, 141
  confirming diagnosis, 132–133
  excised malignancies, 142
  functional activity, 138, 192
  morphology codes (M codes),
    140–141
  prophylactic organ removal, 144
  screenings, 131–132
Neoplasm table, 136t
  benign, 137
  malignant primary, 135
  malignant secondary, 135

uncertain, 137
  unspecified behavior, 137
Neoplasm-related pain, 255
Nephropathy, 189
Nervous system, 13, 240f
  central nervous system (CNS),
    240–242
  dominant and nondominant sides, 240
  peripheral nervous system (PNS),
    242–246
  types of, 239
Neurohypophysis lobes, 183
Neuroleptic drugs, 221
Neurologic disorders
  pain management, 246–247
  treatment, 246–247
Neurologic function assessments, **246**
Neurologic manifestations, 189
Nevus, **420**
Nodule, **420**
Nonmood psychotic disorders, 220–221
Nonpsychotic mental disorders, 225–227
Nonunion, **483**
Nosocomial infections, **102**
Nostrils, 351
Not elsewhere classifiable (NEC)
    notation, 75
Not otherwise specified (NOS) notation, 75
Notations
  See Also, 76
  See Condition, 76
  'and,' 74
  category notes, 74
  code also, 74
  code first, 72–73
  Excludes1, 72, 214
  Excludes2, 72, 214
  Includes, 72
  not elsewhere classifiable (NEC), 75
  not otherwise specified (NOS), 75
  other specified, 75
  See, 76
  unspecified, 75
  use additional code, 74
NSTEMI, **336**
Nucleus pulposus, 470
Nummular psoriasis. *See* Psoriasis vulgaris
Nutritional anemia, 165

O

Obesity, 196
Oblique (O), 18
Oblique fracture, 480
Obliterative bronchiolitis, 356
Observation, preventive care, 614
Obstetrics (OB), **523**
Obstetrics (prenatal) and neonatal exams, 615
Obstruction, **397**
Occipital lobe processes, 241
Oculomotor nerves—cranial nerve III, 242

Olecranon process, 473
Olfactory nerves—cranial nerve I, 242
Onycholysis, 424
Open angle, 281
Open fracture of clavicle, 37
Ophthalmic branch, 242
Ophthalmic manifestations, 188–189
Ophthalmoscopy, 324
Optic nerves—cranial nerve II, 242
Optical system
  anatomy, 268–274
  co-morbidities and underlying
    conditions, 281–283
  diseases of, 276–281
  muscles of, 441f, 441t
  related abbreviations, 274
Ora serrate, 272
Oral cavity, 19, **383**, 383f, 384–385
Orbit, human skull in, **268**, 269f
Organ donation, preventive care, 615–617
Organ of Corti, 296
Organ systems, **13**
Oropharynx, 386
Osgood-Schlatter disease.
    See Osteochondrosis
Ossa coxae, 475, 475f
Osseous tissue, **464, 465**
Ossicles, **296**
Osteoarthritis, 482
Osteochondropathy. *See* Osteochondrosis
Osteochondrosis, 482
Osteoitis deformans, 482
Osteoporosis, 482
Other specified notation, 75
Otitis media, 305
Otosclerosis, 305
Outpatient services, ICD-10-CM codes, **44**
Ovaries, **181, 524**
Overactive thyroid. *See* Hyperthyroidism
Overlapping boundaries, 139
Overweight, 196
Oxytocin (OT), 183

P

Pacemaker, 320
Paget's disease, 446–447. *See also*
    Osteoitis deformans
Pain management
  numeric rating scale for, 254t
  post-procedural, 255
  reporting separately, 254–255
  sequencing pain codes, 255
  site-specific pain codes, 255
Palatine bones, 467
Palatine tonsils, 385
Palpebrae, **273**
Palpebral conjunctiva, **274**
Pancreas, **186**, 187f, **393**
Pancreas, in Alphabetic Index, 41
Pancreatic islets. *See* Islets of Langerhans